THIRD EDITION

MIDDLE RANGE THEORIES

APPLICATION TO NURSING RESEARCH

SANDRA J. PETERSON, PhD, RN

PROFESSOR EMERITA
BETHEL UNIVERSITY
ST. PAUL, MINNESOTA

TIMOTHY S. BREDOW, PhD, RN, NP-C

PROFESSOR
BETHEL UNIVERSITY
ST. PAUL, MINNESOTA

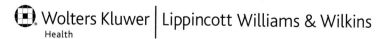

Wolters Kluwer | Lippincott Williams & Wilkins
Health

Philadelphia · Baltimore · New York · London
Buenos Aires · Hong Kong · Sydney · Tokyo

Vice President, Publishing: Julie K. Stegman
Supervising Product Manager: Betsy Gentzler
Editorial Assistant: Jacalyn Clay
Design Coordinator: Holly Reid McLaughlin
Illustration Coordinator: Brett MacNaughton
Manufacturing Coordinator: Karin Duffield
Prepress Vendor: Aptara, Inc.

3rd edition

9 8 7 6 5 4 3 2 1

Printed in China

Library of Congress Cataloging-in-Publication Data
Middle range theories : application to nursing research / [edited by]
Sandra J. Peterson, Timothy S. Bredow. – 3rd ed.
    p. ; cm.
Includes bibliographical references and index.
ISBN 978-1-60831-800-1 (alk. paper)
I. Peterson, Sandra J. II. Bredow, Timothy S.
[DNLM: 1. Nursing Theory. 2. Nursing Research. WY 86]
610.7301—dc23
                              2011040374

CCS1211

For my son, Christopher, daughter, Beth, daughter-in-law, Alisa, and grandchildren, Liam and Jane. You have been a source of wonder, inspiration, joy, and pride.

SANDRA J. PETERSON

I would like to dedicate this third edition to my family who provides me with the love and support to complete a project such as this.
Katherine, Andrea, Ben, and Caroline. To Tiffany, Ben, and also little Kata Grace.

TIMOTHY S. BREDOW

Contributors

Laurel Ash, DNP, CNP, RN
Assistant Professor
College of St. Scholastica
Duluth, Minnesota

Georgene Gaskill Eakes, EdD, RN
Professor Emerita
College of Nursing
East Carolina University
Greenville, North Carolina

Director, Clinical Education
Center for Learning and Performance
Pitt County Memorial Hospital
Greenville, North Carolina

Audrey Gift, PhD, RN, FAAN
Professor Emerita of Nursing
Michigan State University
East Lansing, Michigan

Marion Good, PhD, FAAN
Professor Emerita, Frances Payne Bolton
    School of Nursing
Case Western Reserve University
Cleveland, Ohio

Visiting Professor, Hong Kong University
    School of Nursing
Case Western Reserve FPBSN
Lakewood, Ohio

Joan E. Haase, PhD, RN, FAAN
Holmquist Professor, Pediatric Oncology Nursing
Department of Family Health Nursing
Indiana University
Indianapolis, Indiana

Sonya R. Hardin, PhD, RN, CCRN, NP-C
Professor, School of Nursing
University of North Carolina at Charlotte
Charlotte, North Carolina

Barbara Hoglund, EdD, MSN, RN, FNP-C
Associate Professor of Nursing
Bethel University
St. Paul, Minnesota

Trine Klette, PhD
Associate Professor
Diakonova University College
Oslo, Norway

Katharine Kolcaba, PhD, RN, MSN
Associate Professor
The University of Akron, Ursuline College
Akron, Ohio

Elizabeth R. Lenz, PhD, RN, FAAN
Dean, Professor
College of Nursing
The Ohio State University
Columbus, Ohio

Marjorie Cook McCullagh, PhD, RN,
    APHN-BC, COHN-S
Assistant Professor and Director, Occupational
    Health Nursing Program
School of Nursing
University of Michigan
Ann Arbor, Michigan

Renee A. Milligan, PhD, RN
Associate Professor, School of Nursing
Georgetown University
Washington, DC

Mertie L. Potter, DNP, APRN, BC
Clinical Professor, Nurse Practitioner/Consultant
Massachusetts General Hospital Institute of
    Health Professions
Boston, Massachusetts

Linda C. Pugh, PhD, RNC, CNE, FAAN
Director, Graduate Programs in Nursing
York College of Pennsylvania
York, Pennsylvania

Barbara Resnick, PhD, CRNP, FAAN,
    FAANP
Professor
Sonya Ziporkin Gershowitz Chair in Gerontology
University of Maryland
Baltimore, Maryland

Kristin E. Sandau, PhD, RN
Associate Professor of Nursing
Bethel University
St. Paul, Minnesota

Marjorie A. Schaffer, PhD, MS, BA
Professor of Nursing
Bethel University
St. Paul, Minnesota

Ellen D. Schultz, PhD, RN, CHTP, AHN-BC
Professor of Nursing
Metropolitan State University
St. Paul, Minnesota

Danuta M. Wojnar, PhD, RN, MEd
Associate Professor
Seattle University
Seattle, Washington

Reviewers

Sharon K. Falkenstern, PhD, CRNP, MSN, RN, CNE
Assistant Professor of Nursing
The Pennsylvania State University
University Park, Pennsylvania

Karen Reed Gehrling, PhD, RN
Professor and Director, Graduate Nursing Program
Walsh University
North Canton, Ohio

Leonie Pallikkathayil, PhD, RN, ARNP
Associate Professor, School of Nursing
Kansas University
Kansas City, Kansas

Phyllis Skorga, PhD, RN, CCM
Professor of Nursing
Arkansas State University
Jonesboro, Arkansas

Ida L. Slusher, RN, DSN, CNE
Professor, Nursing Education Coordinator
Department of Baccalaureate and Graduate Nursing
Eastern Kentucky University
Richmond, Kentucky

Mary Ann Stark, PhD, RNC
Associate Professor, Bronson School of Nursing
Western Michigan University
Kalamazoo, Michigan

Cheryl Zambroski, PhD, RN
Associate Professor
College of Nursing
University of South Florida
Tampa, Florida

Preface

Middle range theories have understandably emerged as the focus of knowledge development in nursing with a "broad acceptance of the need to develop middle range theories to support nursing practice" (McEwen, 2007, p. 225). With increasing frequency, middle range theories are being generated and tested through practice-oriented nursing research.

There is a dynamic relationship between theory, research, and practice. Research is a source of theory development and theory is a source of research questions. Theory is used to improve practice and practice is used to shape and refine theories. In this third edition of *Middle Range Theories: Application to Nursing Research,* the authors have attempted to address this dynamic relationship with increased emphasis on applications of middle range theories to practice. We continue to hope that this edition can serve as a resource for nurse scholars, making middle range theories more accessible for their research and practice.

With the increase in the number of middle range theories being developed, determining which to include in this book is a challenge. As for the previous editions, we reviewed published research and practice applications of theories. The goal was to identify those theories that, though in the middle range of abstraction, are not particularly narrow in their possible applications. That process resulted in the addition of two middle range theories, Attachment and the Shuler Nurse Practitioner Practice Model.

ORGANIZATION

PART I

Part I is devoted to an overview of the state of nursing's body of knowledge. In this edition, there is a brief discussion of epistemology with a summary of Carper's conceptualization of nurses' ways of knowing. Chapter 1 considers the hierarchy of nursing knowledge and particularly the place of middle range theory within that hierarchy (i.e., paradigm, philosophy, conceptual framework, and theories). For each component of the hierarchy, the chapter includes a description of its nature, review of its development, a discussion of its contributions to nursing knowledge, consideration of controversies related to its nature or use, and examples of nurse scholars' work. The section devoted to middle range theories includes a table with multiple examples of middle range theories, referenced. As middle range theories continue to be developed, this table has been expanded. Chapter 2 emphasizes the analysis and evaluation of middle range theories, including issues to consider in the selection of a middle range nursing theory for research purposes. This chapter also describes a brief evaluative process that is used as a feature throughout the rest of the chapters. Using this evaluation process, readers can compare and contrast their conclusions about the theory as presented in the chapter with those of a nurse scholar who has also used this evaluation process.

PARTS II TO VI

Parts II to VI are devoted to specific middle range theories. The selected theories are labeled by their developers or by nurse scholars as middle range theories and are ones frequently cited in published nursing research or practice applications. Many of the chapters contain unique nursing theories; some are borrowed from related disciplines, but are, nonetheless, useful to nursing. All theories in the text, however, have the intrinsic capability to be applied to nursing research and practice and address a wide range of phenomena that allow the researcher to consider a variety of nursing research questions and uses in practice. The theories have been organized by categories to reflect the type of research questions or practice applications that could most likely be considered. The categories are not presented as absolute, but more as a guide to direct the user of the book to the theories that might be most relevant to their issue of interest.

- Physiological—Pain: Balance of Analgesia and Side Effects; Unpleasant Symptoms
- Cognitive—Self-efficacy, Reasoned Action
- Emotional—Empathy, Chronic Sorrow
- Social—Social Support, Interpersonal Relations, Attachment

■ Integrative—Modeling and Role-Modeling, Comfort, Heath-Related Quality of Life, Health Promotion, Deliberative Nursing Process, Shuler Nurse Practitioner Practice Model, AACN Synergy Model, Resilience

SPECIAL FEATURES

Each theory chapter provides the nurse researcher with a variety of tools, updated from the earlier editions. Key features include the following:

■ **Definitions of Key Terms** appear at the beginning of each chapter to define concepts and aid the reader's understanding of the theory.
■ **Using Middle Range Theories** boxes provide examples of how the theory has been used in published research.
■ **Research Application** boxes provide a sample application of the theory modeling the research process.
■ **Analysis Exercises** appear at the end of each theory chapter, allowing readers to arrive at their own conclusions about the theory and then compare them to a nurse scholar's evaluation provided in Appendix A.
■ **Critical Thinking Exercises** at the end of each chapter engage readers in analysis of the theory and its application to practice.
■ **Instruments** are discussed in the chapters, with specific examples provided in Appendix B.
■ **Web Resources** to aid readers in their research are provided on thePoint (http://thePoint.lww.com/Peterson3e).

REFERENCE

McEwen, M. (2007). Introduction to middle range nursing theories. In M. McEwen & E. M. Wills (Eds.), *Theoretical basis for nursing* (2nd ed., pp. 224–240). Philadelphia, PA: Lippincott Williams & Wilkins.

Acknowledgments

There is a sense of accomplishment that accompanies the completion of a project such as this text. We would have never been able to experience that rather pleasant sensation without the significant involvement of many others. The quality of the scholarship of the chapter authors will be evident to all those who read the text. Their willingness to invest themselves in this project, consistently providing what was needed in a timely fashion, is much appreciated. Those who completed the Analysis of Theory, found in Appendix A of the book, have added what we believe will be a useful resource to readers, enabling them to clarify their understanding of the theories.

The staff at Lippincott Williams & Wilkins was invaluable. Carrie Brandon, Acquisitions Editor, continued to see this book as a contribution to the body of nursing literature and helped us launch this project. Betsy Gentzler, Supervising Product Manager, expertly coordinated the project. We would also like to thank Karen Ettinger, Project Manager from O'Donnell & Associates for shepherding this project to completion. And finally, we are profoundly grateful for the forbearance of our family and friends (especially husband, Ray Peterson, and wife, Kate Bredow). They helped us have "lives" beyond the scope of completing this book.

Contents

1

Introduction to the Nature of Nursing Knowledge

SANDRA J. PETERSON

DEFINITION OF KEY TERMS

Concept	Symbolic representation of a phenomenon or set of phenomena
Conceptual model	"Set of abstract and general concepts and the propositions" (Fawcett, 1997, pp. 13–14) that represents a phenomenon of interest
Deduction	Reasoning from the general or universal to the particular or specific
Discipline	A field or branch of knowledge that involves research
Domain	Related components or items that reflect the unified subject matter of a discipline
Empiricism	A philosophical theory of knowledge acquisition through experience, observation, and experiment
Ethics	A branch of philosophy concerned with moral principles
Epistemology	A branch of philosophy concerned with the nature and scope of knowledge and the methods used to acquire it
Induction	Reasoning from the individual or particular to the general or universal
Logic	A branch of philosophy concerned with sound reasoning and validity of thought
Logical positivism	Philosophical perspective that espouses logic, objectivity, falseness/truth, observable and operationally defined concepts, and prediction
Metaparadigm	Global concepts specific to a discipline that are philosophically neutral and stable
Metaphysics	A branch of philosophy concerned with the study of ultimate cause and underlying nature of that which exists
Metatheory	A philosophical theory about theories, concerned with "logical and methodological foundations of a discipline" (Beckstrand, 1986, p. 503). Examines "how theory affects and is affected by research and practice within nursing, and philosophy and politics outside nursing" (McKenna, 1997, p. 92)
Ontology	Examination of the nature of being or reality
Paradigm	A worldview, a common philosophical orientation, that serves to define the nature of a discipline
Phenomenon	A designation of an aspect of reality

(Definition of Key Terms continued on next page)

DEFINITION OF KEY TERMS CONTINUED	
Philosophy	(a) A set of beliefs or values; (b) science concerned with the study of reality and the nature of being. Comprised of, but not limited to, aesthetics, epistemology, ethics, logic, and metaphysics
Science	A systematized body of knowledge that has as its main purpose the discovery of "truths about the world" (Jacox, 1974, p. 4), confirmed through empirical investigation
Theory	"Set of interrelated concepts, based on assumption, woven together through a set of propositional statements" (Fitzpatrick, 1997, p. 37) used to provide a perspective on reality

INTRODUCTION

What is knowledge? Attempts to answer that question have been primarily the domain of the branch of philosophy referred to as epistemology. Traditionally, knowledge has been defined as a belief that was justified as true with absolute certainty. This definition requires that for knowledge to exist it must be believed; if not believed, something cannot be known. It also must be true; if not true, even if well justified and believed, it cannot be considered knowledge. Finally, there must be sound reasons for the belief; if there are no sound reasons, it would be more a probable opinion or lucky guess than knowledge. There is no universal agreement about the nature of a sound reason or adequate evidence for a belief.

There are multiple epistemological theories to describe the nature of knowledge and explain its sources, or how something can be known. Examples of epistemological theories include idealism, pragmatism, rationalism, and relativism. The theory of empiricism, most closely associated with natural science, considers knowledge to be a result of human experience. Ideas and theories can then be tested against reality, and accepted or rejected on the basis of how well they are congruent with observable facts.

The traditional ideas about the nature of knowledge are being challenged on an ongoing basis. Edmund Gettier in the 1960s proposed several cases in which a person had a sound justification to believe that something was true; it was true but for reasons other than those believed. The issue then is the nature of the justification of a belief. The two contemporary approaches to consideration of that issue are foundationalism and coherentism. Foundationalism identifies basic beliefs as the justification for a belief. A belief is basic if it is self-evident, providing support for other beliefs. Coherentism rejects the notion of basic beliefs as a form of justification. Instead, this theory of justification claims that it is the interrelationship of a set of beliefs that supports the truth of a belief.

Nurses obviously need knowledge to practice. This discussion of the nature of knowledge is clearly basic but establishes a foundation for consideration of nursing knowledge and the roles that theory and research play in its development.

NURSING KNOWLEDGE

Nurses are fundamentally "knowledge workers" in that they synthesize "a broad array of information and knowledge from a wide variety of sources and bring that synthesis to bear on nursing work" (Porter-O'Grady, 2003, para. 2). The knowledge that nurses need to practice has been conceptualized by Carper (1978) as four distinct patterns: (a) empirics, the science of nursing; (b) aesthetics, the art of nursing; (c) personal knowing, the intra- and interpersonal nature of nursing; and (d) ethics, the moral component of nursing.

Empirical knowing is positivistic science, which means that it is logically determined and based on observable phenomenon. It is knowledge that is systematically organized into general laws and theories that serve to describe, explain, and/or predict the phenomena of interest to nursing (Carper, 1978). The sources of empirical knowledge are research and theory and model development. There is no coherent conceptual structure that is generally accepted as nursing's scientific paradigm, which can lead to the possibility of a confusing and sometimes conflicting knowledge base. For the practicing nurse, empirical knowledge must always be interpreted within the context of specific clinical situations.

Aesthetic knowing is a process of "perceiving or grasping the nature of a clinical situation; interpreting this information in order to understand its meaning for those involved, while envisioning desired outcomes in order to respond with appropriate skilled action; and subsequently reflecting on whether the outcomes were effectively achieved" (Johns, 1995, Aesthetics, para. 1). Aesthetic knowing comes from the nurse's ability to grasp and interpret the meaning of a situation. It makes use of the nurse's intuition and empathy. This type of knowing also involves the nurse's skills in imagining a desired and practical outcome in the actual situation and responding based on an interpretation of the whole situation, analyzing the interrelationships of its various aspects. Unfortunately, aesthetic knowing cannot be articulated; it is not transferable to others. It is based solely on the skill of the nurse in a specific situation. This type of knowing has also been criticized for the role of empathy in nursing knowledge acquisition. White (2004) claims that empathy is a psychological phenomenon that has been uncritically adopted by nursing.

Personal knowing is knowledge of the concrete, individual self; it is not knowledge about the self. It involves encountering and actualization of the self in a way that enables the nurse to transcend the notion of other individuals as objects but instead the nurse engages with others in authentic personal relationships. The type of knowing and the nature of these relationships result in an increasing willingness to accept ambiguity, vagueness, and discrepancy in oneself and others. Personal knowing is the basis of the therapeutic use of self in the nurse–patient relationship. Reflection is the primary means by which personal knowing occurs. It involves three interrelated factors:

1. The perception of the self's feelings and prejudices within the situation
2. The management of the self's feelings and prejudices in order to respond appropriately (to the other)
3. Managing anxiety and sustaining the self (Johns, 1995, The Personal Way of Knowing, para. 2)

Like aesthetic knowing, personal knowing cannot be described, but can only be actualized. In order to escape the problem of self-delusion, there is a need for individual reflection that is informed by the responses of others. But data about self from others can also be problematic in that it can be misperceived. In addition, personal knowing presents the nurse with a dilemma; personal knowledge needs to be integrated or reconciled with the professional responsibility of the nurse to manipulate the environment in order to work toward a desired health outcome (Carper, 1978, p. 19). Personal knowing of all the ways of knowing is the most difficult to teach and to master (White, 2004, p. 253).

Ethical knowing is knowledge of what is right or wrong and the commitment to act on the basis of that knowledge. It involves "judgments of moral value in relation to motives, intentions and traits of character" (Carper, 1978, p. 20) and focuses on obligations, on what ought to be done related to those judgments. Sources of ethical knowledge include the nursing's ethical codes and professional standards. It is also important for the nurse to have an understanding of different philosophical positions as to what is considered good, what is identified as an obligation. Consideration of the philosophical positions can also create confusion since ethical theories of what is good and what constitutes an obligation can conflict. For instance, the teleological perceptive considers what is good on the basis of its production of the greatest good for the greatest number (consequentialism), whereas the deontological perspective identifies good not by the consequences of actions but by the nature of the actions themselves.

Each of the ways of knowing represents a necessary but incomplete representation of the discipline of nursing. There is also an inherent interrelationship between the four patterns. For instance, aesthetic knowing would require empirical knowledge in order to envision what the desired and practical outcomes in a situation might be and what would constitute valid means of helping to bring about that desired outcome. With an acknowledgement of the contributions of all the ways of knowing to the practice of nursing, this book focuses on empirical knowing, on nursing theories, especially those that are considered middle range.

Two claims can be made about the state of empirical knowledge in nursing—it exists in varying degrees of abstraction, and it is characterized by a lack of consistency in the use of its language. Fawcett (2005) recommends what she refers to as a structural "holarchy" of contemporary nursing knowledge to establish the relationships between the various components that comprise nursing's body of knowledge. The components are arranged from most abstract to most concrete in the following order: philosophy/paradigm, conceptual model, and theories. The types of theories available to nurses also exist on a continuum from most abstract to most concrete, with grand theories identified as most abstract, practice theories as most concrete, and middle range theories in the logical middle.

There are few components in the hierarchy that appear consistently in the literature with a single label. The terms *conceptual models, conceptual frameworks,* and *theories* are sometimes used interchangeably. The terms *grand theory, macro theory,* and *general theory* all refer the same level of theory development.

This chapter addresses each component of the conceptual hierarchy, with special emphasis on middle range theories. The nature of the component, its development, its contributions to nursing's body of knowledge, and the debates engaged in by nurses in relation to the component are considered.

PHILOSOPHY

In the nursing literature, the term *philosophy* is used in two distinct ways, as a unique discipline and as set of beliefs of a separate discipline, for example, nursing. As a discipline, it is often defined by its main branches: metaphysics, epistemology, ethics, logic, and aesthetics. Well into the nineteenth century, the classical Greek thought persisted that philosophy represented humanity's total knowledge (Silva, 1997). The scientific revolution, ushered in by a knowledge explosion related to new thinking about survival of species, cause of disease, nature of matter and energy, and the workings of the human mind, came with new ways of knowing and forms of inquiry. This revolution also resulted in new ways of thinking about philosophy and science. Philosophy is concerned with the nature of being, the meaning and purpose of life, and the theory and limits of knowledge, whereas science is more concerned with causality (Silva, 1997). Philosophy is considered discursive, noninvestigative, and dependent on common experience, contrasting with science, which is considered investigative and dependent on special experience (Simmons, 1992, pp. 16–17).

For a discipline, philosophies represent its beliefs and values, and its mindset or worldview. "Nursing philosophy is a statement of foundational and universal assumptions, beliefs, and principles about the nature of knowledge and truth (epistemology)" (Reed, 1995, Nursing Philosophy: Metaparadigms for Knowledge Development, para. 1). Like other disciplines, nursing has and is reflecting the modern, postmodern, and some would include neomodern thinking, or worldview of its time.

DEVELOPMENT

Philosophies emerge as a reflection on the issues of interest to philosophers, primarily logic, ethics, aesthetics, metaphysics, and epistemology. In the twentieth and twenty-first centuries these reflections or philosophies have been often characterized as either modern or postmodern perspectives. Although modernism and postmodernism do not represent singular philosophies but, rather, a collection of philosophies (Burbules, n.d., para. 2), each possesses commonly occurring themes that can serve as points of contrast. The most basic comparison between the schools of thinking is in their perspectives on metanarratives, defined as efforts to offer "general and encompassing accounts of truth, value, and reality" (Burbules, n.d., para. 5). In modernism, the metanarratives are a primary concern. In postmodernism, metanarratives are dismissed. This dismissal is not necessarily rejection or denial but instead doubt and uncertainty about what metanarratives have to offer. These schools of thought also differ in their view of the nature of problems. In modern thinking, problems are to be solved. In postmodern thinking, they are to be deconstructed, requiring a disassembling of the metanarratives that are entangled in values and beliefs that fail to reveal reality or liberate the oppressed (Reed, 1995, Historical Background: Modernism and Postmodernism, para. 3). Reed (1995) also identifies distinctions in epistemology: modernism, concerned with the truth of findings, and postmodernism, concerned with the usefulness of findings. She also suggests a neomodernism perspective, which rejects modernism's logical positivism and postmodernism's radical relativism and lack of coherent vision to focus instead on a plurality of realistic visions of a possible future (Bisk, n.d.). Reed's *Neomodern Perspective for Nursing* embraces the metanarratives of health and the processes of healing but integrates them with the postmodern assumptions that knowledge is value-laden and that context is critical in order to achieve the desired future.

Within these schools of thought—modern, postmodern, and neomodern—a variety of philosophies or philosophical schemes have been used to describe the nature of nursing. Adam (1992) identified the following: (a) Socratic—know self, (b) realism—be self, (c) humanism—give self, (d) rationalism—understand self, (e) naturalism—describe self, (f) pragmatism—prove self, (g) idealism—imagine self, and (h) existentialism—choose self (p. 56).

Another schema, proposed by Lerner (1986), which considered the nature of human development, is useful in categorizing nursing philosophies. Three worldviews of most interest are as follows:

1. Mechanistic, in which the machine is the metaphor for the human being. The whole is equal to the sum of the parts, and the goal is a return to equilibrium.

2. Organistic, in which a biologic organism composed of complex interrelated parts is the basic metaphor. The organism is active in a passive environment. Change is probable, goal-directed, and developmental.

3. Developmental–contextual, in which historical events are the metaphor. The individual is immersed in a dynamic context. Change in the person and the environment is ongoing, irreversible, innovative, and developmental. Chaos and conflict are an energy source for change (Reed, 1995).

USES

Kikuchi (1992) claims that "without an understanding of philosophy in nursing there can be no science of nursing" (p. 45). The branches of philosophy suggest a set of questions with relevance to nursing. For instance, ethical nursing questions would be concerned with what is good to do and to seek to attain nursing's goals (Kikuchi, 1992). Epistemological questions would focus on the structure, scope, and reliability of nursing's knowledge, and ontological questions would relate to the meaning of nurses' and clients' realities (Silva, Sorrell, & Sorrell, 1995). However, these important questions are ones that are best addressed through philosophical inquiry.

The contribution the branches of philosophy make to nursing knowledge is more directly related to research methods than to the nature of the questions generated. Research requires logic in the use of the research process, with a logical progression from problem identification and hypotheses, to methods, and finally to data analyses and conclusions (Silva, 1997). Epistemology leads nurse researchers to consider the nature of not only evidence obtained through research, but also truth and belief. Metaphysics addresses causality, an important issue for nurse researchers. Ethics are of concern to nurse researchers as they consider the ethical implications of research problems, research methods, and dissemination of the research findings.

Philosophy, theory, and research are inextricably linked. "All nursing theory or research derives from or leads to philosophy" (Phillips, 1992, p. 49). Philosophy makes a significant contribution to the development of nursing theories. The conceptual clarification specified by the philosopher of science helps the theorist generate better theories, and the speculation engaged in by the philosopher of science can also suggest the theories of the future (Smart, 1968, p. 17). Analysis of a theory reveals the underlying assumptions and worldview (philosophy). By considering these philosophical statements, nurses can determine the fit between the values and beliefs expressed through the theory and their own. This enables researchers and practitioners to select theories that are philosophically congruent with their own perspectives on nursing. Therefore, philosophy plays a critical role in the formulation of questions important to nursing, the consideration of research methods, and the development of theories and their analysis and use in practice.

CONTROVERSY

The controversy about nursing philosophy centers on the belief systems that exist within the discipline of nursing and the relative value of unity or diversity in nursing thought. Roach (1992) argues that philosophical inquiry in nursing is the pursuit of universal, transcendent principles and suggests metaphysics as the basis for nursing's unity. Others refer to this search for a coherent philosophical foundation in nursing as a pursuit of unity in diversity of thought (Newman, 2002; Phillips, 1992). The diversity of perspectives represented in the variety of existing nursing models requires philosophical inquiry as a means of determining underlying philosophical themes and patterns. This search for the unitary nature of phenomena of concern to nursing will lead to the recognition of core beliefs:

- A holistic view of persons (Phillips, 1992; Roach, 1992)
- A commitment to caring as an expression of the human mode of being (Newman, Sime, & Corcoran-Perry, 1996; Roach, 1992)
- A perspective on education that acknowledges the unity of mind–body–spirit and recognition of the universe of knowledge that is necessary to achieve and makes a contribution to human understanding (Roach, 1992)
- A view of humans in relationship, with awareness of ethical–moral bonds (Roach, 1992).

Although diversity may result in confusion and lack of clarity in nursing's theory development and research agenda, others believe that a philosophy that represents the worldview of all nurse scientists would be diluted to the point of becoming meaningless and useless (Landreneau, 2002). Diversity of philosophies may be viewed as a more accurate representation of reality, a perspective consistent with postmodern thinking, and may have the potential of stimulating greater creativity and variety in the development of nursing models and theories.

PARADIGMS AND METAPARADIGM

The terms *paradigm* and *metaparadigm* are frequently found in the nursing literature. Paradigms provide the basic parameters and framework for organizing a discipline's knowledge. Similar to philosophies, they are an abstract means of expressing that knowledge. Paradigms generally are considered to be discipline specific, philosophical, and mutable. The metaparadigm of a discipline is distinguished from a paradigm in that the metaparadigm is global, philosophically neutral, and fairly stable.

PARADIGMS

Kuhn introduced the term *paradigm* and stimulated interest in its use as a method of defining and analyzing the nature of a discipline. He also acknowledged the existence of multiple and conflicting definitions of the term (Kuhn, 1977, p. 294). Kuhn (1996) included the following as the components of paradigms or, as he later referred to them, disciplinary matrices: (a) symbolic generalizations; the laws accepted by a scientific community and the language used to express them; (b) shared commitments to beliefs in particular models; shared beliefs about and commitment to the prevailing theories of the discipline and the motivation and methods used to create and test them; (c) values—shared values that serve to identify what is significant or meaningful to the scientific community; and (d) exemplars—the specific problems to be solved and the methods used to solve them. Guba (1990) suggested a means of differentiating paradigms. Paradigms can be distinguished by the answers to three questions:

1. *Ontological:* What is the nature of the "knowable"? Or, what is the nature of "reality"?
2. *Epistemological:* What is the nature of the relationship between the knower (the inquirer) and the known (or knowable)?
3. *Methodological:* How should the inquirer go about finding out knowledge (p. 18)?

The components identified by Kuhn and the answers to the questions posed by Guba express the nature of existing paradigms. Before a paradigm is identified, the facts generated by the discipline and the methods used to generate them are disorganized. The discipline is considered to be in a pre-paradigm stage of development.

DEVELOPMENT

Paradigms emerge when they are recognized as a dominant way of thinking about the discipline by its scientific community. Kuhn (1996) refers to the emergence of a new paradigm as a revolution in which the new paradigm replaces an older one. "… scientific revolutions are inaugurated by a growing sense, again often restricted to a narrow subdivision of the scientific community, that an existing paradigm has ceased to function adequately in the exploration of an aspect of nature to which that paradigm itself had previously led the way" (Kuhn, 1996, p. 92).

Shapere (1980) criticized the notion of revolution, noting that scientific advances can be cumulative in that later sciences build on that which was earlier. This is a more evolutionary perspective on paradigm development. Integration has also been proposed as a form of paradigm development. This form of paradigm development describes a pattern in progress that is created "through accommodation, refinement, and collaboration between thoughts, ideas, and individuals (Meleis, 1997, p. 80). Meleis believes paradigm development in nursing is characterized by this approach.

There are multiple paradigms and systems of classifying the paradigms used to express the worldview of the discipline of nursing. Stevens Barnum (1998) suggests a paradigm that focuses on nursing action that is comprised of intervention, conservation, substitution, sustenance/support, and enhancement. Newman et al. (1991) describe three existing paradigms that provide different perspectives on the phenomena of caring and health, identified as the concepts most central to nursing: particulate–deterministic, interactive–integrative, and unitary–transformative. In the particulate–deterministic paradigm, phenomena exist as separate entities, possess properties that can be measured, and relate to each other in predictable and linear ways. Knowledge is identified in terms of facts and universal laws. The interactive–integrative paradigm, an extension of the particulate–deterministic paradigm, considers context and experience from subjective perspectives as a means of understanding the intra-related nature of the properties of phenomena and the reciprocal interrelated nature that exists among phenomena. This paradigm is concerned with probabilistic predictability of interactive–integrative phenomena. The unitary–transformative paradigm is quite distinct, emphasizing the unitary and self-organizing nature of phenomena that exist in a larger but also self-organizing field. Knowledge is derived from both the mutuality that exists between phenomena and those who are observing and focusing on the personal nature of knowledge and pattern recognition.

The classification of nursing paradigms proposed by Parse (1987) is the one most frequently cited in nursing literature. Parse identified two distinct paradigms that describe the relationship between persons and their environments as they relate to health: totality and simultaneity. In the totality paradigm "man is considered a bio-psycho-socio-spiritual organism whose environment can be manipulated to maintain or promote balance" (Parse, 1987, p. 32) and health is viewed as a dynamic state and process of well-being. The goals of nursing are health promotion, illness prevention, and care and cure of the sick. Research from this paradigmatic perspective would be quantitative. In the simultaneity paradigm, man is greater than the sum of parts, a self-initiating being in rhythmical interchanges with environments, living in the "relative Now experiencing what was, is, and will be, all at once" (Parse, 1987, p. 136). Health is the process of becoming, which can be experienced and described only by the individual. "There is no optimum health; health is simply how one is experiencing personal living" (Parse, 1987, p. 136). The goal of nursing in this paradigm is to illuminate meaning and move beyond the immediate or present to changing patterns of health with the person and family. The nurse is considered a guide and the other is the decision maker. Research conducted from this paradigmatic perspective is qualitative in nature.

There are a number of similarities in the paradigms proposed by Newman et al. and Parse, with the particulate–deterministic paradigm sharing features in common with the totality paradigm, and the unitary–transformative paradigm similar to the simultaneity paradigm. There are a number of other classifications of paradigms identified in the literature to describe actual or preferred perspectives of nursing. Many seem to be a renaming of or very similar to the conceptualizations of previously identified paradigms, particularly Parse's. For instance, Monti and Tingen (1999) suggest empiricism and interpretative; Guiliano, Tyer-Viola, and Lopez (2005) identify received view and perceived view; Weaver and Olson (2006) propose positivism/post-positivism and interpretive; and Pilkington and Mitchell (1999; 2003) refer to natural science and human science. A summary of three of the major paradigms is found in Table 1.1.

Uses

One function of a paradigm is to identify the boundary or limits of the subject matter of concern to a discipline (Kim, 1989). A paradigm also provides a summary of the intellectual and social purposes of the

TABLE 1.1 Examples of Nursing's Paradigmatic Schemes

Author	Categorization of perspectives
Parse (1987)	• *Totality.* Man is a total, summative organism, comprised of bio-psycho-social-spiritual features. The environment is a source of external and internal stimuli to which man must adapt in order to maintain balance and achieve goals. • *Simultaneity.* Man is a unitary being in continuous and reciprocal interrelationships with the environment. Health is an unfolding phenomenon.
Newman, Sime, & Corcoran-Perry (1996)	• *Particulate–deterministic.* Phenomena are specific, reducible, measurable entities. Relationships between and within entities are causal and linear. Change, as a result of prior conditions, can be predicted and controlled. • *Interactive–integrative.* Phenomena include experiences and subjective data. Multiple interrelationships that are contextual and reciprocal exist between phenomena. Change is a function of multiple prior conditions and probabilistic relationships. • *Unitary–transformative.* A phenomenon is a unitary, self-organizing field and is identified through pattern recognition and interaction with the larger whole. Change is unidirectional and unpredictable.
Fawcett (1995)	• *Reaction.* Person is viewed as composed of discrete biological, psychological, sociological, and spiritual aspects, who responds in a reactive manner to environmental stimuli. Change occurs when survival is challenged. • *Reciprocal interaction.* Person is holistic, interactive being. Interactions with the environment are reciprocal. Change occurs as a result of multiple factors at varying rates throughout life and can only be estimated, not predicted. • *Simultaneous action.* Person is viewed as a holistic, self-organized field. Person–environment interactions are mutual and rhythmical processes. Change is unpredictable and evolutionary.

Note: These philosophical schemes are also referred to as paradigms.
Source: Fawcett, J. (1995). *Analysis and evaluation of conceptual models of nursing* (3rd ed.). Philadelphia: F. A. Davis Company. (Used with permission.)

discipline. It provides the "perspective with which essential phenomena of concern are conceptualized" (Kim, 1997, p. 32). A paradigm is considered to represent a worldview, "a coherent and common philosophical orientation" (Sarter, 1988, p. 52).

Therefore, paradigms can provide the frames of reference for the construction of nursing theory and the use of nursing and non-nursing theories in nursing research. "The paradigm determines the way in which scientists make sense of the world. Therefore, without it, there is nothing about which to construct theories" (Antiognoli-Toland, 1999, p. 39). Multiple theories generally emerge from a single paradigm. Paradigms also are important to nursing researchers. Researchers need to be assured that what is being studied will contribute to the body of nursing knowledge. By providing definitions of the discipline's boundaries, paradigms provide researchers with a nursing context for their research. Paradigms more specifically suggest the types of research questions that need to be addressed and appropriate methods used to answer the questions (Guiliano et al., 2005). Thus, nursing paradigms function as a means for nurse theorists and researchers to determine the congruence of their work in both focus and methods with the discipline of nursing, as expressed through a particular worldview.

CONTROVERSY

The topic of nursing paradigms is much debated by nurse scholars with differing opinions articulated about which paradigm best serves the discipline's needs in regard to knowledge development. This debate has not always been viewed as particularly constructive. "The paradigm debates have done more to create divisiveness with theoretical nursing than to clearly define our unique mission and facilitate effective communication among nurses" (Thorne et al., 1998, A Unifying Definition, para. 1). The nursing literature reveals four major positions: (a) emergence of a singular dominant paradigm; (b) integration of the most predominant paradigms, that is, totality and simultaneity; (c) the coexistence of multiple paradigms; and (d) avoidance of the issue.

Kikuchi and Simmons (1996), arguing from the perspective of the logic of truth, which holds that "two contradictory positions cannot both be true—one must be true and the other false (p. 8), seem to support the necessity of a single dominant paradigm for the discipline of nursing. It has been argued that a predominant paradigm demonstrates the legitimacy of the science of a discipline. When Parse (1987) labeled and described the totality and simultaneity paradigms, she acknowledged the existence of a dominant paradigm and suggested the emergence of a new and preferred perspective for nursing. She identified the simultaneity paradigm as "an alternative to the traditional predominant worldview in nursing [totality]," one that moves "nursing away from the particulate view of Man" (p. 135) She noted that the simultaneity paradigm was gaining "recognition among scientists and was "beginning to have an impact on research and practice competitive with the totality paradigm" (p. 135). Her use of the term *competition* initiated a debate over a preferred paradigm for nursing that is ongoing. The case for a single dominant paradigm is articulated by Leddy (2000); citing Kim, she concluded that multiple paradigms instead of leading to coherence and patterning, actually results in "chaos, fragmentation, and arbitrariness" (p. 229).

Others support the existence of a single dominant paradigm, one that has not yet been identified. "The dialog is not to determine which [existing] paradigm is, finally, to win out. Rather it is to take us to another level at which all of these paradigms will be replaced by yet another paradigm whose outlines we can see now but dimly, if at all" (Guba, 1990, p. 27). Some nurse scholars have suggested new paradigms. For instance, Georges (2003) recommends a paradigm that claims social justice as the central teleology of its scholarship, is critical of dominant practices, and embraces diversity and the contextual nature of phenomena.

A variation on the position that nursing is best served by a single paradigm is the recommendation made by some nurse scholars that a paradigm integrating both the totality and the simultaneity paradigms become the dominant perspective of the discipline. Rawnsley believes that "constructing new paradigms to complement totality and simultaneity is one way of respecting the contributions of colleagues without compromising philosophical integrity" (Rawnsley, 2003, p. 11). Several nurse scholars have suggested this approach and Winters and Ballou (2004) identified integration as a trend that values not only the traditional scientific worldview, but also the phenomenological and philosophical worldviews (p. 535). Arguing for "a less extreme and more integrated reference point for nursing's theory and practice," Thorne and her coauthors proposed a unifying definition of nursing (Thorne, et al., 1998, p. 1257).

> Nursing is the study of human health and illness processes. Nursing practice is facilitating, supporting, and assisting individuals, families, communities, and/or societies to enhance, maintain and recover health and to reduce and ameliorate the effects of illness. Nursing's relational practice and science are directed toward the explicit outcome of health related quality of life within the immediate and larger environmental contexts. (Thorne et al., 1998, p. 1265)

Engebretson (1997) proposed an integrative paradigm, derived from the Heterdox Explanatory Paradigms Model for health practice. This model consisted of a horizontal axis with a continuum from logical positivism to metaphysics and a vertical axis with mind–body dualistic types of healing. Rawsley (2003) conceptualized two paradigms that she believed promoted an inclusive nursing science, the heuristic paradigm and the complementarity paradigm. The focus of the heuristic paradigm is a valuing of the process of discovery and of the complementarity paradigm a valuing of inclusiveness. Roy is also a proponent of an integrative paradigm, which she refers to as unity in diversity (Guiliano et al., 2005, p. 246). She believes in the existence of universal truths and that knowledge generated from multiple perspectives can and should be unified to serve the needs of nursing practice.

The third position in this debate is that nursing science is best served by a multi-paradigm perspective in which the various paradigms are complementary. As noted by Pilkington and Mitchell (2003) other disciplines exist with multiple and distinctively different paradigms and Barrett (1992) claims that uniformity of perspective is neither possible nor desirable. Other nurse scholars express similar views. Whitehead (2005) claims "that the *real reality* is that there is not single reality or truth in nursing practice and subsequently no one method [for acquiring knowledge] prevails over the next" (p. 144). Fawcett (2003) also acknowledges the contributions of both the totality and the simultaneity paradigms. Those who support the multiple paradigm perspective have concluded that the complexity of the knowledge base that nurses need to practice requires paradigmatic plurality.

Although not as common as the other positions, some nurse scholars are suggesting that the paradigm debate be suspended. Thorne et al. (1998) claim that "paradigm discourse inhibits rather than fosters productive knowledge development within the discipline" (p. 124), certainly a serious indictment. They identify the dichotomies in perspectives (old versus new) that become the focus of discussions on paradigms as unhelpful in synergistic knowledge development. Kikuchi (2003) suggests a rejection of worldviews (i.e., paradigms) in favor of a philosophy of moderate realism with its emphasis on probable not absolute truths and on a belief that reality exists independent of the human mind. This approach to nursing knowledge development is viewed as a public enterprise, one in which: (a) questions are posed that all scholars can answer; (b) questions are answered in a piece-meal fashion; (c) there is both agreement and disagreement regarding the answers proposed; (d) disagreements are resolved using a accepted standards; and (d) scholarly work is cooperative so that the cumulative knowledge can better answer the questions. This avoidance of the paradigm dilemma may be a trend. Cody and Mitchell (2002) noted that there were decreasing numbers of publications addressing the fundamental philosophical issues of nursing (i.e., ontology and epistemology). By definition, paradigms cannot be discussed without consideration of questions of ontology and epistemology.

The paradigm debate remains unresolved. Without the emergence of a single dominant paradigm, nursing is left with multiple paradigms that are either competing or complementary or the need to develop an integrated paradigm that dialectically combines the perspectives of the multiple paradigms. With this state of paradigm confusion, it would be helpful for nurse theorists to identify the paradigmatic perspective from which the theory is developed and nurse researchers to identify the paradigmatic perspective from which the research questions were posed and the research methods chosen.

METAPARADIGM

Metaparadigm is defined as the global concepts specific to a discipline and the global propositions that define and relate the concepts (Fawcett, 2000, p. 4). A metaparadigm transcends all specific philosophical or paradigmatic orientations. There are four requirements for the metaparadigm of any discipline: (a) a domain distinctive from other disciplines, (b) inclusive of all phenomena of interest to the discipline in a parsimonious way, (c) perspective neutral, and (d) international in scope and substance (Fawcett, 1996, p. 94). The metaparadigm is composed of several domains, often referred to as a typology. These domains are a classification system to identify the constructs or phenomena that are the focus of nursing. Several nursing metaparadigms have been suggested. For instance, Kim (2000) suggested a four-domain typology consisting of client, client–nurse, practice, and environment. The client domain is concerned with only those phenomena that pertain to the client. The client–nurse domain focuses on the phenomena that emerge from nurse–client interactions. The practice domain refers to what nurses do as a professional. The environment domain is composed of physical, social, and symbolic components of the client's external world, both past and present. The four-domain typology most frequently cited in nursing literature includes: man/person, health, society/environment, and nursing (Fawcett, 1978; Yura & Torres, 1975). The metaparadigm described by Fawcett is also composed of four nonrelational and four relational propositions. The nonrelational propositions provide the definitions of the four domains and the relational propositions describe the linkages between the domains. (See Table 1.2 for an overview of these propositions.)

DEVELOPMENT

A metaparadigm is not so much constructed as it is identified. This identification process occurs through the analysis of the recurring themes of nursing's theories (Sarter, 1988). This analysis is philosophical in

TABLE 1.2 Fawcett's Relational and Nonrelational Propositions of Metaparadigm

Proposition	Definitions and linkages
Nonrelational	1. Person refers to individuals, families, communities, and other groups who are involved in nursing. 2. Environment refers to the person's social network and physical surroundings and to the setting in which nursing is taking place. It also includes all local, regional, national, cultural, social, political, and economic conditions that might have an impact on a person's health. 3. Health refers to a person's state of well-being at the time of engagement with nursing. It exists on a continuum from high-level wellness to terminal illness. 4. Nursing refers to the definition of the discipline, the actions taken by nurses on behalf and/or with the person, and the goals or outcomes of those actions.
Relational	1. Nursing is concerned with the principles and laws that govern life processes, well-being, and optimal functioning of human beings, sick or well. 2. Nursing is concerned with the patterning of human behavior in the interaction with the environment in normal life events and critical situations. 3. Nursing is concerned with the nursing actions or processes by which positive changes in health status are effected. 4. Nursing is concerned with the wholeness or health of human beings, recognizing that they are in continuous interaction with their environment.

Source: Fawcett, J. (2000). *Analysis and evaluation of contemporary nursing knowledge: Nursing models and theories* (3rd ed., pp. 5–6). Philadelphia, PA: F. A. Davis. Reprinted with permission from F. A. Davis, Philadelphia, PA.

nature and allows for recognition of the "common and coherent philosophical orientation" (p. 52) of the discipline of nursing.

USES

Metaparadigms, or in Kim's (1983) words, a typology, are "boundary-maintaining devices" (p. 19) and as such help delineate nursing's frame of reference. The primary purpose then is to provide a means of focusing on that which is inherently nursing and marginalizing that which is not. This enables nurse practitioners, theorists, and researchers to concentrate their energies on the business of nursing. In addition, the metaparadigm is used for the purpose of analysis, a framework for comparing the perspectives of various nursing theorists (Fawcett, 2005; Fitzpatrick & Whall, 1983; Kim, 1983). For instance, Fitzpatrick and Whall noted that Levine defined health as wholeness, whereas Johnson found health to be a moving state of equilibrium.

CONTROVERSY

By definition, a discipline possesses only one metaparadigm. The controversy involves what that metaparadigm should be. Fawcett (2005) critiqued nine other paradigms using the criteria of distinctiveness, inclusiveness, neutrality, and internationality. The paradigms suggested by Newman; Conway; Kim; Meleis; King; Newman et al.; Malloch, Martinez, Nelson, Predeger, Speakman, Stienbinder, and Tracy; Parse; and Leininger/Watson all failed to meet one or more of the stated criteria. Fawcett's most common criticism was failure of the paradigms to meet the criterion of inclusion. For example, Kim (1983) did not address health; King (1984) eliminated environment and nursing; and Newman et al. (1996) failed to include environment. Obviously, nursing is still in search of a commonly shared metaparadigm and requires further philosophical analysis to arrive at this metaparadigm.

The metaparadigm proposed by Fawcett has also received criticism. It was faulted for using outdated language (Fawcett, 2003), being oriented to a particular paradigm (Fawcett, 2003), providing a limited perspective of the domains (Malone, 2005), and reflecting a cultural bias (Kao, Reeder, Hsu, & Cheng, 2006). Leininger criticized the use of the term *person* as being too individualistic and Fawcett now proposes using the term *persons* (Fawcett, 2003, p. 273). Malone (2005) found the conceptualization of the domain, environment, to be underdeveloped; she believed that greater emphasis is needed on the policy environment. The Western orientation of the metaparadigm is also criticized. In light of the fact that nursing is a global enterprise, this criticism seems warranted. Kao et al. (2006) provided definitions of each of the four domains from the perspective of Chinese philosophies. For instance, the concept person can be defined in part as a social being engaged in ethical relationships, relationships governed by certain rules (p. 93). Fawcett (1996) believes that the nursing metaparadigm that she proposed is the final conceptualization for the discipline. "Indeed, it is anticipated that modifications in the metaparadigm concepts and propositions will be offered as the discipline of nursing evolves" (p. 95). Recent nursing literature reveals only limited consideration of the discipline's metaparadigm.

CONCEPTUAL MODELS

Conceptual models are a "set of interrelated concepts that symbolically represent and convey a mental image of a phenomen[on]" (Fawcett & Alligood, 2005, p. 228). Adam (1992) claims that they are the cornerstone of nursing's development (p. 61). Conceptual models are considered less abstract and more explicit and specific than philosophies but more abstract and less explicit and specific than theories (Adam, 1992; Alligood & Tomey, 2006; Caper, 1986; Fawcett, 2005). The term *conceptual model* has been used interchangeably, accompanied by some controversy, with conceptual framework, theoretical framework, conceptual system (King, 1997), philosophy (Adam, 1992), disciplinary matrix, paradigm (Fawcett, 1992), theory (Dickhoff & James, 1968; Fitzpatrick & Whall, 2005; Meleis, 1997), and macrotheory (Adam, 1992).

Beginning in the 1960s, conceptual models emerged as nursing attempted to distinguish itself from other disciplines, especially medicine (Kikuchi, 1992; Schlotfeldt, 1992). Since the 1960s, nursing models have been developed, proposed, analyzed, critiqued, and refined. Table 1.3 provides examples of the work of nurse scientists that has been labeled as conceptual models.

DEVELOPMENT

Conceptual models are typically developed through the three stages of conceptualization or formulation, model formalization, and validation (Young, Taylor, & Renpenning, p. 11). The process can be empirical or intuitive, deductive or inductive. Empirically, nurse scholars make observations from practice; intuitively, they develop insights; deductively, they combine ideas from a variety of areas of inquiry, particularly other theories (e.g., general systems) and scientific bases; and inductively, they generalize from specific situations or observations. Conceptual nursing models reflect assumptions, beliefs, and values and, according to Adam (1992), are composed of six units, with commonly occurring philosophical perspectives. The following list summarizes the units and philosophical perspectives with examples from Johnson's *Behavioral System Model.*

1. Goal of nursing, generally idealistic, pragmatic, and humanistic; for instance, "fostering effective and efficient behavioral functioning" (Johnson, 1990, p. 24).
2. Conceptualizations of the client, usually existential and humanistic, and almost certainly holistic, as evidenced by Johnson's eight behavioral subsystems (Grubbs, 1974).
3. Social role of nurse, often humanistic and idealistic; for example, nursing is viewed as a service that makes a unique contribution to the health and well-being of individuals—specifically, nurses act to "provide a distinctive service to society" (Grubbs, 1974, p. 160) and "to seek the highest possible level of behavioral functioning [for the patient]" (Grubbs, 1974, p. 161).
4. Source of difficulty, primarily pragmatic, because it identifies the scope of nursing's responsibility; for instance, behavioral disequilibrium and unpredictability, indicating a malfunction in the behavioral system (Grubbs, 1974).
5. Intervention, typically humanistic, idealistic, and pragmatic; for example, restrict (e.g., set limits on dysfunctional behavior), defend (e.g., use isolation techniques), inhibit (e.g., teach new skills), and facilitate (e.g., provide adequate nutrition) (Grubbs, 1974).

TABLE 1.3 Conceptual Models

Model	Selected sources
Johnson's Behavioral System Model	Johnson, D. E. (1959). The nature and science of nursing. *Nursing Outlook, 7*, 291–294. Johnson, D. E. (1980). The behavioral system model for nursing. In J. P. Reihl & C. Roy (Eds.), *Conceptual models for nursing practice* (2nd ed., pp. 207–216). New York: Appleton-Century-Crofts. Johnson, D. E. (1990). The behavioral system model for nursing. In Parker, M. E. (Ed.), *Nursing theories in practice* (pp. 23–32). New York: National League for Nursing.
King's General Systems Framework	King, I. M. (1968). A conceptual frame of reference for nursing. *Nursing Research, 17,* 27–31. King, I. M. (1971). *Toward a theory of nursing: General concepts of human behavior.* New York: Wiley. King, I. M. (1981). *A theory for nursing: Systems, concepts, process.* New York: Wiley.
Levine's Conservation Model	Levine, M. E. (1969). The pursuit of wholeness. *American Journal of Nursing, 69,* 93–98. Levine, M. E. (1991). The conservation model: A model for health. In K. M. Schaefer & J. B. Pond (Eds.), *The conservation model: A framework for nursing practice* (pp. 1–11). Philadelphia: F. A. Davis. Levine, M. E. (1996). The conservation principles: A retrospective. *Nursing Science Quarterly, 9*(1), 38–41.
Neuman's Systems Model	Neuman, B. (1982). *The Neuman systems model: Application to nursing education and practice.* Norwalk, CT: Appleton-Century-Crofts. Neuman, B. (1995). *The Neuman systems model* (3rd ed.). Norwalk, CT: Appleton & Lange. Neuman, B. (1996). The Neuman system model in research and practice. *Nursing Science Quarterly, 9*(1), 67–70.
Rogers' Science of Human Beings	Rogers, M. E. (1980). Nursing: A science of unitary man. In J. P. Reihl & C. Roy (Eds.), *Conceptual models for nursing practice* (2nd ed., pp. 207–216). New York: Appleton-Century-Crofts. Rogers, M. E. (1990). Nursing: A science for unitary, irreducible human beings: Update 1990. In E. A. M. Barrett (Ed.), *Visions of Rogers' science-based nursing* (pp. 5–11). New York: National League for Nursing. Rogers, M. E. (1994). The science of unitary human beings: Current perspectives. *Nursing Science Quarterly, 7,* 33–35.
Roper-Logan-Tierney Model for Nursing	Roper, N., Logan, W., & Tierney, A. (1996). *The elements of nursing: A model for nursing based on a model of living* (4th ed.). Edinburgh: Churchill Livingstone. Roper, N., Logan, W., & Tierney, A. (1983). A nursing model. *Nursing Mirror, 156*(22), 17–19. Roper, N., Logan, W., & Tierney, A. (1997). The Roper-Logan-Tierney model. In P. Hinton-Walker & B. Neuman (Eds.), *Blueprint for use of nursing models.* New York: National League for Nursing.
Roy's Adaptation Model	Roy, C. (1971). Adaptation: A conceptual framework for nursing. *Nursing Outlook, 18*(3), 42–45. Roy, C. (1976). *Introduction to nursing: An adaptation model.* Englewood Cliffs, NJ: Prentice-Hall. Roy, C., & Andrews, H. A. (1999). *The Roy adaptation model: The definitive statement.* Norwalk, CT: Appleton & Lange.

6. Desired consequences, also typically humanistic, idealistic, and pragmatic, as evidenced by Johnson's goal of system balance and stability (Grubbs, 1974; Johnson, 1990).

Although Johnson's *Behavioral System Model* was used as one example of how these components are addressed in a conceptual model, all the conceptual models found in Table 1.3 consider these six components, each from its unique perspective.

Uses

The development of conceptual models is essential to the professional identity of nursing. The conceptual models delineate the goals and scope of nursing and provide frameworks for considering the outcomes of nursing. In general, they can direct a professional discipline's theory development, practice, education, and research.

Conceptual models can give birth to nursing theories. Fawcett (2005, p. 19) claims that "grand theories are derived directly from conceptual models." Because, by definition, conceptual models are considered more abstract and less specific than theories, several can develop from a single conceptual model. For instance, several grand theories were derived from Roger's conceptual model, the *Science of Unitary Human Beings.* The Theory of Power as Knowing Participation in Change (Barrett, 1986) is one example of a theory with its origins in Roger's conceptual model. The alternate view is that conceptual models are "not necessary, and, perhaps, not even important for theoretical growth (Rodman, 1980, p. 436). For instance, Leininger's *Theory of Cultural Care Diversity and Universality* was derived from anthropological concepts, research (the first being a study of the Gadsup people in Papua, New Guinea), and her beliefs about nursing. Peplau's *Theory of Interpersonal Relations* was based on an integration of theories from the field of psychology and the recorded interactions between student nurses and patients.

The relationship between nursing's conceptual models and practice is a reciprocal one. Conceptual models can provide a structure for nursing practice and practice experiences can provide evidence of the credibility of the model (Kahn & Fawcett, 1995). In order for a conceptual model to be considered useful it must demonstrate: (a) social utility—content is understandable and the interpersonal and psychomotor skills needed to apply the model can be mastered; (b) social congruence—nursing activities are culturally congruent with the expectations of the patient, community, and members of the health care team; and (c) social significance—the use of the model provides outcomes of social value, particularly as it relates to patients' health status (Kahn & Fawcett, 1995, p. 189). In practice, the models have most often been used as a framework for implementation of the nursing process (Archibald, 2000, "Nursing Models," para. 2). Assessment based on a conceptual model tends to be more comprehensive, focused, and specific (Hardy, 1986). Because of their level of abstraction, models tend to be less effective in prescribing specific nursing interventions. Instead, the conceptual models suggest general areas of nursing action. The unique focus of each conceptual model also implies criteria for determining when problems have been solved, thus aiding the process of evaluation.

Many schools of nursing used conceptual models as a framework for their curricula. The use of nursing's conceptual models ensured that the focus of the students' education was on nursing, not on medicine. It provided students with a perspective for considering nursing issues and a language for expressing such. Beginning in the 1960s and through the 1990s, schools of nursing have identified the use of specific conceptual models in their curricula, for example, Johnson's *Behavioral System Model* (Harris, 1986), King's *General Systems Framework* (Brown & Lee, 1980), Neuman's *Systems Model* (Kilchenstein & Yakulis, 1984), and Roy's *Adaptation Model* (Brower & Baker, 1976).

Conceptual models can also guide research. "Research is nursing research only if it examines phenomena of special interest to nursing, that is, phenomena that are indicated by one or the other of the conceptual models for nursing" (Adam, 1992, p. 59). Since conceptual models for nursing represent foci of scientific inquiry, they can identify questions for research. For instance, conceptual models generated the following questions: (a) In Johnson's *Behavioral System Model,* what are the effects of the stage of cancer on the eight behavioral subsystems? (Derdiarian, 1988); (b) In King's *General Systems Framework,* what factors interfere with goal attainment? (Kameoda & Sugimori, 1993); and (c), In Neuman's *System Model,* what effect did experience with the model have on the quality of nursing diagnoses? (Mackenzie

& Spence Laschinger, 1995). It is important to note that avenues of questioning suggested by conceptual models are not the same as those of empirical testing, which less abstract theories undergo.

CONTROVERSY

There are some controversies about the use and usefulness of conceptual models. Although conceptual models cannot be tested or validated because of their level of abstractness (Adam, 1992; Downs, 1982), they can and should be evaluated. Evaluation of conceptual models has revealed some general limitations. They have been criticized for the following:

- Their level of abstraction, limiting their usefulness
- Rigidity and inflexibility, which inhibits change
- The subjectivity of perspective, which may not be shared by professional colleagues or clients
- The use of a unique language or jargon, requiring specialized education or resulting in confusing communication
- Potential to be used in inappropriate situations and for incorrect purposes (Adam, 1992; Hardy, 1986; Littlejohn, 2002; Tierney, 1998; Young et al., 2001)

Controversy about the use of conceptual models in relation to theory development is complicated by lack of consistency in labeling the work of nurse scientists. Fawcett's (2005) position is that conceptual models are more abstract and global and less specific than theories. Kramer (1997) identifies conceptual models as a type of theory but claims not all theories are conceptual models. Meleis (1997) concludes that most of the differences between the two are semantic and noted that the nurse scientists themselves referred to their work using a variety of terms. For instance, Rogers called her conceptualization of nursing a science (Science of Unitary Human Beings); Erickson referred to her work as both a theory and a paradigm (Modeling and Role-Modeling: A Theory and Paradigm); and Watson identified her thinking as both philosophy and theory (Watson's *Philosophy and Theory of Human Caring*). In this book, conceptual models and theories have been treated as distinct entities. Although there is some confusion about the term and some limitations regarding their use, conceptual models have proved valuable for the advancement of nursing research and the development of theories.

THEORY: GENERAL ISSUES

Similar to conceptual models, theories are comprised of concepts and propositions. In a theory, the concepts are defined more specifically and the propositions are more narrowly focused. Although theory and paradigm are sometimes used interchangeably, theories differ from both paradigms and philosophies in that they represent what is rather than what should be (Babbie, 1995, pp. 37, 47). A theoretical body of knowledge is considered an essential characteristic of all professions (Johnson, 1974). Therefore, theories serve to further specify the uniqueness or distinctiveness of a profession. "Theories have in fact distinguished nursing from other caring professions by fixing professional boundaries" (Rutty, 1998, Theory, para. 2). The definition of theory by Kerlinger is classic and comprehensive. "Kerlinger (1973) defines theory as follows: A theory is a set of interrelated constructs (concepts, definitions, and propositions) that present a systematic view of phenomena by specifying relations among variables, with the purpose of explaining and predicting phenomena" (King, 1978, p. 11). In addition to explanation and prediction of phenomena Glaser and Straus (1967) identify other uses of theory. They believe that theories by definition should also be able to further advance theory development, guide practice by providing understanding and the possibility of controlling some situations, offer a perspective on behavior, a means of interpreting data, and provide an approach or style for the research of a specific area of human behavior. Theories should be inherently useful.

In addition to considering the development, uses, and controversies surrounding nursing theories, it is important to address the classifications of theories. Theories can be classified in a number of ways, such as by their purposes, sources, and levels. The three major levels of nursing are grand, middle range, and practice, with middle range theory of special interest as it grows in importance in nursing research and practice.

DEVELOPMENT

The development of a theory involves both content and process. Theories are comprised of concepts and their relationships and are constructed through a variety of processes. The history of theory development in nursing helps provide a context for understanding the ongoing work of nurse scientists in the advancement of nursing's body of knowledge.

COMPONENTS

A variety of terms are used to describe concepts and propositions, the two basic elements of a theory. The terms *concept, construct, descriptor,* and *unit* are often used interchangeably, with concept being the most common. Definitions of the concepts can be considered an aspect of the basic element, concept, or as a separate and additional component of a theory. Statements of relationships or propositions refer to the same notion. In addition, some scientists include axioms and postulates as other components of a theory, because, though they are relational statements, they are assertions assumed to be true that lay the groundwork for the propositions (Babbie, 1995, p. 48).

Concepts. Concepts are considered the basic building blocks of theory. Kim (2000, p. 15) defines concepts as "a symbolic statement describing a phenomenon or a class of phenomena." In other words, a concept is a mental image of a phenomenon, an idea, or construct of an object or action (Walker & Avant, 2005, p. 26). Although there are several more complicated classifications of concepts (or units), basically they can be classified on a continuum of abstractness, which some label primitive, abstract, and concrete (Meleis, 1997), and others global, middle range, and empirical (Moody, 1990). They can also be categorized as property or process concepts (Kim, 2000).

Primitive concepts are those that have a culturally shared meaning (Walker & Avant, 2005, p. 26) or are those that are introduced as new in the theory (Meleis, 1997, p. 252). For instance, in culturally derived concepts, a color is usually primitive because it cannot be defined except by giving examples of another color different from the original color. Grass, leaves, and apples would be examples of green, and sky, bark, and grapefruit would be examples of not green. As an original concept in a new theory, role supplementation in the theory of Role Insufficiency and Role Supplementation would be an example of a theory-specific primitive concept (Meleis, 1997, p. 252). Concrete concepts are those that exist in a spatial–temporal reality. They can be defined in terms of primitive concepts. Grass, leaves, apples, sky, bark, and grapefruit would all be examples of concrete concepts. In nursing, touch used by the nurse would be considered a concrete concept. Abstract concepts can be defined by primitive or concrete concepts but are not limited by time or space. "They refer to general cases" (Kim, 2000, p. 16). Communication could be identified as an abstract concept that would be of interest to nursing. Theories can be comprised of both concrete and abstract concepts.

For theories using abstract concepts, operational definitions of those concepts are an important inclusion because the definitions enable the theory to be more easily tested empirically through research. An operational definition "assign[s] explicit meaning to that [abstract] concept" (Duldt & Giffin, 1985, p. 95). Operational definitions can be (a) experimental, providing specific details necessary to manipulate the concept; (b) measurable, describing the means by which the concept can be measured; (c) administrative, including particular information on how to obtain data about the concept; and (d) evaluative, establishing the criteria for operationalizing the concept and the means of determining the degree to which the criteria are met.

The classification of concepts as property or process is significant because it promotes understanding of the concept as defined by the theorist. Property concepts are those that deal with the state of things, and process concepts are those that relate to the way things happen. Stage of grief would be a property concept, whereas, grieving as the means by which an individual deals with loss would be a process concept. A concept can be considered both a property and a process concept, such as communication. In general, theories contain both types of concepts. "The classification system of concepts into property and process types is useful in an analytic sense" (Kim, 2000, p. 18). It provides a clearer sense of the nature of the concepts included in the theory and thus a better understanding of the theory itself.

Propositions. Propositions, defined as statements of the relationships between two or more concepts, provide a theory "with the powers of description, explanation or prediction" (Meleis, 1997, p. 252). Propositional statements can be considered either relational or nonrelational. Relational statements can be either correlational or causal. Nonrelational statements include descriptions of the properties and dimensions of the concept in the definition of the term *proposition* (Meleis, 1997).

In propositional statements that are correlational, the assertion is that two or more concepts exist together or are associated. The associations can be positive, negative, or neutral. Orem's *Self-care Deficit Nursing Theory* provides examples of positive and neutral correlational statements. The nurse affects the movement from the "'present state of affairs' to 'a desirable future state of affairs' by using the 'nursing means' the nurse selects" (Orem, 2001, p. 151) is an example of a positive statement. "Engagement in self-care or dependent-care is affected by persons' valuation of self-care measures with respect to life, development, heath, and well-being" (Orem, 2001, p. 146) is an example of a more neutral or directionless statement.

Causal propositional statements establish cause-and-effect relationships. Examples of causal statements are found in Parse's *Man-Living-Health Theory of Nursing.* "In a nurse–family process, by synchronizing rhythms, the members uncover the opportunities and limitations created by the decisions made in choosing irreplaceable ways of being together. The choices of new ways of being together mobilize transcendence." (Parse, 1987, p. 170). Causal statements are more difficult to establish than correlational statements and therefore more rare.

"Nonrelational statements serve as adjuncts to relational statements"; they are the means by which theorists clarify meanings in the theory (Walker & Avant, 2005, p. 27).

They provide assertions of the existence of concepts or definitions of concepts of a theory and thus help explain the nature of the theory. An example of an existence proposition would be Parse's statement that the practice methodology of her theory is comprised of three dimensions: illuminating meaning, synchronizing rhythms, and mobilizing transcendence (Parse, 1987, p. 167). Parse also provides definitional propositions, for example, "health is Man's unfolding. It is Man's lived experiences, a non linear entity that cannot be qualified by terms as good, bad, more, or less" (Parse, 1987, p. 160).

The nature of the elements of the theory relates to the purposes for which the theory can be used. Theories with only nonrelational prepositional statements serve to describe, whereas theories with relational prepositional statements have the potential to explain (correlational statements) and predict (causal statements).

PROCESS

Theory development can be accomplished by inductive or deductive processes or by a combination of both. The content of a theory comes from other theories, practice, or research, or a combination of two or more of these sources. Using other theories as a source of generating a theory involves a deductive process, whereas using practice experience or research findings for developing a theory requires an inductive process.

Walker and Avant (1995) describe strategies of theory development that include both inductive and deductive processes. Analysis, synthesis, and derivation are applied to concepts, statements, and theories. Analysis is solely an inductive process, whereas synthesis and derivation can involve both inductive and deductive processes (Walker & Avant, 1995, p. 32). Table 1.4 presents a matrix of the purposes of the nine strategies that Walker and Avant (1995) describe in detail in their book, *Strategies for Theory Construction in Nursing.*

This process of theory construction is modeled in the work of Lenz, Suppe, Gift, Pugh, and Milligan (1995), as they collaborated on the development of the middle range theory of unpleasant symptoms. For instance, the researchers used existing literature for concept analysis, examining attributes, characteristics, and dimensions of the concept of dyspnea. The literature review also served as a basis of concept derivation, resulting in the identification of pain as an analog of dyspnea. And through synthesis of the literature and the researchers' own experiences, they conceptualized dyspnea as having five components: sensation, perception, distress, response, and reporting.

Walker and Avant (1995) identify other theories as a source of additional theory development. Theories from other disciplines are one source of nursing theory content. Peplau made use of psychoanalytic theory and Johnson made use of systems theory, informed by their clinical practices, psychiatric and pediatric

TABLE 1.4 Matrix of Approaches to Theory Construction

	Concept	Statement	Theory
Analysis	Distinguish between defining and irrelevant attributes of the concept by breaking a concept into simpler elements and considering similarities and differences	Determine how useful, informative, and logically correct the statements are through an orderly examination	Determine the strengths and weaknesses of theory by applying an analytical framework
Synthesis	Generate new ideas by examining data for new insights	Develop statements about relationships through observations of phenomena	Construct a theory from empirical evidence
Derivation	Generate new ways of thinking about phenomena by developing a new vocabulary based on the relationships between phenomena	Formulate statements about a poorly understood phenomenon by clarifying relationships between phenomena	Explain and predict phenomena, which are poorly understood or for which no methods of study are known, or for which no theory exists

Source: Walker, L. O., & Avant, K. C. (1995). *Strategies for theory construction in nursing* (3rd ed.). Norwalk, CT: Appleton & Lange.

nursing, respectively. Nursing theories and conceptual models often give rise to middle range theory. For instance, from Orem's *Self-care Deficit Theory* came the *Theory of Dependent-care Deficit, Theory of Self-care,* and *Theory of Nursing Systems* (Alligood & Tomey, 2005, p. 53).

"Some theories are driven by clinical practice situations and are inductively developed" (Meleis, 1997, p. 230). This grounded theory approach uses observations and analysis of similarities and differences of observed phenomena to develop concepts and establish their relationships. The works of Peplau, Orlando, Travelbee, and Wiedenbach have been associated with this approach.

Research is often cited as the most common and acceptable source for theory development, most often leading to the development of a middle range theory. "Theories evolve from replicated and confirmed research findings" (Meleis, 1997, p. 231). This is considered an empirical quantitative approach and involves: (a) identifying a phenomenon, listing all its characteristics; (b) measuring these characteristics in a variety of settings; (c) analyzing the results to determine if patterns exist; and (d) formalizing these patterns as theoretical statements (Reynolds, 1971, p. 140). Johnson and Rice's (1974) theory of *Sensory and Distress Components of Pain* was developed using this approach.

Qualitative research is often referred to as theory-generating, with grounded theory and phenomenology often used by nurse scientists to develop theories. Fagerhaugh's (1974) theory of *Pain Expression and Control* is an example of theory developed through qualitative research. Meta-synthesis is emerging as an approach for developing theory, especially middle range theory (Annells, 2005; Walsh & Downe, 2005). This method addresses the criticism that theory development from qualitative research relies on a small number of homogeneous participants (Estbrooks, Field, & Morse, 1994). Meta-synthesis involves aggregation of qualitative data, employing four processes—"comprehending, synthesizing, theorizing, and recontextualizing" (Estabrooks, Field, & Morse, p. 505) with greatest emphasis on theorizing and recontextualizing. Dynamics of hope in adults living with HIV/AIDS: a substantive theory was developed using meta-synthesis (Kylma, 2005). McKenna (1997) noted similarities between the quantitative and qualitative approaches: both use inductive methods, and both generally result in the development of middle range theories.

History

Nursing theory development can trace its roots to the work of Florence Nightingale (Alligood & Tomey, 2005; Dunphy, 2001; Fitzpatrick & Whall, 2005; Meleis, 1997), with her concern for the relationship between health and environment and the nurse's role in that relationship. Hildegard Peplau is credited with being the first contemporary nurse theorist (McKenna, 1997). Other theorists of the 1950s (Henderson [in Henderson and Harmer], 1955; Orem, 1959; Johnson, 1959; Hall, 1959; cited in McKenna, 1997, p. 95) were influenced by Peplau's conceptualization of interpersonal relationships in nursing. Others were influenced by their involvement at Columbia University's Teachers' College and the practical-oriented philosophy of John Dewey, who served on its staff. From Teachers' College in the 1950s, Abdellah, King, Wiedenbach, and Rogers emerged as nurse theorists (Meleis, 1997). Not all of the work of these nurse scientists would be considered theory by today's definition. The theoretical work that did take place in the 1950s focused on what nurses did, not why they did it, and the conceptual frameworks developed at this time were more often used as a basis for the development of curricula than as a guide for practice. The 1950s also saw the introduction of the journal, *Nursing Research,* which provided a forum for the development of nursing theories and their testing.

In addition to continuing development of individual nursing theories, the 1960s brought a more national and coordinated approach to theory development. Federal financial support became available in 1962 to nurses pursuing doctoral education; the American Nurses Association stated in 1965 that theory development was a significant goal for the profession; and in 1967, Case Western Reserve University sponsored a national nursing symposium, a third of which was devoted to nursing theory. The theorists associated with this decade include "Abdellah et al. (1960), Orlando (1961), Wiedenbach (1964), Levine (1966), Travelbee (1966) and King (1968)" (McKenna, 1997, pp. 95, 96). Theorists, particularly Wiedenbach and Orlando, began to consider not only what nurses did, but also what effect it had on patients. Debate, stimulated by the metatheorists, focused on the issue of the types of theories that nursing should develop rather than the content of theories.

Although nursing theorists continued to develop and publish their work, such as Roy (1970), Rogers (1970), Neuman (1972), Riehl (1974), Adam (1975), Patterson and Zderad (1976), Leininger (1978), Watson (1979) and Newman (1979) (McKenna, 1997, p. 97), the questions posed by meta-theorists dominated the 1970s (Meleis, 1997). Efforts were made to determine what is meant by theory; to identify the structural components of theories; and to clarify the methods of analysis and critique of theory. The previously developed theories were criticized for a failure to include explicated propositions and for their lack of empirical testing (McKenna, 1997, p. 97). The development and use of nursing theories were advanced by (a) the adoption by the National League for Nursing of an accreditation criterion requiring a theory base to nursing curricula; (b) the formation of two groups (Nursing Theories Conference Group and Nursing Theory Think Tank) that considered application of theory to practice; and (c) the publication of *Advances in Nursing Science,* a journal dedicated to the development of nursing science.

Alligood and Tomey (2005) refer to the 1980s as the Theory Era, even though few new nursing theories emerged. "Only three new nursing theories were published in the 1980s: the work of Parse (1981), Fitzpatrick (1982) and Erickson, Tomlin and Swain (1983) (McKenna, 1997, p. 97). Fawcett's (1984) explication of a metaparadigm for nursing allowed for the comparative content analysis of theories, and her delineation of the levels of abstraction of nursing knowledge helped nurse scientists and practitioners make the distinctions between grand, middle range, and practice theories. Her work also clarified how nursing grand theory can be derived from nursing conceptual models and how middle range theory can be derived from grand theory. The importance of nursing theory to the profession was well established and the shift by the end of this decade was away from theory development toward theory use (Alligood & Tomey, 2005, p. 9). There was both an increased interest in the relationship between theory and practice and an increased emphasis on the relationship between theory and research.

The 1990s were hallmarked by the development of the middle range and practice theories. These theories are less abstract and therefore more directly applicable to practice and more easily tested empirically by research. Interest in nursing theory was evidenced by the publication of *Nursing Science Quarterly,* edited by Parse, focusing on theory development and testing and by the increasing number of European-based nursing theory conferences.

USES

Nurse scientists have worked on the development of nursing theory as part of the process of establishing nursing as a profession with a unique body of knowledge. Nursing theories provide nurses with the language of nursing, a means of communicating the nature of the discipline within and outside the profession.

In addition, as a component of nursing knowledge considered less abstract than conceptual frameworks, nursing theories generate more specific research questions and provide greater guidance to nursing practice.

Nursing theories provide nursing-specific identifications, definitions, and interrelationships of concepts. This allows the profession to distinguish itself from the medical and behavioral sciences. For example, in nursing, we speak of unitary human beings, self-care, and the centrality of caring. Through analysis of theories, nursing's metaparadigm emerges, providing us with a common and basic frame of reference for communicating about nursing.

The relationship between nursing theory and research is symbiotic. Research provides for both theory generating and theory testing. Qualitative research seeks to identify and define phenomena of interest to nursing, thus serving as a theory-generating tool. By contrast, quantitative research is a means by which the propositions of theories can be substantiated, thus functioning as a theory-testing tool. Theories then serve as a framework for relating the data generated by research, resulting in a more coherent whole nursing body of knowledge than a collection of isolated facts.

In addition, the greater clarification of concepts and their relationships that nursing theories provide allows researchers to formulate more specific and nursing-relevant research questions. The evidence that is generated through the study of these questions, because of the level of specificity and relevance, in turn is more directly applicable to nursing practice. Parse (1999) challenges nurses "to conduct research to ensure that the practice of nursing serves people in a unique way" (Recommendations, para. 1). It is through nursing theories that the profession identifies its unique service to people. The testing of nursing theories also leads to theory-guided evidence-based practice. "Evidence itself refers to evidence about theories. Similarly, theory determines what counts as evidence" (Fawcett, Watson, Neuman, Walker, & Fitzpatrick, 2001). Thus, theory as it guides research has the potential to provide the evidence that makes nursing practice more efficient and more effective.

CONTROVERSY

There are two recurring themes in criticisms of nursing theories: the issue of consistency in labeling and the appropriateness of the sources of the theories used by nurses. The lack of definitional clarity between what is labeled a conceptual model and what is considered a theory is further complicated by confusion over identification of the level of the theory, that is, grand, middle range, or practice. Nurse scientists have not consistently classified the level of the developed theory in the work they publish. This issue is further addressed in the discussion of the middle range level of theory development. In addition, there is some disagreement over the appropriate source of theories to be used by nurses, borrowed or unique. The debate focuses on to what degree nurses can use theories from other disciplines and still advance nursing's unique body of knowledge. The discussion of this issue is integrated into the section on classification of theories by source.

CLASSIFICATIONS

Theories differ in their purposes, sources, and, most importantly, levels of abstraction and scope. These differences lead to classifications. The basic purposes of theory are description, explanation, prediction, and/or control. The sources of theory in nursing include those developed by nurse scientists (unique) and those that are used in nursing but come from other disciplines (borrowed). The terms *theory of nursing* and *theory in nursing* are often used to distinguish between these two sources.

There are multiple terms used to classify the various levels or scope of nursing theories. The broad-scope theories are referred to as *macro, holistic, molar, general, situation,* and, most commonly, *grand.* Narrow-scope theories are called *middle range, circumscribed,* or *situation/factor.* Theories narrowest in scope are labeled *micro, molecular, atomistic, narrow-range, phenomena, prescriptive, factor, situation-specific,* or *practice* (Babbie, 1995; George, 1995; Parker, 2006; Rinehart, 1978). The most common labels for the levels of nursing theory are grand, middle range, and micro or practice. The level is determined primarily by the theory's degree of abstraction. Examination of the level of abstraction of the "purpose, concept, and definitional components of the theory" (Kramer, 1997, p. 65) allows for the identification of the level of the theory.

PURPOSES

Although theories are designed to describe, explain, predict, and/or control, some nurse scientists claim that only theories that enable nurses to control outcomes are legitimate for a practice discipline (Dickhoff & James, 1968). Descriptive theories are limited to naming and classifying characteristics of the phenomenon of interest, which identify what is happening. Peplau's *Theory of Interpersonal Relations* has been labeled a descriptive theory.

Explanatory theories expand the knowledge base by delineating the relationships between characteristics of the phenomenon, clarifying why it is happening. Watson's *Theory of Human Caring* is considered an explanatory theory. But predictive theories provide the conditions that can result in a preferred outcome, determining how it can intentionally happen. Orlando's *Theory of the Deliberative Nursing Process* is an example of a predictive theory. Theories whose purpose is to control, often referred to as prescriptive theories, guide action to create an intended result. The three ingredients for this type of theory are content of goal, primary prescription for activity to achieve goal, and list of additional recommendation of activity (Dickhoff & James, 1968, p. 201).

The existence of descriptive and explanatory theories is a necessary precursor for the development of predictive and prescriptive theories. "Predictive theory presupposes the prior existence of more elementary types of theories" (Dickhoff & James, 1968, p. 200). The relationship between the purposes of a theory has been conceptualized in some instances as a hierarchy:

1. Factor-isolating theories (descriptive)
2. Factor-relating theories (descriptive/explanatory)
3. Situation-relating theories (explanatory/predictive)
4. Situation-producing theories (prescriptive) (Dickhoff & James, 1968, pp. 200–201)

SOURCES

The source of theory refers to the discipline from which it developed. The possibilities include theories unique to nursing, theories borrowed from other disciplines, and theories from other disciplines adapted for nursing. A borrowed theory is one in which the knowledge "is developed in the main by other disciplines and is drawn upon by nursing" (Johnson, 1986, p. 118). The distinctions between these three sources are difficult to make since "the man-made, more-or less arbitrary divisions between the sciences are neither firm nor constant" (Johnson, 1986, p. 117).

Given that the differences between the sources of theory may be less than perfectly precise, unique theory can be defined "as that knowledge derived from the observation of phenomena and the asking of questions unlike those which characterized other disciplines" (Johnson, 1986, p. 118). Many argue that nursing's identity as a profession and, ultimately, its ability to improve nursing practice are dependent on the existence of nursing theories unique to the discipline. Wald and Leonard (1964), the most frequently cited proponents of this position, claimed that to become an independent discipline, nursing was required to develop its own theories rather than borrow theories or apply principles from other disciplines. They expressed concern about nursing's reliance on these borrowed theories.

Wald and Leonard's concerns seem validated by Jacobson's (1987) findings. When nurses with advanced degrees were asked to identify "conceptual models of nursing," responses included Selye's stress model, Piaget's theory of cognitive development, general system's theory, problem solving, and Maslow's hierarchy of needs. All of these examples would be considered borrowed rather than knowledge unique to nursing.

As recently as 2001, the literature reveals continued reliance on theories from fields other than nursing. Fawcett and Bourbonniere (2001) found that of 90 research studies published in two clinical journals, *Geriatric Nursing* and *Nurse Practitioner,* and two research journals, *Nursing Research* and *Research in Nursing and Health,* only nine (10%) used nursing conceptual models or theories (p. 314). The borrowed theories or models used in these studies came from psychology, sociology, medicine, dentistry, physiology, biology, education, decision sciences, economics, ethics, epidemiology, management sciences, marketing, and communications.

Borrowed theories continue to be used with some frequency as the theoretical foundation of nursing research. Of the 47 research articles published in *Nursing Research* in 2006, only four (8.5%) used existing nursing theories, all in the middle range. The theory of unpleasant symptoms was the only nursing theory tested in more than one study. Borrowed middle range theories were cited in 17 studies (36.2%), with social support, health-related quality of life, and self-efficacy the most commonly identified theories. There were no theories identified in 15 (31.9%) of the studies and in 11 (23.4%) studies, models were created specifically for the research study from a variety of conceptual models and theories.

In past decades, the practice of borrowing theories seemed to be the result of a belief in the superiority of theories "imported" from other disciplines (Meleis, 1997). This perspective was reinforced by nurses whose advanced degrees were in fields other than nursing. Theories from sociology, psychology, education, ecology, physiology, and others were and still are borrowed. The argument for borrowed theories seems to be that theorists and practitioners should not place boundaries on any knowledge that might be useful to nursing because "knowledge does not innately 'belong' to any field of science" (Johnson, 1986, p. 117). Borrowing theories from other disciplines is sometimes referred to as theory adoption and involves the unchanged use of a theory developed from a field other than nursing. The use of unmodified theories from physiology, for instance, acid–base balance, is an example of a completely borrowed theory. Although the need for adopted borrowed theories does exist, there is concern about their prevalence. The preferred approach for the use of borrowed theories seems to be to adapt them to a distinctively nursing perspective.

Adaptation refers to altering the content or structure of a theory that was initially developed for application to a discipline other than nursing. Borrowing and altering theory is seen as necessary "to acquire a means of explanation and prediction about some phenomena that is currently poorly understood, or for which there is no present means to study it, or for which there is no theory at all" (Walker & Avant, 1995, p. 172). Walker and Avant provide a process called theory derivation, which allows nurses to modify the concepts and structures of a theory from another discipline to create a new theory more relevant to nursing. The steps of the process are not considered strictly linear; they are repeated as necessary until the theory being developed is sufficiently complete. Box 1.1 summarizes the steps in theory derivation.

The debate about the value of borrowed theories continues. Fawcett and Bourbonniere (2001) identify premises necessary for a healthy future for the nursing profession. They claim that "the discipline of nursing can survive only if we celebrate our own heritage and utilize nursing knowledge" (p. 311). This premise and the future it suggests is challenged by the ongoing dependence of nurses on perspectives of nursing that are grounded in the knowledge of other disciplines. The solution they suggest is to end nursing's "romance" with borrowed theories. Few would argue that nursing needs to attend to the ongoing development of its unique body of knowledge; perhaps not for the sole purpose of divorcing itself from other disciplines, but for creating a body of knowledge that could be shared across disciplines. Thus, nursing theory could be borrowed.

Box 1.1   Steps in the Process of Theory Derivation

1. Become acquainted with the literature that addresses the phenomenon. Evaluate theory in nursing for its adequacy.
2. Read extensively in related fields. Look for unusual relationships between the knowledge in those fields and the phenomenon of interest to nursing.
3. Choose a parent theory as a source of the derivation. Focus on the theory, or parts of the theory, that best explains or predicts the phenomenon.
4. Select the relevant concepts and/or structures. Eliminate those aspects of the theory that are not useful.
5. Develop, refine, or redefine the concepts, statements, and structures from the parent theory to develop a theory more meaningful for nursing. This requires reflection and creativity.

Source: Walker, L. O., & Avant, K. C. (1995). *Strategies for theory construction in nursing* (3rd ed., pp. 172–173). Norwalk, CT: Appleton & Lange.

GRAND THEORY

Grand theories, as the most abstract of the three identified levels, attempt "to create a view of the whole of nursing" (Liehr & Smith, 1999, Juxtaposition with Grand Nursing theory, para. 1). They address the nature, mission, and goals of nursing care (Meleis, 1997) in a general fashion and are created through the observations and/or insights of the theorist. The development of grand theories served to differentiate the discipline of nursing from the medical model, stimulated the expansion of nursing knowledge (McKenna, 1997), and provided a general "structure for the organization of nursing knowledge" (Orem, 2001, p. 139). Orem also claimed that the unstructured nature of grand or general theories allows for a wide range of knowledge available to practitioners and scholars within a nursing-specific frame of reference. McKenna (1997) outlined the benefits of grand theories to include: (a) a guide for practice as an alternative to practicing solely by tradition or intuition, (b) a framework for education by suggesting a focus and a structure for curricula, and (c) an aid to the professionalization of nursing by providing a basis of practice.

More than 50 grand theories have been identified (McKenna, 1997, p. 93), although that number may vary based on the label assigned to the work. Because of their level of abstraction, there has been some difficulty in distinguishing between grand theories, philosophies, and conceptual models. Examples of nursing theories that have been designated as grand include Leininger's *Theory of Culture Care Diversity and Universality,* *Newman's Theory of Health as Expanding Consciousness,* and Parse's *Theory of Human Becoming* (Fawcett & Bourbonniere, 2001; Fawcett, 2005; Parker, 2006). Parker (2006) also identifies Orem's *Self-care Deficit,* *Roger's Science of Human Beings,* and Roy's *Adaptation Model* as theories, whereas Fawcett (2005) and Alligood and Tomey (2005) label these nursing scientists' work as conceptual models. Orem (2001) refers to her work as a general theory. Table 1.5 provides sources of information about specific grand theories.

The level of abstraction makes it difficult to test grand theories empirically. In fact, Donnelly (2001), citing the work of Lundh, Soder, and Waerness (1988), claimed that because the theories were abstract and normative "rather than facilitating research development [they] actually made research development in nursing 'more difficult'" (p. 337). This conclusion is supported in part by the findings of Moody et al. (1988) that in nursing practice research published from 1977 to 1986, fewer than 13% of the 720 studies identified were linked to one of the grand theories.

Grand theories seem better able to serve as a basis for the development of the more specific theories of the middle and practice range, which can undergo empirical testing. For instance, the middle range theory, "A Theory of Sentient Evolution" was derived from Roger's *Science of Unitary Human Beings* (Parker, 1989). In addition, grand theories have fulfilled the important functions of distinguishing nursing from other helping professions and providing legitimization to its science. But because of their success in fulfilling these functions, grand theories have become less necessary and the focus of theory development has changed to the middle range theories (Suppe, 1996a).

MIDDLE RANGE THEORY

Compared to grand theories, middle range theories are less abstract. Merton (1968), whose work served to promote the development of middle range theories, described them as lying between "the minor but necessary working hypotheses that evolve in abundance during day to day research and the all-inclusive systematic efforts to develop a unified theory . . ." (p. 39). Consistent with Merton's conceptualization, nurse authors have described middle range theories in comparison to grand theories as follows:

- Narrower in scope (Fawcett, 2005; Liehr & Smith, 1999; McKenna, 1997; Meleis, 1997; Parker, 2001; Walker & Avant, 1995)
- Concerned with less abstract, more specific phenomena (Fawcett, 2005; Meleis, 1997)
- Comprised of fewer concepts and propositions (Fawcett, 2005; McKenna, 1997; Walker & Avant, 1995)
- Representative of a limited or partial view of nursing reality (Jacox, 1974; Liehr & Smith, 1999; Young, et al., 2001)
- More appropriate for empirical testing (Liehr & Smith, 1999; McKenna, 1997; Meleis, 1997; Parker, 2006; Walker & Avant, 1995)

TABLE 1.5 Examples of Grand Theories with Sources of Information

Theory	Primary sources of information
King's Theory of Goal Attainment	King, I. M. (1981). *A theory of goal attainment: Systems, concepts, process.* New York: Wiley. King, I. M. (1990). Health the goal for nursing. *Nursing Science Quarterly, 3,* 123. King, I. M. (1992). King's theory of goal attainment. *Nursing Science Quarterly, 5,* 19. King, I. M. (1994). Quality of life and goal attainment. *Nursing Science Quarterly, 7,* 29. King, I. M. (1996). The theory of goal attainment in research and practice. *Nursing Science Quarterly, 9,* 61. King, I. M. (1997). King's theory of goal attainment in practice. *Nursing Science Quarterly, 10,* 180–185.
Leininger's Theory of Culture Care and Universality	Leininger, M. M. (1970). *Nursing and anthropology: Two worlds blend.* New York: Wiley. Leininger, M. M. (1978). *Transcultural nursing: Concepts, theories, and practices.* New York: Wiley. Leininger, M. M. (1985). Transcultural care diversity and universality: A theory of nursing. *Nursing and Health Care, 6,* 208–212. Leininger, M. M. (1988). Leininger's theory of nursing: Cultural care diversity and universality. *Nursing Science Quarterly, 1,* 152–160. Leininger, M. M. (1991). *Cultural care diversity and universality: A theory of nursing.* New York: National League for Nursing. Leininger, M. M. (1995). *Transcultural nursing: Concepts, theories, research, and practice.* Columbus, OH: McGraw Hill College Custom Series.
Newman's Theory of Health as Expanding Consciousness	Newman, M. A. (1986). *Health as expanding consciousness.* St. Louis, MO: Mosby. Newman, M. A. (1990). Newman's theory of health as praxis. *Nursing Science Quarterly, 3,* 37–41. Newman, M. A. (1994). *Health as expanding consciousness* (2nd ed.). Boston, MA: Jones & Bartlett. Newman, M. A. (1997). Evolution of a theory of health as expanding consciousness. *Nursing Science Quarterly, 10,* 22–25.
Orem's Self-care Deficit Theory	Orem, D. E. (1971). *Nursing: Concepts of practice* (2nd ed.). New York: McGraw Hill. Orem, D. E. (1983). *The self-care deficit theory of nursing.* New York: Wiley. Orem, D. E. (1987). *Orem's general theory of nursing.* Philadelphia, PA: Saunders. Orem, D. E., & Taylor, S. G. (1986). *Orem's general theory of nursing.* New York: National League for Nursing. Orem, D. E. (2001). Nursing: *Concepts of practice* (6th ed.). New York: McGraw Hill.
Parse's Theory of Human Becoming	Parse, R. R. (1981). *Man-living-health: A theory of nursing.* New York: Wiley. Parse, R. R. (1987). *Nursing science: Major paradigms, theories, and critiques.* Philadelphia, PA: Saunders. Parse, R. R. (1992). Human becoming: Parse's theory of nursing. *Nursing Science Quarterly, 5,* 35–42. Parse, R. R. (1994). Quality of life: Sciencing and living the art of human becoming. *Nursing Science Quarterly, 7,* 16–21. Parse, R. R. (1996). Reality: A seamless symphony of becoming. *Nursing Science Quarterly, 9,* 181–183. Parse, R. R. (1997). The human becoming theory: There was, is, and will be. *Nursing Science Quarterly, 10,* 32–38. Parse, R. R. (1998). *The human becoming school of thought.* Thousand Oaks, CA: Sage.

■ More applicable directly to practice for explanation and implementation (McKenna, 1997; Walker & Avant, 1995; Young et al., 2001)

These attributes make middle range theories attractive to nurses who wish to engage in theory-based research and practice.

The appeal of these theories to nurse researchers and practitioners is demonstrated by their proliferation in the past 15 years. Lenz (1996) identified a number of the middle range theories developed in the 1980s and 1990s. Table 1.6 provides a partial listing of theories used by nurses in research and/or practice that have been considered to be middle range. Included in the table are middle range theories in various stages of development and testing, most of which focus on patient care phenomena. There has been a modest trend toward the development and use of theories applicable to the education and practice of nurses. The table also includes one reference for each theory.

DEVELOPMENT OF MIDDLE RANGE THEORY

Liehr and Smith (1999) outlined the relationships between the intellectual processes and the sources of content related to the development of middle range theories, which included the following:

■ Inductive theory, building theory through research
■ Deductive theory, building from grand nursing theories
■ Combining existing nursing and non-nursing theories
■ Synthesizing theories from published research findings
■ Developing theories from clinical practice guidelines (Approaches for Generating Middle Range Theory, para. 1)

Qualitative research, particularly phenomenological and grounded theory studies, has served as a source of middle range theory development. Ten qualitative studies conducted through the Nursing Consortium for Research on Chronic Sorrow provided a foundation for the development of the middle range theory of chronic sorrow (Eakes, Burke, & Hainsworth, 1998). The research findings of these and of other studies underwent concept analysis as part of the process of developing this theory. A major source of middle range theory development is the qualitative research produced by nursing's Ph.D. students and presented in their doctoral dissertations.

Several conceptual models and grand theories have served as the foundation for the development of middle range theories. Seiloff and Frey's (2007) book, *Middle Range Theory Development Using King's Conceptual System* describes King's conceptual system and theory of goal attainment as a source for middle range theory development. A number of other grand theories have provided a foundation for further theory development. For instance, the middle range theory of homecare effectiveness was based on Roy's *Adaptation Model* (Smith et al., 2002). The work of the theorists resulted in increased specificity of the conceptualization of Roy's interdependence mode. Other examples of middle range theories derived directly and specifically from nursing's major conceptual models and grand theories are found in Table 1.7. Middle range theories have been developed from Johnson's *Behavioral System Model,* Levine's *Conservation Principles,* Roger's *Science of Unitary Beings,* and Roy's *Adaptation Model* (Alligood & Tomey, 2005).

Theories from nursing have been combined with those from other disciplines to create middle range theories. Mercer used Rubin's work on maternal role attainment (i.e., attachment and role identity during pregnancy and early infancy) and integrated role and developmental theories from the field of psychology to arrive at her *Theory of Maternal Role Attainment* (Meighan, 2006). She also conducted a number of research studies on the subject, the findings of which were reflected in the theory.

Published research findings have been cited as the most common source for constructing middle range theories of nursing (Lenz, 1998). The development of *Online Social Support Theory* is an example of this approach (LaCoursiere, 2001). Synthesized research findings from various patient populations (e.g., patients diagnosed with cancer or cardiovascular illness) that reflected the perspectives of those involved with the use of online social support (i.e., patient, caregiver, and nurse) served as a foundation for LaCoursiere's theory.

Clinical practice and clinical practice guidelines are sources of middle range theory development. Peplau is credited with introducing the use of clinical data in the development of her theory, the Theory of Interpersonal

TABLE 1.6 Examples of Middle Range Theories

Theory	Reference
Physiological	
Acute pain	Good, M. A. (1998). A middle range theory of acute pain management: Use in research. *Nursing Outlook, 46,* 120–124.
Chronotherapeutic intervention for postsurgical pain	Auvil-Novak, S. E. (1997). A mid-range theory of chronotherapeutic intervention of postsurgical pain. *Nursing Research, 46,* 66–71.
Dyspnea	Gift, A. G. (1992). Dyspnea. *Northern Clinics of North America, 25,* 955–965.
Perimenopausal process	Quinn, A. A. (1991). A theoretical model of the perimenopausal process. *Journal of Nurse-Midwifery, 36*(1), 25–29.
Sensing presence and sensing space	Orticio, L. P. (2007). Sensing presence and sensing space: A middle range theory of nursing. *Insight: The Journal of American Society of Ophthalmic Registered Nurses, 32*(4), 7–11.
Unpleasant symptoms	Lenz, E. R., Pugh, L. C., Milligan, R. A., Gift, A. G., & Suppe, F. (1997). The middle range theory of unpleasant symptoms: An update. *Advances in Nursing Science, 19,* 14–27.
Cognitive	
Facilitated sensemaking	Davidson, J. E. (2010). Facilitated sensemaking a strategy and new middle range theory to support families of intensive care unit patients. *Critical Care Nurse, 30*(6), 28–39.
Health belief[a]	Champion, V. L. (1985). Use of the health belief model in determining frequency of breast self-examination. *Research in Nursing Health, 8,* 373–379.
Nursing intellectual capital	Covell, C. L. (2008). The middle range theory of nursing intellectual capital. *Journal of Advanced Nursing Practice, 63,* 94–103.
Social learning theory[a]	Bandura, A. (1986). *Social foundations of thought and action: A social cognitive theory.* Englewood Cliffs, NJ: Prentice-Hall.
Story theory	Smith, M. J., & Liehr, P. (2005). Story theory: Advancing nursing practice scholarship. *Holistic Nursing Practice, 19*(6), 272–276.
Emotional	
Caregiver stress	Tsai, P. (2003). A middle range theory of caregiver stress. *Nursing Science Quarterly, 16*(2), 137–145. doi: 10.1177/0894318403251789.
Chronic sorrow	Eakes, G. G., Burke, M. L., & Hainsworth, M. A. (1998). Middle range theory of chronic sorrow. *Image, 30,* 179–184.
Chronic stress	Peters, R. M. (2006). The relationship of racism, chronic stress emotions, and blood pressure. *Journal of Nursing Scholarship, 38,* 234–240.
Empathy	Olson, J., & Hanchett, E. (1997). Nurse expressed empathy, patient outcomes, and development of a middle range theory. *Image, 29,* 71–76.
Fulfillment	Kylma, J., & Vehvilainen-Julkunen, K. (1995). Hope in nursing research: A meta-analysis of the ontological and epistemological foundations of research on hope. *Journal of Advanced Nursing, 25*(2), 364–371.
Grief	Chapman, K. J., & Pepler, C. (1998). Coping, hope and anticipatory grief in family members with palliative home care. *Cancer Nursing, 21*(4), 226–234.
Hope	Morse, J. M., & Doberneck, B. (1995). Delineating the concept of hope. *Image, 27*(4), 277–285.

TABLE 1.6 Examples of Middle Range Theories *(continued)*

Theory	Reference
Personal risking	Hitchcock, J. M., & Wilson, H. S. (1992). Personal risking: Lesbian self-disclosure of sexual orientation to professional health care providers. *Nursing Research, 41,* 178–183.
Postpartum depression	Beck, C. T. (1993). The lived experience of postpartum depression: A substantive theory of postpartum depression. *Nursing Research, 42,* 42–48.
Resilience	Polk, L. V. (1997). Toward a middle range theory of resilience. *Advances in Nursing Science, 19,* 1–13.
Uncertainty	Mishel, M. H. (1991). Reconceptualization of the uncertainty in illness theory. *Image, 2,* 256–261.
Uncertainty of illness	Deane, K. A., & Degner, L. F. (1998). Information needs, uncertainty, and anxiety in women who had a breast biopsy with benign outcome. *Cancer Nursing, 21*(2), 117–126.
Social	
Bureaucratic caring	Ray, M. (1989). The theory of bureaucratic caring for nursing practice in the organizational culture. *Nursing Administrative Quarterly, 13*(2), 31–42.
Caring through relation and dialogue	Sanford, R. C. (2000). Caring through relation and dialogue: A nursing perspective for patient education. *Advances in Nursing Science, 22*(3), 1–15.
Coercion in the development of behavior[a]	Patterson, G. R. (1982). *Coercive family process.* Eugene, OR: Castalia.
Department (group power)	Sieloff, C. L., & Dunn, K. (2008). Factor validation of an instrument measuring group power. *Journal of Nursing Measurement, 16*(2), 113–124.
Entry into nursing home as a status passage	Chenitz, W. C. (1983, March/April). Entry into a nursing home as status passage: A theory to guide nursing practice. *Geriatric Nursing,* 92–97.
Home care	Smith, C. E., Pace, K., Kochinda, C., Kleinbeck, S., Koehler, J., & Popkess-Vawter, S. (2002). Caregiver effectiveness model evolution to a midrange theory of home care: A process for critique and replication. *Advances in Nursing Science, 25*(1), 50–64.
Humor	McCreaddie, M., & Wiggins, S. (2009). Reconciling the good patient personal with problematic and non-problematic humor: A grounded theory. *International Journal of Nursing Studies, 46,* 1079–1091.
Informed caring	Swanson, K. M. (1993). Nursing as informed caring for the well-being of others. *Image, 25*(4), 352–357.
Maternal role attainment	Mercer, R. T. (1986). *First time motherhood: Experiences from teens to forties.* New York: Springer.
Negotiating partnerships	Powell-Cope, G. M. (1994). Family caregivers of people with AIDS: Negotiating partnerships with professional health care providers. *Nursing Research, 43,* 324–330.
Quality of family caregiving	Phillips, L. R., & Rempusheski, V. F. (1986). Caring for the frail elderly at home: Toward a theoretical explanation of the dynamics of poor quality family caregiving. *Advances in Nursing Science, 8*(4), 62–84.
Self-transcendence	Reed, P. (1991). Toward a nursing theory of self-transcendence: Deductive reformulation using developmental theories. *Advances in Nursing Science, 12,* 64–74.

continued

TABLE 1.6 Examples of Middle Range Theories *(continued)*

Theory	Reference
Spiritual empathy	Chism, L. A., & Magnan, M. A. (2009). The relationship of nursing students' spiritual care perspectives to their expressions of spiritual empathy. *Journal of Nursing Education, 48,* 597–605.
Super-link system	Chen, H., & Boore, J. R. P. (2007). Establishing a super-link system: Spinal cord injury rehabilitation nursing. *Journal of Advanced Nursing, 57,* 639–648.
Waiting theory model	Trimm, D. R., & Sanford, J. T. (2010). The process of family waiting during surgery. *Journal of Family Nursing, 16,* 435–461. doi: 10.1177/1074840710385691.
Integrative	
Adapting to diabetes mellitus	Whittemore, R., & Roy, C. (2002). Adapting to diabetes mellitus: A theory synthesis. *Nursing Science Quarterly, 15,* 311–317.
Adolescent vulnerability to risk behaviors	Cazzell, M. (2008). Linking theory, evidence, and practice in assessment of adolescent inhalant use. *Journal of Addictions Nursing, 19*(1), 17–25.
Career persistence	Hodges, H. F., Troyan, P. J., & Keeley, A. C. (2010). Career persistence in baccalaureate-prepared acute care nurses. *Journal of Nursing Scholarship, 42,* 83–91.
Experiencing transitions	Meleis, A. I., Sawyer, L. M., Im, E., Messias, D. K., & Schumacher, K. (2000). Experiencing transitions: An emerging middle range theory. *Advances in Nursing Science, 23*(1), 12–28.
Health promotion	Pender, N. J. (1987). *Health promotion in nursing practice.* Norwalk, CT: Saunders.
Illness constellation	Morse, J. M., & Johnson, H. K. (1991). *In The Illness Experience: Dimensions of Suffering.* Newbury Park, CA: Sage.
Interaction model of client behavior	Cox, C. L. (1982). An interaction model of client behavior: A theoretical prescription for nursing. *Advances in Nursing Science, 5*(1), 41–56.
Music, mood, and movement	Murrock, C. J., & Higgins, P. A. (2009). The theory of music, mood, and movement to improve health outcomes. *Journal of Advanced Nursing, 65,* 2249–2257.
Self-care management for vulnerable populations	Dorsey, C. J., & Murdaugh, C. L. (2003). *Journal of Theory Construction & Testing, 7*(2), 43–49.
Symptom management	Linder, L. (2010). Analysis of the UCSF Symptom Management Theory: Implications for pediatric oncology nursing. *Journal of Pediatric Oncology Nursing, 6,* 316–324. doi:10.1177/1043454210368532.

*a*Theories used in nursing research that are not nursing-developed theories.

Relations. She based her understanding of the stages of the nurse–patient relationship on the observations of interactions between student nurses and psychiatric patients. The guidelines established by the Agency for Health Care Policy and Research for the management of acute pain were used by Good and Moore in the development of the theory of a balance between analgesia and side effects in the management of pain.

It is important to note that most of the nurses involved in the development of middle range theories used more than one approach. As part of arriving at the creation of the middle range theory, often findings from previous research studies were reviewed and analyzed, conceptual models and theories were considered, and additional research was conducted that targeted the phenomenon of most interest.

TABLE 1.7 Middle Range Theories Derived from Conceptual Models

Conceptual model	Middle range theory
Johnson's Behavioral System Model	Theory of a Restorative Subsystem Theory of Sustenal Imperatives
Levine's Conservation Principles	Theory of Redundancy Theory of Therapeutic Intention
Rogers' Science of Unitary Human Beings	Theory of Perception of Dissonant Pattern
Roy's Adaptation Model	Theory of the Physiologic Mode Theory of the Self-concept Mode Theory of the Interdependence Mode Theory of the Role Function Mode

Source: Alligood, M. R., & Tomey, A. M. (2002). *Nursing theory: Utilization & application* (pp. 46–54). St. Louis, MO: Mosby. With permission from Elsevier Science.

USES OF MIDDLE RANGE THEORY

Middle range theory has been found to be useful in both research and practice. "Theory can serve a heuristic function to stimulate and provide the rationale for studies, as well as help guide the selection of research questions and variables" (Lenz, 1998, p. 26). Middle range theories also can assist practice by facilitating understanding of client's behavior, suggesting interventions, and providing possible explanations for the degree of effectiveness of the interventions.

Reviews of published studies reveal a fairly extensive use of middle range theory in nursing research. Through the 1990s, most often, middle range theories from other disciplines (Lenz, 1998) were used. This was particularly evident when comparing how frequently middle range theories and grand theories of nursing are cited in the nursing research literature. Of 173 studies included in *Nursing Research* from January 1994 through June 1997, only 79 (45.7%) identified any theory. Of the 79 studies that identified a theory, 25 were nursing theories and 54 were middle range theories borrowed from other disciplines, most frequently from psychology. Of the 25 using nursing theories, middle range theories accounted for most of the nursing theories used in the studies, 22 of the 25 (Lenz, 1998, p. 27). A more recent review of published research reveals that an increasing number of nurse researchers are identifying the theoretical foundation of their research, with most using middle range nursing theories.

Although middle range theory has great potential for guiding nursing practice, the nursing literature suggests that the potential has not been fully realized. Many authors note a gap between theory and practice. And when applications of theory to practice are included in the literature, it is more likely to be a grand rather than a middle range theory (Lenz, 1998). An informal survey of 10 clinical nurse specialists and five staff nurses, conducted by Lenz, revealed few who were able to identify theories they were using in their practice. She attributes this to several factors: (a) the busyness of practicing nurses that does not allow time for consideration of the theoretical bases for their actions; (b) educational programs that do not help students learn the connections between theory and practice; (c) clinical environments that do not value theory-based practice; and (d) the lack of availability and usability of information on middle range theories. Nurse theorists need to address the last factor by producing literature describing their theories in understandable terms, identifying the theories' implications for practice, and placing that information in practice-oriented journals.

CONTROVERSY SURROUNDING MIDDLE RANGE THEORY

The identification of middle range theories is not unambiguous. For instance, Chenitz, primary author of Entry into a Nursing Home as Status Passage, labeled it as practice theory, whereas others considered it middle range theory (Liehr & Smith, 1999). "The question about what constitutes theory at the middle range is not a black and white issue for which a precise and clear definition can be offered. Middle range theory holds to a given level of abstraction. It is not too broad nor too narrow, but somewhere in the middle" (Liehr & Smith, 1999, p. 85). To reduce confusion, nurse theorists are encouraged to clearly identify their work as middle range and provide a name that represents its conceptual components (Liehr & Smith, 1999; Sanford, 2000).

The imprecision of what constitutes a middle range theory is only one of several criticisms of middle range theory. In addition to lack of definitional clarity, middle range theory has been criticized for distinguishing itself from grand theories by its ability to be tested, using a logical positivistic idea of testability. Suppe (1996b) suggests an alternative approach to considering the testability of middle range theory. He rejects the widely accepted notion of theories as a set of propositions and proposes the idea that theories are "state-transitions systems modeling the behaviors of real world systems within the theory's scope" (Suppe, 1996b, p. 10). By this conceptualization of theories, operational concepts become descriptors; the values of these concepts become state specifications; and the propositions become specifications of state-transition relations (Suppe, 1996b, p. 11). The purpose of testing using this understanding of the nature of theories is delineating the scope of the middle range theory rather than subjecting a hypothesis to statistical analysis or qualitative data to coding. The basic research question is for what systems does the theory work and for what systems does it not, a question of scope. This type of research question is well suited to the testing of middle range theories.

Since Merton (1968) first promoted the notion of middle range theories, they have been criticized as being intellectually unambitious. Critics argue that their scope and suggested methods of inquiry are too limited. Merton countered that middle range theory was addressing just the questions that the discipline of sociology was asking, and that middle range theories can undergo the same systematic empirical testing that both more and less abstract theories can (pp. 63–64).

Another criticism of middle range theories is that their increasing numbers can lead to fragmentation of nursing's knowledge base into unrelated and distinct theories. This claim could be as legitimately made about either grand or micro theories. Merton acknowledged that risk and proposed consolidating theories to create groups of like theories at the middle range (Whall, 1996). Nurse scientists have addressed this issue. The identification of a metaparadigm is an attempt to create some conceptual cohesion for nursing's knowledge base. In addition, there has been an intentional effort to relate middle range theories to nursing's conceptual models, grand theories, and taxonomies. For instance, the middle range theory of therapeutic intention is clearly linked to Levine's *Conservation Principles*. Nurse scientists have proposed anchoring middle range theories to nursing's taxonomies of: (a) diagnoses, NANDA International; (b) interventions, Nursing Interventions Classification (NIC); and (c) outcomes, Nursing Outcomes Classification (NOC) (Blegan & Tripp-Reimer, 1997) and have identified a structure to accomplish that linkage (Tripp-Reimer, Woodworth, McCloskey, & Bulechek, 1996). Others consider these taxonomies as types of middle range theories rather than frameworks for categorizing the theories because they consist of concepts, definitions of concepts, propositional statements, and assumptions (Whall, 1996). As taxonomies, these middle range theories could not be considered unrelated and fragmented aspects of nursing's knowledge base. Nurse scientists continue to recommend persistence in efforts to "create an association between the proposed theory and a disciplinary perspective in nursing" (Liehr & Smith, 1999).

Nurse researchers have been denounced for making use of middle range theories from disciplines other than nursing. This was certainly true of nursing research published from the mid-1970s to the mid-1980s. During this period, more than half of the studies made use of theories or models from disciplines other than nursing (Moody et al., 1988). The increasing number of nursing middle range theories is reversing that trend. Liehr and Smith (1999) found 22 middle range nursing theories published in the decade from 1988 to 1999 through a CINAHL search. These theories met a number of criteria, including identification by the author that the theory was of the middle range. The criticism that nurse researchers use middle range theories from disciplines other than nursing is also being addressed by a call to continue to develop theories in the midlevel of scope and abstractness. "Situating middle range theory at the forefront for practice and research is critical to epistemologic and ontologic growth in nursing" (Sanford, 2000, Recommendation 5, para. 1).

PRACTICE THEORY/MICRO THEORY/ SITUATION-SPECIFIC THEORY

The literature includes a confusing variety of terms to refer to the level of theory that is considered less abstract, more specific, and narrower in scope than middle range theory. *Practice theory* seems to be the most commonly used term (Jones, 2001; McKenna, 1997; Walker & Avant, 1995). Suppe (1996b), Kramer (1997), and Parker (2006) referred to both practice and micro theory, and Suppe discussed some of the distinctions between the two terms. The term *micro theory* was also used by Kim (2000), Duldt and Giffin (1985), Chinn and Kramer (1999, 2004), and by George (1995) and Young et al. (2001), who both cited Chinn and Kramer. The most recently introduced term is *situation-specific theory* (Im & Meleis, 1999; Meleis & Im, 2001).

Practice theory can trace its origin to the work of metatheorists Dickhoff and James (1968). Its position is that because nursing is a profession, its theory must have an action orientation that can shape reality to create a desired goal. "The major contention here is that theory exists finally for the sake of practice" (p. 199).

Several authors have provided a list of the components of a practice theory. As stated earlier, Dickhoff and James referred to this goal-oriented theory as "situation-producing" and identified its essential elements as: "1) goal-content specified as aim for activity; 2) prescriptions for activity to realize the goal-content; and 3) a survey list to serve as a supplement to present prescription and preparation for future prescription for activity toward the goal-content" (p. 201). Jones (2001, p. 376) interprets these elements to include the use of nursing diagnosis and outcomes classification systems as components of practice theory. Walker and Avant (1995) and Kramer (1997) referred to these three components in their definitions of practice theory and both suggested additional considerations. Walker and Avant claim that without a basis in situation-relating (predictive) theories, it would require a liberal definition of theory to identify practice or situation-producing theory as theory. They suggest that it would be more legitimate to refer to practice theory as nursing practices (pp. 12–13). Kramer identifies a similar issue, the importance of connecting practice theory to the more encompassing knowledge structures of nursing as identified by metatheory. To the traditional understanding of practice theory she adds theory about nursing practice (e.g., administrative and educational theories). This is not a commonly occurring use.

Like other levels of theory, practice theories as situation producing are derived from middle range theories, practice experiences, and empirical testing. Middle range theories are the source of the prescriptions that are directed at the specified goal (McKenna, 1997; Parker, 2006; Walker & Avant, 1995) and if not specifically derived from these middle range theories, at the very least, practice theories should identify how the concepts from both levels of theory are interrelated. Practice theory also develops from the clinical experiences of nurses that have been subjected to the process of reflection. Reflection on practice leads to insights that can serve as a foundation for developing theory. It provides a real world basis for the creation of practice theory. Research is also an important source of practice theories. Walker and Avant (1995) note the contributions of the Conduct and Utilization of Research in Nursing project in the formulation of practice theories. This project, initiated in 1975, identified a need for change in practice and summarized the relevant research to arrive at research-based principles for nursing interventions. There were 10 practice theories or protocols that were considered during the project. Examples of the protocols that were developed include: (a) lactose-free diet, (b) sensation information: distress, (c) intravenous cannula-change regiment, and (d) prevention of decubitus by means of small shifts of body weight (Haller, Reynolds, & Horsley, 1979, p. 47).

Micro theory, a term sometimes identified as interchangeable with practice theory, is included in the writings of Kim (2000), Suppe (1996b), and Chinn and Kramer (2005). Kim's (1983) definition of micro theory as a set of "theoretical statements, usually hypotheses, that deal with narrowly defined phenomena" (p. 13) suggests a research-based theory. Suppe (1996b) also identifies hypothesis testing as a primary feature of micro theories and claims that this fact provides the primary distinction between micro theory and middle range theory, both of which could be considered practice theories (pp. 12–13). According to Suppe, the term *micro theory* is found with increasing frequency in the literature to refer to theories that are too limited in scope to be considered middle range. He provided a hypothetical example of a micro theory of pain management for a hospitalized patient with acute postamputation pain, who was treated with PCA morphine, with possible Valium potentiation, focusing on pain intensity and addiction outcomes (Suppe, 1996b, p. 12). Kim (1983) provided examples of what she labeled as micro theories, that is, maternal attachment, pressure sores, wound healing, and positioning. Other examples of this level of theory development found in the literature include alcoholism recovery in lesbian women (Hall, 1990), quality of care (Nielson, 1992), milieu therapy for short-stay units (LeCuyer, 1992), caring for patients with chronic skin disease (Kirkevold, 1993), therapeutic touch (Green, 1998), exercise as self-care (Ulbrich, 1999), and ecological view of protection (Shearer, 2002).

Im and Meleis (1999) use the term *situation-specific* to refer to that level of nursing theory that focuses on specific nursing phenomena with direct application to nursing practice. There are a number of features that distinguish situation-specific theories from either grand or middle range theories. They exhibit "(1) a lower level of abstraction, (2) reflection of specific nursing phenomenon, (3) context, (4) readily accessible connection to nursing research and practice, (5) reflection of diversities in nursing phenomena, and (6) limitation of generalization" (*Properties of Situation-Specific Theories,* para. 1). A somewhat unique quality of situation-specific theories is their emphasis on sociopolitical, cultural, and historical contexts, demonstrated by the theory of menopausal transition of Korean immigrant women described by Im and Meleis.

In addition to the debate on the term to use in referring to this level of theory, the controversies about practice theory center on whether it is a theory, and if so, whether it is needed. Walker (1986) suggests that, based on a definition of practice theory as sets of principles or directives, the terms *policy, procedure,* or *principles of practice* might be more appropriate. Her conclusion is based on an understanding of theory as a "systematic description and explanation" (p. 28). Walker's position seems consistent with the increasingly popular phenomena of research utilization and evidence-based practice. Berkstrand's (1986) contention is that practice theory is unnecessary. She claims that "all the theoretical knowledge relevant to practice can be discovered within existing systems of knowledge such as metatheory, philosophy, science, and ethics." Collins and Fielder (1986) respond to Beckstrand's conclusion by emphasizing the unique issues that nursing theories must address. They assert that Beckstrand's position does not consider the nurse's responsibility for caring for the client as a "particular" individual. Nursing still has a need for "a nursing theory that will set out the kinds of nursing practice and the particular set of moral ideals that nursing practice seeks to bring about" (Collins & Fielder, 1986, p. 510). The increasing number of practice theories or their semantic equivalent identified in the literature in the 1990s seems to be supporting, if not a need, at least an interest in this level of theory development.

SUMMARY

The development of nursing knowledge is an ongoing process, though debates continue on the direction that this development should take. For instance, there are differences of opinion on whether diversity or unity of paradigms and philosophies is preferred. The language of nursing science is not firmly established or used consistently; there still is not consensus on the use of some of the terms that refer to the components of the structural hierarchy of nursing knowledge. One term used fairly consistently in the literature is *middle range theory,* and it is the development of this level of theory verified by research and useful for practice that is the focus of the efforts of many nurse scientists.

CRITICAL THINKING EXERCISES

1. In the debate on nursing paradigms, which of the currently proposed considerations—emergence of a single paradigm, coexistence of complementary paradigms, or creation of an integrated paradigm from the two most prominent paradigms—seems to best serve the advancement of nursing knowledge? What would be the implications of the chosen perspective on paradigms for the development of nursing knowledge?

2. Make a case for the ongoing development and use of nursing grand theories. Conversely, make a case for the obsolescence of nursing grand theories for today's practice and research.

3. Identify a research topic or develop a research question. Refer to the table *Examples of Middle Range Theories.* Which middle range theory might be applicable to the research topic or question? If none seems appropriate, why might that be?

WEB RESOURCES

Visit **http://thePoint.lww.com/Peterson3e** for helpful web resources related to this chapter.

REFERENCES

Adam, E. (1992). Contemporary conceptualization of nursing: Philosophy or science? In J. F. Kikuchi & H. Simmons (Eds.), *Philosophic inquiry in nursing* (pp. 55–63). London: Sage.

Alligood, M. R., & Tomey, A. M. (2005). *Nursing theory: Utilization and application* (3rd ed.). St. Louis, MO: Mosby.

Annells. M. (2005). Guest editorial: A qualitative quandary: Alternative representations and meta-synthesis. *Journal of Clinical Nursing, 14*(5), 535–536.

Antiognoli-Toland, P. L. (1999). Kuhn and Reigel: The nature of scientific revolutions and theory construction. *The Journal of Theory Construction & Testing, 3*(2), 38–41.

Archibald, G. (2000). A postmodern nursing model. *Nursing Standard, 14*(34), 40–42.

Babbie, E. (1995). *The practice of social research* (7th ed.). Belmont, CA: Wadsworth.

Barrett, E. (1986). Investigation of the principle of helicy: The relationship of human filed motion and power, In V. Mailinski (Ed.), *Explorations on Martha Rogers' science of unitary human beings* (pp. 173–184). Norwalk, CT: Appleton-Century-Crofts.

Barrett, E. A. M. (1992). Diversity reigns. *Nursing Science Quarterly, 5*(4), 155–157.

Berkstrand, J. (1986). A critique of several conceptions of practice theory in nursing. In L. H. Nicholl (Ed.), *Perspectives on nursing theory* (pp. 494–504). Boston, MA: Little, Brown and Company.

Bisk, T. (n.d.). Utopianism come to age: From postmodernism to neo-modernism. Retrieved August 16, 2006 from http://www.wfs.org/bisk.htm.

Blegan, M. A., & Tripp-Reimer, T. (1997). Implications of nursing taxonomies for middle range theory development. *Advances in Nursing Science, 19*(3), *37*(13). Retrieved December 14, 1999 from Health Reference Center–Academic database.

Brower, H. T. F., & Baker, B. J. (1976). Using the adaptation model in a practitioner curriculum. *Nursing Outlook, 24*, 686–689.

Brown, S. T., & Lee, B. T. (1980). Imogene King's conceptual framework: A proposed model for continuing nursing education. *Journal of Advanced Nursing, 5*, 467–473.

Burbules, N. C. (n.d). *Postmodern doubt and philosophy of education.* Retrieved June 6, 2002, from University of Illinois at Urbana-Champaign Web site: http://www.ed.uiuc.edu/EPS/PES-Yearbook/95_docs/burbules.html

Caper, C. F. (1986). Some basic facts about models, nursing conceptualizations, and nursing theories. *The Journal of Continuing Education in Nursing, 16*(5), 149–154.

Chinn, P. L., & Kramer, M. K. (1999). *Theory and nursing: Integrated nursing knowledge* (5th ed.). St. Louis, MO: Mosby.

Chinn, P. L., & Kramer, M. K. (2005). *Theory and nursing: Integrated nursing knowledge* (6th ed.). St. Louis, MO: Mosby.

Cody, W. C., & Mitchell, G. J. (2002). Nursing knowledge and human science revisited: Practical and political considerations. *Nursing Science Quarterly, 15*(1), 4–13.

Collins, R. C., & Fielder, J. H. (1986). Beckstrand's concept of practice theory: A critique. In L. H. Nicholl (Ed.), *Perspectives on nursing theory* (pp. 505–511). Boston, MA: Little, Brown.

Derdiarian, A. K. (1988). Sensitivity of the Derdiarian behavioral system model instrument to age, sit, and stage of cancer: A preliminary validation study. *Scholarly Inquiry for Nursing Practice, 2*, 103–121.

Dickhoff, J., & James, P. (1968). A theory of theories: A position paper. *Nursing Research, 17*(3), 197–203.

Donnelly, E. (2001). An assessment of nursing theories as guides to scientific inquiry. In N. L. Chaska (Ed.), *The nursing profession: Tomorrow and beyond.* (pp. 331–344). Thousand Oaks, CA: Sage.

Downs, F. S. (1982). A theoretical question. *Nursing Research, 3*, 259.

Duldt, B. W., & Giffin, K. (1985). *Theoretical perspectives for nursing.* Boston, MA: Little, Brown.

Dunphy, L. H. (2001). Florence Nightingale care actualized: A legacy for nursing. In M. E. Parker, *Nursing theories and nursing practice* (pp. 31–53). Philadelphia, PA: F. A. Davis.

Eakes, G. G., Burke, M. L., & Hainsworth, M. A. (1998). Middle range theory of chronic sorrow. *Image, 30*(2), 179–184.

Engebretson, J. (1997). A multiparadigm approach to nursing. *Advances in Nursing Science, 20*(1), 21–33. Retrieved June 3, 2002 from CINAHL/OVID database.

Estabrooks, C. A., Field, P. A., & Morse, J. M. (1994). Aggregating qualitative findings: An approach to theory development. *Qualitative Health Research, 4*(4), 503–511.

Fagerhaugh, S. Y. (1974). Pain expression and control on a burn care unit. *Nursing Outlook, 22*, 645–650.

Fawcett, J. (1978). The what of theory development. In National League for Nursing, *Theory development: What, why, how?* (pp. 106–122). New York: National League for Nursing.

Fawcett, J. (1984). *Analysis and evaluation of conceptual models in nursing.* Philadelphia, PA: F. A. Davis.

Fawcett, J. (1992). Contemporary conceptualizations of nursing: philosopsy or science? In J. F. Kikuchi, *Philosophic inquiry in nursing* (pp. 64–70). Thousand Oaks, CA: Sage.

Fawcett, J. (1996). On the requirements for a metaparadigm: An invitation to dialogue. *Nursing Science Quarterly, 9*(3), 94–97.

Fawcett, J. (1997). The structural hierarchy of nursing knowledge: Components and their definitions. In I. M. King & J. Fawcett. (Eds.), *The language of nursing theory and metatheory* (pp. 11–17). Indianapolis, IN: Sigma Theta Tau.

Fawcett, J. (2003). Critiquing contemporary nursing knowledge: A dialogue. *Nursing Science Quarterly, 16*(3), 273–276.

Fawcett, J. (2005). *Contemporary nursing knowledge: Analysis and evaluation of nursing models and theories* (2nd ed.). Philadelphia, PA: F.A. Davis.

Fawcett, J., & Alligood, M. R. (2005). Influences on advancement of nursing knowledge. *Nursing Science Quarterly, 18*(3), 227–232.

Fawcett, J., & Bourbonniere, M. G. (2001). Utilization of nursing knowledge and the future of the discipline. In N. L. Chaska (Ed.), *The nursing profession: Tomorrow and beyond.* (pp. 311–320). Thousand Oaks, CA: Sage.

Fawcett, J., Watson, J., Neuman, B., Walker, P. H., & Fitzpatrick, J. J. (2001). On nursing theories and evidence. *Journal of Nursing Scholarship, 33*(2), 115–119.

Fitzpatrick, J. J. (1997). Nursing theory and metatheory. In I. M. King and J. Fawcett (Eds.), *The language of nursing theory and metatheory* (pp. 37–39). Indianapolis, IN: Sigma Theta Tau.

Fitzpatrick, J., & Whall, A. (2005). *Conceptual models of nursing: Analysis and Application* (4th ed.). Bowie, MD: Robert J. Brady.

George, J. B. (1995). *Nursing theories: The base for professional nursing practice* (4th ed.). Norwalk, CT: Appleton & Lange.

Georges, J. M. (2003). An emerging discourse: Toward epistemic diversity in nursing, *Advances in Nursing Science, 26*(1), 44–52.

Glaser, B. G., & Straus, A. L. (1967). *The discovery of grounded theory: Strategies for qualitative research.* Chicago, IL: Aldine.

Green, C. A. (1998). Critically exploring the use of Rogers' nursing theory of unitary beings as a framework to underpin therapeutic touch practice. *European Nurse, 3*(3), 158–169.

Grubbs, J. (1974). An interpretation of the Johnson behavioral system model for nursing practice. In J. P. Riehl & C. Roy, *Conceptual models for nursing practice* (pp. 160–206). New York: Appleton-Century-Crofts.

Guba, E. G. (1990). *The paradigm dialog.* Newbury Park, CA: Sage.

Guiliano, K. K., Tyer-viola, L., & Lopex, R. P. (2005). Unity of knowledge in the advancement of nursing knowledge. *Nursing Science Quarterly, 18*(3), 242–248.

Hall, J. M. (1990). Alcoholism recovery of lesbian women: A theory in development. *Scholarly Inquiry for Nursing Practice, 4*(2), 109–122.

Haller, K. B., Reynolds, M. A., & Horsley, J. A. (1979). Developing research-based innovation protocols: Process, criteria, and issues. *Research in Nursing and Health, 2*, 45–51.

Hardy, L. K. (1986). Janforum: Identifying the place of theoretical frameworks in an evolving discipline. *Journal of Advanced Nursing 11*, 103–107.

Harris, R. B. (1986). Introduction of a conceptual model into a fundamental baccalaureate course. *Journal of Nursing Education, 25*, 66–69.

Im, E. O., & Meleis, A. (1999). Situation-specific theories: Philosophical roots, properties, and approach. *Advances in Nursing Science, 22*(2), 11–24. Retrieved June 3, 2002 from CINAHL/OVID database.

Jacobson, S. F. (1987). Studying and using conceptual models of nursing. *Image: Journal of Nursing Scholarship, 19*(2), 78–82.

Jacox, A. (1974). Theory construction in nursing: An overview. *Nursing Research, 23*(1), 4–13.

Johns, J. (1995). Framing learning through reflection within Carper's fundmental way of knowing in nursing. *Journal of Advanced Nursing, 22*(2), 226–234.

Johnson, D. E. (1974). Development of theory: A requisite for nursing as a primary health profession. *Nursing Research 23*(5), 372–377.

Johnson, D. E. (1986). Theory in nursing: Borrowed and unique. In L. H. Nicholl (Ed.), *Perspectives on nursing theory* (pp. 117–121). Boston, MA: Little, Brown.

Johnson, D. E. (1990). The behavioral system model for nursing. In M. E. Parker (Ed.), *Nursing theories in practice* (pp. 23–32). New York: National League for Nursing.

Johnson, J. E., & Rice, V. H. (1974). Sensory and distress components of pain. *Nursing Research, 23*, 203–209.

Jones, D. A. (2001). Linking nursing language and knowledge development. In N. L. Chaska (Ed.), *The nursing profession: Tomorrow and beyond* (pp. 373–386). Thousand Oaks, CA: Sage.

Kahn, S., & Fawcett, J. (1995). Critiquing the dialogue: A response to Draper's critique of Fawcett's "Conceptual models and nursing practice: The reciprocal relationship." *Journal of Advanced Nursing, 22*(1), 188–192.

Kameoda, T., & Sugimori, M. (1993, June). *Application of King's goal attainment theory in Japanese clinical setting.* Paper presented at the meeting of Sigma Theta Tau International's Sixth International Nursing Research Congress, Madrid, Spain.

Kao, H. S., Reeder, F. M., Hsu, M., & Cheng, S. (2006). A Chinese view of the western metaparadigm. *Journal of Holistic Nursing, 24*(2), 92–101.

Kikuchi, J. F. (1992). Nursing questions that science cannot answer. In J. F. Kikuchi & H. Simmons (Eds.), *Philosophic inquiry in nursing* (pp. 26–37). Newbury Park, CA: Sage.

Kikuchi, J. F. (2003). Nursing knowledge and the problem of worldviews. *Research & Theory for Nursing Practice, 17*, 7–17.

Kikuchi, J. F., & Simmons, H. (1996). The whole truth and progress in nursing knowledge development. In J. F. Kikuchi, H. Simmons & D. Romyn (Eds.), *Truth in nursing inquiry* (pp. 5–18). Newbury Park, CA: Sage.

Kilchenstein, L., & Yakulis, I. (1984). The birth of a curriculum: Utilization of the Neuman health care system model in an integrated baccalaureate program. *Journal of Nursing Education, 23,* 126–127.

Kim, H. S. (1983). *The nature of theoretical thinking in nursing.* Norwalk, CT: Appleton-Century-Crofts.

Kim, H. S. (1989). Theoretical thinking in nursing: Problems and perspectives. *Recent Advances in Nursing, 24,* 106–122.

Kim, H. S. (1997). Terminology in structuring and developing nursing knowledge. In I. M. King & J. Fawcett (Eds.), *The language of nursing theory and metatheory* (pp. 27–35). Indianapolis, IN: Sigma Theta Tau.

Kim, H. S. (2000). *The nature of theoretical thinking in nursing* (2nd ed.). New York: Springer.

King, I. M. (1978). The "why" of theory development. In *National League for Nursing, Theory development: What, why, how?* (pp. 11–16). New York: National League for Nursing.

King, I. M. (1984). Philosophy of nursing education: A national survey. *Western Journal of Nursing Research, 6,* 387–406.

King, I. M. (1997). Knowledge development for nursing: A process. In I. M. King & J. Fawcett (Eds.), *The language of nursing theory and metatheory* (pp. 19–25). Indianapolis, IN: Sigma Theta Tau.

Kirkevold, M. (1993). Toward a practice theory of caring for patients with chronic skin disease. *Scholarly Inquiry for Nursing Practice, 7*(1), 37–57.

Kramer, M. K. (1997). Terminology in theory: Definitions and comments. In I. M. King & J. Fawcett (Eds.), *The language of nursing theory and metatheory* (pp. 61–71). Indianapolis, IN: Sigma Theta Tau.

Kuhn, T. S. (1977). *The essential tension.* Chicago, IL: Chicago University Press.

Kuhn, T. S. (1996). *The structure of scientific revolutions* (3rd ed.). Chicago, IL: Chicago University Press.

Kylma, J. (2005). Dynamics of hope in adults living with HIV/AIDS: A substantive theory. *Journal of Advanced Nursing, 52*(6), 620–630.

LaCoursiere, S. P. (2001). A theory of online social support. *Advances in Nursing Science, 24*(1), 60–77.

Landreneau, K. J. (2002). Response to: The nature of philosophy of science, theory and knowledge relating to nursing and professionalism. *Journal of Advanced Nursing, 38*(3), 283–285. Retrieved November 6, 2002 from CINAHL/OVID database.

LeCuyer, E. A. (1992). Milieu therapy for short stay units: A transformed practice theory. *Archives of Psychiatric Nursing, 6*(2), 108–116.

Leddy, S. K. (2000). Toward a complementary perspective on worldviews. *Nursing Science Quarterly, 13*(3), 225–233.

Lenz, E. R. (1996). *Role of middle range theory for research and practice.* Paper presented at the Proceedings of the Sixth Rosemary Ellis Scholars' Retreat, Frances Payne Bolton School of Nursing, Case Western Reserve University, Cleveland, OH.

Lenz, E. R. (1998). Role of middle range theory for nursing research and practice. Part 1. Nursing research. *Nursing Leadership Forum, 3*(1), 24–33.

Lenz, E. R., Suppe, F., Gift, A. G., Pugh, L. C., & Milligan, R. A. (1995). Collaborative development of middle-range theories: Toward a theory of unpleasant symptoms. *Advances in Nursing Science, 17*(3), 1–13.

Lerner, R. M. (1986). *Concepts and theories of human development* (2nd ed.). New York: Random House.

Liehr, P., & Smith, M. J. (1999). Middle range theory: Spinning research and practice to create knowledge for the new millennium. *Advances in Nursing Science, 21*(4), 81–91. Retrieved June 11, 2002, from CINAHL/OVID database.

Littlejohn, C. (2002). Are nursing models to blame for low morale? *Nursing Standard, 16*(17), 39–41.

Mackenzie, S., & Spence Laschinger, H. (1995). Correlates of nursing diagnoses in public health nursing. *Journal of Advanced Nursing, 21*(4), 772–777.

Malone, R. E. (2005). Assessing the policy environment. *Policy, Politics, & Nursing Practice, 6*(2), 135–143.

McKenna, H. (1997). *Nursing theories and models.* London: Routledge.

Meighan, M. (2006). Mercer's becoming a mother theory in nursing practice. In M. R. Alligood & A. M. Tomey (Eds.), *Nursing theory: Utilization & application.* (3rd ed., pp. 399–411). St. Louis, MO: Mosby.

Meleis, A. I. (1997). *Theoretical nursing: Development and progress* (3rd ed.). Philadelphia, PA: Lippincott-Raven.

Meleis, A. I., & Im, E. (2001). From fragmentation to integration in the discipline of nursing: Situation-specific theories. In N. L. Chaska (Ed.), *The nursing profession: Tomorrow and beyond* (pp. 881–891). Thousand Oaks, CA: Sage.

Merton, R. K. (1968). *On social theory and social structure.* New York: Free Press.

Monti, E. J., & Tingen, M. S. (1999). Multiple paradigms in nursing. *Advances in Nursing Science, 21*(4), 64–80.

Moody, L. E. (1990). *Advancing nursing science through research* (Vol. 1). Newbury Park, CA: Sage.

Moody, L. E., Wilson, N. E., Smyth, K., Schwartz, R., Tittle, M., & Van Cott, M. L. (1988). Analysis of a decade of nursing practice research: 1977–1986. *Nursing Research, 37*(6), 374–379.

Newman, M. (2002). The pattern that connects. *Advances in Nursing Science, 24*(3), 1–7.

Newman, M. A., Sime, A. M., & Corcoran-Perry, S. A. (1996). The focus of the discipline of nursing. In J. W. Kenney (Ed.), *Philosophical and theoretical perspectives for advanced nursing practice* (pp. 297–301). Boston, MA: Jones and Bartlett.

Nielson, P. A. (1992). Quality of care: Discovering a modified practice theory. *Journal of Nursing Care Quality, 6*(2), 63–76.

Orem, D. E. (2001). *Nursing: Concepts of practice* (6th ed.). St. Louis, MO: Mosby.

Parker, K. P. (1989). The theory of sentience evolution: A practice-level theory of sleeping, waking, and beyond waking patterns based on the science of unitary human beings. *Rogerian Nursing Science News, 2*(1), 4–6.

Parker, M. E. (2006). *Nursing theories and nursing practice* (2nd ed.). Philadelphia, PA: F. A. Davis.

Parse, R. R. (1987). *Nursing science: Major paradigms, theories, and critiques.* Philadelphia, PA: Saunders.

Parse, R. R. (1997). The language of nursing knowledge: Saying what we mean. In King, I. M. & Fawcett, J. (Eds.) *The language of nursing theory and metatheory* (pp. 73–77). Indianapolis, IN: Sigma Theta Tau.

Parse, R. R. (1999). Nursing science: the transformation of practice. *Journal of Advanced Nursing, 30*(6), 1383–1387. Retrieved November 6, 2002, from Ovid/CINAHL database.

Phillips, J. R. (1992). The aim of philosophical inquiry in nursing: Unity or diversity of thought. In J. F. Kikuchi & H. Simmons (Eds.), *Philosophic inquiry in nursing* (pp. 45–50). Newbury Park, CA: Sage.

Pilkington, F. B., & Mitchell, G. J. (1999). A dialogue on the comparability of research paradigms—and other theoretical things. *Nursing Science Quarterly, 12*(4), 283–289.

Pilkington, F. B., & Mitchell, G. J. (2003). Mistakes across paradigms. *Nursing Science Quarterly, 16*(2), 102–108.

Porter-O'Grady, T. (2003). Nurses as knowledge workers. *Creative Nursing, 9*(2), 6–9.

Rawnsley, M. M. (2003). Dimensions of scholarship and the advancement of nursing science: Articulating a vision. *Nursing Science Quarterly, 16*(1), 5–15.

Reed, P. G. (1995). A treatise on nursing knowledge development for the 21st century: Beyond postmodernism. *Advances in Nursing Science 17*(3), 70–84. Retrieved June 3, 2002, from CINAHL/OVID database.

Reynolds, P. D. (1971). *A primer for theory construction.* Indianapolis, IN: Bobbs-Merrill.

Rinehart, J. M. (1978). The "how" of theory development in nursing. In *National league for nursing, theory development: What, why, how?* (pp. 67–74). New York: National League for Nursing.

Roach, M. S. (1992). The aim of philosophical inquiry in nursing: Unity or diversity of thought. In J. F. Kikuchi & H. Simmons (Eds.), *Philosophic inquiry in nursing* (pp. 38–44). Newbury Park, CA: Sage.

Rodman, H. (1980). Are conceptual frameworks necessary for theory building? The case of family sociology. *The Sociology Quarterly, 21*, 429–441.

Rutty, J. E. (1998). The nature of philosophy of science, theory and knowledge relating to nursing and professionalism. *Journal of Advanced Nursing, 28*(2),

243–250. Retrieved July 16, 2002, from Ovid/CINAHL database.

Sanford, R. C. (2000). Caring through relation and dialogue: A nursing perspective for patient education. *Advances in Nursing Science, 22*(3), 1–15. Retrieved April 15, 2002, from CINAHL/OVID database.

Sarter, B. (1988). Philosophical sources of nursing theory. *Nursing Science Quarterly, 1*(2), 52–59.

Schlotfeldt, R. M. (1992). Answering nursing's philosophical questions: Whose responsibility is it? In J. F. Kikuchi & H. Simmons (Eds.), *Philosophic inquiry in nursing* (pp. 97–104). Newbury Park, CA: Sage.

Seiloff, C. L., & Frey, M. A. (2007). *Middle range theory development using king's conceptual system.* New York: Springer.

Shapere, D. (1980). The structure of scientific revolutions. In G. Gutting (Ed.), *Paradigms & revolutions* (pp. 27–38). Notre Dame, IN: University of Notre Dame Press.

Shearer, J. E. (2002). The concept of protection: A dimensional analysis and critique of a theory of protection. *Advances in Nursing Science, 25*(1), 65–78.

Silva, M. C. (1997). Philosophy, science, theory, interrelationships and implications for nursing research. *Image: Journal of Nursing Scholarship, 29*(3), 210–213. Retrieved June 7, 2002, from CINAHL/OVID database.

Silva M. C., Sorrell, J. M., & Sorrell, C. D. (1995). From Carper's ways of knowing to ways of being: An ontological philosophical shift. *Advances in Nursing Science, 18*(1), 1–13.

Simmons, H. (1992). Philosophic and scientific inquiry: The interface. In J. F. Kikuchi & H. Simmons (Eds.), *Philosophic inquiry in nursing* (pp. 9–25). Newbury Park, CA: Sage.

Smart, J. J. C. (1968). *Between science and philosophy.* New York: Random House.

Smith, C. E., Pace, K., Kochinda, C., Kleinbeck, S., Koehler, J., & Popkess-Vawter, S. (2002). Caregiver effectiveness model evolution to a midrange theory of home care: A process for critique and replication. *Advances in Nursing Science, 25*(1), 50–64.

Stevens-Barnum, B. J. (1998). *Nursing theory: Analysis, application, evaluation* (5th ed.). Philadelphia, PA: Lippincott Williams & Wilkins.

Suppe, F. (1996a, May). *Middle range theory: Nursing theory and knowledge development.* Paper presented at the Proceedings of the Sixth Rosemary Ellis Scholars' Retreat, Frances Payne Bolton School of Nursing, Case Western Reserve University, Cleveland, OH.

Suppe, F. (1996b, July). *Middle range theories: Historical and contemporary perspectives.* Available from Institute for Advanced Study, Indiana University, Poplars 335, Bloomington, IN.

Thorne, S., Canam, C., Dahinten, S., Hall, W., Henderson, A., & Kirkham, S. R. (1998). Nursing's metaparadigm concepts: Disimpacting the debates. *Journal of Advanced Nursing, 27*(6), 1257–1268.

Tierney, A. J. (1998). Nursing models: Extant or extinct? *Journal of Advanced Nursing, 28*(1), 77–85. Retrieved June 3, 2002, from CINAHL/OVID database.

Tripp-Reimer, T., Woodworth, G., McCloskey, J. C., & Bulechek. (1996). The dimensional structure of nursing interventions. *Nursing Research, 45*(1), 10–17.

Ulbrich, S. L. (1999). Nursing practice theory of exercise as self-care. *Image, 31*(1), 65–70. Retrieved August 1, 2002, from CINAHL/OVID database.

Wald, F. S., & Leonard, R. C. (1964). Towards development of nursing practice theory. *Nursing Research, 13*, 309–313.

Walker, L. O. (1986). Toward a clearer understanding of the concept of nursing theory. In L. H. Nicholl (Ed.), *Perspectives on nursing theory* (pp. 26–38). Boston, MA: Little, Brown.

Walker, L. O., & Avant, K. C. (1995). *Strategies for theory construction in nursing* (3rd ed.). Norwalk, CT: Appleton & Lange.

Walker, L. O., & Avant, K. C. (2005). *Strategies for theory construction in nursing* (4th ed.). Upper Saddle River, NJ: Pearson/Prentice Hall.

Walsh, D., & Downe, S. (2005). Meta-synthesis method for qualitative research: A literature review. *Journal of Advanced Nursing, 50*(2), 204–211.

Weaver, K., & Olson J. K. (2006). Understanding paradigms used for nursing research. *Journal of Advanced Nursing, 53*(4), 459–468.

Whall, A. L. (1996, May). *Overview of middle range theory.* Paper presented at the Proceedings of the Sixth Rosemary Ellis Scholars' Retreat, Frances Payne Bolton School of Nursing, Case Western Reserve University, Cleveland, OH.

White, J. (2004). Patterns of knowing: Review, critique, and update. In P. G. Reed, N. C. Shearer, and L. H. Nicoll (eds.), *Perspectives in nursing theory* (6th ed., pp. 247–258). Philadelphia: PA: Lippincott Williams & Wilkins.

Whitehead, D. (2005). Guest editorial: Empirical or tacit knowledge as a basis for theory development. *Journal of Clinical Nursing, 14*(2), 143–144.

Winters, J., & Ballou, K. A. (2004). The idea of nursing science. *Journal of Advanced Nursing, 45*(5), 533–535.

Young, A., Taylor, S. G., & Renpenning, K. (2001). *Connections: Nursing research, theory, and practice.* St. Louis, MO: Mosby.

Yura, H., & Torres, G. (1975). Today's conceptual frameworks within baccalaureate nursing programs. In *National League for Nursing, Faculty-curriculum development part III: Conceptual frameworks—its meaning and functioning* (pp. 17–30). New York: National League for Nursing.

2

Analysis, Evaluation, and Selection of a Middle Range Nursing Theory

TIMOTHY S. BREDOW

DEFINITION OF KEY TERMS

Adequacy	Determines how completely the theory addresses the topics it claims to address. Establishes if there are holes or gaps that need to be filled in by other work or further refinement of the theory. Addresses if the theory accounts for the subject matter under consideration
Clarity	Addresses if the theory clearly states the main components to be considered. Determines if it is easily understood by the reader
Complexity	Reviews how many concepts are involved as key components in the theory. Decides how complicated the description of the theory is, and if it can be understood without lengthy descriptions and explanations: considers the number of variables being addressed, and exists on a continuum from parsimony–limited number of variables to complex–extensive number of variables
Consistency	Addresses whether the theory maintains the definitions of the key concepts throughout the explanation of the theory. Determines if it has congruent use of terms, interpretations, principles, and methods throughout
Discrimination	Addresses whether the hypothesis generated by the theory led to research results that could not be arrived at using some other nursing theory. Determines how unique the theory is to the area of nursing that it addresses. Decides if it has precise and clear boundaries and definitive parameters of the subject matter
External criticism	Considers the fit between the theory and criteria external to the theory, such as the social environment and the prevailing views on the nursing metaparadigm. Criticism here is dependent on individual preference. It depends on reasonableness and perceptions of the evaluator
Internal criticism	Deals with the criteria concerning the inner workings (internal dimensions) of the theory and how the theory's components fit with each other
Logical development	Resolves the questions, does the theory logically follow a line of thought of previous work that has been shown to be true or does it launch out into unproven territory with its assumptions and premises? Do the conclusions proceed in a logical fashion? Are the arguments well supported?

(Definition of Key Terms continued on next page)

DEFINITION OF KEY TERMS (CONTINUED)

Nursing metaparadigm	Global concepts that identify the phenomena of nursing, including person, environment, health, and nursing (Fawcett, 1995)
Pragmatic	Determines if the theory can be operationalized in real-life settings
Reality convergence	Determines if the theory's underlying assumptions ring true. Decides if the theory's assumptions represent the real world, and if it represents the real world of nursing. Does the theory reflect the real world as understood by the reader?
Scope	Determines how broad or narrow is the range of phenomena that this theory covers. Does it stay in a narrow range of scope to keep it a middle range theory? (Narrower implies more applicable to practice; wider implies more global and all-encompassing.)
Significance	Will the result of the research that is conducted because of the hypotheses generated by the theory have any impact on the way nurses carry out nursing interventions in the real world, or does it merely describe what nurses do? Does the theory address essential, not irrelevant, issues to the discipline?
Theory analysis	Systematic examination of exactly what was written by the theory author(s)
Theory evaluation	The identification of component parts of a theory and the judgment of them against a set of predetermined criteria
Utility	Determines if the theory can be used to generate hypotheses that are researchable by nurses

INTRODUCTION

Middle range nursing theories can help nurses and graduate nursing students alike meet and accomplish their goals of carrying out sound nursing research. When nursing theories are analyzed and evaluated in a thorough, systematic fashion, it is easier to determine which middle range nursing theory will provide the proper guidance and direction for the research under consideration. This chapter should help graduate student nurses and research nurses deal with the problem of how to analyze, evaluate, and choose a middle range nursing theory for their assignments, and apply it to their research interests.

Theory analysis is the systematic examination of what was personally written over time by the theory author(s) about the theory. When performing a middle range theory analysis, the component parts are identified and the relationships of these components to each other and to the whole theory are examined. This analysis can provide the nurse researcher a thorough understanding about the theory. Theory evaluation is the identification of the theory's same components and judging them against a set of predetermined criteria. The criteria used for judging theories are not standardized within the field of nursing, but, rather, have evolved over time and are different depending on who is presenting the evaluation. Nonetheless, a thorough evaluation of a middle range theory will help the nurse researcher determine the robustness of the theory and the goodness of fit for application to a particular research project.

Over the years, nursing theorists have emerged with different theoretical positions and theories proposing how various nursing concepts and the nursing metaparadigm are uniquely linked. Most of these theorists have constructed theories of nursing that could be termed grand theories, while later theorists have constructed middle range nursing theories. There are now more than 50 different grand nursing theories (McKenna, 1997) and several dozen middle range nursing theories for nursing researchers to choose from.

HISTORICAL BACKGROUND

Historically, nursing theorists worked hard to explain the nature of nursing, carving out a differentiated scientific field to call their own. At the same time, nursing researchers wanted nursing theory to be constructed to aid the generation of testable research hypotheses and also have the ability to affect the practice of nursing. As nursing theory developed and progressed through different stages of maturity, so did the evaluation process of what constitutes sound nursing theory.

In the past, nurses had Nightingale's environmental model, the medical model, and borrowed theories to use as a basis for nursing research. Through the 1960s, 1970s, and 1980s, several different grand nursing theories and some middle range theories were developed for nurses to use as a basis for their research. In the 1990s and beyond, many more middle range theories have emerged, allowing nurses to move away from using the Nightingale, the medical model, borrowed theories, and grand nursing theories. When compared to grand theories, middle range theories contain fewer concepts, with relationships that are adaptable and concrete enough to be tested. Middle range theories have a particular substantive focus and consider only a limited aspect of reality. For example, Orem's Self-Care Deficit grand nursing theory would consider patients who are unable to carry out the activities of daily living and provide nursing care necessary to aid them back to a level of living where they were able to provide self-care. The middle range theory of unpleasant symptoms would use this same situation and consider the actual unpleasant symptom that was causing the problem for the patient. It would address the patient's symptom as a consideration for a multidimensional approach to health care symptom management. Kolcaba states that "for these reasons middle range theories are particularly cogent as nursing science addresses the challenges of the 21st century" (2001, p. 86). The use of many different middle range nursing theories for research purposes became a relatively new and exciting possibility for nurses during the 1990s. Now, researchers are expanding the knowledge base of nursing by enhancement of nursing's frameworks and theories (Parse, 2001). Because of this evolutionary process of theory building, nurses need to understand the historical roots for the analysis and evaluation of grand and middle range nursing theories. In addition, understanding the process of analysis and evaluation provides insight to the evaluator about the strengths and weaknesses of the individual theory itself, as well as its possible use and application to nursing research and practice.

Meleis (1997, p. 245) states that "nurses have always evaluated theories." She provides the reasons why evaluation of theory is an essential component of nursing research:

- To decide which theory is more appropriate to use as a framework for research
- To identify effective theories for guiding a research project
- To compare and contrast different explanations of the same phenomenon
- To identify epistemological approaches of a discipline through attention to the sociocultural context of the theorist and the theory
- To assess the ontological beliefs and schools of thought in a discipline
- To define research priorities (Meleis, 1997)

THEORY ANALYSIS

THEORY ANALYSIS BY EARLY AUTHORS

The analysis of nursing theory has evolved over time as nurses have proposed increasingly sophisticated methods for reviewing and analyzing nursing theory. Three "early approaches" to theory analysis by Duffy and Muhlenkamp, Hardy, and Chinn and Jacobs will be discussed followed by a discussion of "recent approaches" by Barnum, Meleis, and Fawcett.

In 1974, Duffy and Muhlenkamp wrote that nursing theory should be examined using four distinct questions. They suggested looking at the origin of the problem, the methods used in the pursuit of knowledge, the subject matter, and the kind of outcomes of testing generated by this theory.

These four questions when used alone to examine a nursing theory provided a fairly good evaluation of the theory; however, additional evaluation questions were proposed when the theory was used for research. Their additional questions for analyzing a nursing theory for nursing research included:

- Does it generate a testable hypothesis, and is it complete in terms of subject matter and perspective?
- Are the biases or values underlying the theory made explicit?
- Are the relationships among the propositions made explicit, and are they parsimonious?

With all of these questions in hand, a nurse could do what was thought, at the time, to be a thorough and complete assessment of any particular nursing theory to be used for nursing research.

During the same period of time, Hardy (1974) developed another way to analyze nursing theories. Her analysis method contained some unique criteria when compared to Duffy and Muhlenkamp's and included more criteria related to the process and outcome of theory evaluation. Her evaluation criteria identified the need for the theory to have adequacy, meaning, logic, and pragmatism. She wanted the theory to provide empirical evidence, have the ability to be generalized, contribute to further understanding, and be able to predict outcomes.

These two positions within the same historical time period contain some unique as well as overlapping criteria for the analysis and evaluation of nursing theory.

In the 1980s, Chinn and Jacobs (1983) proposed a combination of the previous two positions and recommended five brief criteria for evaluating nursing theories. They stated that a theory could be evaluated by asking if it had clarity, simplicity, generality, empirical applicability, and consequences. Clarity was further expanded to include semantic clarity, semantic consistency, structural clarity, and structural consistency. Apparently they felt that semantics and clarity were becoming issues in the nursing community, and they were attempting to address these particular issues.

RECENT APPROACHES TO THEORY ANALYSIS

In addition to consideration of criteria for evaluation of theories, nursing theorists have proposed steps for the analysis process of nursing theories. Barnum, Meleis, and Fawcett all present several steps for the analysis of a nursing theory.

Recognizing the underlying assumptions of a theoretical work is an analyst's first task in understanding the theory (Barnum, 1998; Meleis, 1997). These assumptions may not be stated but may be inferred by the reader on the basis of other statements made about the given nursing theory in other publications and writings. However, recognizing underlying assumptions may not be possible for some middle range theories, because many of these middle range theories are not constructed by any one particular nursing author but are the work of multiple authors. It then becomes difficult to understand all of the different assumptions from a variety of publications written by them. In addition, not all middle range theories are named after some nursing author or even have a particular author's name attached to the theory. For example, most of the middle range theories contained in this text do not have a theorist name attached to them, yet they have proved useful in the furtherance of nursing understanding. In addition, there are middle range theories such as Quality of Life or Reasoned Action that are borrowed from other disciplines unrelated to nursing but are used by nurses to describe and build the understanding of nursing. Nonetheless, there are some middle range theories that do have information available about the underlying assumptions, and for them, it is important to understand and relate these assumptions to the research problem.

Barnum (1990, p. 22) asserts that analysis of a theory demands that the analyst "dig beneath the surface for a deeper insight into a thesis in all its meaning and implications." This "reading between the lines" work may be difficult for some nurses because they may not be comfortable with criticism at this level. Meleis (1997) would like to see reviews of theorists; their education, experience, and professional network; and the sociocultural context of their theories. Because theory development in nursing did not take place in a vacuum, Meleis (1997) feels that it is important to carefully consider the paradigmatic origins of the theory through careful analysis of the references and citations cited by the author. In addition, she wants the analysis to include a thorough review of the assumptions, concepts, propositions, and hypothesis that the author employed, and she wants the theory to be examined for beginnings. Analysis of beginnings looks at where the theory started. Did it begin in the mind of the theorist as an attempt to explain what ought to be, or did it arise out of experience and explain what it is? Fawcett (1995) suggests that analysis needs to include a thorough review of all the author's original works and presentations. However, for some middle range theories, because they are relatively new to the field of nursing, there may not be enough published work produced by a particular author or group of authors for the analyst to read and grasp this level of understanding about the theory's meaning and implications.

Barnum believes that the analyst should determine who or what performs an activity within the theory, as well as to determine who or what is the recipient of the activity. A third area that should be evaluated in each theory is in what context the activity is performed and what the end point of the activity is. Two additional concepts that need to be addressed include the procedures that guide the activity and the energy source of the activity. Other concepts Barnum considered essential for theory analysis include nursing acts, the patient, and health (1998). Also included for good theory analysis are the relationship of nursing acts to the patient, the relationship of nursing acts to health, and the relationship of the patient to health. These concepts from Barnum are closely associated with the nursing metaparadigm that includes the concepts of nursing, person, health, and environment.

Barnum presents several devices for theory analysis. These devices use common nursing concepts to define nursing theory elements and their interrelationships. They also include determination of the level of theory development, descriptive or explanatory, and the need to discriminate nursing acts from nonnursing acts. Barnum (1990) adds that every nursing theory is based upon one or more dominant principles. These dominant principles contain an idea that is essential for stating or explaining a theory. It is important to identify and consider the nature of each key principle. A principle is a fundamental or basic concept with an explanatory function. It explains the basis upon which the theory rests. The theorist's interpretation of reality, if it is given, should be analyzed by asking, "What is reality like?" Many of these considerations were geared toward the analysis of grand theories and have to be adapted for use when considering middle range theories. For example, if a middle range theory has been formulated over time by several authors, then it will be difficult, if not impossible, to determine the theorist's interpretation of reality.

Meleis includes internal dimensions as a criterion of her method of theory analysis. Internal dimensions include assumptions and concepts upon which the theory is built. She includes several units of analysis as part of this inquiry. Her units of analysis include content, context, and methods, and are similar to the units of analysis contained in Barnum's list. Other items unique to Meleis include the rationale, the system of relations, beginnings, scope, goals, and abstractness. Examining the rationale of a theory's construction provides clarification of how the elements of the theory are united. Meleis wants the analyst to discover the theory's system of relations. This is accomplished by asking the question, "Do relations explain elements or do the elements explain relations?" (Meleis, 1997, p. 258). The scope of a theory determines how broad or narrow is the range of phenomena that the theory covers. Middle range theories keep their scope narrow, helping to make the theory more applicable to research and practice. The scope of a theory also deals with the breadth of the explanations it attempts to accomplish. The scope is narrower, more specific, and more concrete for middle range theories than it is for grand theories (Fawcett, 1999).

The goals of a theory also need to be examined. Does the theory attempt to describe, explain, predict, or prescribe? Each theory must attempt to accomplish at least one of these goals. Middle range theories can be classified as falling into three distinct categories. These categories are descriptive, explanatory, and predictive (Fawcett, 2000). These three categories are closely aligned with the definition given by Meleis (1997) for a grand theory that includes describing, explaining, and predicting different phenomena.

Abstractness is another point that Meleis says is necessary to examine when analyzing a theory. Analyzing abstractness is an attempt to determine the width of the gaps between the theories, propositions, concepts, and reality. In middle range theories, this gap should be small, or nonexistent, since middle range theories deal with what is and not with what ought to be.

Fawcett (2000) has several recommendations for theory analysis that are similar to Meleis' and Barnum's. She has two additional components to consider. They are theory context and theory content. Theory context is the environment in which the theory's nursing action takes place. It tells about the nature of the nurses' world and may describe the nature of the client environment. Theory context is also concerned with which nursing metaparadigm concepts are addressed by the theory (Fawcett, 2000). In middle range theories, the focus of the theory may be purposefully limited to just one of the nursing metaparadigm concepts, such as in pain theory.

Theory content identifies the theory elements that are the subject matter of the theory. The content is stated through the concepts and propositions (Fawcett, 2000). Middle range theories should have their content well defined and their concepts clearly stated in the description of the theory.

A theory's process refers to the activities that either the nurse or the client has to perform to implement the theory. This should be the strength of middle range theories as they give clear direction to some process or activity carried out in the application of the theory in research or practice.

THEORY EVALUATION

BARNUM'S THEORY EVALUATION RECOMMENDATIONS

Barnum (1990, p. 20) states that "a thorough criticism (both analysis and evaluation) of a theory requires that attention be given to both aspects of internal and external criticism." Internal criticism refers to the internal construction of how the components of the theory fit together, while external criticism considers the theory and its relationship to people, nursing, and health. Internal criticism requires the reviewer to answer the following questions:

■ Given the theorist's underlying assumptions, does the theory logically follow?
■ Is the theory consistent with and logical in light of the underlying assumptions?

For external criticism, the reviewer would ask the following questions:

■ Do the theory's underlying assumptions ring true?
■ Do the assumptions represent the "real world" out there, especially the real world of nursing?

Barnum's criteria for evaluating theories include both internal and external criticism based on specific criteria. Her criteria for judging theories for internal criticism include clarity, consistency, adequacy, logical development, and level of theory development. Her criteria for judging theories using external criticism include reality convergence, utility, significance, discrimination, scope of theory, and complexity (Barnum, 1998).

Internal criticism is first evaluated by deciding the clarity of the theory. Two questions should be answered to determine clarity:

■ Does the theory clearly state the main components to be considered?
■ Is it easily understood by the reader?

Next on Barnum's list is consistency. Two more questions help to determine if the theory is consistent:

■ Does the description of the theory continue to maintain the definitions of the key concepts throughout the explanation of the theory?
■ Does it have congruent use of terms, interpretations, principles, and methods?

The next criterion is adequacy. Three questions help to determine if the theory is adequate:

■ How completely does the theory speak to the topics it claims to address?
■ Are there holes or gaps that need to be filled in by other work or further refinement of the theory?
■ Does it account for the subject matter under consideration?

Her fourth criterion is logical development. The quality of this criterion is determined by asking three questions:

■ Does the theory logically follow a line of thought of previous work that has been shown to be true or does it launch out into unproven territory with its assumptions and premises?
■ Do the conclusions proceed in a logical fashion?
■ Are the arguments well supported?

The final criterion for evaluating the internal portion of the theory is the level of theory development, which can be determined by asking the following questions:

■ Is it in early development, just at the stage of naming its elements, or has it been around a long time and is able to explain or even predict outcomes?
■ How often have different nurse researchers conducted independent research studies applying the theory to different situations and reported the findings in the literature?

Barnum (1998, p. 178) states that "external criticism evaluates a nursing theory as it relates to the real world of man, of nursing, and of health." She recommends that the following criteria should be considered: reality convergence, utility, significance, and capacity for discrimination. In addition, two other criteria may be included: scope and complexity (Barnum, 1998).

Reality convergence deals with how well the theory builds upon the premises from which it is derived and then relates that to reality. Some nursing theorists build on past work and remain within the framework of traditional thinking. Other nurse theorists deconstruct the past and develop a new framework to build upon. These theorists are termed *deconstructionists*. Deconstructionists start with a different set of presuppositions than the historical nursing leaders did, and the resulting nursing theories may not represent the same worldview of nursing as described in the past. At this point, the person doing the evaluation may choose to disagree as to whether a particular theory achieves reality convergence, based primarily on the differences between the beliefs and the values that he or she holds to be true and those proposed by the theory. This part of theory evaluation may have more applicability to grand theories than middle range theories, but is an important point to consider, as new and different middle range theories are developed in future.

Utility simply requires that the theory be useful to the nurse researcher employing it. It should suggest subject material that could be investigated and lent itself to methods of inquiry. Middle range theories generally lend themselves to a greater ease of usefulness by nurse researchers than grand nursing theories. This is because they tend to be very narrow in scope and focused on specific concepts, like health promotion, pain, and quality of life.

The significance of a nursing theory depends upon the extent to which it addresses the phenomena of nursing and lends itself to further research.

Discrimination is the capacity to differentiate nursing from other health-related disciplines through the use of well-defined boundaries. The boundaries need to be clear and precise so that judgments can be made about any given action performed by a nurse.

Barnum includes the scope of a theory as a necessary criterion for external criticism. Important questions to consider here are, does it have a narrow range of scope to help identify it as a middle range theory, and does that narrow focus make it easier to use in a research setting?

Complexity is the final criterion in Barnum's list. Complexity is at the opposite pole from the criterion of parsimony. The level of complexity is determined by the number of variables. Middle range nursing theories are less complex than grand nursing theories because they deal with fewer variables, resulting in a fewer number of relationships between the concepts.

MELEIS' THEORY EVALUATION RECOMMENDATIONS

Meleis (1997) provides a complex model for theory evaluation. It includes several integral parts: theory description, theory support, theory analysis, and theory critique. She proposes that this complete model represents the necessary elements needed to thoroughly evaluate a theory. Meleis begins the description of her model by listing two criteria that help describe the theory. These two criteria are structural and functional components. Within the criterion of structural components, there are separate units of analysis to consider. The first is assumptions. Assumptions are "givens" in the theory and are based on the theorist's values. They are not subject to testing but lead to the set of propositions that are to be tested. In nursing theories, there are many assumptions made about the concepts included in the nursing metaparadigm and, additionally, to the concepts of human behavior, life, death, and illness. Again, it must be stated that it will not be possible to find the assumptions of all middle range theories.

Another part of Meleis' theory description includes functional components. A functional assessment of a theory carefully considers the anticipated consequences of the theory and its purposes. The units of analysis of the functional components are the theory's focus, that is, the client, nursing, health, nurse–patient interactions, the environment, nursing problems, and nursing therapeutics (p. 251).

Meleis offers several questions to ask when considering the functional components of a nursing theory (p. 254). They include the following:

1. Whom does the theory act upon?
2. What definitions does the theory offer for the elements of the nursing metaparadigm?

3. Does the theory offer a clear idea of what the sources of nursing problems are?

4. Does the theory provide interventions for nurses?

5. Are there guidelines for intervention modalities?

6. Does it provide guidelines for the role of the nurse?

7. Are the consequences of the nurse's actions articulated?

Meleis feels that these criteria are consistent with the ones offered by Barnum.

Another major area of theory evaluation for Meleis is theory support. She includes theory testing in this area. Theory testing consists of four separate tests: tests of utility, tests of nonnursing propositions, tests of concepts, and tests of propositions.

A final area of evaluation in the model is what Meleis calls theory critique. Theory critique is made up of several criteria. Many of her criteria are similar to the ones developed by Barnum, but some are unique to Meleis. The duplicated criteria similar to Barnum's are clarity, consistency, simplicity/complexity, and usefulness. Some unique criteria are tautology/teleology and diagrams.

Tautology considers evaluating the needless repetition of an idea in separate parts of the theory. Overuse of repetition can confuse a reader and make the theory explanation unclear.

Teleology is assessed by considering the extent to which causes and consequences are kept separate in the theory. Meleis (1997) says teleology occurs when the theorist defines concepts by consequences and then introduces totally new concepts, rather than getting to the definitions of the original concepts. As this process continues, there is never a clear definition of the theory's concepts, and the theory remains unclear.

Diagrams are useful to visually see the interrelationship of the concepts to each other before doing research. They can be especially useful for reviewing the strength of statistical correlations between the theory's concepts.

FAWCETT'S THEORY EVALUATION RECOMMENDATIONS

Fawcett (2000) made the following recommendations to be used for the evaluation of nursing theories. Her criteria include significance, internal consistency, parsimony, testability, empirical adequacy, and pragmatic adequacy. She also recommends that the evaluation of a theory requires judgments to be made about the extent to which a theory satisfies the criteria.

Significance may be determined by asking the following questions: Are the metaparadigm concepts and propositions addressed by the theory explicit? In middle range theories, all aspects of the metaparadigm for nursing are not always covered, and that should not detract from its use by nursing researchers. Are the philosophical claims on which the theory is based explicit? Here again, some middle range theories will be devoid of philosophical claims. Is the conceptual model from which the theory was derived explicit? Are the authors of antecedent knowledge from nursing and adjunctive disciplines acknowledged, and are bibliographical citations given? (Fawcett, 2000, p. 504).

Fawcett's second criterion of internal consistency requires that all the elements of the theory be congruent. These elements may include conceptual model and theory concepts and propositions. In addition, Fawcett suggests that semantic clarity and consistency are required for internal consistency to be maintained. She proposes that the following questions be asked when evaluating the internal consistency of a theory: Are the content and the context of the theory congruent? Do the concepts reflect semantic clarity and consistency? Do the theory propositions reflect structural consistency? (Fawcett, 2000).

Parsimony is concerned with whether the theory is stated clearly and concisely. This criterion is met when the statements clarify rather than obscure the topic of interest. This is as important in middle range theory as it is in grand theory. Even though the scope of the theory may be narrow in a middle range theory, it is still important to be clear and concise in the explanations of the concepts.

The goal of theory development in nursing is the empirical testing of interventions that are specified in the form of middle range theories (Fawcett, 2000). The concepts of a middle range theory should be observable and the propositions measurable. Fawcett (2000, p. 506) suggests that the following questions should be asked when evaluating the testability of a middle range theory: Does the research methodology reflect the middle range theory? Are the middle range theory concepts observable through instruments that are appropriate empirical indicators of those concepts? Do the data analysis techniques permit measurement of the middle range theory propositions?

Empirical adequacy is the fifth step that Fawcett says is necessary in the evaluation of nursing theories. This step requires that assertions made by the theory are congruent with empirical evidence found through studies done using the theory as a basis for research. It usually takes more than one research study to establish empirical adequacy. The end result of using empirical adequacy is to establish the level of confidence in the theory from the best studies yielding empirical results. The question to be considered here is, are the middle range theory's assertions harmonious with the research studies' empirical results?

The final and sixth step in Fawcett's framework for evaluation of nursing theories is the criterion of pragmatic adequacy. This criterion evaluates the extent of how well the middle range theory is utilized in clinical practice. The criterion also requires that nurses fully understand the full content of the theory. In addition, the theory should help move resulting nursing action toward favorable client outcomes. Ask the following questions when evaluating a theory for pragmatic adequacy:

- Do nurses need special education and skill training to apply the theory in clinical practice?
- Is it possible to derive clinical protocols from the theory?
- How often has the theory been used as the basis of nursing research?
- Do favorable outcomes result from using the theory as a basis for nursing actions? (Fawcett, 2000)

KOLCABA'S THEORY EVALUATION RECOMMENDATIONS

A recent contribution to this discussion of theory evaluation comes from Kolcaba. According to Kolcaba (2001), there are several criteria that determine a good middle range theory. Her criteria involve evaluation and do not mention steps for theory analysis. They include questions concerning the theory's concepts and propositions, and whether or not they are specific to nursing. She also wants to determine if the theory has components that are readily operationalized and can be applied to many situations. She asserts that a middle range theory's propositions can range from causal to associative, depending on their application. The assumptions provided fit the middle range theory. The theory should be relevant for the potential users. The middle range theory should be oriented to outcomes that are important for patients and not merely describe what nurses do. Finally, Kolcaba thinks that middle range theory should describe nursing-sensitive phenomena that are readily associated with the deliberate actions of nurses.

An interesting review process of the Synergy Middle Range Theory (see Chapter 5, Synergy Model) took place during its development. A committee of experts in the analysis of theoretical and conceptual frameworks was assembled to review this theory in order to identify its strengths and weaknesses, and to obtain recommendations regarding the refinement of the model (Sechrist, Berlin, & Biel, 2000. This review committee was made up of the following nurse leaders: Barbara Stevens Barnum, RN, PhD; Marion Broome, RN, PhD; Rose Constantino, RN, PhD; Jacqueline Fawcett, RN, PhD; Edna Menke, RN, PhD; Carolyn Murdaugh, RN, PhD; Patricia Moritz, RN, PhD; Bonnie Rogers, DPH, COHN-S; and Marilyn Frank-Stromborg, EdD, JD, ANP. This esteemed committee developed a review instrument that was organized into six criteria. These criteria included the headings of clarity, consistency, adequacy, utility, significance, and summary. When compared to the recommended criteria listed in this chapter, the expert review committee decided to evaluate the synergy theory on fewer criteria. Their evaluation left out "logical development" and "determining the level of theory development" in the appraisal of internal theory analysis. When determining which criteria to include for the external middle range theory analysis, they chose to reduce the list to just three criteria, leaving out complexity, discrimination, reality convergence, pragmatic, and scope. They did add one new criterion, which may act as a "catch all" for the criteria left out, which they called the summary. In a PowerPoint presentation that was posted on the World Wide Web, Fawcett has suggested an even smaller set of criteria to evaluate middle range theories. Her list is short and includes just four total criteria: significance, internal consistency, and two new criteria, parsimony and testability (Fawcett, 2005).

It is evident that there are several distinct differences between the analysis and evaluation process for grand theories and middle range theories. At the same time, there are several similarities. Many of the principles applied to the analysis and evaluation of grand theories can be readily applied to middle range theories and, with some minor modification, can be used to determine the adequacy of a middle range theory. With this in mind, the next section will address the selection of a middle range theory for use in nursing research.

SELECTING A THEORY FOR NURSING RESEARCH

Before starting to write a proposal, Fawcett (1999) suggests that each investigator become familiar with the research topic and the conceptual model that will guide the study. She reiterates that this is done by an immersion into the literature and a thorough study of the research topic. In addition, a comprehensive literature search should be done several months before making a proposal of the study. This much time must be given to allow the proper amount of time for reading and thinking about both the content of the proposed study and the conceptual model to provide the basis for the study. It is during this time that the most appropriate middle range theory can be decided upon for use in the research.

As nurse researchers shift away from using grand nursing theories and begin to consider using middle range theories, the philosophical underpinnings of the theory itself become of decreased importance. The emphasis shifts from the philosophical basis of the nursing theory to how the middle range theory is applied in research and practice. Thus, time previously spent with the philosophy and background of the theorist can now be devoted to ensuring the proper fit between the research questions to be studied and the middle range theory. Each nurse researcher should ask the following questions about the middle range theory proposed for use in his or her research:

- Does the theory seem to fit the research that you wish to do?
- Is it readily operationalized?
- What has been the primary application for this theory in the past?
- Where has the theory in question been applied and used before?
- How well has the theory performed at describing, predicting, and/or explaining the phenomena that it relates to?
- Does the theory relate to and address the research hypothesis in its description and explanation?
- Does the hypothesis flow from the research problem?
- Does the theory address the primary and secondary research questions?
- Are the theory's assumptions congruent with the assumptions that are made for this research?
- Is it oriented to outcomes that are critical to patients and does not describe what nurses perform?
- Are tools available to test relationships of the theory or do they need to be developed?

The nurse researcher should consider several different middle range theories as possibilities for use. A thorough analysis and evaluation of these theories in question should be done before selecting one. Subsequently, the nurse researcher should become familiar with all aspects of the theory, using the questions provided in the discussion above. It is essential to have a sound understanding and be in total agreement with the theory selected before beginning the study. This is accomplished by becoming immersed in the literature about the middle range theory in question and arriving at a thorough and complete understanding of the theory before using it. The nurse researcher should try to understand the middle range theory by identifying all the major concepts. The definitions of these concepts, in turn, should be studied for this particular theory, to make sure that the meanings have not been changed slightly over time as they are described in the literature.

In addition, the major concepts should be examined to determine how they relate to each other. Next, the researcher needs to decide if he or she can accept the premises, rationale, and presuppositions that the nursing theory is based upon before adopting it for use (McKenna, 1997). Finally, it is necessary to determine what means of measurement have been used with previous studies employing this theory. It will be important to know if new measurement tools need to be obtained or if similar tools can be employed for the study at hand.

It is evident that to decide upon and use a middle range theory effectively in nursing research, the potential nurse researcher must do a thorough analysis and evaluation of the middle range nursing theory.

The following analysis exercise will provide the guidance for conducting an evaluation of a middle range theory before selecting it for use in a research study.

MIDDLE RANGE THEORY EVALUATION PROCESS

This evaluation process, to be applied at the end of each subsequent chapter as an intellectual educational exercise, is a synthesis of the works of the authors reviewed in this chapter. After careful review of the theory presented in each chapter, taking into consideration the examples given where the middle range theory is applied in practice and the case study provided, the reader should be able to carry out this theory evaluation, taking into account the following criteria listed here with their definitions. Answer the questions posed for each criterion. Summarize the findings in a concluding paragraph for both internal and external criticism. Finally, make a judgment as to whether this theory could be adapted for use in research. Start the process by evaluating internal criticism.

Internal Criticism

Adequacy: How completely does the theory address the topics it claims to address? Are there holes or gaps that need to be filled in by other work or further refinement of the theory? Does it account for the subject matter under consideration?

Clarity: Does the theory clearly state the main components to be considered? Is it easily understood by the reader?

Consistency: Does the description of the theory address whether it maintains the definitions of the key concepts throughout the explanation? Does it have congruent use of terms, interpretations, principles, and methods?

Logical development: Does the theory logically follow a line of thought of previous work that has been shown to be true, or does it launch out into unproven territory with its assumptions and premises? Do the conclusions proceed in a logical fashion? Are the arguments well supported?

Level of theory development: Is it consistent with the conceptualization of middle range theory?

External Criticism

Complexity: How many concepts are involved as key components in the theory? How complicated is the description of the theory? Can it be understood without lengthy descriptions and explanations? (considers the number of variables being addressed, exists on a continuum from parsimony–limited number of variables to complex–extensive number of variables).

Discrimination: Is this theory able to produce hypotheses that will lead to research results that could not be arrived at using some other nursing theory? How unique is this theory to the area of nursing that it addresses? Does it have precise and clear boundaries and definitive parameters of the subject matter?

Reality convergence: Do the theory's underlying assumptions ring true? Do these assumptions represent the real world? Do they represent the real world of nursing? Does the theory reflect the real world as understood by the reader?

Pragmatic: Can the theory be operationalized in real-life settings?

Scope: How broad or narrow is the range of phenomena that this theory covers? Does it stay in a narrow range of scope to keep it a middle range theory? (Narrower implies more applicable to practice; wider implies more global and all-encompassing.)

Significance: Will the result of the research that is conducted because of the hypothesis generated by the theory have any impact on the way nurses carry out nursing interventions in the real world, or does it merely describe what nurses do? Does the theory address issues essential, not irrelevant, to the discipline?

Utility: Is the theory able to be used to generate hypotheses that are researchable by nurses?

After completing the evaluation based on the criteria listed above, compare and contrast responses to the ones done by contributors for each chapter listed in Appendix A at the end of the text.

CRITICAL THINKING EXERCISES

1. Recently groups of nurses and nurse theorists alike have migrated to an abbreviated process for middle range theory analysis. What information about the theory is not available from this abbreviated review?

2. Do you think that the shorter method of analysis results in a "good enough" analysis of any one middle range theory? Why or why not?

3. If you were going to use a particular middle range theory for your own research study, would you be satisfied with the abbreviated method of analysis before you begin the project?

WEB RESOURCES

Visit **http://thePoint.lww.com/Peterson3e** for helpful web resources related to this chapter.

REFERENCES

Barnum, B. (1990). *Nursing theory, analysis application, evaluation* (3rd ed.). Glenview, IL: Scott, Foresman, Little Brown.

Barnum, B. (1998). *Nursing theory: Analysis, application and evaluation* (5th ed.). Philadelphia: Lippincott Williams & Wilkins.

Chinn, P., & Jacobs, M. (1983). *Theory and nursing: A systematic approach.* St. Louis, MO: Mosby.

Duffy, M., & Muhlenkamp, A. (1974). A framework for theory analysis. *Nursing Outlook, 22*(9), 570–574.

Fawcett, J. (1995). *Analysis and evaluation of conceptual models of nursing* (3rd ed.). Philadelphia: F.A. Davis.

Fawcett, J. (1999). *The relationship of theory and research* (3rd ed.). Philadelphia: F.A. Davis.

Fawcett, J. (2000). *Analysis and evaluation of contemporary nursing knowledge: Nursing models and theories.* Philadelphia: F.A. Davis.

Fawcett, J. (2005). Evaluating conceptual-theoretical-empirical structures for science of unitary human beings-based research. Retrieved July 2005 from http://medweb.uwcm.ac.uk/martha/Repository/Fawcett2005.ppt#398,1.

Hardy, M. (1974). Theories: Components, development, evaluation. *Nursing Research, 23*(2), 100–107.

Kolcaba, K. (2001). Evolution of the middle range theory of comfort for outcomes research. *Nursing Outlook, 49*(2), 86–92.

McKenna, H. (1997). *Nursing theories and models.* London: Routledge.

Meleis, A. (1997). *Theoretical nursing: Development & progress* (3rd ed.). Philadelphia: Lippincott-Raven.

Parse, R. (2001). Rosemary Rizzo Parse the human becoming school of thought. In M. Parker (Ed.), *Nursing theories and nursing practice.* Philadelphia: F.A. Davis.

Sechrist K., Berlin, L., & Biel, M. (2000). The synergy model: Overview of theoretical review process. *Critical Care Nurse, 20*(1), 85–86.

BIBLIOGRAPHY

Alligood, M. R., & Marriner-Tomey, A. M. (2002). *Nursing theory: Utilization & application* (2nd ed.). St. Louis, MO: Mosby.

Barns, B. (1999). *Nursing theories' conceptual and philosophical foundations.* New York: Springer Publishing Company.

Chinn, P., & Kramer, M. (1995). *Theory and nursing: A systematic approach* (4th ed.). St. Louis, MO: Mosby.

Chinn, P., & Kramer, M. (1999). *Theory and nursing: Integrated knowledge development* (5th ed.). St. Louis, MO: Mosby.

Dubin, R. (1978). *Theory building.* New York: The Free Press.

Fawcett, J. (1993). *Analysis and evaluation of nursing theories.* Philadelphia: F.A. Davis.

Fawcett, J. (1994). Analysis and evaluation of nursing theories. In V. Malinski & E. Barrett (Eds.), *Martha E. Rogers: Her life and her work.* Philadelphia: F.A. Davis.

Fawcett, J. (1995). *Analysis and evaluation of conceptual models of nursing* (3rd ed.). Philadelphia: F.A. Davis.

Fawcett, J. (1999). *The relationship of theory and research* (3rd ed.). Philadelphia: F.A. Davis.

Fawcett, J. (2000). *Analysis and evaluation of contemporary nursing knowledge: Nursing models and theories.* Philadelphia: F.A. Davis.

George, J. (1995). *Nursing theories: The base for professional nursing practice* (4th ed.). Norwalk, CT: Appleton & Lange.

Gift, A. (1997). *Clarifying concepts in nursing research.* New York: Springer Publishing Company.

Greenwood, J. (Ed.). (2000). *Nursing theory in Australia: Development and application.* Sydney: Harper Collins.

Huck, S., & Cormier, W. (1996). *Reading statistics & research.* New York: Harper Collins College Publishers.

Kim, H., Kollak, I., & Parker, M. (Eds.). (1990). *Nursing theories in practice.* New York: National League for Nursing, Publ. #15-2350.

McKenna, H. (1997). *Nursing models and theories.* London: Routledge.

McQuiston, C., & Webb, A. (Eds.). (1995). *Foundations of nursing theory.* Thousand Oaks, CA: Sage Publications.

Meleis, A. I. (1997). *Theoretical nursing: Development and progress* (3rd ed.). Philadelphia: Lippincott-Raven.

Nicoll, L. H. (1992). *Perspectives on nursing theory.* Philadelphia: J. B. Lippincott.

Nolan, M., & Grant, G. (1992). Middle range theory building and the nursing theory-practice gap: A respite case study. *Journal of Advanced Nursing, 17,* 217–223.

Parker, M. (Ed.). (1990). *Nursing theories in practice.* New York: National League for Nursing.

Parker, M. (Ed.). (1993). *Patterns of nursing theories in practice.* New York: National League for Nursing, Publ. #15-2548.

Parker, M. E. (2000). *Nursing theories and nursing practice.* Philadelphia: F.A. Davis.

Tomey, A. M., & Alligood, M. R. (Eds.). (2002). *Nursing theorists and their work* (5th ed.). St. Louis, MO: Mosby.

Walker, L. O., & Avant, K. C. (1997). *Strategies for theory construction in nursing.* New York: Appleton-Century-Crofts.

Wesley, R. L. (1995). *Nursing theories and models* (2nd ed.). Springhouse, PA: Springhouse.

Whall, A. (1996). The structure of nursing knowledge: Analysis and evaluation of practice, middle range and grand theory. In J. Fitzpatrick & A. Whall (Eds.), *Conceptual models of nursing: Analysis and application* (3rd ed.). Norwalk, CT: Appleton & Lange.

Winstead-Fry, P. (Ed.). (1986). *Case studies in nursing theory.* New York: National League for Nursing.

Young A., Taylor, S. G., & Renpenning, K. (2001). *Connections: Nursing research, theory and practice.* St. Louis, MO: Mosby.

3

Pain: A Balance Between Analgesia and Side Effects

MARION GOOD

DEFINITION OF KEY TERMS

Analgesia	Pain relief
Balance between analgesia and side effects	Patient satisfaction with relief of pain and relief or absence of side effects
Identification of lack of pain or relief of side effect	Pain intensity greater than the mutual goal; side effects of opioids reported by the patient or observed by the nurse
Intervention, reassessment, and reintervention	Immediate intervention for pain and side effects; reassessment when peak effect is expected, and reintervention if pain and side effects are still unacceptable
Mutual goal-setting	Mutually agreed-upon, safe, realistic goals for relief
Nonpharmacological adjuvant	Complementary nursing therapies for pain relief (relaxation, music, imagery, massage, and cold)
Pain	An unpleasant sensory and affective experience associated with tissue damage
Patient teaching	Patient instruction encouraging attitudes, expectations, and action in reporting pain; obtaining medication, preventing pain during activity, and use of complementary therapies
Pharmacological adjuvant	Analgesic given as a supplement
Potent pain medication	Opioid analgesic or local anesthetic given systemically or by epidural for acute pain
Regular assessment of pain and side effects	Report of pain and side effects every 2 hours until under control, and then every 4 hours
Side effects	Unpleasant sensory and affective experiences associated with adverse effects of pain medication

INTRODUCTION

Pain is the most common reason for people to seek health care, and although pain is known to be a part of life, it is compelling in its unpleasantness and is sometimes overwhelming in its effect. Patients who are in pain endure considerable suffering and are at risk for long-term adverse effects that include slower wound healing, down-regulation of the immune system, and metastasis of tumor cells (Page, 1996). There are many different types of pain: acute pain of injury, surgery, labor, and sickle cell crisis; chronic pain of

51

musculoskeletal or gastrointestinal disorders; procedural pain of lumbar puncture, venipuncture, and chest tube removal; cancer pain from the enlarging tumor, its metastases, or its treatment; and pain in infants, the critically ill, and at the end of life. Health care professionals today have a duty and an obligation to identify the source, to treat the cause, and to relieve the pain. Theories have been developed to explain and manage pain, and researchers have an obligation to test interventions for relief.

To study pain, researchers can experimentally induce it in animals and humans using noxious stimuli such as heat, cold, constriction, and sharpness, or they can study the pain of humans who are ill. In animal research, surgically exposed pain pathways provide information about the transmission of noxious impulses to the thalamus, sensory cortex, and limbic system, but the affective component of pain is difficult to discern. When studying humans, the patients can report both the sensory and affective components of pain, but experimentally induced pain does not have the holistic physical and emotional impact over time that clinical pain does. The pain of illness and surgery can limit life functions and arouse existential fears. The emotional impact of these limitations is intense and it interacts with the sensory pain. Therefore, clinical studies are needed. To measure pain in alert adults who can communicate, clinicians and researchers must ask their patients to indicate a number on a scale. Further, they must believe the number that their patients tell them. Only the person in pain can tell them what their pain is like, and describe it in terms of intensity, quality, duration, and trajectory. Therefore, patient reports of pain are valid.

HISTORICAL BACKGROUND

THEORIES OF PAIN MECHANISM

Beginning in the 17th century, scientists proposed various theories of the way pain events are transmitted to the brain and felt. Early pain theories included direct transmission, proposed by Descartes (Melzack & Wall, 1962), specificity theory (von Frey, 1895), and pattern theories (reviewed in Melzack & Wall, 1965). Evidence of affective pain was dramatically demonstrated by Beecher (1959), who showed that pain had a psychological component that could attenuate the transmission of impulses. The gate control theory was a major watershed or paradigm shift in pain theory (Melzack & Wall, 1965). It unified several sensory pain theories and added the affective, motivational, and central control elements, which could modify pain by descending mechanisms from the brain to the dorsal horn.

Discoveries of endogenous opiates in the periaqueductal gray area of the brain, opioid receptors in the central nervous system, and also catecholamines, serotonin, and neuropeptide receptors all produced new theories that scientists viewed as either supporting or refuting the gate control theory. Finally, Melzack presented his new neuromatrix theory of pain that encompassed existing knowledge about the complexity of pain in humans (Melzack, 1996). Nurses have created middle range descriptive and predictive theories of pain from the perspective of both patients and expert nurses (Im, 2006; Lenz, Pugh, Milligan, Gift, & Suppe, 1997; Morse, Bottorff, & Hutchinson, 1995; Mahon, 1994; Tsai, Tak, Moore, & Palencia, 2003; Simon, Baumann, & Nolan, 1995). However, all these theories describe and explain only the *mechanisms and manifestations* of pain. They propose the way pain occurs, is modulated, and its associated conditions, and although very useful, they do not specify effective interventions. Therefore, they are not the prescriptive theories needed by nurses for providing and testing interventions (Dickhoff & James, 1968).

SHIFT TO THEORIES OF PAIN RELIEF

A second watershed in pain theory was a paradigm shift from theories of the mechanisms of pain to theories of relief. These included prescriptive and explanatory theories of opioids and of nonopioids such as local anesthetics and nonsteroidal anti-inflammatory drugs (NSAIDs). Opioids, whether taken orally or injected into blood vessels, muscles, or the epidural space, provides potent relief for moderate to severe pain. The explanatory theory (mechanism) for this effect was later found to be that opioids attach to mu and kappa opioid receptors in the central nervous system. NSAIDs, including aspirin, ibuprofen, acetaminophen, cyclooxygenase-2 (COX-2) inhibitors, and ketorolac, have different mechanisms from centrally acting opioids. NSAIDs act at the site of the tissue injury to decrease the release of inflammatory substances that sensitize the nerve fibers to respond to the painful stimuli. When they are used as adjuvants, NSAIDs can be opioid sparing but may also interfere with blood clotting.

DEVELOPMENT OF INTEGRATED PRESCRIPTIVE APPROACHES

A third paradigm shift was the notion that pain alleviation by nurses requires an *integrated* prescriptive approach, proposed in Good and Moore's theory of a balance between analgesia and side effects (Good, 1998; Good & Moore, 1996). Integrated prescriptive pain theories specify the actions that nurses must take to deliver both medical and nursing interventions, for example, pharmacological and nonpharmacological therapies, for relief. There is an integrative pain alleviation theory for adults (Good & Moore, 1996) and also one for children that adds prescriptions for assessment of developmental level, coping strategies, and cultural background (Huth & Moore, 1998). Recent evidence-based acute pain management guidelines are consistent with the nursing theory of a balance between analgesia and side effects, proposed by Good and Moore in 1996. Examples are guidelines published by the American Society of Anesthesiologists on Pain Management (2004), the American Pain Society (2005), and the Joint Commission. The principles of the Good and Moore theory have stood these tests of time and interdisciplinary agreement and are therefore current for guiding nurses when caring for patients.

DEFINITION OF THEORY CONCEPTS

The major concepts of the theory, a balance between analgesia and side effects, are found in Table 3.1, along with theoretical definitions and examples of operational definitions that can be used in research. In addition, Figure 3.1 is a graphic representation of the theory. Acute pain is conceptualized as a multidimensional phenomenon that occurs after surgery or trauma and includes sensory and affective dimensions. Pain in alert adults is what the person reports. The sensory component of pain following damage to body tissues is the localized physical perception of hurt. It is ordinarily termed "sensation of pain" (Good et al., 2001). The affective component of pain is the unpleasant emotion associated with the sensation and has been named "distress of pain" (Good et al., 2001), "anxiety" (Good, 1995a), or "unpleasantness" (Price, McGrath, Rafii, & Buckingham, 1983). The sensory and affective components of pain affect each other (Casey & Melzack, 1967; Johnson & Rice, 1974) and can be measured in terms of intensity magnitude (Good et al., 2001).

The concept of *potent pain medication* refers to the major method used for relief. This may be opioids delivered by patient-controlled analgesia (PCA) or by subcutaneous, intramuscular, or intravenous injection. However, opioid analgesics have side effects of nausea, vomiting, drowsiness, urinary retention, and respiratory depression. In addition, dependence can also occur. To avoid these side effects, patients often take less analgesic than is needed for adequate relief (Acute Pain Management Guideline Panel, 1992). Epidural analgesia can be achieved with the use of opioids, local anesthetics, or both; these are injected into the epidural space of the spinal cord. Side effects of epidural analgesia include lower extremity numbness. Other techniques may include postincisional infiltration with local anesthetics, intra-articular analgesia, and peripheral nerve blocks (American Society of Anesthesiologists Task Force on Pain Management, 2004). As these methods often provide insufficient analgesia and uncomfortable side effects, adjuvants are often recommended.

Pharmacological adjuvants may be given because their unrelated mechanism of action increases relief, yet can "spare" the use and the side effects of strong analgesics. The American Society of Anesthesiologists Task Force on Pain Management (2004) reports that the literature suggests that two routes of administration may be more effective and recommends several combinations, such as (a) epidural opioid analgesia combined with oral or systemic analgesics and (b) intravenous opioids combined with oral NSAIDs such as ibuprofen; COX-2 inhibitors (COXIBs) such as celecoxib; or acetaminophen.

Nonpharmacological adjuvants to analgesic medication can include relaxation techniques, music, hypnosis, guided imagery with self-efficacy messages, or guided imagery with pleasant image messages (Box 3.1). Music can be soft, soothing, sedative instrumental music (Good et al., 2000) and can be combined

TABLE 3.1 Concepts with Theoretical and Operational Definitions

Concepts	Theoretical definitions	Operational definitions (examples)
Outcomes		
Balance between analgesia and side effects	Patient satisfaction with relief of pain and relief or absence of side effects	Patient report of safe and satisfying pain relief with few or no side effects
Pain	An unpleasant sensory and affective experience associated with tissue injury following surgery or trauma	Pain intensity on a visual analogue scale
Side effects	Unpleasant sensory and affective experiences associated with pain medication	Opioid Side Effects Scale (Good et al., 2001–2005)
Proposition 1		
Potent pain medication	Opioid analgesic or local anesthetic given systemically or by epidural for acute pain	Drug, dose, frequency, route, and method of administration
Pharmacological adjuvant	Analgesic given as a supplement	Drug, dose, frequency, route, and method of administration
Nonpharmacological adjuvant	Complementary nursing therapies: relaxation, music, imagery, massage, or cold for pain relief	Technique, dose, frequency given, and mastery of use
Proposition 2		
Regular assessment of pain and side effects	Report of pain and side effects every 2 h until under control, and then every 4 h	Pain rating scale Patient report or nurse observation of side effects of opioids
Identification of inadequate relief of pain and side effects	Pain/side effect intensity greater than mutual goal	Number and intensity of side effects that are unacceptable to patient/nurse
Intervention, reassessment, and reintervention	Immediate intervention for pain and side effects; reassessment when peak effect is expected, and reintervention if pain and side effects are still unacceptable	Nurse documentation
Proposition 3		
Patient teaching	Patient instruction, encouraging attitudes, expectations, and action in reporting pain, obtaining medication, preventing pain during activity, and using complementary therapies	Documentation of nurse instruction, or patient use of audio/videotape
Mutual goal setting	Mutually agreed-upon, safe, realistic, goals for relief	Nurse discussions with patient daily, including documentation

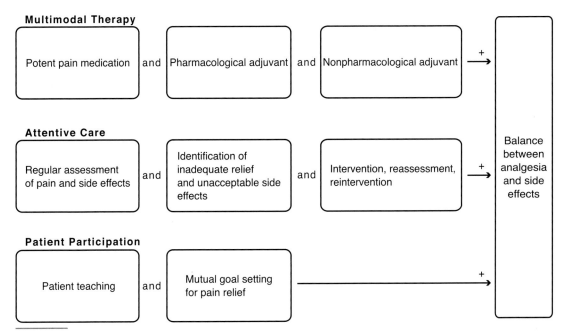

Figure 3.1 The middle range theory of a balance between analgesia and side effects prescribes nursing actions to encourage patient participation in using multimodal therapy with attentive care. (Adapted from Good, M. [1998]. A middle range theory of acute pain management: Use in research. *Nursing Outlook, 46*[3], 120–124.)

with relaxation or guided imagery. Nonpharmacological adjuvants have been studied during emergency treatment, following surgery and trauma, during labor, and during painful procedures. Nonpharmacological music interventions have also been found to be effective in cancer, arthritis, and other types of chronic pain.

Regular pain and side effect assessments are actions nurses take to identify patient symptoms. The theory then prescribes that nurses treat these symptoms, rather than simply recording them. *Identification of inadequate pain relief and side effects* directs the nurse to believe the patient's report and to know

---

Box 3.1 Nonpharmacological Adjuvants

Relaxation
Jaw relaxation (Good et al., 1999)
Autogenic phrases (Green, Green, & Norris, 1979)
Progressive muscle relaxation (Pestka, Bee, & Evans, 2010)
Systematic relaxation (Roykulcharoen & Good, 2004)
Slow rhythmic breathing

Guided imagery
Self-efficacy imagery (Tusek, Church, Strong, Grass, & Fazeo, 1997)
Pleasant imagery (Locsin, 1988; Huth, Broome, & Good, 2004; Lewandowski, 2004)
Hypnosis (Olness, 1981)

Music
Sedative music (Good et al., 1999, 2010; Siedlecki & Good, 2006)
Favorite music (Siedlecki & Good, 2006)
Tempos (fast or slow)
Instruments

what intensity is less than adequate relief, considering norms in the postoperative nursing unit and the wide variations in patient responses to pain and analgesics. In hospitals, nurses can request and use rescue orders and dose ranges (e.g., 1–2 mg), when the usual dose is insufficient (Gordon et al., 2004). The nurse can also encourage the use of nonpharmacological interventions. All interventions should be followed by *reassessment* when the greatest effect is expected, and then *reintervention* if pain is still not relieved.

Patient teaching and mutual goal setting will assist patients in their important role in managing their own pain. It is proposed that nurses teach patients effective attitudes and accurate expectations of pain. Nurses also teach patients to report pain, obtain medication, and use adjuvants. It is proposed that nurses initiate dialogue for mutual goal setting to set realistic relief goals that are acceptable to their patients.

When testing a middle range theory, more specific concepts and testable hypotheses can be deducted from the more general concepts and prepositions (Good, 1998). A balance between analgesia and side effects is the general outcome. To deduct more specific concepts, the researcher would think of components of the concept and state their relationships to the general concept. For example, the concept of side effects is a subset of the balance between analgesia and side effects. Less sensation and distress of pain can be deducted from analgesia and studied individually (Good, 1998). Any part of the theory can be examined in research: one concept, new relationships between concepts, part of a proposition, all of a proposition, or the whole theory. In addition, the application to nursing practice or education can be studied.

DESCRIPTION OF THE THEORY OF PAIN: A BALANCE BETWEEN ANALGESIA AND SIDE EFFECTS

The theory of a balance between analgesia and side effects is the first integrative prescriptive middle range pain management theory. Even though it is based on pain management guidelines and is consistent with them, the theory provides a broader and more parsimonious overview. Its general principles of acute pain management are a framework for research and a guide for nursing practice and education. The theorists expect practitioners to use the overall principles, along with the detailed knowledge contained in the adult acute pain guidelines and any current empirical evidence. These overall principles can be used in practice. They are called "propositions" when referring to the theory or testing them in research. This terminology is a matter of function: principles for practice and theoretical propositions for research. With the idea that the purpose of theory is research and the purpose of research is theory, but the purpose of both is practice, this theory with its principles/propositions is organized to stimulate additional research and to organize the teaching and communicating pain management information to nurses. Furthermore, the theory presents a new perspective that the best pain management practice is an integrated one that combines analgesic medications with nonpharmacological adjuvants, careful nursing care, and patient participation. The goal of the theory is to achieve a more holistic relief outcome than analgesia alone, that is, to balance greater pain relief with fewer side effects of opioids by using the principles.

SCOPE

The scope for the theory is fairly narrow, encompassing acute postoperative pain or trauma in hospitalized adults. The assumptions of the theory are presented in Box 3.2. They are fairly narrow so that prescriptions can be specific. The theorists meant the theory to be used clinically and tested in adults who have moderate

Box 3.2 Assumptions of the Theory of a Balance Between Analgesia and Side Effects
1. The nurse and the physician collaborate to effectively manage acute pain.
2. Systemic opioid analgesics or epidural opioids or anesthetic agents are indicated.
3. Medication for side effects is given as needed.
4. Patients are adults with ability to learn, set goals, and communicate symptoms.
5. Nurses have current knowledge of pain management.

to severe acute pain after surgery or trauma. The theory has limits; it does not address the treatment of pain in children, elders, or those with special kinds of acute pain. However, middle range theories have been or can be developed for these phenomena as well.

PROPOSITIONS

The theory has three prescriptive propositions that can be summarized as follows: In acute pain, patient participation, multimodal interventions, and attentive care are needed for a balance between analgesia and side effects.

The first proposition is about multimodal intervention. It proposes that nurses use potent pain medication plus pharmacological and nonpharmacological adjuvants to achieve a balance between analgesia and side effects. The effect on pain has empirical support published by the Acute Pain Management Guideline Panel (1992) and Good and colleagues (Good et al., 1999; Good, Anderson, Stanton-Hicks, Grass, & Makii, 2002; Good, Anderson, Ahn, Cong, & Stanton-Hicks, 2005; Good et al., 2010).

The second proposition is about attentive care. It proposes that nurses assess, intervene, reassess, and reintervene to achieve a balance between analgesia and side effects. The effect on pain is supported by 30 years of research showing that pain is inadequately treated and by findings that regular assessment alone does not produce relief (Good, Auvil-Novak, & Group, 1994). Intervention, reassessment after a strategic interval, and reintervention by increasing the dose of analgesic and/or adding an adjuvant are needed and should continue until a satisfactory balance is attained (Good & Moore, 1996).

The third proposition is about patient participation. It proposes that patient teaching and goal setting contribute to a balance between analgesia and side effects (see Fig. 3.1). This proposition is supported by meta-analyses for patient teaching (Devine, 1992; Devine & Cook, 1986; Shuldham, 1999) and expert opinion for goal setting (Acute Pain Management Guideline Panel, 1992). Patient teaching is a key concept to consider when trying to improve outcomes. It should include ways to obtain medication, report pain, and use a nonpharmacological adjuvant.

APPLICATIONS OF THE THEORY

The theory is useful for clinical intervention research with experimental designs, called randomized controlled trials (RCTs). It is useful in alert adult populations in which acute pain is incompletely controlled by medication alone, and side effects may prevent increasing analgesic medication. The theory has been adopted by postsurgical nursing units as the basis for their postoperative pain management program. It has been used many times to teach graduate nursing students the usefulness and composition of a focused, concrete nursing theory. It can also be used to teach acute pain management to undergraduate students, using the three principles with current practice guidelines that add the details.

RESEARCH SUPPORT FOR THE THEORY

The first proposition of the theory was partially, but directly tested in two studies of abdominal surgical patients. Both studies tested and compared nonpharmacological adjuvants. Pharmacological adjuvants (NSAIDs) were not tested, as that was not standard postoperative practice in the five hospitals we used. Both studies were funded by the National Institute of Nursing Research (NINR). This level of funding for a program of nursing research demonstrates national interest and support for studying nonpharmacological adjuvants for pain management. In the first study, relaxation, music, and their combination provided up to 31% more relief than PCA alone, following major abdominal surgery (Good et al., 1999). When subgroups of gynecological and intestinal surgical patients were examined from this database, the percent relief compared to opioids alone was even greater (Good et al., 2002, 2005).

In the second study, both the first and the third propositions of the theory were partially tested. The relaxation/music intervention was compared to a patient-teaching tape that was specific to pain management, and a third tape that combined relaxation/music and patient teaching. Pharmacological adjuvants and goal setting were not tested. The patient-teaching tape was intended to supplement the relief provided by relaxation/music and opioids as found in Good et al., 1999. It taught patients to let go of fears of opioid dependency, to use their PCA system, and to tell their nurse about their pain until relief was obtained. Postoperative abdominal surgery patients were encouraged to use the tapes as much as possible the first two days. Pain and side effects were measured four times a day and at five pre- and posttests of the 20-minute interventions. Three of the five tests showed that relaxation music lowered pain significantly more than the control condition, but independent use did not result in less pain at other times during the day. There was no clear evidence of duration (Good et al., 2010). The study demonstrated once again in a more diverse sample that relaxation combined with music, in addition to pharmacological interventions, reduced pain during the first two postoperative days, giving patients more options and a small to medium amount of relief. The patient-teaching method used did not reduce pain in any of the five tests or at eight other times during the first two days. Neither intervention reduced opioid intake or the side effects of analgesics (Good et al., 2010).

The concept of nonpharmacological adjuvant has been tested and supported in other populations, therefore, extending this portion of the theory. For example, music has reduced chronic (Siedlecki & Good, 2006), labor (Phumdoung & Good, 2003), arthritis (McCaffrey & Freeman, 2003), and cancer pain (Huang, Good, & Zausniewski, 2010), whereas guided imagery has reduced chronic pain (Lewandowski, 2004; 2006) and massage reduced back pain after surgery in Asian patients who remain on bed rest after surgery (Chin, 1999).

In addition, reviews have aggregated the results of many studies of relaxation, music, and guided imagery for acute postoperative pain. Authors of a Cochrane Review of music for pain report heterogeneity in the 14 postoperative studies with 510 participants exposed to music and 493 controls. They found that there was 0.5 units (0–10 scale) lower pain intensity in those who listened to adjuvant music. Only four music-for-pain studies reported the proportion of participants in each group who achieved at least 50% pain relief. Based on the four studies, the number of patients needed to treat (NNT) was five, in order to have one patient who received 50% relief (that they would not have had if they had not listened to music). The authors recommended that future studies report proportions in each group (Cepeda, Carr, Lau, & Alvarez, 2006). However, scientists are still establishing the correct method of determining the clinical effect of a nonpharmacological adjuvant to opioids that are already providing considerable relief (Good et al., 2010). One issue is that 35% relief is meaningful in people with moderate pain, such as patients treated with analgesics (Cepeda, Africano, Polo, Alcala, & Carr, 2003). Another issue is that people with pain less than 3 on a 0 to 10 scale may not need an adjuvant. Perhaps investigators should select only patients with pain ≥3/10 and report proportions of those in each group with 35% and 50% or greater relief (Good et al., 2010, Supplemental Digital Content 3, http://links.lww.com/NRES/A24).

Subsequent systematic reviews of music for perioperative pain reported relief in most of the studies. Nilsson (2008) reported that in 42 perioperative studies, half found that music interventions relieved anxiety and pain, whereas Engwall and Dupplis (2008) found that 15 of 18 studies (83%) had a significant positive effect for music on postoperative pain. In addition, three of four individual studies since 2008 found that music reduced postoperative pain. The largest was Good et al., 2010; music was combined with relaxation and was effective in three of five pre- and posttests in 517 abdominal surgical patients but not at other times during the day. Good and Ahn 2008 found that choice of Korean or American music reduced pain after gynecological surgery in Korea. Music was also successfully tested intraoperatively during total knee arthroplasty in a randomized, blind, placebo-controlled clinical trial. The result was less pain in the music group at 3 and 24 hours postoperatively (Simcock et al., 2008). The results also revealed that listening to music during bone marrow biopsy and aspiration resulted in lower state anxiety and pain scores (Shabanloei et al., 2010). Music is an intervention that is available, is low cost, does not add side effects, in most cases, and improves patient satisfaction.

Reviews of randomized trials for relaxation support part of the first proposition. In 1996, an interdisciplinary Technology Assessment Panel at NIH reported strong evidence for the use of relaxation techniques in reducing chronic pain (NIH Technology Assessment Panel, 1996). An early review of relaxation for postoperative pain reported that 9 of 11 RCTs (82%) found significantly less pain sensation and/or pain distress (Good, 1996). Another review found weaker evidence to support use of relaxation for pain. Using only RCTs, three of seven demonstrated significantly less pain sensation and/or pain distress in those who had relaxation (Sears & Carroll, 1998). A third review reported support for jaw relaxation and systematic relaxation for pain relief after surgery (Kwekkeboom & Gretarsdottir, 2006). Jaw relaxation for postopera-tive pain has been shown to be effective for pain at the second postoperative ambulation, recovery from ambulation, and at rest (Good et al., 1999, 2010) but not during the first ambulation/recovery after major abdominal surgery (Good, 1995a). However, a whole body relaxation technique has shown promise and should be used when the patient is resting in bed, rather than during ambulation. A Thai nurse researcher used a systematic (whole body) relaxation technique with 102 abdominal surgical patients and found that it relieved pain by 55% compared to controls during 15 minutes of recovery in bed from the first ambula-tion after surgery (Roykulcharoen & Good, 2004). A later RCT compared jaw relaxation and total body relaxation for postoperative pain at rest and on movement. These researchers found significant posttest reductions for both the relaxation groups and the attention control group, but no between-group differ-ences, perhaps because the study was underpowered (Seers, Crichton, Tutton, Smith, & Saunders, 2008). Comparisons of jaw relaxation and systematic whole body relaxation should continue with attention to patient acceptance and duration of effect.

The use of massage and cold therapy has initial support for the effect of nonpharmacological interven-tions, consistent with the first proposition. Five early studies found that massage reduced postoperative pain (Forchuk et al., 2004; Kshettry, Carole, Henly, Sendelbach, & Kummer, 2006; Piotrowski et al., 2003; Taylor et al., 2003; Wang & Keck, 2004), and no ineffective massage studies were found. Although the use of cold therapy is the oldest analgesic still being used clinically, its postoperative testing seems limited to sports and to prevention of edema-related pain in orthopedic surgeries and trauma. Findings are mixed; six studies found an effect of cold on pain (Chou & Liu, 2008; Cohn, Draeger, & Jackson, 1989; Scheffler, Sheitel, & Lipton, 1992; Webb, Williams, Ivory, Day, & Williamson, 1998; Chailler, Ellis, Stolarik, & Woodend, 2010; Shin, Lim, Yun, & Park, 2009), while three others did not (Edwards, Rimmer, & Keene, 1996; Forouzanfar, Sabelis, Ausems, Baart, & van der Waal, 2008; Whitelaw, DeMuth, Demos, Schepsis, & Jacques, 1995). A reviewer reported that there was insufficient evidence to support cryotherapy for pain in soft tissue injuries (Collins, 2008). Principles, techniques, and nursing care involved in cryotherapy are reviewed by McDowell, McFarland, and Nalli (1994).

Patient teaching for pain management after surgery informs and empowers patients by increasing their knowledge and self-efficacy for engaging in postoperative care activities and PCA (Chumbley, Ward, Hall, & Salmon, 2004; Ong, Miller, Appleby, Allegretto, & Gawlinski, 2009; Pellino et al., 1998). Older meta-analyses have shown that patient teaching resulted in less pain (Devine, 1992; Shuldham, 1999), but the interventions were long, not pain specific, and not relevant to current analgesic delivery systems. Two brief interventions for PCA use had no effect on pain, whether delivered by pamphlet (Chumbley et al., 2004) or anesthetists' teaching and demonstration (Lam, Chan, Chen, & Ngan Kee, 2001).

Our recent study ($N = 517$) tested patient teaching for pain management, based on the third proposition of the theory of a balance between analgesia and side effects. The results showed that this patient-teaching intervention for pain management was not effective for postoperative pain at five pre- and posttests and at eight other time points in the first two days (Good et al., 2010). The intervention consisted of audiotaped patient teaching for pain management that included information on expected pain sensations, reporting pain, obtaining analgesics, preventing pain, modifying attitudes, managing pain during activity, and being a participant in their own pain management. The same instructions were played at all the posttests, which may have been a little repetitive to the patients. Nurses usually do more interactive teaching and instruct patients appropriately when individual patients need either positive reinforcement or additional informa-tion and emphasis. In addition, there may have been variation in individual patient interpretation of the instructions, as well as persistent beliefs about self-efficacy and addiction to opioids. Interpretations and beliefs can be potent influences on patient decisions to press the PCA button (Chumbley et al., 2004).

SUGGESTIONS FOR ADDITIONAL RESEARCH

The time has come to conduct studies of translation of music, relaxation, and/or their combination to nursing practice for adjuvant pain management. Choices of music that are culturally and age appropriate should be offered. Doctoral students have developed Korean (Good and Ahn, 2008) and Taiwanese music tapes (Huang and Good, 2010) to appeal to patients in those countries. Studies are needed to compare

sedative music for pain with music with faster tempos and also to compare the effects of various musical instruments or the presence of lyrics. Cultural preferences in music for pain need to be developed for
the many countries and cultures in the world and nurses need to become aware of those in their patient
populations.

The whole body systematic relaxation technique should be tested in a replication study and then recom-
pared to jaw relaxation after surgery. Culturally congruent relaxation scripts and voices can be developed
and used in research. An excellent example can be obtained from Josepha Campinha-Bacote, an
African–American nurse who is an expert on culturally competent nursing care. She and her husband have
developed a taped Culturally Specific Africentric Relaxation Exercise, which is accompanied by music
that is congruent with the African–American culture (Campinha-Bacote, Campinha-Bacote, & Allbright,
1992). Nurses could develop such tapes for other cultures, incorporating the linguistic characteristics and
musical tastes of their people.

The second proposition to provide attentive care and to intervene until pain is relieved may be incorporated into practice better today than 15 years ago when the theory was first published. Today, there is
greater attention to pain relief due to requirements of the Joint Commission. However, nurses in hospitals
in which attentive care for pain is not practiced may want to provide in-service education on pain management and measure the results in knowledge and practice.

The third proposition is to provide patient teaching and to set pain goals with patients. New methods
of pharmacological patient teaching for postoperative pain management are needed for greater relief and
the most promising teaching interventions should be tested in research. In addition, an effective patient-
teaching intervention for PCA use is needed. Setting comfort-function goals as discussed by Pasero and
McCaffrey (2004) could be compared to usual care. Methods of teaching patients to use nonpharmacological methods to use as adjuvants also need testing. Researchers can use the pain scales listed in Table 3.2.
Research Application 3.1 provides an example of a study designed to further test the theory.

USE OF THE THEORY IN PRACTICE

Nurses have written to the author saying that they use the theory as a basis of practice on their postoperative unit. However, examples of use of the entire theory were not found in the literature. There are
publications describing how nurses can use parts of the theory, that is, complementary therapies in addition to analgesics, and patient teaching and goal setting for pain relief. Using Middle Range Theories 3.1
provides several examples of use of the theory.

It would be ideal if an entire postoperative nursing unit would implement the complete theory in caring
for their patients. They could first assign readings from this chapter and then hold educational sessions
for the nursing staff on pain management, the theory, and the advantages of using evidence-based theories
and interventions. In these sessions, nurses could discuss the concepts of the theory and learn what could
be offered in terms of analgesics (American Pain Society, 2008) and range orders (Gordon et al., 2004),
nonpharmacological adjuvants, patient teaching, and goal setting. They could discuss the day-to-day relief
goals and comfort-function goals that they think would be realistic on their unit as patients recover. They
could discuss the meaning of attentive care (e.g., intervention, reassessment, and reintervention, until a
comfort-function goal is met) (Pasero & McCaffrey, 2003, 2004). Since Good et al. found that a specific
patient teaching for pain management intervention was not effective for pain reduction (2010), nurses on
the unit should use current information to teach patients to use their PCA effectively (McCaffrey
& Pasero, 1999; Greenwich Hospital http://www.greenhosp.org/pe_pdf/pain_PCA.pdf). Nurses should
ensure that quality improvement procedures are in place to verify that the principles are carried out. To
use music clinically, nurses would need to secure a small amount of funding to provide a modest library on
the unit containing music, guided imagery, and relaxation exercises on audiotapes or compact discs. They
would also need equipment for playing that could be used by patients. Practice information on using a
music intervention for pain can be found in Good et al. (2000), and information on using a relaxation intervention can be found in Good (1995b). Practitioners can use the Numeric Pain Intensity Scale (Table 3.2)
to measure pain regularly in adult patients and any of the children's pain scales in pediatric patients.

TABLE 3.2 Instruments to Measure Pain

Category	Abbreviation	Name of scale and citation
Pain	VAS	Visual Analogue Scale[a]
Sensory pain	—	VAS Sensation of Pain Scale[b]
Sensory pain	—	Numeric Pain Intensity Scale[c]
Sensory pain	—	Descriptive Pain Intensity Scale[d]
Affective pain	—	VAS Distress of Pain Scale[e]
Affective pain	—	Numeric Pain Distress Scale[f]
Affective pain	—	Descriptive Pain Distress Scale[g]
Affective pain	—	VAS Unpleasantness Scale[h]
Affective pain	—	VAS Anxiety of Pain Scale[i]
Affective pain	MPQ	McGill Pain Questionnaire[j]
Total pain	MPQ-PRI	Pain Rating Index (PRI)
Sensory pain	PRI-sensory	Sensory subscale
Affective pain	PRI-affective	Affective subscale
Pain intensity	MPQ-NWC	Number of Words Chosen
Pain intensity	MPQ-PPI	Present Pain Index
Pain intensity	MPQ-VAS	Visual Analogue Scale
Total, sensory, and affective pain	MPQ-SF	McGill Pain Questionnaire–Short Form[k]
Chronic pain	UAB	University of Alabama–Birmingham Pain Behavior Scale[l]
Chronic pain	WHYMPI	West Haven–Yale Multidimensional Pain Inventory[m]
Cancer pain	BPI	Brief Pain Inventory[n]
Cancer pain, relief, mood	MPAC	Memorial Pain Assessment Card[o]
24-h time-intensity	–	Keele's Pain Chart[p]
Labor pain	–	Behavioral Index for Assessment of Labor Pain[q]
Children's pain	–	Poker Chip Scale[r]
Children's pain	–	Word-Graphic Rating Scale[s]
Children's pain	–	Oucher Scale[t]
Children's pain	–	Wong-Baker FACES Scale[u]
Young children's pain	FLACC	Faces, legs, activity, cry, consolability[v]

– = No abbreviation.
[a,b,e]Good et al. (2001), [b,c,d,e,f,g,r,s]Acute Pain Management Guideline Panel (1992), [h]Price et al. (1983), [c]McCormack et al. (1988), [s,j,k]Melzack (1975), [f]Richards et al. (1982), [m]Kerns, Turk, & Rudy (1985), [n]Daut, Cleeland, & Flanery (1983), [o]Fishman et al. (1987), [p]Keele (1948), [q]Bonnel & Boureau (1985), [t]Beyer, Denyes, & Villarruel (1992), [u]Wong & Baker (1988), [v]Merkel, Voepel-Lewis, Shayevitz, & Malviya (1997).

Research Application

A nurse researcher conducted a study in which the research question is "What is the effect of relaxation and music, patient teaching for pain management, and the combination of both on postoperative pain, side effects of opioids, stress, and secretory immunoglobulin A?" Using an RCT, the researcher reviews the surgery schedule each day to identify males and females scheduled for major abdominal surgery who meet the criterion for age (18–75 years) and are expecting to receive general anesthesia and PCA.

The researcher arrived at the hospital at 6:00 AM and introduced herself to Mr. Green, who had been admitted to the surgical waiting area for a 7:30 AM colectomy for cancer, but has not yet received any premedication that would compromise his ability to give consent.

After obtaining written informed consent, the nurse conducted a brief interview and teaches Mr. Green to use the Sensation and Distress of Pain Visual Analogue Scales (Good et al., 2001). The researcher used a computerized minimization program to randomly assign Mr. Green to one of four groups, while balancing the groups on potentially confounding variables such as age, sex, race, type of surgery, chronic pain, smoking, alcohol use, and time of surgery. The groups were: (a) relaxation and music; (b) patient teaching for pain management; (c) the combination of the two; and (d) the control group, which receives the usual care. Mr. Green's assignment was the combination of relaxation, music, and patient teaching. He then listened to the 9-minute teaching tape giving him instruction in using the jaw relaxation technique and offering him a choice among six types of sedative instrumental music (Gaston, 1951). He listened to 20 seconds of each type of music: synthesizer, harp, piano, orchestra, jazz, and inspirational. Mr. Green chose the inspirational music.

After surgery, Mr. Green was taken to his postoperative room, and the nurse researcher went to the bedside to conduct the first pretest–posttest. She asked him to rate the intensity of his sensation and distress of pain on the dual VAS scales, and then she obtained pulse and respirations. She gave him the tape and recorder and played his assigned tape for 20 minutes. The tape reviewed his role in pain management, guided him in the use of a relaxation technique, and played soft inspirational music for 20 minutes. The researcher asked him to rate his pain again for the posttest and recorded his pulse and respirations. She showed Mr. Green, his wife, and daughter how to use the tape recorder and encouraged him to use it as much as possible for the rest of the day, evening, and even during the night. The idea was to get pain under control early in the postoperative period and keep it controlled.

For the next two days at 8 AM, 12 noon, 4 PM, and 8 PM, a research nurse or graduate student came to the bedside to ask about pain and side effects of opioids. In addition, at 10 AM and 2 PM each day, the research nurse conducted 20-minute pre- and posttests. On day 2, she also collected pre- and posttest saliva specimens. The patient's chart was reviewed at each visit for medications and other factors that could confound the outcome. At 8 AM on the third day, the research nurse conducted a structured interview, asking about demographics and information on contextual variables that might confound the outcome. Mr. Green was thanked for participating in the study and for his contribution to nursing knowledge about pain management. A $20 gift certificate was mailed to subjects who completed the study.

The data recorded on the questionnaire was coded and entered into an SPSS statistical program file by graduate student assistants who were learning to become researchers. The principal investigator and the project manager analyzed the data to determine whether or not the interventions reduce pain, side effects of opioids, stress, and/or improve immunity. The findings were written in a manuscript and will be sent to a peer-reviewed research journal for publication.

SUMMARY

Pain is a universal human experience that has been known since the first human experienced illness, trauma, or labor. Although pain has been studied descriptively for more than a century, it has only recently been studied from a prescriptive nursing perspective. The middle range prescriptive pain management theory of a balance between analgesic and side effects reflects the nursing mission to intervene effectively and holistically to relieve pain, suffering, and to prevent their long-term effects. There is increasing empirical support and nurse researchers can continue to test and to provide support and creative extensions of the theory. Practicing nurses are using the evidence-based principles for effective relief of acute pain in their patients.

Nurses' use of relaxation for postoperative pain, which includes general instructions and specific relaxation techniques is described in Good (1995b). The empirically tested jaw relaxation technique is included, because it is easy for patients to remember after surgery. When recorded on an audiotape, soft relaxing music could be added. More recently, nurses' use of relaxation for pain management in nursing practice was carefully described by Schaffer and Yucha (2004). They provide a sample of a full body relaxation script that nurses can read to patients or record on an audiotape for the patient to use independently. They also review the empirical literature that supports the use of relaxation techniques for pain and provide two clinical case studies that illustrate the use of relaxation for neck, back, and headache pain.

Nurses' use of soft music to ease the pain of clinical patients is based on nursing studies in postoperative patients, and in patients with the pain of labor, osteoarthritis, cancer, and chronic pain. Based on Nightingale's framework, Mc Caffrey discussed nurses' use of music as a healing environment for older adults having surgical, arthritis, and other kinds of pain (2008). She recommends that nurses be given educational sessions to understand the use of music as an intervention in various settings. She encourages assessing preferences, offering a variety of types of music for patients to choose from, use of iPods® with downloaded music, bringing music from home, and she lists some composers and CDs that have been used in her studies. Others describe the use of music for labor pain, recommending that women be advised during prenatal childbirth classes of the efficacy of music for pain and relaxation (Zwelling, Johnson, & Allen, 2006). Music should be chosen and obtained in advance, and women should bring their own playing equipment, if it is not available in the hospital. Zwelling et al. give recommendations for use of complementary therapies in general, including educating the labor and delivery nurses in their use.

The third principle of the theory is that patient teaching and goal setting contribute to balance between analgesia and side effects. Nurses at the bedside can use current guidelines to teach patients to manage pain pharmacologically (McCaffery & Pasero, 1999). An example of a patient and family information sheet for PCA can be found at http://www.greenhosp.org/pe_pdf/pain_PCA.pdf. Setting goals with patients is described in detail by Pasero and McCaffrey (2003, 2004). Teaching patients to use a pain rating scale is the first step, and the next step is establishing a comfort-function goal. Examples of comfort-function goals for postoperative patients are given in Pasero and McCaffrey (2003). The goal should be documented on the chart, close to the pain scores; if the goal is not met, the pain rating should be addressed with interventions to relieve it. Nurses should consider whether an analgesic can be given, or whether to use the range of doses ordered by the physician, call the physician for further orders, and/or add a nonpharmacological therapy. She should then reassess pain and side effects at a time when they are expected to be effective and reintervene if necessary. The health care team's achievement of the comfort-function goals should be monitored in quality improvement plans. Nurses can help patients establish realistic comfort-function goals and should discuss them during shift report and rounds. Pasero and McCaffrey (2004) emphasize that pain assessment does not necessarily mean pain relief.

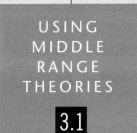

USING MIDDLE RANGE THEORIES

3.1

ANALYSIS OF THEORY

Using the criteria presented in Chapter 2, critique the theory of Pain: A Balance Between Analgesia and Side Effects. Compare your conclusions about the theory with those found in Appendix A. An experienced nurse has completed the analysis found in Appendix A.

Internal Criticism

1. Clarity
2. Consistency
3. Adequacy
4. Logical development
5. Level of theory development

External Criticism

1. Reality convergence
2. Utility
3. Significance
4. Discrimination
5. Scope of theory
6. Complexity

CRITICAL THINKING EXERCISES

1. Compare two scenarios or scripts for nurses and patients engaging in mutual goal setting for pain management after a specific surgical procedure. With peers, analyze each for advantages and disadvantages to the patient and to those who provide care.

2. Analyze the trajectory of patients undergoing a specific surgical procedure and the places they receive nursing care, from the surgeon's office and the decision for surgery, through the pre- and postoperative hospitalization, to recovery at home. Plan the most effective times, amounts of information, and ways nurses can introduce and reinforce the elements of patient teaching for pain management. *The elements are to encourage attitudes, expectations, and actions in reporting pain, obtaining medication, preventing pain during activity, and using complementary therapies.* Describe ways by which this nursing care, delivered in several places, could be streamlined and coordinated with the surgeon's patient teaching.

3. Envision yourself as a leader who is introducing this nursing theory as the basis of postoperative pain management on your unit. Create introductory scripts with arguments for its usefulness to be delivered to the nursing and medical staff. Describe how you would begin to demonstrate its usefulness. Explain your method of presenting its current evidence base. Give the main points of a clinically useable protocol for your unit.

WEB RESOURCES

Visit **http://thePoint.lww.com/Peterson3e** for helpful web resources related to this chapter.

ACKNOWLEDGMENTS

This chapter was supported in part by the National Institute of Nursing Research (NINR) Grant Number R01 NR3933 (1994–2005), to M. Good, PhD, Principal Investigator, and by the General Clinical Research Center, Case Western Reserve University.

REFERENCES

Acute Pain Management Guideline Panel. (1992). *Acute pain management: Operative or medical procedures and trauma. Clinical practice guideline* (Vol. AHCPR No. 92–0032). Rockville, MD: Agency for Health Care Policy and Research, Public Health Service, U.S. Department of Health and Human Services. Retrieved January 16, 2007, from http://www.ncbi.nlm.nih.gov/books/bv.fcgi?rid=hstat6.chapter.8991

American Pain Society. (2008). *Principles of analgesic use in the treatment of acute pain and cancer pain* (6th ed.). Skokie, IL: American Pain Society.

American Pain Society Quality of Care Task Force. (2005). American Pain Society Recommendations for improving the quality of acute and cancer pain management. *Archives of Internal Medicine, 165,* 1574–1580.

American Society of Anesthesiologists. (2004). Practice guidelines for acute pain management in the perioperative setting: An updated report by the American Society of Anesthesiologists Task Force on Acute Pain Management. *Anesthesiology, 100,* 1573–1581.

Beecher, H. K. (1959). *Measurement of subjective responses: Quantitative effects of drugs.* New York: Oxford University Press.

Beyer, J. E., Denyes, M. J., & Villarruel, A. M. (1992). The creation, validation, and continuing development of the Oucher: A measure of pain intensity in children. *Journal of Pediatric Nursing, 7*(5), 335–346.

Bonnel, A. M., & Boureau, F. (1985). Labor pain assessment: Validity of a behavioral index. *Pain, 22*(1), 81.

Campinha-Bacote, J., Campinha-Bacote, D., & Allbright, R.J. (1992). **C.A.R.E. I** (*Culturally-specific Africentric Relaxation Exercise*). A culturally specific relaxation audio cassette produced by Twin Hills Recording Studio; California, Ohio. This tape is based on Africentric & Ethnomusic Therapy principles (flute and narrative composition arranged by J. Campinha-Bacote). Dr. Josepha Campinha-Bacote.

Casey, K. L., & Melzack, R. (1967). Neural mechanisms of pain: A conceptual model. In E. L. Way (Ed.), *New concepts in pain and its clinical management* (pp. 13–31). Philadelphia, PA: F.A. Davis.

Cepeda, M. S., Africano, J. M., Polo, R., Alcala, R., & Carr, D. B. (2003). What decline in pain intensity is meaningful to patients with acute pain? *Pain, 105*(1–2), 151–157.

Cepeda, M. S., Carr, D. B., Lau, J., & Alvarez, H. (2006). Music for pain relief. *Cochrane Database Systematic Review,* (2), Art No. CD004843.

Chailler, M., Ellis, J., Stolarik, A., & Woodend, K. (2010). Cold therapy for the management of pain associated with deep breathing and coughing post-cardiac surgery. *Canadian Journal of Cardiovascular Nursing, 20*(2), 18–24.

Chin, C-C. (1999). *Effects of back massage on surgical stress responses and postoperative pain.* Unpublished doctoral dissertation, Case Western Reserve University, Cleveland, OH.

Chou, S. Y., & Liu, H. E. (2008). Comparison of effectiveness between moist and dry cryotherapy in reducing discomfort after orthognathic surgery. *Journal of Clinical Nursing, 17*(13), 1735–1741.

Chumbley, G. M., Ward, L., Hal, G. M., & Salmon, P. (2004). Pre-operative information and patient-controlled analgesia: Much ado about nothing. *Anaesthesia, 59*(4), 354–358.

Cohn, B. T., Draeger, R. I., & Jackson, D. W. (1989). The effects of cold therapy in the postoperative management of pain in patients undergoing anterior cruciate ligament reconstruction. *American Journal of Sports Medicine, 17*(3), 344–349.

Collins, N. C. (2008). Is ice right? Does cryotherapy improve outcome for acute soft tissue injury? *Emergency Medicine Journal, 25*(2), 65–68.

Daut, R. L., Cleeland, C. S., & Flanery, R. C. (1983). Development of the Wisconsin brief pain questionnaire to assess pain in cancer and other diseases. *Pain, 17*, 197–210.

Devine, E. C. (1992). Effects of psychoeducational care for adult surgical patients: A meta-analysis of 191 studies. *Patient Education and Counseling, 19*, 129–142.

Devine, E. C., & Cook, T. D. (1986). Clinical and cost saving effects of psychoeducational interventions with surgical patients: A meta analysis. *Research in Nursing and Health, 9*, 89–105.

Dickhoff, J., & James, P. (1968). A theory of theories: A position paper. *Nursing Research, 17*(3), 197–203.

Edwards, D. J., Rimmer, M., & Keene, G. C. (1996). The use of cold therapy in the postoperative management of patients undergoing arthroscopic anterior cruciate ligament reconstruction. *American Journal of Sports Medicine, 24*(2), 193–195.

Engwall, M., & Duppils, G. S. (2009). Music as a nursing intervention for postoperative pain: A systematic review. *Journal of Perianesthesia Nursing, 24*(6), 370–383.

Fishman, B., Pasternak, S., Wallenstein, S. L., Houde, R.W., Holland, J. C., & Foley, K. M. (1987). The Memorial Pain Assessment Card: A valid instrument for the evaluation of cancer pain. *Cancer, 60*(5), 1151–1158.

Forchuk, C., Baruth, P., Prendergast, M., Holliday, R., Bareham, R., Brimner, S., et al. (2004). Postoperative arm massage: A support for women with lymph node dissection. *Cancer Nursing, 27*(1), 25–33.

Forouzanfar, T., Sabelis, A., Ausems, S., Baart, J. A., & van der Waal, I. (2008). Effect of ice compression on pain after mandibular third molar surgery: A single-blind, randomized controlled trial. *International Journal of Oral Maxillofacial Surgery, 37*(9), 824–830.

Gaston, E. T. (1951). Dynamic music factors in mood changes. *Music Educators Journal, 37*, 42–44.

Good, M. (1995a). A comparison of the effects of jaw relaxation and music on postoperative pain. *Nursing Research, 44*(1), 52–57.

Good, M. (1995b). Relaxation techniques for surgical patients. Complementary modalities/Part 2, Continuing education two hours. *American Journal of Nursing, 95*(5), 39–43.

Good, M. (1996). Effects of relaxation and music on postoperative pain: A review. *Journal of Advanced Nursing, 24*, 905–914.

Good, M. (1998). A middle range theory of acute pain management; use in research. *Nursing Outlook, 46*(3), 120–124.

Good, M., & Ahn, S. (2008). Korean and American music reduces pain in Korean women after gynecologic surgery. *Pain Management Nursing, 9*(3), 96–103.

Good M., Albert J. M., Anderson G. C., Wotman S., Cong X., Lane D., et al. (2010). Supplementing relaxation and music for pain after surgery. *Nursing Research, 59*(4), 259–269.

Good, M., Anderson, G. C., Ahn, S., Cong, X., & Stanton-Hicks, M. (2005). Relaxation and music reduce pain following intestinal surgery. *Research in Nursing and Health, 28*(3), 240–251.

Good, M., Anderson, G., Stanton-Hicks, M., Grass, J., & Makii, M. (2002). Relaxation and music reduce pain following gynecological surgery. *Pain Management Nursing, 3*(2), 61–70.

Good, M., Anderson, G. C., Ahn, S., Cong, X., & Stanton-Hicks, M. (2005). Relaxation and music reduce pain following intestinal surgery. *Research in Nursing and Health, 28*(3), 240–251.

Good, M., Auvil-Novak, S., & Group, M. (1994). Pain and its management: One year after the guidelines. Paper presented at the AHSR & FSHR Annual Conference, June 12–14. San Diego, CA: Health Services Research.

Good, M., & Moore, S. M. (1996). Clinical practice guidelines as a new source of middle-range theory: Focus on acute pain. *Nursing Outlook, 44*(2), 74–79.

Good, M., Picot, B., Salem, S., Chin, C., Picot, S., & Lane, D. (2000). Cultural responses to music for pain relief. *Journal of Holistic Nursing, 18*(3), 245–260.

Good, M., Stanton-Hicks, M., Grass, J. M., Anderson, G. C., Choi, C. C., Schoolmeesters, L., et al. (1999). Relief of postoperative pain with jaw relaxation, music, and their combination. *Pain, 81*(1–2), 163–172.

Good, M., Stiller, C., Zauszniewski, J., Stanton-Hicks, M., Grass, J., & Anderson, G. C. (2001). Sensation and distress of pain scales: Reliability, validity and sensitivity. *Journal of Nursing Measurement, 9*(3), 219–238.

Gordon, D. B., Dahl, J., Phillips, P., Frandsen, J., Cowley, C., Foster, R. L., et al. (2004). The use of "as-needed" range orders for opioid analgesics in the management of acute pain: A consensus statement of the American Society for Pain Management Nursing and the American Pain Society. *Pain Management Nursing, 5*(2), 53–58.

Green, E. E., Green, A. M., & Norris, P. A. (1979). Preliminary observation on a new-drug method for control of hypertension. *Journal of the South Carolina Medical Association, 75*(11), 575–582.

Huang, S. T., Good, M., & Zauszniewski, J. A. (2010). The effectiveness of music in relieving pain in cancer patients: a randomized controlled trial. *International Journal of Nursing Studies, 47*(11), 1354–1362.

Huth, M. M., Broome, M. E., & Good, M. (2004). Imagery reduces children's post-operative pain. *Pain, 110*(1–2), 439–448.

Huth, M. M., & Moore, S. M. (1998). Prescriptive theory of acute pain management in infants and children. *Journal of the Society of Pediatric Nursing, 3*(1), 23–32.

Im, E. O. (2006). A situation-specific theory of Caucasian cancer patients' pain experience. *ANS Advances in Nursing Science, 29*(3), 232–244.

Johnson, J. E., & Rice, V. H. (1974). Sensory and distress components of pain: Implications for the study of clinical pain. *Nursing Research, 23*, 203–209.

Keele, K. D. (1948). The pain chart. *Lancet, 2*, 6–8.

Kerns, R. D., Turk, D. C., & Rudy, T. E. (1985). The West Haven–Yale Multidimensional Pain Inventory (WHYMPI). *Pain, 23*(4), 345.

Kshettry, V. R., Carole, L. F., Henly, S. J., Sendelbach, S., & Kummer, B. (2006). Complementary alternative medical therapies for heart surgery patients: Feasibility, safety, and impact. *Annuals of Thoracic Surgery, 81*(1), 201–205.

Kwekkeboom, K. L., & Gretarsdottir, E. (2006). Systematic review of relaxation interventions for pain. *Journal of Nursing Scholarship, 38*(3), 269–277.

Lam, K. K., Chan, M.T., Chen, P. P., Ngan Kee, W. D. (2001). Structured preoperative patient education for patient-controlled analgesia. *Journal of Clinical Anesthesia, 13*(6), 465–469.

Lenz, E. R., Pugh, L. C., Milligan, R. A., Gift, A., & Suppe, F. (1997). The middle-range theory of unpleasant symptoms: An update. *Advances in Nursing Science, 19*(3), 14–27.

Lewandowski, W. A. (2004). Patterning of pain and power with guided imagery. *Nursing Science Quarterly, 17*(3), 233–241.

Locsin, R. (1988). Effects of preferred music and guided imagery music on the pain of selected postoperative patients. *ANPHI Papers, 23*(1), 2–4.

Mahon, S. M. (1994). Concept analysis of pain: Implications related to nursing diagnoses. *Nursing Diagnosis, 5*(1), 14–25.

McCaffery, M., & Pasero, C. (1999). *Pain: Clinical manual* (2nd ed.). St. Louis, MO: Mosby.

McCaffrey, R. (2008). Music listening: Its effects in creating a healing environment. *Journal of Psychosocial Nursing and Mental Health Services, 46*(10), 39–44.

McCaffrey, R., & Freeman, E. (2003). Effect of music on chronic osteoarthritis pain in older people. *Journal of Advanced Nursing, 44*(5), 517–524.

McCormack, H. M., Horne, D. J., & Sheather, S. (1988). Clinical applications of visual analogue scales: A critical review. *Psychological Medicine, 18*(4):1007–1019.

McDowell, J. H., McFarland, E. G., & Nalli, B. J. (1994). Use of cryotherapy for orthopaedic patients. *Orthopedic Nursing, 13*(5), 21–30.

Melzack, R. (1975). The McGill Pain Questionnaire: Major properties and scoring methods. *Pain, 1*, 277–299.

Melzack, R. (1996). Gate control theory. *Pain Forum, 5*(2), 128–138.

Melzack, R., & Wall, P. D. (1962). On the nature of cutaneous sensory mechanisms. *Brain, 85*, 331.

Melzack, R., & Wall, P. D. (1965). Pain mechanisms: A new theory. *Science, 150*(3699), 971–979.

Merkel, S. I., Voepel-Lewis, T., Shayevitz, J. R., & Malviya, S. (1997). The FLACC: A behavioral scale for scoring postoperative pain in young children. *Pediatric Nursing, 23*(3), 293–297.

Morse, J. M., Bottorff, J. L., & Hutchinson, S. (1995). The paradox of comfort. *Nursing Research, 44*(1), 14–19.

NIH Technology Assessment Panel. (1996). Integration of behavioral and relaxation approaches into the treatment of chronic pain and insomnia. *JAMA, 276*(4), 313–318.

Nilsson, U. (2008). The anxiety- and pain-reducing effects of music interventions: a systematic review. *AORN Journal, 87*(4), 780–807.

Olness, K. (1981). Self-hypnosis as adjunct therapy in childhood cancer: Clinical experience with 25 patients. *American Journal of Pediatric Hematology Oncology, 3*, 313–321.

Ong, J., Miller, P.S., Appleby, R., Allegretto, R., & Gawlinski, A. (2009). Effect of a preoperative instructional digital video disc on patient knowledge and preparedness for engaging in postoperative care activities. *Nursing Clinics of North America, 44*(1), 103–115, xii.

Page, G. G. (1996). The medical necessity of adequate pain management. *Pain Forum, 5*(4), 227–233.

Pasero, C., & McCaffery, M. (2003). Accountability for pain relief: Use of comfort-function goals. *Journal of Perianesthesia Nursing, 18*(1), 50–52.

Pasero, C., & McCaffery, M. (2004). Comfort-function goals: A way to establish accountability for pain relief. *American Journal of Nursing, 104*(9), 77–78, 81.

Phumdoung, S., & Good, M. (2003). Music reduces sensation and distress of labor pain. *Pain Management Nursing, 4*(2), 54–61.

Pellino, T., Tluczek, A., Collins, M., Trimborn, S., Norwick, H., Engelke, Z. K., et al. (1998). Increasing self-efficacy through empowerment: Preoperative education for orthopaedic patients. *Orthopedic Nursing, 17*(4), 48–51, 54–49.

Pestka, E. L., Bee, S. M., & Evans, M. M. (2010). Relaxation therapies. In M. Snyder & R. Lindquist (Eds.), *Complementary and alternative therapies in nursing* (6th ed., pp. 382–396). New York: Springer.

Piotrowski, M. M., Paterson, C., Mitchinson, A., Kim, H. M., Kirsh, M., & Hinshaw, D. B. (2003). Massage as adjuvant therapy in the management of acute postoperative pain: A preliminary study in men. *Journal of the American College of Surgeons, 197*(6), 1037–1046.

Price, D. D., McGrath, P. A., Rafii, A., & Buckingham, B. (1983). The validation of visual analogue scales as ratio scale measures for chronic and experimental pain. *Pain, 17*(1), 45–56.

Richards, J. S., Nepomuceno, C., Riles, M., & Suer, Z. (1982). Assessing pain behavior: The UAB pain behavior scale. *Pain, 14*(4), 393.

Roykulcharoen, V., & Good, M. (2004). Systematic relaxation relieves postoperative pain in Thailand. *Journal of Advanced Nursing, 48*(2), 1–9.

Scheffler, N. M., Sheitel, P. L., & Lipton, M. N. (1992). Use of Cryo/Cuff for the control of postoperative pain and edema. *Journal of Foot Surgery, 31*(2), 141–148.

Sears, K., & Carroll, D. (1998). Relaxation techniques for acute pain management: A systematic review. *Journal of Advanced Nursing, 27*, 466–475.

Seers K, Crichton N, Tutton L, Smith L, & Saunders T. (2008). Effectiveness of relaxation for postoperative pain and anxiety: Randomized controlled trial. *Journal of Advanced Nursing, 62*(6), 681–688.

Shabanloei, R., Golchin, M., Esfahani, A., Dolatkhah, R., & Rasoulian, M. (2010). Effects of music therapy on pain and anxiety in patients undergoing bone marrow biopsy and aspiration. *AORN Journal, 91*(6), 746–751.

Shin, Y. S., Lim, N. Y., Yun, S. C., & Park, K.O. (2009). A randomised controlled trial of the effects of cryotherapy on pain, eyelid oedema and facial ecchymosis after craniotomy. *Journal of Clinical Nursing, 18*(21), 3029–3036.

Shuldham, C. (1999). A review of the impact of preoperative education on recovery from surgery. *International Journal of Nursing Studies, 36*(2), 171–177.

Siedlecki, S., & Good, M. (2006). Effect of music on power, pain, depression and disability. *Journal of Advanced Nursing, 54*(5), 553–562.

Simcock, X.C., Yoon, R.S., Chalmers, P., Geller, J.A., Kiernan, H.A., & Macaulay, W. (2008). Intraoperative music reduces perceived pain after total knee arthroplasty: a blinded, prospective, randomized, placebo-controlled clinical trial. *Journal of Knee Surgery, 21*(4), 275–278.

Simon, J. M., Baumann, M. A., & Nolan, L. (1995). Differential diagnostic validation: Acute and chronic pain. *Nursing Diagnosis, 6*(2), 73–79.

Taylor, A. G., Galper, D. I., Taylor, P., Rice, L. W., Andersen, W., Irvin, W., et al. (2003). Effects of adjunctive Swedish massage and vibration therapy on short-term postoperative outcomes: A randomized, controlled trial. *Journal of Alternative and Complementary Medicine, 9*(1), 77–89.

Tsai, P. F., Tak, S., Moore, C., & Palencia, I. (2003). Testing a theory of chronic pain. *Journal of Advanced Nursing, 43*(2), 158–169.

Tusek, D. L., Church, J. M., Strong, S. A., Grass, J. A., & Fazio, V. W. (1997). Guided imagery: A significant advance in the care of patients undergoing elective colorectal surgery. *Diseases of the Colon and Rectum, 40*(2), 172–178.

Wang, H. L., & Keck, J. F. (2004). Foot and hand massage as an intervention for postoperative pain. *Pain Management Nursing, 5*(2), 59–65.

Webb, J. M., Williams, D., Ivory, J. P., Day, S., & Williamson, D. M. (1998). The use of cold compression dressings after total knee replacement: a randomized controlled trial. *Orthopedics, 21*(1), 59–61.

Whitelaw, G. P., DeMuth, K. A., Demos, H. A., Schepsis, A., & Jacques, E. (1995). The use of the Cryo/Cuff versus ice and elastic wrap in the postoperative care of knee arthroscopy patients. *American Journal of Knee Surgery, 8*(1), 28–30; discussion 30–31.

Wong, D. L., & Baker, C. M. (1988). Pain in children: Comparison of assessment scales. *Pediatric Nursing, 14*(1), 9–17.

Zwelling, E., Johnson, K., & Allen, J. (2006). How to implement complementary therapies for laboring women. *MCN The American Journal of Maternal/Child Nursing, 31*(6), 365–370.

4

Unpleasant Symptoms

ELIZABETH R. LENZ

AUDREY GIFT

LINDA C. PUGH

RENEE A. MILLIGAN

DEFINITION OF KEY TERMS

Performance	Performance is the multifaceted outcome or effect of the symptom experience. It includes functional and cognitive activities. Functional performance includes activities of daily living (ADLs), social interaction, and role performance. Cognitive performance includes knowledge and ability to learn, solve problems, and think abstractly and logically. Quality of life (QoL) can be considered to be an indicator of performance, because it incorporates both functional and cognitive ability.
Physiological factors	Physiological factors are the normal or abnormal functioning of bodily systems. They may include diseases and dysfunctions, physiological and anatomical abnormalities, comorbidities, diet and nutritional balance, hydration, and amount of exercise.
Psychological factors	Psychological factors include mental state or mood, affective reaction to illness, and the degree of uncertainty and knowledge about the symptoms and their possible meaning, based on earlier symptom experiences.
Situational factors	Situational factors include aspects of the social and physical environment that surround the person and may influence the experience and reporting of symptoms. They include environmental factors, such as heat, humidity, noise, light, safety, and air and water quality. They may include socioeconomic factors, marital status, social support, and treatments, such as medication regimens or therapies that may influence the individual's physiology and the experience of symptoms.
Unpleasant symptoms	Symptoms are the perceived indicators of change in normal functioning as experienced by patients. They are the subjective indicators of threats to health. Generally, they are experienced as unpleasant sensations.

INTRODUCTION

The theory of unpleasant symptoms (TOUS) is a middle range nursing theory that was developed and intended for application and use by nurses and clinical researchers. The original concept paper appeared in 1995 and was revised in 1997. The theory allows for the presence of multiple symptoms that interact and/or are multiplicative. It implies that management of one symptom will contribute to the management of other symptoms.

HISTORICAL BACKGROUND

In 1993, two efforts emerged from clinical practice and empirical research that led to the development of the TOUS. Linda Pugh and Audrey Gift, clinical researchers studying a single symptom (fatigue and dyspnea, respectively), developed a model that included elements believed to be common to both symptoms. Pugh's practice and research specialty was intrapartum fatigue. She teamed with Renee Milligan whose practice and research specialty was postpartum fatigue. Together, they developed a framework for childbearing fatigue that identified common factors related to fatigue across the childbearing period. Both the model and the framework linked antecedent or influencing factors to the symptom of interest and the way in which it is reported by patients. In addition, the symptom was conceptualized as an experience that influences performance outcomes. In addition to noting that the models for the two symptoms were similar, Gift and Pugh realized that similar interventions, such as the use of progressive muscle relaxation, had been proposed and tested for both dyspnea and fatigue. These management techniques were consistent with those proposed for the management of pain.

Both symptom models were usable, but there was a need for a more abstract and inclusive model that could encompass these and other symptoms. Elizabeth Lenz was familiar with the work of all three researchers and had offered critique and support regarding their studies and the theoretical implications. Lenz took the lead to call the collaborators together to further develop the more inclusive model. The team was joined by Frederick Suppe, an eminent philosopher of science with a wealth of experience related to nursing science. The authors began meeting regularly to develop the model, assign writing tasks, and discuss each other's work. The more abstract model that resulted was presented to the nursing scholarly community as an exemplar of a middle range nursing theory (Lenz, Suppe, Gift, Pugh, & Milligan, 1995).

During the next few years, interest in the development of middle range theories increased considerably in the nursing literature. In a later revision and amplification of the TOUS, the authors refined the model to be more realistic, that is, more accurately to reflect the complexity and dynamism of clinical situations (Lenz, Pugh, Milligan, Gift, & Suppe, 1997). The multiplicative nature of symptoms, the interaction among the influencing factors, and the feedback among the factors, symptoms, and performance were integrated into the theory.

In summary, the TOUS originated from clinical observations, empirical research, and teamwork among investigators. Refining the theory and communicating those ideas to the nursing community required the collaboration of those with an in-depth understanding of a clinical population who regularly experienced symptoms, those who knew the research literature related to at least one symptom, and those with expertise in theory development and skill in writing theoretical articles.

THE THEORY OF UNPLEASANT SYMPTOMS

Most models of symptoms focus on one symptom and specifically on the intensity of the symptom, not on its other features, such as quality, distress, or duration. The TOUS was one of the earliest to portray multiple symptoms occurring together and relating to each other in a multiplicative manner, potentially catalyzing each other. Thus, this theory, which allows for the presence of multiple symptoms and implies that management of one symptom will contribute to the management of other symptoms is consistent with the large body of current literature that addresses symptom clusters, which are multiple symptoms that occur simultaneously and are related to one another (Barsevick, Dudley, & Beck, 2006; Dirksen, Belyea, & Epstein, 2009; Dodd, Miaskowski, & Lee, 2004; Fox & Lyon, 2007; Jurgens et al., 2009).

DESCRIPTION OF THE THEORY OF UNPLEASANT SYMPTOMS

The TOUS addresses the symptom experience and allows a focus on either multiple symptoms occurring together or a single symptom. It has been used as the theoretical framework to guide several studies of the symptom experience associated with a variety of illnesses, including cancer, chronic obstructive pulmonary disease, heart failure, and gastric and transplant surgery, as well as with pregnancy and the

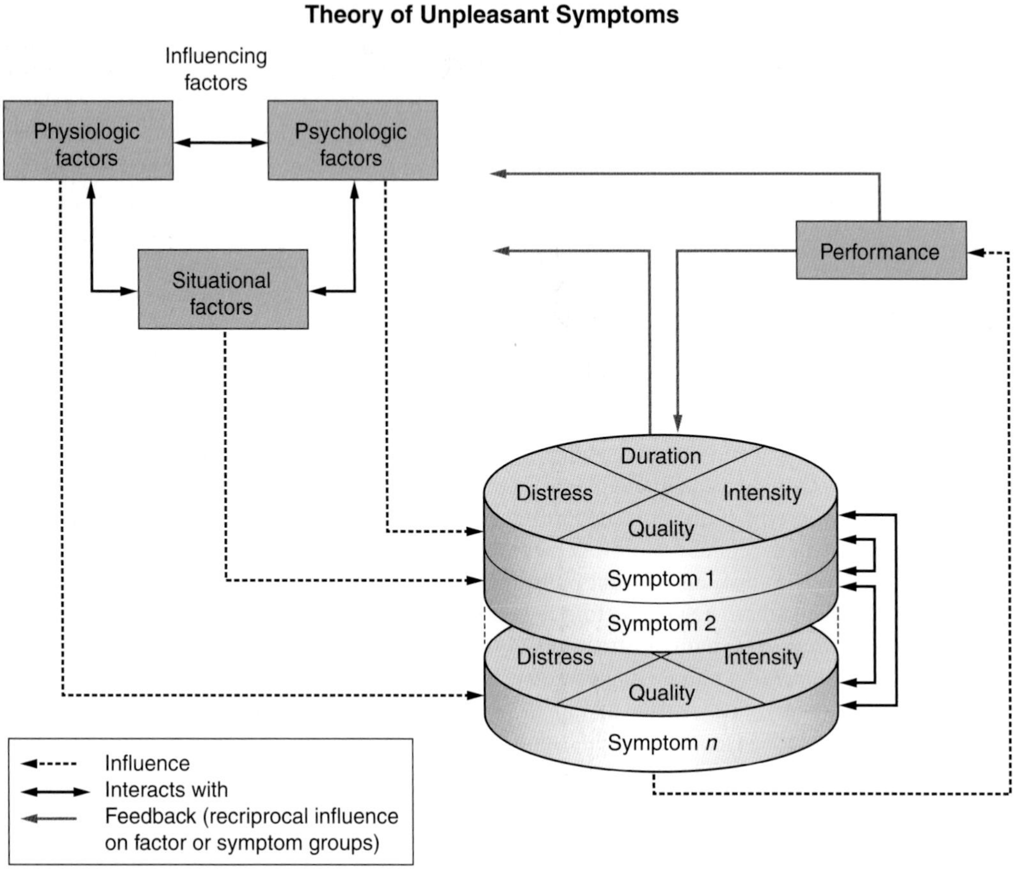

Theory of Unpleasant Symptoms

Figure 4.1 Theory of unpleasant symptoms. (From Lenz, E. R., Pugh, L. C., Milligan, R. A., Gift, A., & Suppe, F. (1997). The middle-range theory of unpleasant symptoms: An update. *Advances in Nursing Science, 19*[3], 14–27. Copyright 1997 by Lippincott Williams & Wilkins.)

postpartum (e.g., Dirksen et al., 2009; Hicks & Spector, 2003; Jurgens et al., 2009; Kapella et al., 2006). The symptoms are viewed as having a multiplicative, rather than an additive relationship to one another. Symptoms have antecedent factors that are physiological, psychological, and environmental. These antecedents are interactive and reciprocal as they relate to one another and to the symptom(s) (Fig. 4.1).

Symptoms have the measurable dimensions of intensity (severity), timing (frequency, duration, repetition pattern if the symptom is recurrent, and relationship of onset to precipitating events), distress (the person's reaction to the sensation), and quality (descriptors used to characterize the way the symptom feels and/or its location). The quality dimension may be especially difficult to measure, depending on the culture and language of the patient and the number of symptoms experienced at the same time.

The antecedent factors are categorized as physiological, psychological, or situational. Physiological antecedents may include individual's age, precipitating illness(es) or dysfunction(s) with severity and stage, or normal developmental stage (e.g., menopause). In addition, other physiological antecedents can be an event (e.g., pregnancy), individual comorbidities, abnormal blood values, or any other physiological findings that can be attributed to the illness or its treatment (e.g., medication, surgery, or radiation therapy). Psychological factors affecting the symptom experience may include the person's mood or emotional state, affective reaction to disease, degree of perceived uncertainty regarding the symptoms or the illness, level of perceived self-efficacy, and the meaning ascribed to the symptoms by the patient. Situational factors refer to aspects of the social and physical environment that may affect

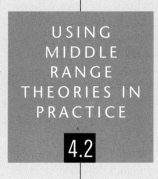

The TOUS has been used as a theoretical framework with which to guide an analysis of symptoms of cardiac failure in adults. Jurgens et al. (2009) used nine symptom-specific questions from the 21-item Minnesota Living with Heart Failure Questionnaire for secondary analysis of data from 687 heart failure patients. Factor analysis of the nine items revealed three symptom clusters that can be indicative of impending physiologic decompensation: acute volume overload (shortness of breath, fatigue, and sleep disturbance); chronic volume overload (swelling, shortness of breath on exertion, and emotional distress); and the emotional factor cluster (depression, worry, and loss of memory). The clusters explained 46%, 13%, and 9% of the variance in symptom impact, respectively. The importance of the TOUS in understanding cardiac failure is that the construct highlights the reality that disease symptoms may manifest in multiples (groupings) within various physical or mental domains. Single symptom recognition can be highly nonspecific for heart failure and individual symptoms with slow insidious presentations such as fatigue or dyspnea may be ignored over time as they become an "accepted" annoyance of the disease. Patient self-identification of symptom group clusters may improve chances of early treatment and prevent hospital admission.

USING MIDDLE RANGE THEORIES IN RESEARCH

4.1

Source: Jurgens, C., Moser, D., Armola, R., Carlson, B., Sethares, K., & Riegel, B. (2009). Symptom clusters of heart failure. *Research in Nursing and Health, 32*, 551–560.

patients' symptom experiences and their reporting of those experiences, including social support, marital status, cultural background, occupation, family and work demands, and available resources.

In the TOUS, symptoms are hypothesized to affect performance, which could be functional and/or cognitive. Functional performance refers to an individual's ability to perform physical activity and the degree to which he or she is able to perform social and personal roles. Cognitive performance is one's ability to concentrate, learn, solve problem, reason, and/or think. There is empirical support for relationships between patterns of cognition and levels of symptoms experienced (Barsevick et al., 2006; Lee, 2005).

In the most recent version of the theory (Lenz, Pugh et al., 1997), multiple symptoms are conceptualized as potentially occurring simultaneously and interacting with one another, as are antecedent factors (see Fig. 4.1 for a model of the TOUS). Interactive and reciprocal relationships among the antecedent factors and symptoms are also hypothesized. Symptoms are hypothesized to influence performance. Performance, likewise, reciprocally affects the symptom experience and also possibly changes the antecedent factors (see Using Middle Range Theories 4.1, 4.2, and 4.3 for examples of the use of the theory).

The TOUS has been shown to be useful as a theoretical construct in the care of bariatric surgical patients. Tyler and Pugh (2009) presented a case study of an actual patient viewed through the lens of the TOUS. They concluded that clinicians should apply the TOUS theoretical framework when assessing the needs of the postoperative bariatric patient. It is imperative to survey the overall clinical picture and consider all factors that may influence the physiological, psychological, and situational components of postsurgical recovery to decrease the possibility of morbidity and mortality following bariatric surgery. To bring about optimal recovery from bariatric surgery, the bariatric postoperative patient and clinician must recognize that symptom management for gastric motility issues such as nausea, vomiting, and constipation is as important as the management of food cravings, and procurement of reliable social support.

USING MIDDLE RANGE THEORIES IN PRACTICE

4.2

Source: Tyler, R., & Pugh, L. (2009). Application of the theory of unpleasant symptoms in bariatric surgery. *Bariatric Nursing and Surgical Patient Care, 4*, 271–276.

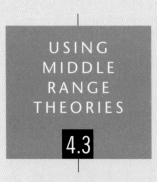

The number of Korean women diagnosed with breast cancer has increased rapidly, making it currently the most common type of cancer in Korean women. Treatment for this disease produces multiple symptoms that interfere with the patient's activities and social functioning. Researchers examined the relationships among the situational factor of social support, the psychological factor of mood disturbance, and symptoms. They found that while mood disturbance was positively correlated with the symptom experience, this relationship was moderated by social support. Women with a higher level of mood disturbance were at greater risk for experiencing symptoms when the level of social support was low. Thus, the nurse is advised to be especially attentive to evaluate the patient's social support along with mood disturbance when planning interventions to reduce symptoms, especially in Korean women with breast cancer.

USING MIDDLE RANGE THEORIES 4.3

Source: Lee, E. H., Chung, B. Y., Park, H. B., & Chun, K. H. (2004). Relationships of mood disturbance and social support to symptom experience in Korean women with breast cancer. *Journal of Pain and Symptom Management, 27*(5), 425–433.

MODELS THAT EXPAND OR MODIFY THE THEORY OF UNPLEASANT SYMPTOMS

In 2009, Brant, Beck, and Miaskowski conducted a systematic review of models related to symptoms or symptoms management. The two seminal models they identified were the TOUS and the theory of symptom management (TSM; Humphreys et al., 2008), an outgrowth of the Symptom Management Model (SMM; Larson et al., 1994). Models that have expanded or modified the TOUS include the Symptoms Experience Model (SEM; Armstrong, 2003) and Symptoms Experience in Time Model (SET; Henly, Kallas, Klatt, & Swenson, 2003). In addition to the models that have been developed to expand the TOUS, a number of investigators have tested aspects of the theory and, based on their findings, have suggested modifications (see Lenz & Pugh, 2008). It has also been used as a basis for investigator-generated models, which are then tested using path analytic techniques (e.g., Hoffman et al., 2009).

ARMSTRONG MODEL OF SYMPTOM EXPERIENCE

Armstrong (2003) proposed a symptom model that builds on the TOUS but focuses attention on the meaning or perception of the symptom as well as its expression. Multiple co-occurring symptoms can interact and affect the patient's perception of the symptom as a new or recurring event and his/her perception of the ability to deal with the situation. Armstrong further extends the TOUS to include the existential meaning of the symptom(s) to the patient, that is, his/her own feelings of vulnerability and mortality related to the symptom. Alternatively, existential meaning can be positive, such as when a treatment is working or when a patient's illness has forced a family to reunite. In Armstrong's modification, antecedents are reorganized as demographic, disease, and individual characteristics. Symptom dimensions are frequency, intensity, and distress (consistent with the TOUS), and the descriptor of symptom meaning. In the TOUS, the patient's interpretation of the meaning of the symptom experience is, to some extent, captured in the individual's description of the level of distress. The consequences of the symptom experience are expanded beyond physical, social, and role performance (or cognitive functioning) to include emotional consequences. The Armstrong Model of Symptom Experience is appropriate to use when symptom meaning is the focus of the investigation and/or when one is examining the emotional consequences of the symptom experience (Armstrong, 2003).

SYMPTOM EXPERIENCE IN TIME MODEL

The SET model was conceptualized by combining the TOUS and the SMM (now the TSM) with a time model for the purpose of examining symptom flow (Henly et al., 2003). In this model, the symptom is initiated by a precipitating event that leads to the onset of the symptom(s). The influencing factors of the TOUS are broadened to include nursing metaparadigm concepts such as person, health, and environment that either mediate or moderate the symptom. Every symptom has an onset, an experience, a cognitive evaluation, and an emotional response. Symptom dimensions of timing, intensity, distress, and quality are retained from the TOUS. The cognitive evaluation determines whether the symptom is serious, unpleasant, and/or inexplicable. Each symptom is also evaluated as being chronic or treatable. If treatable, symptom management can take the form of either self-care or help-seeking behavior. The outcomes of these strategies can be changes in the symptom itself, as well as changes in the person, his/her health, and/or environment.

Time, a factor determining the patterning of a symptom experience, may serve as input to the symptom experience, or as output from the symptom management process (Henly et al., 2003). It may also be a component of an intervention. Time is discussed as having different patterns whether considering per- ceived time, biological/social time, or clock/calendar time. Transcendence is the qualitative repositioning in time and is beyond time. The value of the SET model is that it provides a conceptual framework from which to study changes in symptoms over the course of time.

ASSESSMENT OF SYMPTOMS

The TOUS is relevant to practice, and can be used as a framework for nursing assessment or care decisions. Symptom experience is subjective; thus, assessment must be tempered by the notion that the distress asso- ciated with a symptom reflects the individual's interpretation of that symptom experience. A sensation of the same magnitude might be interpreted quite differently (therefore, rated or described differently) by two individuals. Appropriate symptom assessment and management depend on understanding the symptom involved, the underlying disease or causative factor, the stage of the illness, and the patient's prognosis.

The medical history is an important part of symptom assessment (Bickley, 2008). The TOUS framework can provide a guide for the medical history, because physiological, psychological, and situational factors provide a framework for identifying symptom antecedents. For instance, physiological factors identified from history taking could include physical sequelae of past illness or injury, or the history of an individual's medication use to decrease symptom effects. Psychological factors identified in history taking could include recent or previous depressive incidents or mood changes. Situational factors potentially identified in the history could include family/caregiver issues and living situations. Symptoms should be characterized by assessing their time and rate of onset (sudden or gradual) relative to any precipitating or alleviating factors, as well as their frequency and duration. Other symptom characteristics to report are the intensity and quality of the symptom, as well as the symptom-related distress felt by the patient (Bickley, 2008). This history should be carefully validated by physical examination focusing on possible underlying causes of the symptoms.

Diagnostic tests that are specific for helping to determine the etiology of the symptom are advised (Ferri, 2011). Since many symptoms are contextual and related to movement or exercise, it is important to assess these parameters as well.

INSTRUMENTS USED IN EMPIRICAL TESTING

Symptom measures can either focus on one symptom (e.g., Gift, Moore, & Soeken, 1992; Pugh & Milligan, 1998) or include multiple symptoms that are commonly seen in a specific disease entity, the most frequently studied being cancer (e.g., Dirksen et al., 2009; Fox & Lyon, 2007). Some symptom measures focus only on physical symptoms, while others include both physical and emotional symptoms. Symptom measures may focus only on presence or absence, intensity or frequency, rather than all the dimensions described in the TOUS. Many instruments have been used to measure the other components of the TOUS as well. Among the most commonly used are those that address performance, particularly functional performance measures, which use individuals' reports of their activities of daily living and roles, or observations of activity measures (e.g., ability to walk a given distance, grip strength, or range of motion achieved). Many activity measures are limited in use, because they cannot be used for patients who are in critical care or at the end stage of life. In addition to the self-report and activity measures, some investigators have also used physiological mea- sures, such as spirography or blood values to measure severity of illness. A few examples of the self-report symptom measures that have been used in applying or testing the TOUS are described briefly in Table 4.1.

SELECTION OF INSTRUMENTS

The use of a particular instrument to measure symptom(s), performance, or influencing factors in research or in clinical practice will largely depend upon what the researcher needs to answer the research questions

TABLE 4.1 Examples of Self-report Instruments Used to Apply TOUS in Research and Practice

Instrument	Concept(s) measured	TOUS component measured	Description
Profile of Mood States (POMS)[a]	Fatigue/inertia (intensity), depression	Symptoms (separate subscales for specific symptoms), psychological factors; cognitive performance	Long form is comprised of 65 adjectives; for each, respondents are asked to indicate the extent to which they are currently experiencing the emotion described. Subscales measure tension-anxiety, depression-dejection, anger-hostility, fatigue-inertia, vigor-activity, and confusion-bewilderment. A short form exists.
Visual Analog Scale[b,c]	Most symptoms (e.g., fatigue, pain, dyspnea); has been used primarily to measure symptom intensity, but also other dimensions such as and associated distress	Symptoms (single symptom measured at a time)	Subject places mark along a 100-mm line anchored by descriptors (polar opposites) to reflect the intensity of the symptom. Scoring involves measuring the distance from the lowest or left end of the line to the mark.
Numeric Rating Scale[d,e]	Most symptoms; most often used to measure intensity; commonly used in clinical practice, especially in pain measurement	Symptoms (single symptom measured at a time)	Subject is asked to describe the level of the symptom being experienced on a numerical range (e.g., 1–10, with 1 = no pain and 10 = the worst pain possible). Score is the numerical value. Telephone pads have been used to measure responses in phone interviews.
McGill Pain Questionnaire[f]	Pain	Symptom (single)	Measures sensory, affective and evaluative dimensions of pain, including the relative intensity of each dimension. Current pain intensity is rated on a 0–5 scale.
Brief Fatigue Inventory[g]	Fatigue	Symptom (single)	Measures severity of fatigue in last 24 h, and degree of interference with the patient's daily functioning. Items (9) are rated on a 10-point scale. Originally developed for cancer-related fatigue has also been used in patients with kidney failure.
Minnesota Living with Heart Failure Questionnaire[h]	Quality of life; physical and emotional symptoms impacting QoL in HF patients	Disease-specific symptoms (9); Performance	A 21-item Likert-type scale measuring quality of life in patients with heart failure. Patients rate impact of each of six physical and three emotional symptoms on living during the previous month.
Short Form-36[i]	Symptoms of pain, depressive symptoms, fatigue; performance (functional health) general health status	Symptoms (separate subscales for specific symptoms); physiological and psychological factors; performance	36 items that measure general health; subscales measure mental health, vitality, bodily pain, social functioning, mental health, role limitations, vitality and perception of general health. Responses are based on how individual reports feeling over past 4 weeks.

TABLE 4.1 Examples of Self-report Instruments Used to Apply TOUS in Research and Practice (*Continued*)

Instrument	Concept(s) measured	TOUS component measured	Description
CES-D[j]	Depressive symptoms	Symptoms, psychological factors	Respondents indicate the frequency in the past week with which they experienced each of 20 beliefs and emotions. Designed for use in the general population; should not be viewed as diagnostic of depression.
Memorial Symptom Assessment Scale[k,l]	Physical and psychological symptoms	Symptoms (multiple)	Presence, frequency, intensity, and distress associated with each of 24 symptoms. Scoring consists of a global distress score, physical and psychological distress scores, and total MSAS score. Originally developed for use with cancer patients, it has also been used to measure symptoms in patients with heart failure. A short form with 19 symptoms has been developed for patients with COPD.
Fox Simple Quality of Life Scale[m]	Quality of life	Performance	25-item scale in which respondents are asked to respond on a Likert-type scale to items addressing cognitive and affective aspects of QoL. Total score is used as the measure of QoL.

[a]McNair, Lorr, & Droppelman (1992). [b]Waltz, Strickland, & Lenz (2010). [c]Gift, Plaut, & Jacox (1986). [d]Kapella et al. (2006). [e]Cleeland et al. (2000). [f]Melzack (1983). [g]Mendoza et al. (1999). [h]Rector, Kubo, & Cohn (1987). [i]Ware & Sherbourne, C (1992). [j]Radloff (1977). [k]Portenoy et al. (1994). [l]Jablonski, Gift, & Cook (2007). [m]Fox (2004).

being studied and/or the needs and limitations imposed by a particular clinical setting. In general, it is preferable to select an existing instrument than to develop a new one, provided it has not only a good fit to the situation in which it will be used, but also established reliability and validity (see Waltz, Strickland, & Lenz, 2010). Research Application 4.1 provides an example of how the TOUS may be used, and how symptoms can be assessed using a single-symptom assessment measure.

Research Application   4.1

A nurse researcher is interested in studying ways to reduce pain postoperatively in hip-replacement patients. The researcher decides to use the TOUS to structure an experimental preoperative teaching class. The class has components related to all aspects of the model, such as physiological factors that can be controlled to reduce pain postoperatively, psychological factors, and social or environmental factors that will help patients manage their pain postoperatively. Patients are taught to characterize their pain according to the intensity, frequency, distress, and quality of the sensation, and to record the sensation, so that they can note the changes that occur following medication and over time as they recover. They are taught to note other symptoms that may accompany the pain. In addition, patients are told what to expect related to their performance after surgery, and how gradually and safely to increase their activity as the pain decreases. The effectiveness of this preoperative teaching is assessed by having patients rate their pain using a visual analogue pain scale during the postoperative period and comparing it to pain ratings in those not exposed to the teaching.

SUMMARY

Having symptoms as the focus of nursing care, rather than simply being an indication of the underlying "cause" or indication of another problem, is somewhat new to the nursing literature. The use of middle range theories to guide the management of symptoms has been gaining considerable momentum. They serve the useful purpose of guiding the practitioner to focus on more than the sensation and its intensity but, rather, to have a more comprehensive approach, including the context in which the symptom occurs. The situational aspects that contribute to the symptom experience need further study. We know that there are environmental, social, and cultural factors that play a part in the interpretation of symptoms, but more detail is needed to guide the clinician in planning nursing care. Although the symptom models advocate the assessment of multiple symptoms rather than only one (such as pain), few clinical settings implement the assessment in their routine patient care.

The effects of symptoms on patient performance are just beginning to be identified. This chapter has endeavored to identify how symptoms may affect all aspects of individual performance. Nursing management of symptoms can be expected to affect patients physically, psychologically, and socially; thus, it is important for nurses to operate within a scientific framework to better assess and manage unpleasant symptoms.

ANALYSIS OF THEORY

Using the criteria presented in Chapter 2, critique the TOUS. Compare your conclusions about the theory with those found in Appendix A. An experienced nurse has completed the analysis found in Appendix A.

Internal Criticism

1. Clarity
2. Consistency
3. Adequacy
4. Logical development
5. Level of theory development

External Criticism

1. Reality convergence
2. Utility
3. Significance
4. Discrimination
5. Scope of theory
6. Complexity

CRITICAL THINKING EXERCISES

1. Using the theory of unpleasant symptoms as your guide, what would you look for in an assessment tool for patient symptoms?

   a. Do you monitor all symptom dimensions, such as how distressing the symptom is, or do you only ask about symptom severity/intensity?

   b. Do you monitor only one symptom or multiple symptoms?

2. In your patient assessment, how would you include the antecedents to symptoms?

3. How would you use the theory of unpleasant symptoms to plan a comprehensive intervention to alleviate symptoms?

   a. What interventions might you plan that would target the antecedents?

   b. What would you do to intervene regarding symptom distress?

4. What outcome would you use to assess the effectiveness of your interventions?

   a. Would you use an outcome measure that focuses on the physical, role, and/or cognitive performance outcome of symptoms? If so, what measure(s) would that be, specifically?

   b. If you were to have symptom alleviation as your outcome measure, which specific measurement tool would you use?

WEB RESOURCES

Visit **http://thePoint.lww.com/Peterson3e** for helpful Web resources related to this chapter.

REFERENCES

Armstrong, T. S. (2003). Symptoms experience: A concept analysis. *Oncology Nursing Forum, 30*, 601–605.

Barsevick, A. M., Dudley, W. N., & Beck, S. L. (2006). Cancer-related fatigue, depressive symptoms, and functional status: A mediation model. *Nursing Research, 55*, 366–372.

Bickley, L. S. (2008). *Bates guide to physical examination and history taking* (10th ed.). New York: Lippincott.

Cleeland, C. S., Mendoza, T., Wang, X. S., Chou, C., Harle, M. T., & Morrissey, M. (2000). Assessing symptom distress in cancer patients. *Cancer, 89*, 1634–1645.

Dirksen, S. R., Belyea, M. J., & Epstein, D. R. (2009). Fatigue-based subgroups of breast cancer survivors with insomnia. *Cancer Nursing, 32*, 404–411.

Dodd, M., Miaskowski, C., & Lee, K. A. (2004). Occurrence of symptom clusters. *Journal of the National Cancer Institute, 32*, 76–78.

Fox, S. (2004). Preliminary psychometric development of the Fox simple quality of life scale. *Journal of Neuroscience Nursing, 36*, 157–166.

Fox, S. W., & Lyon, D. (2007). Symptom clusters and quality of life in survivors of ovarian cancer. *Cancer Nursing, 30*, 354–361.

Gift, A. G., Plaut, S. M., & Jacox, A. K. (1986). Psychologic and physiologic factors related to dyspnea in subjects with chronic obstructive pulmonary disease. *Heart & Lung, 15*, 595–602.

Henly, S. J., Kallas, K. D., Klatt, C. M., & Swenson, K. K. (2003). The notion of time in symptom experiences. *Nursing Research, 52*, 410–417.

Hoffman, A. J., von Eye, A., Gift, A. G., Given, B. A., Given, C. W., & Rothert, M. (2009). Testing a theoretical model of perceived self-efficacy for cancer-related fatigue self-management and optimal physical functional status. *Nursing Research, 58*, 32–41. doi:10.1097/NNR.0b013e3181903d7b

Humphreys, J., Lee, K., Carrieri-Kohlman, V., Puntillo, K., Faucett, J., Janson, S., et al. (2008). Theory of symptom management. In M. J. Smith & P. R. Liehr (Eds.), *Middle range theory for nursing* (pp. 145–158). New York: Springer.

Jablonski, A., Gift, A. G., & Cook, K. E. (2007). Symptom assessment of patients with chronic obstructive pulmonary disease. *Western Journal of Nursing Research, 29* (7), 845–863.

Jurgens, C. Y., Moser, D. K., Armola, R., Carlson, B., Sethares, K., Riegel, B., & The Heart Failure Quality of Life Trialist Collaborators. (2009). Symptom clusters of heart failure. *Research in Nursing and Health;32*, 551–560.

Kapella, M. C., Larson, J. L., Patel, M. K., Covey, M. K., & Berry, J. K. (2006). Subjective fatigue, influencing variables, and consequences in chronic obstructive pulmonary disease. *Nursing Research, 55*, 10–17.

Larson, P., Carrieri-Kohlman, V., Dodd, M., Douglas, M., Faucett, J., Froelicher, E., et al. (1994). A model for symptom management. *Image: Journal of Nursing Scholarship, 26*, 272–276.

Lenz, E. R., & Pugh, L. C. (2008). The theory of unpleasant symptoms. In M. J. Smith & P. Liehr (Eds.), *Middle range theory for nursing* (2nd ed.) New York: Springer.

Lenz, E. R., Pugh, L. C., Milligan, R. A., Gift, A., & Suppe, F. (1997). The middle range theory of unpleasant symptoms: An update. *Advances in Nursing Science, 19*(3), 14–27.

Lenz, E. R., Suppe, F., Gift, A. G., Pugh, L. C., & Milligan, R. A. (1995). Collaborative development of middle-range nursing theories: Toward a theory of unpleasant symptoms. *Advances in Nursing Science,17*, 1–13.

McNair, D. M., Lorr, M., & Droppelman, M. F. (1992). *The profile of mood states.* San Diego, CA: Educational Testing Service.

Melzack, R. (1983). The McGill pain questionnaire. In R. Melzack (Ed.), *Pain measurement and assessment* (pp. 41–47). New York: Raven Press.

Mendoza, T. R., Wang, X. S., Cleeland, C. S., Morrissey, M., Johnson, B. A., Wendt, J. K., et al. (1999). The rapid assessment of fatigue severity in cancer patients: Use of the Brief Fatigue Inventory. *Cancer, 85*, 1186–1196.

Portenoy, R. K., Thaler, H. T., Kornblith, A. B., Lepore, J. M., Friedlander-Klar, H., & Kiyasu, E. (1994). The Memorial Symptoms Assessment Scale: An instrument for the evaluation of symptom prevalence, characteristics and distress. *European Journal of Cancer, 30A*, 1326–1336.

Pugh, L. C., & Milligan, R. A. (1998). Nursing intervention to increase the duration of breastfeeding. *Applied Nursing Research, 11*, 190–194.

Radloff, L. S. (1977). The CES-D scale: A self-report depression scale for research in the general population. *Applied Psychological Measurement, 1*, 385–401.

Rector, T. S., Kubo, S. H., & Cohn, J. N. (1987). Patients' self-assessment of their congestive heart failure, part 2: Content, reliability and validity of a new measure of the Minnesota Living with Heart Failure Questionnaire. *Heart Failure, 3*, 198–209.

Tyler, R., & Pugh, L. C. (2009). Application of the theory of unpleasant symptoms in bariatric surgery. *Bariatric Nursing and Surgical Patient Care, 4*, 271–276.

Waltz, C. F., Strickland, O. L., & Lenz, E. R. (2010). *Measurement in nursing and health research* (4th ed.). New York: Springer.

Ware, J., & Sherbourne, C. (1992). The MOS 36-item short form health survey (SF-36): Conceptual framework and item selection. *MedicaL Care, 30,* 473–483.

Zambroski, C. H., Moser, D. K., Bhat, G., & Ziegler, S. (2005). Impact of symptom prevalence and symptom burden on quality of life in patients with heart failure. *European Journal of Cardiovascular Nursing, 4,* 198–206.

BIBLIOGRAPHY

Aaronson, L. S., Teel, C. S., Cassmeyer, V., Neuberger, G. B., Pallikkathayil, L., Pierce, J., et al. (1999). Defining and measuring fatigue. *Image, 31*(1), 45–50.

Acheson, A., & MacCormack, D. (1997). Dyspnea and the cancer patient—An overview. *Canadian Oncology Nursing Journal, 7,* 209–213.

Aitken, R. C. B. (1969). Measurement of feelings using visual analogue scales. *Proceedings of Research Social Medicine, 62,* 989–993.

Algase, D. L., Newton, S. E., & Higgins, P. A. (2001). Nursing theory across curricula: A status report from Midwest nursing schools. *Journal of Professional Nursing, 17,* 248–255.

Armstrong, T. S., Cohen, M. Z., Eriksen, L., & Cleeland, C. (2005). Content validity of self-report measurement instruments: An illustration from the development of the brain tumor module of the M.D. Anderson Symptom Inventory. *Oncology Nursing Forum, 32,* 669–676.

Armstrong, T. S., Cohen, M. Z., Eriksen, L., & Hickey, J. V. (2004). Symptom clusters in oncology patients and implications for symptom research in people with primary brain tumors. *Journal of Nursing Scholarship, 36,* 197–206.

Blegen, M. A., & Tripp-Reimer, T. (1997). Implications of nursing taxonomies for middle-range theory development. *Advanced Nursing Science, 19*(3), 37–49.

Brant J. M., Beck, S., & Miaskowski, C. (2010). Building dynamic models and theories to advance the science of symptom management research. *Journal of Advanced Nursing, 66,* 228–240.

Bredin, M., Corner, J., Krishnasamy, M., Plant, H., Bailey, C., & A'Hern, R. (1999). Multicentre randomized controlled trial of nursing intervention for breathlessness in patients with lung cancer. *British Medical Journal, 318,* 901–904.

Carrieri-Kohlman, V., Gormley, J. M., Douglas, M. K., Paul, S. M., & Stulbarg, M. S. (1996). Differentiation between dyspnea and its affective components. *Western Journal of Nursing Research, 18,* 626–642.

Cella, D., Passik, S., Jacobsen, P., & Breitbart, W. (1998). Progress toward guidelines for the management of fatigue. *Oncology, 12*(11A), 369–377.

Cody, W. K. (1999). Middle-range theories: Do they foster the development of nursing science? *Nursing Science Quarterly, 12*(1), 9–14.

Cooley, M. E. (2000). Symptoms in adults with lung cancer: A systematic research review. *Journal of Pain and Symptom Management, 19,* 137–153.

Corwin, E. J., Brownstead, J., Barton, N., Heckard, S., & Morin, K. (2005). The impact of fatigue on the development of postpartum depression. *Journal of Obstetric Gynecologic and Neonatal Nursing, 34,* 577–586.

Corwin, E. J., Klein, L. C., & Rickelman, K. (2002). Predictors of fatigue in healthy young adults: Moderating effects of cigarette smoking and gender. *Biologic Research in Nursing, 3,* 222–233.

Dabbs, A. D., Dew, M. A., Stilley, C. S., Manzetti, J., Zullo, T., McCurry, K. R., et al. (2003). Psychosocial vulnerability, physical symptoms and physical impairment after lung and heart-lung transplantation. *Journal of Heart and Lung Transplantation, 22,* 1268–1275.

Dabbs, A. D., Hoffman, L. A., Swigart, V., Happ, M. B., Iacono, A. T., & Dauber, J. H. (2004). Using conceptual triangulation to develop an integrated model of the symptom experience of acute rejection after lung transplantation. *Advances in Nursing Science, 27*(2), 138–149.

Deets, C. (1998). Nursing—A maturing discipline? *Journal of Professional Nursing, 14*(2), 65.

Dodd, M., Janson, S., Facione, N., Faucett, J., Froelicher, E. S., Humphreys, J., et al. (2001). Advancing the science of symptom management. *Journal of Advanced Nursing, 33,* 668–676.

Dodd, M., Miaskowski, C., & Paul, S. (2001). Symptom clusters and their effect on the functional status of patients with cancer. *Oncology Nursing Forum, 28,* 465–470.

Drevdahl, D. (1999). Sailing beyond: Nursing theory and the person. *Advanced Nursing Science, 21*(4), 1–13.

Ducharme, F., Ricard, N., Duquette, A., Levesque, L., & Lachance, L. (1998). Empirical testing of a longitudinal model derived from the Roy adaptation model. *Nursing Science Quarterly, 11*(4), 149–159.

Dudley-Brown, S. L. (1997). The evaluation of nursing theory: A method for our madness. *International Journal of Nursing Studies, 34*(1), 76–83.

Eakin, E., Prewitt, L. M., Ries, A., & Kaplan, R. (1994). Validation of the UCSD shortness of breath questionnaire. *Journal of Cardiopulmonary Rehabilitation, 14,* 322–323.

Eakin, E., Sassi-Dambron, D. E., Ries, A., & Kaplan, R. (1995). Reliability and validity of dyspnea measures in patients with obstructive lung disease. *International Journal of Behavioral Medicine, 2*(2), 118–134.

Eller, L. S., Lev, E. L., Gejerman, G., Colella, J., Esposito, M., Lanteri, V., et al. (2006). Prospective study of quality of life of patients receiving treatment for prostate cancer. *Nursing Research, 55,* S28–S36.

Ferri, F. (2011). *Ferri's differential diagnosis: A practical guide to the differential diagnosis of symptoms, signs, and clinical disorders.* Providence, RI: Mosby.

Gift, A. G. (1989). Validation of a vertical visual analogue scale as a measure of clinical dyspnea. *Rehabilitation Nursing, 14*, 323–325.

Gift, A. G., Jablonski, A., Stommel, M., & Given, C. W. (2004). Symptom clusters in elderly patients with lung cancer. *Oncology Nursing Forum, 31*, 203–210.

Gift, A. G., Moore, T., & Soeken, K. (1992). Relaxation to reduce dyspnea and anxiety in COPD patients. *Nursing Research, 41*, 242–246.

Gift, A. G., & Narsavage, G. (1998). Validity of the numeric rating scale as a measure of dyspnea. *American Journal of Critical Care, 7*, 200–204.

Gift, A. G., Stommel, M., Jablonski, A., & Given, W. (2003). A cluster of symptoms over time in patients with lung cancer. *Nursing Research, 52*, 393–400.

Given, C. W., Stommel, M., Given, B., Osuch, J., Kurtz, M. E., & Kurtz, J. C. (1993). The influence of cancer patients' symptoms and functional status on patients' depression and family caregivers' reaction and depression. *Health Psychology, 12*, 277–285.

Good, M. (1998). A middle-range theory of acute pain management: Use in research. *Nursing Outlook, 46*(3), 120–124.

Hann, D., Jacobson, P., Azzarillo, M., & Martin, S. (1998). Measurement of fatigue in cancer patients: Development and validation of the fatigue symptom inventory. *Quality of Life Research, 7*, 301–311.

Hicks, F. D., & Spector, N. M. (2003). The life after gastric surgery index. *Gastroenterology Nursing, 27*, 50-54.

Higgins, P. A. (1998). Patient perception of fatigue while undergoing long-term mechanical ventilation: Incidence and associated factors. *Heart & Lung, 27*(3), 177–183.

Higgins, P. A., & Moore, S. M. (2000). Levels of theoretical thinking in nursing. *Nursing Outlook, 48*, 179–183.

Hopp, J. P., & Duffy, S. A. (2000). Racial variations in end-of-life care. *Journal of the American Geriatrics Society, 48*, 658–663.

Hupcey, J. A., Morse, J. M., Lenz, E., & Tason, M. C. (1996). Wilsonian methods of concept analysis: A critique. *Scholarly Inquiry for Nursing Practice, 10*, 185–210.

Hutchinson, S. A., & Wilson, H. S. (1998). The theory of unpleasant symptoms and Alzheimer's disease. *Scholarly Inquiry for Nursing Practice: An International Journal, 12*, 143–158.

Huth, M. M., & Broome, M. E. (2007). A snapshot of children's postoperative tonsillectomy outcomes at home. *Journal for Specialists in Pediatric Nursing, 121*, 86–95.

Hwang, S. S., Chang, V. T., Cogswell, J., & Kasimis, B. S. (2002). Clinical relevance of fatigue levels in cancer patients at a Veterans Administration Medical Center. *Cancer, 94*, 2481–2489.

Jenkins, P. C. (2007). The relationship between dyspnea and blood pressure in chronic obstructive pulmonary disease. *Journal of Cardiovascular Nursing, 22*, 351–358.

Kim, H. J., McGuire, D. B., Tulman, L., & Barsevick, A. M. (2005). Symptom clusters: Concept analysis and clinical implications for cancer nursing. *Cancer Nursing, 28*, 270–282.

Lee, E. H. (2005). Relationships of mood disturbance, symptom experience, and attentional function in women with breast cancer based upon the theory of unpleasant symptoms. *Taehan Kanho Hakhoe Chi, 35*, 728–736.

Lee, E. H., Chung, B. Y., Park, H. B., & Chun, K. H. (2004). Relationships of mood disturbance and social support to symptom experience in Korean women with breast cancer. *Journal of Pain and Symptom Management, 27*, 425–433.

Liehr, P., & Smith, M. J. (1999). Middle range theory: Spinning research and practice to create knowledge for the new millennium. *Advance Nursing Science, 21*(4), 81–91.

Liu, H. E. (2006). Fatigue and associated factors in hemodialysis patients in Taiwan. *Research in Nursing and Health, 29*(1), 40–50.

Mahler, D. A., Harver, A., Lentine, T., Scott, J. A., Beck, K., & Schwartzstein, R. M. (1996). Descriptors of breathlessness in cardiorespiratory diseases. *American Journal of Respiratory and Critical Care Medicine, 154*, 1357–1363.

Mahler, D. A., & Jones, P. W. (1997). Measurement of dyspnea and quality of life in advanced lung disease. *Clinical Chest Medicine, 18*, 457–469.

Mahler, D. A., & Wells, C. K. (1988). Evaluation of clinical methods for rating dyspnea. *Chest, 93*(3), 580–586.

Mancini, I., & Body, J. J. (1999). Assessment of dyspnea in advanced cancer patients. *Supportive Care in Cancer, 7*, 229–232.

McCann, K., & Boore, J. (2000). Fatigue in persons with renal failure who require maintenance haemodialysis. *Journal of Advanced Nursing, 32*, 1132–1142.

McCarley, C. (1999). A model of chronic dyspnea. *Image: Journal of Nursing Scholarship, 31*, 231–236.

McCorkle, R., & Young, K. (1978). Development of a symptom distress scale. *Cancer Nursing, 1*, 373–378.

Meek, P. M., Lareau, S. C., & Anderson, D. (2001). Memory for symptoms in COPD patients: How accurate are their reports? *European Respiratory Journal, 18*, 1–8.

Meek, P. M., Schwartzstein, R. M., Adams, M. M., Altose, M. D., Breslin, E. H., Carrieri-Kohlman, V., et al. (1999). Dyspnea: Mechanisms, assessment, and management: A consensus statement. *American Journal of Respiratory and Critical Care Medicine, 159*, 321–340.

Melzack, R. (1975). The McGill Pain Questionnaire: Major properties and scoring methods. *Pain, 1*, 277–299.

Morse, J. M., Hupcey, J., Mitcham, C., & Lenz, E. (1996). Concept analysis in nursing research: A critical appraisal. *Scholarly Inquiry for Nursing Practice, 10,* 257–281.

Morse, J. M., Hutchinson, S. A., & Penrod, J. (1998). From theory to practice: The development of assessment guides from qualitatively derived theory. *Qualitative Health Research, 8,* 329–340.

Morse, J. M., Mitcham, C., Hupcey, J. E., & Tason, M. C. (1996). Criteria for concept evaluation. *Journal of Advanced Nursing, 24,* 385–390.

Motl, R. W., & McAuley, E. (2009). Symptom cluster as a predictor of physical activity in multiple sclerosis: Preliminary evidence. *Journal of Pain and Symptom Management, 38,* 270–280. doi:10.1016/j.jpainsymman.2008.08.004.

Myers, J. S. (2009). A comparison of the theory of unpleasant symptoms and the conceptual model of chemotherapy-related changes in cognitive function. *Oncology Nursing Forum, 36*(1), E1–E10.

Nield, M. (2000). Dyspnea self-management in African Americans with chronic lung disease. *Heart & Lung, 29,* 50–55.

Otte, J. L., & Carpenter, J. S. (2009). Theories, models, and frameworks related to sleep-wake disturbances in the context of cancer. *Cancer Nursing, 32,* 90-104.

Parker, K. P., Kimble, L. P., Dunbar, D. B., & Clark, P. C. (2005). Symptom interactions as mechanisms underlying symptom pairs and clusters. *Journal of Nursing Scholarship, 37,* 209–215.

Parshall, M. B., Welsh, J. D., Brockopp, D. Y., Heiser, R. M., Schooler, M. P., & Cassidy, K. B. (2001). Dyspnea duration, distress, and intensity in emergency department visits for heart failure. *Heart & Lung, 30,* 47–56.

Piper, B., Dibble, S., Dodd, M., Weiss, M., Slaughter, R., & Paul, S. (1998). The Revised Piper Fatigue Scale: Psychometric evaluation in women with breast cancer. *Oncology Nursing Forum, 25,* 677–684.

Pugh, L. C., Milligan, R., Parks, P. L., Lenz, E. R., Kitzman, H. (1999). Clinical approaches in the assessment of childbearing fatigue. *Journal of Obstetric Gynecologic and Neonatal Nursing, 28*(1), 74–80.

Redeker, N. S., Lev, E. L., & Ruggiero, J. (2000). Insomnia, fatigue, anxiety, depression and quality of life of cancer patients undergoing chemotherapy. *Scholarly Inquiry for Nursing Practice, 14,* 275–290.

Reishtein, J. L. (2005). Relationship between symptoms and functional performance in COPD. *Research in Nursing and Health, 28*(1), 39–47.

Robinson, J., Bunting-Perry, L., & Moriarty, H. (2007). An explanatory study of the lower urinary tract symptom experience and quality of life in men with Parkinson's disease. *JWOCN, 34*(3S), S4.

Ruland, C. M., & Moore, S. M. (1998). Theory construction based on standards of care: A proposed theory of the peaceful end of life. *Nursing Outlook, 46,* 169–175.

Rychnovsky, J. D. (2007). Postpartum fatigue in the active-duty military woman. *Journal of Obstetric Gynecologic and Neonatal Nursing, 36*(1), 38–46.

Sarna, L., & Brecht, M. (1997). Dimensions of symptom distress in women with advanced lung cancer: A factor analysis. *Heart & Lung, 26*(1), 23–30.

Schneider, R. (1998). Reliability and validity of the Multidimensional Fatigue Inventory (MFI-20) and the Rhoten Fatigue Scale among rural cancer outpatients. *Cancer Nursing, 21,* 370–373.

Schwartz, A. (1998). The Schwartz Cancer Fatigue Scale: Testing reliability and validity. *Oncology Nursing Forum, 25,* 711–717.

Shih, F. J., & Chu, S. H. (1999). Comparisons of American-Chinese and Taiwanese patients' perceptions of dyspnea and helpful nursing actions during the intensive care unit transition from cardiac surgery. *Heart & Lung, 28,* 41–54.

Smith, C. E., Pace, K., Kochinda, C., Kleinbeck, S. V. M., Koehler, J., & Popkess-Vawter, S. (2002). Caregiving effectiveness model evolution to a midrange theory of home care: A process for critique and replication. *Advances in Nursing Science, 25*(1), 50–64.

Smith, M. C. (1999). Caring and the science of unitary human beings. *Advanced Nursing Science, 21*(4), 14–28.

Spector, N. M., Hicks, F. D., & Pickleman, J. (2002). Quality of life and symptoms after surgery for gastroesophageal cancer: A pilot study. *Gastroenterology Nursing, 25,* 120-125.

Steele, B., & Shaver, J. (1992). The dyspnea experience: Nociceptive properties and a model for research and practice. *Advances in Nursing Science, 15*(1), 64–76.

Teel, C. S., Meek, P., McNamara, A. M., & Watson, L. (1997). Perspectives unifying symptom interpretation. *Image: Journal of Nursing Scholarship, 29,* 175–181.

University of California at San Francisco, School of Nursing, Symptom Management Faculty Group. (1994). A model for symptom management. *Image: Journal of Nursing Scholarship, 26,* 272–276.

Vainio, A., Aurinen, A., & Members of the Symptom Prevalence Group. (1996). Prevalence of symptoms among patients with advanced cancer: An international collaborative study. *Journal of Pain and Symptom Management, 12*(1), 3–10.

Wolfe, J., Grier, H. E., Klar, N., Levin, S. B., Ellenbogen, J. M., Salem-Schatz, S., et al. (2000). Symptoms and suffering at the end of life in children with cancer. *The New England Journal of Medicine, 342,* 326–333.

Woods, S. J., Kozachik, S. L., & Hall, R. J. (2010). Subjective sleep quality in women experiencing intimate partner violence: Contributions of situational, psychological, and physiological factors*. *Journal*

of Traumatic Stress, 23, 141–150. doi:10.1002/
jts.20495

Yeh, C. H. (2002). Life experience of Taiwanese adolescents with cancer. *Scandinavian Journal of Caring
Sciences, 16,* 232–239.

Zeppetella, G. (1998). The palliation of dyspnea in terminal disease. *The American Journal of Hospice and
Palliative Care, 15,* 322–330.

5

Self-Efficacy

BARBARA RESNICK

DEFINITION OF KEY TERMS

Mastery experience	The most influential of self-efficacy information is the interpreted result of one's previous performance or mastery experience. Individuals engage in tasks and activities, interpret the results of their actions, use the interpretations to develop beliefs about their capability to engage in subsequent tasks or activities, and act in concert with the beliefs created.
Outcome expectations	The belief that if a specific behavior is completed, there will be a certain outcome. Bandura postulates that because the outcomes an individual expects are the result of the judgments of what he/she can accomplish, outcome expectations are unlikely to contribute to predications of behavior.
Self-efficacy	People's judgments of their capabilities to organize and execute courses of action required to attain designated types of performances. Self-efficacy beliefs provide the foundation for human motivation, well-being, and personal accomplishment.
Social persuasions	Individuals also create and develop self-efficacy beliefs as a result of the social persuasions they receive from others. These persuasions can involve exposure to verbal judgments of others.
Somatic and emotional states	Somatic and emotional states, such as anxiety, stress, arousal, and mood, also provide information about efficacy beliefs. People can gauge their degree of confidence by the emotional state they experience as they contemplate an action.
Vicarious experience	In addition to interpreting the results of their actions, people acquire their self-efficacy beliefs through the vicarious experience of observing others perform tasks. This source of information is weaker than mastery experience in helping to create self-efficacy beliefs but when people are uncertain about their own abilities or when they have limited prior experience, they are more likely to be influenced by observation reactions.

INTRODUCTION

Self-efficacy is defined as an individual's judgment of his or her capabilities to organize and execute courses of action. At the core of self-efficacy theory is the assumption that people can exercise influence over what they do. Through reflective thought, generative use of knowledge and skills to perform a specific behavior, and other tools of self-influence, a person will decide how to behave (Bandura, 1977, 1986, 1995, 1997). To determine self-efficacy, an individual must have the opportunity for self-evaluation or the ability to compare individual output to some sort of evaluative criterion. It is this comparison process that enables an individual to judge performance capability and establish self-efficacy expectation.

HISTORICAL BACKGROUND

Self-efficacy theory is based on social cognitive theory and conceptualizes person–behavior–environment interaction as triadic reciprocality, the foundation for reciprocal determinism (Bandura, 1977, 1986, 1995, 1997). In the initial study (Bandura, 1977) that led to the development of self-efficacy theory, 33 subjects with snake phobias were randomly assigned to three different treatment conditions: (1) enactive attainment, which included actually touching the snakes; (2) role modeling, or seeing others touch the snakes; and (3) the control group. Results suggested that self-efficacy was predictive of subsequent behavior, and enactive attainment resulted in stronger and more generalized (to other snakes) self-efficacy expectations. This early self-efficacy research used an ideal controlled setting in that the individuals with snake phobias were unlikely to seek out opportunities to interact with snakes when away from the laboratory setting. Therefore, there was controlled input of efficacy information. While this ideal situation is not possible in the clinical setting, the theory of self-efficacy has been used to study and predict health behavior change and management in a variety of settings.

DEFINITION OF THEORY CONCEPTS

Bandura, a social scientist, differentiated between two components of self-efficacy theory: self-efficacy and outcome expectations. Self-efficacy expectations are judgments about personal ability to accomplish a given task. Outcome expectations are judgments about what will happen if a given task is successfully accomplished. Self-efficacy and outcome expectations were differentiated because individuals can believe that a certain behavior will result in a specific outcome; however, they may not believe that they are capable of performing the behavior required for the outcome to occur.

The types of outcomes people anticipate generally depend on their judgments of how well they will be able to perform the behavior. Those who consider themselves to be highly efficacious in accomplishing a given behavior will expect favorable outcomes for that behavior. Expected outcomes are dependent on self-efficacy judgments. Therefore, Bandura postulated that expected outcomes may not add much on their own to the prediction of behavior. Bandura (1997) does state, however, that there are instances when outcome expectations can be dissociated from self-efficacy expectations. This occurs either when no action will result in a specific outcome, or the outcome is loosely linked to the level or quality of the performance. For example, if Mrs. White knows that *even if she* regains functional independence by participating in rehabilitation she will still be discharged to a skilled nursing facility rather than back home; her behavior is likely to be influenced by her outcome expectations (discharge to the skilled nursing facility). In this situation, no matter what Mrs. White's performance is, the outcome is the same; thus, outcome expectancy may influence her behavior independent of her self-efficacy beliefs.

Expected outcomes are also partially separable from self-efficacy judgments when extrinsic outcomes are fixed. For example, when a nurse provides care to six patients during an 8-hour shift, the nurse receives a certain salary. When the same nurse cares for 10 patients during the same shift, she receives the same salary. This could negatively impact performance. It is also possible for an individual to believe that he/she is capable of performing a specific behavior, but does not believe that the outcome of performing that behavior is worthwhile. For example, older adults in rehabilitation may believe that they are capable of performing the exercises and activities involved in the rehabilitation process, but may not believe that performing the exercises will result in improved functional ability. Some older adults believe that resting rather than exercising will lead to recovery. In this situation, outcome expectations may have a direct impact on performance.

Outcome expectations are particularly relevant to older adults. These individuals may have high self-efficacy expectations for exercise, but if they do not believe in the outcomes associated with exercise, for example, improved health, strength, or function, then it is unlikely that there will be adherence to a regular exercise program.

SOURCES OF SELF-EFFICACY JUDGMENT

Bandura (1986) suggested that judgment about one's self-efficacy is based on four informational sources: (1) enactive attainment, which is the actual performance of a behavior; (2) vicarious experience or visualizing other similar people perform a behavior; (3) verbal persuasion or exhortation; and (4) physiological state or physiological feedback during a behavior, such as pain or fatigue. The cognitive appraisal of these factors results in a perception of a level of confidence in the individual's ability to perform a certain behavior. The positive performance of this behavior reinforces self-efficacy expectations (Bandura, 1995).

ENACTIVE ATTAINMENT

Enactive attainment has been described as the most influential source of self-efficacy information (Bandura, 1977, 1986). There has been repetition in empirical verification that actually performing an activity strengthens self-efficacy beliefs. Specifically, self-efficacy and outcome expectations play an influential role in the performance of functional activities (Resnick, Galik, Gruber-Baldini, & Zimmerman, 2009; van den Akker-Scheek et al., 2007), adoption and maintenance of exercise behavior (Hays, Pressler, Damush, Rawl, & Clark, 2010; Lee, Arthur, & Avis, 2008; Resnick, Luisi, & Vogel, 2008; Resnick, Shaughnessy, et al., 2009), and optimal self-management of numerous clinical problems such as congestive heart failure (Hiltunen et al., 2005; Padula, Yeaw, & Mistry, 2009), diabetes (Utz et al., 2008), peritoneal dialysis (Su, Lu, Chen, & Wang, 2009), depression (Weng, Dai, Wang, Huang, & Chiang, 2008), and back pain (Göhner & Schlicht, 2006). Enactive attainment generally results in greater strengthening of self-efficacy expectations than do informational sources.

However, performance alone does not establish self-efficacy beliefs. Other factors, such as preconceptions of ability, the perceived difficulty of the task, the amount of effort expended, the external aid received, the situational circumstance, and past successes and failures all impact the individual's cognitive appraisal of self-efficacy (Bandura, 1995). An older adult who strongly believes that he/she is able to bathe and dress independently because he/she has been doing so for 90 years will not likely alter self-efficacy expectations if he/she wakes up with severe arthritic changes one morning and is consequently unable to put on a shirt. However, repeated failures to perform the activity will impact self-efficacy expectations. The relative stability of strong self-efficacy expectations is important; otherwise, an occasional failure or setback could severely impact both self-efficacy expectations and behavior.

VICARIOUS EXPERIENCE

Self-efficacy expectations are also influenced by vicarious experiences or seeing other similar people successfully performing the same activity. There are some conditions, however, which impact the influence of vicarious experience. If the individual has not been exposed to the behavior of interest, or has had little experience with it, vicarious experience is likely to have a greater impact. In addition, when clear guidelines for performance are not explicated, self-efficacy will be more likely to be impacted by the performance of others. Likewise, self-modeling has been noted to influence self-efficacy and outcome expectations and specifically was not to strengthen self-efficacy expectations and related behavior in older adults with diabetes. Such things are kept as personal records of behavior (Resnick, Shaughnessy et al., 2009; Siebolds, Gaedeke, Schwedes, & SMBG Study Group, 2006).

VERBAL PERSUASION

Verbal persuasion involves telling an individual that he/she has the capabilities to master the given behavior. Empirical support for the influence of verbal persuasion has been documented since Bandura's early research of phobias (Bandura, 1977). Verbal persuasion has proven effective in supporting recovery from chronic illness and in health promotion research. Persuasive health influences lead people with a high sense of self-efficacy to intensify efforts at self-directed change of risky health behavior. For example, in rehabilitation settings, verbal persuasion by a nurse had a positive impact on self-efficacy expectations and participation in rehabilitation (Hiltunen et al., 2005), as well as participation in exercise (Galik et al., 2008; Resnick, Gruber-Baldini, Zimmerman, et al., 2009). In nursing, educational interventions are often used as a way to provide verbal encouragement. Multiple examples of this exist in areas such as diabetes management (Fisher, 2006; Utz et al., 2008) and breast-feeding and infant care (Noel-Weiss, Rupp, Cragg, Bassett, & Woodend, 2006).

PHYSIOLOGICAL FEEDBACK

Individuals rely in part on information from their physiological state in order to judge their abilities. Physiological indicators are especially important in relation to coping with stressors, physical accomplishments, and health functioning. Individuals evaluate their physiological state, or arousal, and if aversive, they may avoid performing the behavior. For example, if the older adult has a fear of falling or getting hurt when walking, a high arousal state associated with the fear can limit performance, and decrease the individual's confidence in ability to perform the activity. Likewise, if the rehabilitation activities result in fatigue, pain, or shortness of breath, these symptoms may be interpreted as physical inefficacy, and the older adult may not feel capable of performing the activity.

Interventions can be used to alter the interpretation of physiological feedback and help individuals cope with physical sensations, enhancing self-efficacy and resulting in improved performance. Interventions include things such as elimination of pain, fear of falling, or shortness of breath associated with physical activity (Landsman-Dijkstra, Van Wijck, & Groothoff, 2006; Resnick, Pretzer-Aboff et al., 2008).

RELATIONSHIPS AMONG THE CONCEPTS: THE MODEL

The theory of self-efficacy was derived from social cognitive theory and must be considered within the context of reciprocal determinism. The four sources of experience (direct experience, vicarious experience, judgments by others, and derivation of knowledge by inference) that can potentially influence self-efficacy and outcome expectations interact with characteristics of the individual and the environment. Ideally, self-efficacy and outcome expectations are strengthened by these experiences and subsequently moderate behavior. Since self-efficacy and outcome expectations are influenced by performance of a behavior, it is likely that there is a reciprocal relationship between performance and efficacy expectations.

USE OF THE THEORY IN NURSING RESEARCH

The theory of self-efficacy has been used in nursing research, focusing on clinical aspects of care, education, nursing competency, and professionalism. There have been hundreds of articles in nursing journal using self-efficacy to guide interventions and predict behavior. While the focus of the articles ranges from management of chronic illnesses to education of nurses and parental training, the majority have been related to chronic health problems and participation in health-promoting activities such as exercise, smoking cessation, and weight loss.

The majority of these studies are descriptive in nature, exploring the relationship between self-efficacy expectations and behavior. Although more and more intervention studies are being guided by self-efficacy expectations (Resnick, Galik et al., 2009; Resnick et al., 2007; Siebolds et al., 2006; Utz et al., 2008), the interventions continue to focus mainly on mastery experiences and verbal encouragement usually through education. Although limited, there is some work that is beginning to address the impact of dose effect of the intervention in terms of strengthening self-efficacy (Oka, DeMarco, & Haskell, 2005; Resnick, et al., 2007) or testing the impact of different sources of efficacy information (Resnick, et al., 2007). Oka et al. (2005), for example, reported that self-efficacy was not strengthened following only a single treadmill exercise activity that continued in an exercise program. In addition, mastery alone was not noted to be more effective than verbal encouragement, physiological feedback, and cueing with self-modeling (Resnick, et al., 2007). The most important factor with regard to the use of the theory of self-efficacy in nursing research is that the researcher maintains the behavioral specificity by developing a specific fit between the behavior that is being considered and the efficacy and outcome expectations. If the behavior of interest is walking for 20 minutes every day, the self-efficacy measure should focus on the challenges related to this specific behavior (time, fatigue, pain, or fear of falling).

SELF-EFFICACY STUDIES RELATED TO HEALTH BEHAVIORS

Self-efficacy has been used to improve and understand health behaviors with regard to exercise (Chang, Fang, & Yang, 2006; Hays et al., 2010; Lee et al., 2008; Murrock & Madigan, 2008; Resnick, Luisi et al., 2008; Resnick, Michael et al., 2008; Resnick, Shaughnessy et al., 2009; van den Akker-Scheek et al., 2007). Specifically, these nursing studies considered the impact of motivational interventions and engaging individuals in exercise activities on self-efficacy expectations and explored relationships between self-efficacy and outcome expectations and exercise behavior. In contrast to Bandura's earlier findings (Bandura, 1997), which stressed that self-efficacy expectations were better predictors of behavior than outcome expectations, in several nursing studies, outcome expectations, rather than self-efficacy expectations, were predictive of exercise behavior (Murrock & Madigan, 2008; Resnick, Luisi et al., 2008).

Self-efficacy theory has also been used to address health behaviors such as healthy eating in rural women (Walker, Pullen, Hertzog, Boeckner, & Hageman, 2006), health-promoting behaviors in incarcerated men (Loeb, Steffensmeier, & Lawrence, 2008), osteoporosis screening (Hsieh, Wang, McCubbin, Zhang, & Inouye, 2008), Papanicolaou (Pap) testing (Tung, Nguyen, & Tran, 2008) in Asian adult samples, and smoking cessation (Kim, 2006). Across all of these studies, there were significant positive relationships between self-efficacy and behavior of interest.

SELF-EFFICACY AND CULTURAL AND NURSING CARE COMPETENCE

Cultural competence in nurses has been considered by using a measure of knowledge of cultural concepts, knowledge of cultural life patterns for specific ethnic groups, and self-efficacy in performing cultural nursing skills (Hagman, 2006). Findings indicated that nurses were moderately efficacious in cultural knowledge and abilities. Self-efficacy expectations associated with dementia care management have also been considered (Connor et al., 2009), as self-efficacy for providing restorative care (Resnick, Galik et al., 2008), self-efficacy for knowledge of use of assistive devices (Roelands, Van Oost, Depoorter, Buysse, & Stevens, 2006), and self-efficacy for professional nursing behavior (Manojlovich, 2005). Self-efficacy either directly influenced outcome behaviors or mediated these behaviors.

SELF-EFFICACY AND FUNCTIONAL PERFORMANCE

Self-efficacy has been considered with regard to functional performance, particularly with regard to adults undergoing orthopedic interventions (Resnick, Galik et al., 2009; van den Akker-Scheek et al., 2007). Although interventions did not always strengthen self-efficacy with regard to functional behaviors, there was an association between these beliefs and performance of function.

SELF-EFFICACY AND PATIENT SELF-MANAGEMENT

Nursing research frequently uses self-efficacy theory to address self-care and self-management across a variety of clinical problems. For example, self-efficacy has been used with regard to self-care management of post-acute cardiac events and associated with congestive heart failure (Hiltunen et al., 2005; Padula et al., 2009), diabetes self-care management (Utz et al., 2008), and self-management for peritoneal dialysis (Su et al., 2009), managing depression (Weng et al., 2008), back pain (Göhner & Schlicht, 2006), and birth control. Nursing interventions intended to improve adherence to self-care behaviors were guided by self-efficacy theory in these studies, and findings indicated that there were improvements in self-efficacy as well as anticipated behaviors. Research Application 5.1 provides a description of a study that uses self-efficacy for the framework to improve outcomes in individuals with heart failure. More recently, self-efficacy-based interventions have been used to help adults manage multiple

Research Application 5.1

This study, using self-efficacy as a theoretical framework, compared the effectiveness of home-based inspiratory muscle training (IMT) to educational materials in improving IM strength, reducing dyspnea, improving self-efficacy for breathing, and higher levels of health-related quality of life. Subjects were recruited from physician's offices, home care agencies, provider referral, and newspaper advertisements. To be included in the study, subjects had to be adult, community dwelling, medically stable, and without coexisting pulmonary disease or cognitive impairment. Thirty-six subjects out of the 288 that were screened were found to be eligible and of those 36, 32 agreed to participate. The study employed a two-group quasi-experimental design with subjects diagnosed with heart failure and dyspnea randomly assigned via a coin toss to one of two groups, the treatment group, which received individual training to improve breathing or the control group, which received standard educational materials. The treatment group was comprised of 15 subjects and the control group of 17 subjects.

The individual training consisted of a demonstration of the threshold device by a nurse research assistant with return demonstration. The subjects then trained with the device daily, 10–20 minutes/day for a week. The control group received a booklet that addressed basic anatomy and physiology of the heart, health regimes related to diet, medication, sleep and rest, and activity patterns. It also advised on what and when to report to their physician and incorporated principles of self-efficacy.

The two groups were compared to inspiratory muscle strength (IMS) measured by pulmonary inspiration score; dyspnea, using the Borg scale and the Chronic Respiratory Disease Questionnaire (CRDQ); and self-efficacy with the COPD Self-Efficacy scale. Data were collected over a 12-week period. The training group experienced increased IM strength (48.72 ± 25.69 to 78.5 ± 37.08), whereas the educational group remained unchanged (52.25 ± 27.32 to 52.61 ± 28.25). There was a statistically significant difference in the experience of dyspnea between the two groups as measured by rankings on shortness of breath with three activities at baseline, 6 weeks, and 12 weeks. Between 6 and 12 weeks $p = 0.027$. There were no statistically significant differences in COPD Self-Efficacy scale scores between the two groups.

Self-efficacy provided the framework for both the individual training of subjects and the education materials created and provided to subjects. The study did conclude that nurse-coached, home-based IMT is a safe and effective approach to improving IMS.

Source: Padula, C. A. Yeaw, E., & Mistry, S. (2009). A home-based nurse-coached inspiratory muscle training intervention in heart failure. *Applied Nursing Research*, 22(1), 18–25.

chronic illnesses. Specifically, education during a 2-hour workshop focused on management of chronic illness by building patient-directed skills such as medication management was noted to improve health and quality of life among older adults with multiple chronic illnesses (Hochhalter, Song, Rush, Sklar, & Stevens, 2010).

SELF-EFFICACY AND BREAST-FEEDING AND INFANT CARE

Another common use of self-efficacy theory in nursing research is around the area of mothering, specifically with regard to breast-feeding and infant care (Noel-Weiss et al., 2006; Padula et al., 2009; Prasopkittikun, Tilokskulchai, Sinsuksai, & Sitthimongkol, 2006). Self-efficacy expectations were shown to be associated with breast-feeding and infant care, and interventions to strengthen self-efficacy associated with these behaviors improved adherence to nursing behaviors.

SELF-EFFICACY AND CANCER CARE

Nurse researchers in the area of oncology identified relationships among self-efficacy, cancer prevention, and adaptation to cancer. Strong self-efficacy expectations predict behaviors such as intention to quit smoking, increased participation in screening programs, and adjustment to cancer diagnosis (Griffiths, Kidd, Pike, & Chan, 2010; Jennings-Sanders, 2009; Park, Song, Hur, & Kim, 2009). Increased self-efficacy is associated with increased adherence to treatment, increased self-care behaviors, and decreased physical and psychological symptoms.

SELF-EFFICACY FOR BONE HEALTH

Self-efficacy interventions have been used to increase adherence to behaviors that are consistent with good bone health such as high calcium diets and exercise (Aree-Ue, Pothiban, Belza, Sucamvang, & Panuthai, 2006; Nahm et al., 2010). These studies have been both descriptive and have used education and mastery experiences to strengthen self-efficacy expectations in exercise focused on bone strengthening, adherence to bone building medications, and diet.

SELF-EFFICACY FOR FALL PREVENTION

Self-efficacy interventions have been used to strengthen self-efficacy expectations related to fear of falling (Zijlstra, Tennstedt, van Haastregt, van Eijk, & Kempen, 2006). This focus of self-efficacy for fear of falling is based on the assumption that individuals vary in terms of how much they fear engaging in certain activities. Strengthening fear of falling is assumed to result in increased performance of the behavior of interest.

SELF-EFFICACY FOR EXERCISE

Resnick (Galik et al., 2008; Resnick, Galik et al., 2009; Resnick, Gruber-Baldini, Zimmerman, et al., 2009), using combined quantitative and qualitative approaches, demonstrated that self-efficacy and outcome expectations influence older adults' participation in functional activities and exercise. Based on these findings, interventions were developed to strengthen self-efficacy and outcome expectations related to these activities. Overall, this work uses self-efficacy theory to encourage healthy behaviors such as engaging in regular exercise. The work by Resnick and her interdisciplinary team was started with qualitative research to explore factors that influenced motivation to engage in such behaviors (Resnick, Luisi et al., 2008; Resnick & Spellbring, 2000). Once identified through qualitative study, specific challenges and benefits of performing exercise were used to develop the self-efficacy and outcome expectation scales that were appropriate for this behavior. Development of self-efficacy expectation measures was based on Bandura's (1977) early work with snake phobias. This approach included a paper and pencil measure that listed activities, from least to most difficult, in a specific behavioral domain. Respondents were given a 100-point scale, divided into 10-unit intervals ranging from 0, which is completely uncertain, to 10, which is completely certain, to identify the extent of confidence they had in performing a particular activity (strength of self-efficacy) given the existence of a challenge or benefit. An example of items on a self-efficacy scale for exercise follows:

How confident are you right now that you could exercise three times per week for 20 minutes if:

	Not confident		Very confident
1. The weather was bothering you	0	1 2 3 4 5 6 7 8 9	10
2. You were bored by the program or activity	0	1 2 3 4 5 6 7 8 9	10

The development of appropriate self-efficacy and outcome expectation measures enables the testing of interventions designed to help participants believe in the benefits and overcome the challenges of performing selected activities. Examples of how this has been done are demonstrated in the WALC (Walk, Address unpleasant symptoms, Learn about exercise, Cueing to exercise) intervention and the Exercise Plus Program (Resnick et al., 2007), the Senior Exercise Self-efficacy Project (Resnick, Luisi et al., 2008), PRAISEDD, and exercise intervention program for minority older adults living in senior housing (Resnick, Shaughnessy et al., 2009) and multiple function-focused care interventions in nursing homes (Galik et al., 2008; Resnick, Gruber-Baldini, Galik et al., 2009; Resnick, Gruber-Baldini, ZImmerman et al., 2009). All of these interventions incorporate the four sources of information known to influence self-efficacy and outcome expectations. Specifically, they both use verbal encouragement, decreasing unpleasant sensations, cueing and role modeling, and the actual performance of the behavior.

In addition, self-efficacy theory has been used as a foundation for programs that encourage functional and physical activity in older adults (Resnick, 2002; Resnick, Luisi, & Vogel, 2008; Phillips, 2006; Pretzer-Aboff, Galik, & Resnick, 2009; Resnick, Galik et al., 2009; Resnick, Gruber-Baldini, Zimmerman et al., 2009), and increase direct care worker (DCW) performance of function-focused care, or care that optimizes function and physical activity among older adults. A detailed description of this intervention, referred to as function-focused care, is provided in Box 5.1.

Box 5.1 Function-Focused Care in Assisted Living (FFC-AL) Intervention

Following pilot testing (Resnick, et al., 2009), FFC-AL was tested using a cluster-randomized controlled trial with a repeated measure design (Resnick, Galik, Gruber-Baldini et al., in press). The intervention persisted and participants were followed over a 12-month period. A total of four AL communities were matched on ownership and all were similar in size, staffing, and services. A total of 171 residents and 96 DCWs were recruited from these sites.

The FFC-AL intervention was coordinated and implemented by a research Function-Focused Care Nurse (FFCN) with support from an interdisciplinary research team that included advanced practice nurses, social work, and physical therapy. The FFCN worked with the intervention sites 15 hours per week for the first 6 months of the intervention, 8 hours a week for the next 3 months, and 4 hours a week for the final 3 months of the intervention. To assure sustainability of the function-focused care philosophy, each treatment site identified a staff champion who worked with the FFCN, learned the four components necessary to implement and sustain the function-focused care philosophy, and helped to institutionalize function-focused care within the community. Working with the champion, the FFCN implemented the four components of FFC-AL: (1) environment and policy/procedure assessments, (2) education, (3) developing function-focused goals, and (4) mentoring and motivating.

Components were implemented sequentially although overlapped in that once initiated they continued throughout the course of the intervention. Component 1 involved having the FFCN evaluate the environment and community policies and procedures to determine if they presented barriers to implementation of a function-focused care approach. Environments, for example, were evaluated for pleasant walking areas, destination sites, and appropriate bed and chair heights. Findings were discussed during the course of the 12-month study period with AL administrative staff to facilitate appropriate changes. Component 2, the education component, was then implemented and all staff were invited to attend a 30-minute session on implementing a function-focused care approach (e.g., benefits of FFC, motivational strategies to engage residents, and recommendations for how to incorporate FFC into routine care activities).

Component 3, individual goal setting, was initiated by the FFCN working closely with the resident, staff champion, and DCWs. Residents' physical capability was evaluated using a Physical Capability Assessment form. This assessment evaluated cognitive status and functional ability (e.g., range of motion and balance) of residents. Goals included things such as walking to the dining room, going to exercise classes, or engaging in personal care activities. Once individual goals were established for all participants, Component 4, mentoring and motivating, was initiated. This involved the FFCN and community champion mentoring DCWs and helping them motivate residents to work toward goal achievement. Motivational interventions were used to reward and recognize staff for providing function-focused care and residents for participating in exercise-related activities. Ongoing informal education and positive role modeling at the bedside related to function-focused care was provided by the FFCN and staff champion throughout the course of the 12-month intervention.

AL communities randomized to control received FFC-Education only. All staff in these communities were invited to attend an educational session on function-focused care. The education material was identical to that provided to the treatment group, with the exclusion of motivational techniques to engage residents in functional and physical activity.

Study Results

The majority of the DCWs were female ($n = 95$; 99%) and black ($n = 59$; 62%), with a mean age of 41.7 years (SD = 13.8). The residents were mostly female (80%), white (93%), and widowed (80%) with a mean age of 87.7 years (SD = 5.7). Outcomes for residents included psychosocial domains (mood, resilience, and self-efficacy and outcome expectations for function and physical activity), function, gait, and balance, and actigraphy. Outcomes for DCWs included knowledge, performance, and beliefs associated with function-focused care.

(continued)

> ### Box 5.1   Function-Focused Care in Assisted Living (FFC-AL) Intervention (*Continued*)
>
> Based on observations, DCWs in treatment sites provided more function-focused care by 12 months than those in the control sites. The treatment group increased from providing function-focused care during 76% of observed care interactions at baseline to 82% at 4 months, and 90% at 12 months ($p = 0.001$) compared to the control group which provided function-focused care during 75% of care interactions at baseline and 4 months and then this decreased to 69% of care interactions at 12 months.
>
> Residents in treatment sites demonstrated less decline in function, a greater percentage returned to ambulatory status, and there were positive trends demonstrating more time in moderate level physical activity at 4 months and more overall counts of activity at 12 months when compared to residents in control sites. Specifically, the control group declined 6.95 points versus 4.33 points for the treatment group, $p = 0.01$ in overall function based on the Barthel Index (scores range from 0 to 100 with higher scores indicative of more independent function). From baseline to 12 months, 13 (17%) residents in the treatment group versus 2 (4%) residents in the control group resumed walking functional distances versus remaining wheelchair dependent (chi square = 4.94, $p = 0.026$). Although not significantly different, residents in the intervention group showed a greater increase in the amount of time spent in moderate level physical activity at 4 months ($p = 0.08$). Specifically, the treatment group increased from 0.43 at baseline to 1.00 minute of moderate level physical activity with 24 hours versus the control group, which had a decline from 0.51 to 0.35 minutes. In addition, the treatment group had an increase in counts of activity from 40,668 at 4 months to 46,960 at 12 months, while the control group declined from 36,834 at 4 months to 32,563 at 12 months ($p = 0.07$). There were no treatment effects on residents' self-efficacy or outcome expectations, mood, resilience, balance, or gait.
>
> This study supports the use of FFC-AL to change care behaviors among DCWs and suggests that FFC-AL may help prevent some of the persistent functional decline and sedentary behavior commonly noted in these settings.

Source: Resnick, B., Galik, E., Gruber-Baldini, A., & Zimmerman, S. (2009). Implementing a restorative care philosophy of care in assisted living: Pilot testing of Res-Care-AL. *Journal of the American Academy of Nurse Practitioners, 21*(2), 123–133.

USE OF THE THEORY IN NURSING PRACTICE

Translation of research findings into practice is not often done in a timely fashion. This is particularly true of research findings that focus on behavior change. There is, however, evidence to demonstrate that the theory of self-efficacy can help direct nursing care. The theory has been particularly helpful with regard to motivating individuals to participate in health-promoting activities such as regular exercise, smoking cessation, weight loss, and going for recommended cancer screenings.

The ultimate goal of any intervention implemented in a research setting is to maintain the intervention over time and persist in day-to-day clinical practice. Function-focused care interventions are developed so as to be integrated into routine care and continue even at the end of the research activities. It has been demonstrated that function-focused care interventions persist in clinical settings.

In clinical practice, function-focused care, like any innovative intervention, requires a champion. The champion can be self-identified or identified by administrative staff to take on the project or focus of care. Assisted Living (AL) communities that have successfully implemented function-focused care have been identified as such a champion. This individual varied in terms of professional level and administrative position. The individual, however, believed in the benefit of optimizing function and physical activity among older adults and was passionate about helping other caregivers to achieve that type of care. Using Middle Range Theories 5.1 provides a description of the theory applied to a restorative care activity.

EVALUATION OF THE ENVIRONMENT AND POLICIES

The first step in the implementation of a function-focused care approach is to evaluate the current environment and policies within the community. Policy and environmental changes should be established to facilitate implementation of function-focused care approaches with staff and residents. The communities altered their environments to optimize function in simple ways by doing such things as setting up pleasant and safe

The theory of self-efficacy served as the foundation for the development of a restorative care intervention (Res-Care) that was used to teach and motivate nursing assistants to provide restorative care to residents of nursing homes. This particular project was implemented in 12 nursing homes in the greater Baltimore area. Nursing assistants attended a 6-week in-service program that introduced them to: (a) the philosophy of restorative care in this program, contrasting it to more traditional approaches; (b) motivational strategies based on the theory of self-efficacy; (c) integration of restorative care activities with personal care activities (bathing, dressing, and feeding); (d) integration of restorative care activities (exercise) during transfers and ambulation; (e) documentation of time spent in restorative care activities; and (e) overcoming challenges in providing restorative care. Specific examples of restorative care were provided. For instance, to promote bed mobility, the resident was instructed to move in bed and given time to accomplish the task and/or was given step-by-step instructions on how to move in bed.

The effectiveness of this approach was evaluated using a number of outcome measures. It was determined that the intervention accounted for some improvement in balance and mobility and less decline in gait but not in overall function, contractures, and muscle strength.

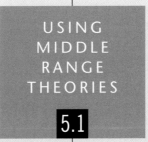

USING MIDDLE RANGE THEORIES

5.1

Source: Resnick, V., Gruber-Baldini, A. L., Zimmerman, S., Galik, E., Pretzer-Aboff, I., & Hebel, J. R. (2009). Nursing home resident outcomes from the Res-Care Intervention. *Journal of the American Geriatric Society, 57*, 1156–1165.

walking areas, so there were chairs for residents to sit in to rest, clutter was removed from residents' living spaces to encourage ambulation, and new exercise-focused classes were developed for resident activities to replace sedentary activities. Policy changes included new Service Plan Forms, which are required in AL communities, that included function-focused care goals for all residents. The function-focused care goals delineated what the resident was required to do with regard to function and physical activity and how the DCW would help the resident achieve those goals (e.g., remind the individual to go to exercise class).

Self-efficacy-based mentoring and motivation of staff occurs via ongoing formal and informal education of DCWs. Following basic education of all staff during a single 30-minute in-service program, all new staff must go through a function-focused care training module and pass the function-focused care knowledge test with an 80% or greater, or repeat the module. The champion provides monthly oversight to DCWs in these communities during monthly observations of an interaction between a DCW and a resident and provides positive feedback regarding ways in which the DCW encouraged and facilitated function and physical activity. Verbal encouragement is provided to the DCW to continue these positive interventions and examples, and role modeling provided to increase functional engagement and physical activity of the resident during routine care activities.

Reward systems are established within clinical settings for the DCWs and the residents. DCWs are recognized with gold stars on a bulletin board to indicate their exemplary performance of function-focused care during observations. Rewards for residents include a program called "Gifts of the Heart." Residents receive tokens or tickets for participating in function-focused care activities (e.g., a resident who walked to the dining room or attended an exercise class). Residents collect their tokens and then trade them for prizes from a glass display case of gifts.

Taken together, the verbal encouragement through education and goal setting, role modeling, ongoing awareness and changes in the environment and policies to eliminate unpleasant sensations around function and physical activity (e.g., providing places for the residents to rest), and the strengthening of self-efficacy that occurs as DCWs and residents engage in function-focused care activities assure that this innovative philosophy of care persists in the clinical setting.

SUMMARY

The studies done by nurse researchers using the theory of self-efficacy provide support for the importance of self-efficacy and outcome expectations with regard to behavior change. They also provide support for the effectiveness of specific interventions that have been tested to strengthen both self-efficacy and outcome expectations and thereby improve behavior. It is important to note, however, that these studies have also demonstrated that self-efficacy and outcome expectations may not be the only predictors of behavior.

Other variables such as tension/anxiety, barriers to behavior, and other psychosocial experiences impact behavior. Bandura (1986) recognized that expectations alone would not result in behavior change if there was no incentive to perform, or if there were inadequate resources or external constraints. Certainly, an individual may believe that he/she can participate in a rehabilitation program, but may not have the resources (i.e., transportation or money) to do so. Moreover, increasingly, it is recognized that use of a comprehensive social ecological model (SEM) approach, which incorporates intrapersonal, interpersonal (including social networks), environmental, and policy factors, is needed to positively influence preventive health behaviors (Sallis et al., 2006).

Self-efficacy theory is situation specific. It is difficult, therefore, to generalize an individual's self-efficacy from one type of behavior to another. If an individual has high self-efficacy with regard to diet management, this may or may not generalize to persistence in an exercise program. Future nursing research needs to focus on the degree to which specific self-efficacy behaviors can be generalized. To what degree is self-efficacy a dimension of individual humanness, distinct for each person, but consistent across a range of related behaviors for one person?

Measurement of self-efficacy and outcome expectations requires the development of situation-specific scales with a series of activities listed in order of increasing difficulty, or by a contextual arrangement in non-psychomotor skills such as dietary modification (Resnick, 2002; Resnick, Luisi, & Vogel, 2008; Phillips, 2006). It is important to carefully construct these scales and establish evidence of reliability and validity. These scales, which are behavior specific, can be used as the foundation for assessing an individual's self-care abilities in a particular area. Interventions can then be developed that are relevant for that individual.

Current research, as part of the Patient Reported Outcomes Measurement Information System (PROMIS) Program, will hopefully add to the knowledge of measurement of self-efficacy by assuring that the full spectrum of behaviors associated with management of chronic illness and the challenges encountered by patients with regard to those behaviors (e.g., confidence driving at night) are addressed. This type of exciting program of research will be useful for guiding future nursing interventions in this area.

A major problem with the use of the theory of self-efficacy in nursing research has been the lack of consideration of outcome expectations. In particular, with regard to exercise in older adults, outcome expectations have been noted to be better predictors of exercise behavior than self-efficacy expectations (Ferrier, Dunlop, & Blanchard, 2010; Resnick, 2002; Resnick, Luisi, & Vogel, 2008; Phillips, 2006; Sirur, Richardson, Wishart, & Hanna, 2009). Consideration also needs to be given to the influence of self-efficacy expectations beyond the initiation of behavior to focus more on long-term adherence. Clearly, social cognitive theory and the theory of self-efficacy have helped guide nursing research related to behavior change. Ongoing studies are needed to continue to evaluate the impact of both self-efficacy and outcome expectations on behavior change, as well as develop and test interventions that strengthen these expectations.

ANALYSIS OF THEORY

Using the criteria presented in Chapter 2, critique the theory of Self-Efficacy. Compare your conclusions about the theory with those found in Appendix A. A researcher who has worked with the theory completed the analysis found in the appendix.

Internal Criticism	External Criticism
1. Clarity	1. Reality convergence
2. Consistency	2. Utility
3. Adequacy	3. Significance
4. Logical development	4. Discrimination
5. Level of theory development	5. Scope of theory
	6. Complexity

CRITICAL THINKING EXERCISES

1. As a nurse on a medical surgical unit you are getting ready to discharge a patient home who has just had a hip fracture and a right hemiorthoplasty to repair the fracture. She is independent with ambulation using her walker and will have some home physical therapy. Of note, however, she had a bone density scan that indicated severe osteoporosis and has been started on a bisphosphonate and calcium. Your goal at discharge is to increase the likelihood that she will adhere to taking these medications. Address the interventions you would do to ensure this.

2. You have just moved to New Mexico and are very concerned about working with a large percentage of Spanish-speaking older adults. You know little about their culture. Address what interventions you might do for yourself to facilitate this transition in your nursing career.

3. You have just started working on a maternity ward and noted that the mothers admitted who are younger than 20 years of age have a great deal of difficulty with the idea of breast-feeding and how to begin to breast-feed. Develop an intervention that you could implement to optimize your nursing interventions with these individuals.

WEB RESOURCES

Visit **http://thePoint.lww.com/Peterson3e** for helpful web resources related to this chapter.

REFERENCES

Aree-Ue, S., Pothiban, L., Belza, B., Sucamvang, K., & Panuthai, S. (2006). Osteoporosis preventive behavior in Thai older adults: Feasibility and acceptability. *Journal of Gerontological Nursing, 32*(7), 23–30.

Bandura, A. (1977). Self-efficacy: Toward a unifying theory of behavioral change. *Psychological Review, 84,* 191–215.

Bandura, A. (1986). *Social foundations of thought and action.* Englewood Cliffs, NJ: Prentice Hall.

Bandura, A. (1995). *Self-efficacy in changing societies.* New York: Cambridge University Press.

Bandura, A. (1997). *Self-efficacy: The exercise of control.* New York: W.H. Freeman.

Chang, S., Fang, M., & Yang, Y. (2006). The effectiveness of a health promotion programme for women in southern Taiwan. *International Journal of Nursing Practice, 15*(5), 252–259.

Connor, K., McNeese-Smith, D., van Servellen, G., Chang, B., Lee, M., Cheng, E., et al. (2009). Insight into dementia care management using social-behavioral theory and mixed methods. *Nursing Research, 58*(5), 348–358.

Ferrier, S., Dunlop, N., & Blanchard, C. (2010). The role of outcome expectations and self-efficacy in explaining physical activity behaviors of individuals with multiple sclerosis. *Behavioral Medicine, 36*(1), 7–11.

Fisher, K. (2006). School nurses' perceptions of self-efficacy in providing diabetes care. *School Nurse, 22*(4), 223–228.

Galik, E., Resnick, B., Gruber-Baldini, A., Nahm, E., Pearson, K., & Pretzer-Aboff, I. (2008). Pilot testing of the restorative care intervention for the cognitively impaired. *Journal of the American Medical Directors Association, 9*(7), 516–522.

Göhner, W., & Schlicht, W. (2006). Preventing chronic back pain: Evaluation of a theory-based cognitive-behavioural training programme for patients with sub-acute back pain. *Patient Education and Counseling, 64*(1–3), 87–95.

Griffiths, M., Kidd, S., Pike, S., & Chan, J. (2010). The tobacco addiction recovery program: Initial outcome findings. *Archives of Psychiatric Nursing, 24*(4), 239–246.

Hagman, L. (2006). Cultural self-efficacy of licensed registered nurses in New Mexico. *Journal of Cultural Diversity, 13*(2), 105–112.

Hays, L., Pressler, S., Damush, T., Rawl, S., & Clark, D. (2010). Exercise adoption among older, low-income women at risk for cardiovascular disease. *Public Health Nursing, 27*(1), 79–88.

Hiltunen, E., Winder, P., Rait, M., Buselli, E., Carroll, D., & Rankin, S. (2005). Implementation of efficacy enhancement nursing interventions with cardiac elders. *Rehabilitation Nursing, 30*(6), 221–229.

Hochhalter, A., Song, J., Rush, J., Sklar, L., & Stevens, A. (2010). Making the Most of Your Healthcare intervention for older adults with multiple chronic illnesses (includes abstract). *Patient Education & Counseling, 81*(2), 201–213.

Hsieh, C., Wang, C., McCubbin, M., Zhang, S., & Inouye, J. (2008). Factors influencing osteoporosis preventive behaviours: Testing a path model. *Journal of Advanced Nursing, 63*(3), 336–345.

Jennings-Sanders, A. (2009). Measuring self efficacy for mammography screening in older African American women. *ABNF Journal, 20*(2), 49–52.

Kim, Y. (2006). Adolescents' smoking behavior and its relationships with psychological constructs based on transtheoretical model: A cross-sectional survey. *International Journal of Nursing Studies, 43*(4), 439–446.

Landsman-Dijkstra, J., Van Wijck, R., & Groothoff, J. (2006). The long term lasting effectiveness on self-efficacy, attribution style, expression of emotions and quality of life of a body awareness program for chronic a-specific psychosomatic symptoms. *Patient Education and Counseling, 60*(1), 66–79.

Lee, L., Arthur, A., & Avis, M. (2008). Using self-efficacy theory to develop interventions that help older people overcome psychological barriers to physical activity: a discussion paper. *International Journal of Nursing Studies, 45*(11), 1690–1699.

Loeb, S., Steffensmeier, D., & Lawrence, F. (2008). Comparing incarcerated and community-dwelling older men's health. *Western Journal of Nursing Research, 30*(2), 234–249.

Manojlovich, M. (2005). Promoting nurses' self-efficacy: A leadership strategy to improve practice. *Journal of Nursing Administration, 35*(5), 271–278.

Murrock, C., & Madigan, E. (2008). Self-efficacy and social support as mediators between culturally specific dance and lifestyle physical activity. *Research Theory and Nursing Practice, 22*(3), 192–204.

Nahm, E., Barker, B., Resnick, B., Covington, B., Magaziner, J., & Brennan, P. (2010). Effects of a social cognitive theory-based hip fracture prevention web site for older adults. *Computers, Informatics, Nursing, 28*(6), 371–377.

Noel-Weiss, J., Rupp, A., Cragg, B., Bassett, V., & Woodend, A. (2006). Randomized controlled trial to determine effects of prenatal breastfeeding workshop on maternal breastfeeding self-efficacy and breastfeeding duration. *Journal of Obstetrics and Gynecological Neonatal Nursing, 35*(5), 616–624.

Oka, R., DeMarco, T., & Haskell, W. (2005). Effect of treadmill testing and exercise training on self-efficacy in patients with heart failure. *European Journal of Cardiovascular Nursing, 4*(3), 215–219.

Padula, C., Yeaw, E., & Mistry, S. (2009). A home-based nurse-coached inspiratory muscle training intervention in heart failure. *Applied Nursing Research, 22*(1), 18–25.

Park, S., Song, H., Hur, H., & Kim, G. (2009). Effects of a cognition-oriented breast self-examination intervention for Korean women and their spouses. *Public Health Nursing, 26*(3), 259–268.

Phillips, R. (2006). An examination of the impact of self-efficacy interventions versus outcome expectation interventions on efficacy beliefs, expectancy beliefs, participation, and functional performance in a population of medical rehabilitation patients. *Clinical Psychology*. The Fielding Institute, 182.

Prasopkittikun, T., Tilokskulchai, F., Sinsuksai, N., & Sitthimongkol, Y. (2006). Self-Efficacy in Infant Care Scale: Development and psychometric testing. *Nursing Health Science, 8*(1), 44–50.

Pretzer-Aboff, I., Galik, E., & Resnick, B. (2009). Parkinson's disease: Barriers and facilitators to optimizing function. *Rehabilitation Nursing, 34*(2), 55–63.

Resnick, B. (2002). Testing the impact of the WALC intervention on exercise adherence in older adults. *Journal of Gerontological Nursing, 28*(6), 32–40.

Resnick, B., Galik, E., Gruber-Baldini, A., & Zimmerman, S. (2009). Implementing a restorative care philosophy of care in assisted living: Pilot testing of Res-Care-AL. *Journal of the American Academy of Nurse Practitioners, 21*(2), 123–133.

Resnick, B., Galik, E., Gruber-Baldini, A., & Zimmerman, S. (In press). Testing the impact of function focused care in assisted living. *Journal of the American Geriatrics Society*.

Resnick, B., Galik, E., Pretzer-Aboff, I., Rogers, V., & Gruber-Baldini, A. (2008). Testing the reliability and validity of self-efficacy and outcome expectations of restorative care performed by nursing assistants. *Journal of Nursing Care Quality, 23*(2), 162–169.

Resnick, B., Gruber-Baldini, A., Galik, E., Pretzer-Aboff, I., Russ, K., Hebel, J., et al. (2009). Changing the philosophy of care in long-term care: Testing of the restorative care intervention. *The Gerontologist 49*(2), 175–184.

Resnick, B., Gruber-Baldini, A., Zimmerman, S., Galik, E., Pretzer-Aboff, I., Russ, K., et al. (2009). Nursing home resident outcomes from the Res-Care intervention. *Journal of the American Geriatrics Society, 57*(7), 1156–1165.

Resnick, B., Luisi, D., & Vogel, A. (2008). Testing The Senior Exercise Self-efficacy Pilot Project (SESEP) for use with urban dwelling minority older adults. *Public Health Nursing, 25*(3), 221–234.

Resnick, B., Michael, K., Shaughnessy, M., Nahm, E., Kopunek, S., Whitall, J., et al. (2008). Inflated perceptions of physical activity after stroke: Pairing self-report with physiologic measures. *Journal of Physical Activity and Health, 5*(2), 308–318.

Resnick, B., Orwig, D., Yu-Yahiro, J., Hawkes, W., Shardell, M., Hebel, J., et al. (2007). Testing the effectiveness of the exercise plus program in older women post hip fracture. *Annals of Behavioral Medicine, 34*(1), 67–76.

Resnick, B., Pretzer-Aboff, I., Galik, E., Russ, K., Cayo, J., Simpson, M., et al. (2008). Barriers and benefits to implementing a restorative care intervention in nursing homes. *Journal of the American Medical Directors Association, 9*(2), 102–108.

Resnick, B., Shaughnessy, M., Galik, E., Scheve, A., Fitten, R., Morrison, T., et al. (2009). Pilot testing of the PRAISEDD intervention among African American and low income older adults. *Journal of Cardiovascular Nursing 24*(5), 352–361.

Resnick, B., & Spellbring, A. (2000). Understanding what motivates older adults to exercise. *Journal of Gerontological Nursing, 26*(3), 34–42.

Roelands, M., Van Oost, P., Depoorter, A., Buysse, A., & Stevens, V. (2006). Introduction of assistive devices: Home nurses' practices and beliefs. *Journal of Advanced Nursing, 54*(2), 180–188.

Sallis, J., Cervero, R., Ascher, W., Henderson, K., Kraft, M., & Kerr, J. (2006). Ecological approach to creating active living communities. *Annual Review of Public Health, 27,* 297–322.

Siebolds, M., Gaedeke, O., Schwedes, U., & SMBG Study Group. (2006). Self-monitoring of blood glucose-psychological aspects relevant to changes in HbA1c in type 2 diabetic patients treated with diet or diet plus oral antidiabetic medication. *Patient Education Counseling, 62,* 104–110.

Sirur, R., Richardson, J., Wishart, L., & Hanna, S. (2009). The role of theory in increasing adherence to prescribed practice. *Physiotherapy Canada, 61*(2), 68–77.

Su, C., Lu, X., Chen, W., & Wang, T. (2009). Promoting self-management improves the health status of patients having peritoneal dialysis. *Journal of Advanced Nursing, 65*(7), 1381–1389.

Tung, W., Nguyen, D., & Tran, D. (2008). Applying the transtheoretical model to cervical cancer screening in Vietnamese-American women. *International Nursing Review, 55*(1), 73–80.

Utz, S., Williams, I., Jones, R., Hinton, I., Alexander, G., Yan, G., et al. (2008). Culturally tailored intervention for rural African Americans with type 2 diabetes. *Diabetes Education, 34*(5), 854–865.

van den Akker-Scheek, I., Zijlstra, W., Groothoff, J., van Horn, J., Bulstra, S., & Stevens, M. (2007). Groningen orthopaedic exit strategy: Validation of a support program after total hip or knee arthroplasty. *Patient Education and Counseling, 65*(2), 171–179.

Walker, S., Pullen, C., Hertzog, M., Boeckner, L., & Hageman, P. (2006). Determinants of older rural women's activity and eating. *Western Journal of Nursing Research, 28*(4), 469–474.

Weng, L., Dai, Y., Wang, Y., Huang, H., & Chiang, Y. (2008). Effects of self-efficacy, self-care behaviours on depressive symptom of Taiwanese kidney transplant recipients. *Journal of Clinical Nursing, 17*(13), 1786–1794.

Zijlstra, G., Tennstedt, S., van Haastregt, J., van Eijk, J., & Kempen, G. (2006). Reducing fear of falling and avoidance of activity in elderly persons: the development of a Dutch version of an American intervention. *Patient Education and Counseling, 62*(2), 220–227.

6

Chronic Sorrow

GEORGENE GASKILL EAKES

INTRODUCTION

The middle range theory of chronic sorrow, first documented in the literature in 1998 by Eakes, Burke, and Hainsworth, offers a framework for explaining how individuals may respond to both ongoing and single loss events. Moreover, the theoretical model of chronic sorrow provides an alternative way of viewing the experience of grief. The theory of chronic sorrow was inductively derived and subsequently validated from an extensive review of the literature and from the data gathered through 10 qualitative research studies conducted by members of the Nursing Consortium for Research on Chronic Sorrow (NCRCS). Using the Burke/NCRCS Chronic Sorrow Questionnaire, adapted from a guide developed by Burke (1989), as an interview guide, these nurse researchers interviewed 196 individuals who shared their loss experiences as people with chronic conditions, as family caregivers of the chronically ill or disabled, or as bereaved family members.

HISTORICAL BACKGROUND

The term *chronic sorrow* was introduced into the literature 40 years ago to characterize the recurring episodes of grief experienced by parents of children with disabilities (Olshansky, 1962). This recurring sadness appeared to persist throughout the lives of these parents, although its intensity varied from time to time, from situation to situation, and from one family member to another. Rather than viewing this phenomenon as pathological, Olshansky described chronic sorrow as a normal response to an ongoing loss situation. Professionals were encouraged to recognize the presence of this phenomenon when working with a parent of a disabled child and to support parents' expressions of feelings. Although the term gained wide acceptance in the professional literature, almost two decades passed before there was any documented research on chronic sorrow.

Initial research conducted in the 1980s validated the occurrence of chronic sorrow among parents of disabled young children. Several investigators suggested that the never-ending nature of the loss of the "perfect" child prevented resolution of grief (Burke, 1989; Damrosh & Perry, 1989; Fraley, 1986; Kratochvil and Devereux, 1988; Wikler, Wasow, & Hatfield, 1981). Moreover, it was this inability to bring closure to the loss experience that was thought to precipitate periodic episodes of re-grief labeled as chronic sorrow. These early studies refined and operationalized the definition of chronic sorrow as a pervasive sadness that was permanent, periodic, and progressive in nature.

CURRENT RESEARCH ON CHRONIC SORROW

More recent research supports the fact that chronic sorrow is a common experience among family caregivers (Bettle & Latimer, 2009; Bowes, Lowes, Warner & Gregory, 2009; Clubb, 1991; Copley & Bodensteiner, 1987; Doornbos, 1997; Eakes, 1995; Eakes, Burke, Hainsworth, & Lindgren, 1993; Fraley, 1990; George & Vickers, 2006–2007; Golden, 1994; Gordon, 2009; Hainsworth, 1995; Hainsworth, Busch, Eakes, & Burke, 1995; Hobdell, 2004; Hobdell et al., 2007; Hummel & Eastman, 1991; Johnsonius, 1996; Keamy & Griffin, 2001; Krafft and Krafft, 1998; Liedstrom, Isaksson, & Ahlstrom, 2008; Lindgren, 1996: Lowes & Lyne, 2000; Mallow & Bechtel, 1999; Mayer, 2001; Northington, 2000; Patrick-Ott & Ladd, 2010; Phillips, 1991; Rosenberg, 1998; Seideman & Kleine, 1995; Shumaker, 1995). The caregivers studied represent parents of young children with various disabilities, spouses of individuals diagnosed with chronic illnesses, and parents of adult children with debilitating conditions.

The NCRCS, established in 1989 (Eakes, Hainsworth, Lindgren, & Burke, 1991), expanded research on chronic sorrow and explored the relevance of the concept of chronic sorrow among individuals experiencing a variety of loss situations. This group of nurse researchers not only conducted research on chronic sorrow among family caregivers, but also investigated individuals affected with chronic conditions and bereaved individuals. Among those diagnosed with a chronic condition, 83% evidenced chronic sorrow (Burke et al., 1992; Eakes, 1993; Hainsworth, 1994; Hainsworth, Eakes, & Burke, 1994; Lindgren, 1996). Others have since been validated by the experience of chronic sorrow among those diagnosed with a chronic condition (Isaksson, Gunnarsson, & Ahlstrom, 2007; Lichtenstein, Laska, & Clair, 2002; Smith, 2009).

The NCRCS also conducted research studies designed to investigate the occurrence of chronic sorrow among individuals who had experienced a single loss event rather than an ongoing loss. Toward the end, people who had experienced the death of a significant other a minimum of 2 years prior to the study were interviewed. This time lapse was to allow for acute grief to have subsided. Findings revealed that a vast majority (97%) of those interviewed evidenced chronic sorrow (Eakes, Burke, and Hainsworth, 1999). These findings lead to further modification of the defining characteristics of chronic sorrow, with recognition that it was ongoing disparity associated with the loss, rather than the ongoing nature of the loss experience as originally thought, that was the antecedent to chronic sorrow. Consequently, chronic sorrow was redefined as permanent, periodic recurrence of pervasive sadness or other grief-related feelings associated with ongoing disparity resulting from significant loss (Eakes, Burke, & Hainsworth, 1998). The necessary antecedent event is involvement in an experience of significant loss. This loss may be ongoing in nature with no predictable end, such as with the birth of a disabled child or diagnosis of a debilitating illness, or it may be more circumscribed as with the death of a loved one. Disparity is created by a loss/situation when an individual's current reality differs markedly from the idealized or when a gap exists between the desired and the actual reality. This lack of closure sets the stage for grief to be periodically reexperienced. That is, the chronic sorrow experience is cyclical and continues as long as the disparity created by the loss remains.

MIDDLE RANGE NURSING THEORY OF CHRONIC SORROW

The middle range theory of chronic sorrow (Eakes et al., 1998) was inductively derived and validated through the qualitative studies described above as well as a critical review of existing literature (see Fig. 6.1). Chronic sorrow was reconceptualized based on these findings and is now defined as

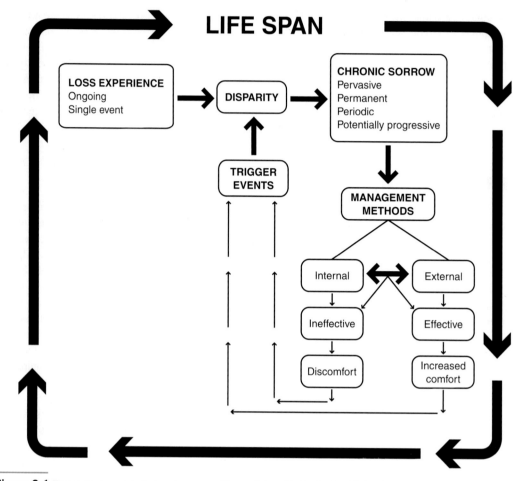

Figure 6.1 Theoretical model of chronic sorrow. (From Eakes, G. G., Burke, M. L., & Hainsworth, M. A. (1998). Middle range theory of chronic sorrow. *Image: The Journal of Nursing Scholarship, 30*[2], 179–184.)

"the periodic recurrence of permanent, pervasive sadness or other grief-related feelings associated with ongoing disparity resulting from a loss experience" (Eakes, et al., 1998, p. 180, 1999). Moreover, chronic sorrow is characterized as pervasive, permanent, periodic, and potentially progressive in nature and continues to be viewed as a normal response to loss. Indeed, the theory of chronic sorrow purports that the periodic return of grief among individuals and caregivers whose anticipated life course has been interrupted continues throughout one's lifetime as long as the disparity created by the loss remains.

The middle range theory of chronic sorrow provides a framework for understanding the reactions of individuals to various loss situations and offers a new way of viewing the experience of bereavement. Although chronic sorrow is viewed as a normal response to the ongoing disparity or void created by significant loss, it is important to note that normalization of the experience in no way diminishes the validity or the intensity of the feelings experienced. At times, feelings can be intense and distressing for the individual experiencing chronic sorrow.

Involvement in an experience of significant loss is the necessary antecedent to the development of chronic sorrow. This may be a loss with no predictable end, such as the birth of a disabled child or diagnosis of a chronic illness, or a more clearly defined loss event such as the death of a loved one. The second antecedent to chronic sorrow is ongoing disparity resulting from the loss. That is, a gap exists between the desired and the actual reality. The lack of closure associated with ongoing disparity sets the stage for chronic sorrow, with the loss experienced in bits and pieces over time. The defining characteristics of chronic sorrow borne out by the research are pervasiveness, permanence, periodicity, and the potential for progressivity. As graphically represented in the theoretical model of chronic sorrow, the experience of chronic sorrow may occur at any point across the life span.

Trigger events, also referenced as milestones, are those situations or circumstances that bring the disparity created by the loss into focus, thereby triggering the grief-related feelings associated with chronic sorrow. Triggers of chronic sorrow have been shown to vary depending on the nature of the loss experience. For affected individuals, chronic sorrow is most commonly triggered when individuals confront disparity with established norms, whether, social, development, or personal in nature (Eakes, 1993; Eakes et al., 1993; Hainsworth, 1994; Isaksson & Ahlstrom, 2008; Isaksson et al., 2007). For example, when someone diagnosed with a chronic illness is unable to engage in an activity that they once enjoyed due to exacerbation of their condition.

The most frequent trigger of chronic sorrow among parents of young children with disabilities is disparity associated with developmental milestones (Bowes et al., 2009; Burke, 1989; Clubb, 1991; Damrosch & Perry, 1989; Fraley, 1986, 1990; George & Vickers, 2006–2007; Golden, 1994; Hobdell, 2004; Hobdell et al., 2007; Hummel & Eastman, 1991; Kafft & Krafft, 1998; Mallow & Bechtel, 1999; Olshansky, 1962; Patrick-Ott & Ladd, 2010; Phillips, 1991; Seideman & Kleine, 1995; Shumaker, 1995; Wikler et al., 1981). The chronic sorrow of other family caregivers is often triggered by crises associated with management of the family member's illness and by recognition of the never-ending nature of the caregiving activities (Bettle & Latimer, 2009; Bowes et al., 2009; Eakes, 1995; Eakes et al., 1993; George & Vickers, 2006–2007; Hainsworth, 1995; Hainsworth et al., 1995; Isaksson & Ahlstrom, 2008; Liedstrom at al., 2008; Lindgren, 1996; Patrick-Ott & Ladd, 2010).

The chronic sorrow experience of bereaved individuals is triggered by those situations and circumstances that magnify the "presence of the absence" of the deceased, such as anniversaries and other special occasions (Eakes et al., 1998, p. 182). In addition, changes in roles and responsibilities necessitated by the death of a loved one may trigger chronic sorrow.

Another key element of the theoretical model of chronic sorrow is management methods. This term is used to refer to both personal coping strategies used by individuals during the chronic sorrow experience (internal) and supportive interventions provided by helping professionals (external). As depicted in the theoretical model, effective internal and external management methods lead to increased comfort and may serve to extend the time between episodes of chronic sorrow.

Effective internal management strategies used by those with chronic sorrow are consistent across the various loss situations. Action-oriented strategies that increase feelings of control are most frequently used to cope with the recurrence grief-related feelings of chronic sorrow (Burke, 1989; Eakes, 1993, 1995; Hainsworth, 1995; Hainsworth et al., 1994, 1995; Hobdell et al., 2007; Lindgren, 1996). Examples of action-oriented coping include continuing to pursue involvement in interests and activities, gathering information specific to one's loss experience and seeking out respite opportunities. Other types of coping strategies identified as helpful in dealing with the chronic sorrow experience are labeled as cognitive and interpersonal. Cognitive strategies include adopting a "can do" attitude and focusing on the positive elements of one's life (Burke, 1989; Eakes, 1993, 1995; Hainsworth, 1995; Hainsworth et al., 1994, 1995; Isaksson & Ahlstrom, 2008). Interpersonal ways of coping include talking with someone close or a trusted professional and interacting with others in a similar situation such as in a support group (Burke, 1989; Eakes, 1993, 1995; Fraley, 1990; Hainsworth, 1995; Hainsworth et al., 1994, 1995; Wikler et al., 1981).

Interventions provided by health care professionals, referred to as external management methods, must be based upon the premise that chronic sorrow is a normal response to a significant loss situation. As long as disparity created by a loss experience remains, one can anticipate that the individual will likely experience chronic sorrow. Indeed, normalization of the periodic re-grief of chronic sorrow is foundational to all other interventions. It is important for professionals to recognize that individuals who have experienced a significant loss may evidence the periodic recurrence of grief-related feelings defined as chronic sorrow. Armed with this awareness, anticipatory guidance may be provided regarding the situations and circumstances likely to trigger episodes of chronic sorrow. Personal coping mechanisms (internal management methods) can be assessed, strengthened, and supported.

In addition, specific interventions provided by heath care professionals, categorized as roles, have been noted as helpful by those experiencing chronic sorrow (Burke, 1989; Copley & Bodensteiner, 1987; Eakes, 1993, 1995; Eakes et al., 1993; Fraley, 1990; Hobdell et al., 2007; Hainsworth, 1995; Hainsworth et al., 1995; Hummel & Eastman, 1991; Isaksson & Ahlstrom, 2008; Wikler et al., 1981). Family caregivers with chronic sorrow derive the most benefit from professional interventions labeled as the role of "teacher/ expert." More specifically, these actions include providing situation-specific information in a manner that can be easily understood and giving practical tips for managing care-giving responsibilities (Burke, 1989; Clubb, 1991; Eakes, 1995; Fraley, 1990; Hainsworth, 1995; Hainsworth et al., 1995; Hummel & Eastman, 1991; Warda, 1992, Wikler et al., 1981). Actions associated with the professional role of "empathetic presence" characterized by taking time to listen, offering support, focusing on feelings, and recognizing uniqueness of each individual are also helpful to those who were in a caregiver role (Burke, 1989; Clubb, 1991; Eakes, 1995; Fraley, 1990; George & Vickers, 2006-2007; Gordon, 2009; Hainsworth, 1995; Hummel & Eastman, 1991; Isaksson & Ahlstrom, 2008; Olshansky, 1962; Phillips, 1991; Teel, 1991; Warda, 1992).

For those individuals affected with a chronic or life-threatening condition as well as bereaved persons, the professional role of "empathetic presence" discussed above is perceived as most helpful in dealing with the periodic episodes of chronic sorrow. In addition, the complementary role of "caring professional," evidenced by sensitivity, respectfulness and nonjudgmental acceptance, and interventions associated with the role of "teacher/expert" are described as beneficial (Burke, 1989; Eakes, 1993; Eakes et al., 1993; Hainsworth et al., 1995, Isaksson & Ahlstrom, 2008).

RESEARCH APPLICATIONS OF CHRONIC SORROW

Chronic sorrow has research applications among a variety of populations and across a myriad of loss situations. Identification of the presence of chronic sorrow among affected individuals, family caregivers, and bereaved individuals can alert professionals to potential triggers of the recurrent grief and lead to the identification and reinforcement of effective coping mechanisms for those experiencing chronic sorrow.

EXAMPLE

Isaksson and Ahlstrom (2008) utilized the theoretical model of chronic sorrow as a framework for exploring coping strategies of 38 individuals diagnosed with multiple sclerosis. The subjects, identified in an earlier study as experiencing chronic sorrow, were interviewed using the questions on the NCRCS Chronic Sorrow Questionnaire that focused on management strategies. Qualitative content analysis was conducted on verbatim transcripts with identification of both internal and external management methods. Coping strategies were further categorized as "effective" or "ineffective."

Findings were consistent with the theoretical model of chronic sorrow, revealing the use of both internal and external management methods by those experiencing chronic sorrow. Moreover, when effective internal management methods were used, individuals experienced increased comfort; conversely, when episodes of chronic sorrow were not managed effectively, subjects described increased discomfort. Effective internal management methods were captured in the recurring theme of "mastering with realistic awareness" and included distraction, allowing and sharing emotions, having a "can do" attitude and taking care of oneself. Effective external management methods were categorized under the theme of "endorsing management" represented by a caring and supportive family/friends and confirmation from health care professionals. Ineffective internal coping was described as "struggling with vulnerability," while ineffective external management was classified under the theme of "deficient affirmation." These strategies are reflective of those identified in the research underpinning the theoretical model of chronic sorrow.

The researchers concluded that the theoretical model of chronic sorrow provided an empirically trustworthy framework for interpretation of data and was useful in increasing both knowledge and understanding of chronic sorrow.

NCRCS CHRONIC SORROW INSTRUMENT DEVELOPMENT

Historically, research on chronic sorrow has employed qualitative methods with open-ended interview guides used in both face-to-face and telephone interviews with study participants. The Burke/NCRCS Chronic Sorrow Questionnaire (Burke, 1989; with versions adapted for individuals affected with chronic conditions, for family caregivers and for bereaved individuals, has been used for the majority of studies documented in the literature. This interview guide is comprised of 11 open-ended questions that explore feelings experienced at the time of the loss and whether or not they have been reexperienced. Moreover, questions focus on circumstances or situations that trigger recurrence of the grief-related feeling and identification of effective coping mechanisms.

In 2001, two of the original members of the NCRCS undertook the development of a quantitative assessment tool. Questions for the instrument were developed based on the theoretical model and findings from the qualitative studies previously conducted by members of the NCRCS and other researchers. Face and content validity were established by using Lynn's (1986) methodology for establishing validity of an instrument. Once face and content validity of the Burke/Eakes Chronic Sorrow Assessment Tool were established, test–retest reliability studies were conducted. Subjects participating in this aspect of instrument development represented each of the populations previously studied (family caregivers, affected individuals, and bereaved persons). Test–retest correlations for items 4 through 9 (the first three questions assess demographic data) were at acceptable levels, ranging from 0.72 to 0.93. Questions 10 and 11 allow for little variability in responses and the restricted response range resulted in more marginal test–retest correlations on these items (0.62 and 0.56, respectively) (see Box 6.1).

Box 6.1 Burke/Eakes Chronic Sorrow Assessment Tool

The questions below are about the impacts of certain life events or situations on people over a period of time so that helping professionals can better meet their needs. In answering these questions, please focus on the impacts that these life events or situations continue to have on your life. There are no right or wrong answers. You do not have to answer any or all of the questions and can stop without penalty of any kind. Thank you for taking the time to answer these questions.

1. Which of the following best describes your situation? (Please check only one.)

   (a) Parent of disabled child
       (please specify the disability) _____

   (b) Person with a chronic condition
       (please specify the condition) _____

   (c) Caregiver of someone with a chronic or life-threatening illness
       (please specify the condition) _____

   (d) Bereaved person
       (please specify the relationship of deceased to you) _____

2. I have been dealing with this situation/loss for _____ years (please write in number of years).

3. Please provide the following information about yourself:

   (a) Sex: _____ male _____ female

   (b) Age: _____ years

   (c) Marital status: _____ single _____ married _____ widowed _____ divorced _____ separated

   (d) Religion: _____ Protestant _____ Catholic _____ Jewish
       Other (please specify) _____

   (e) Ethnic origin: ____ Caucasian ____ Hispanic ____ African-American ____ American Indian ____ Asian
       Other (please specify) _____

(continued)

Box 6.1 Burke/Eakes Chronic Sorrow Assessment Tool *(Continued)*

(f) Please indicate your highest level of education:

    a. Below high school

    b. High school graduate

    c. Associate/technical degree

    d. Bachelor's degree

    e. Master's degree

    f. PhD/MD or equivalent

(g) Total family income per year from all sources before taxes:

    a. Below $5,000

    b. $5,001–10,000

    c. $10,001–15,000

    d. $15,001–20,000

    e. $20,001–25,000

    f. $25,001–30,000

    g. $30,001–40,000

    h. Over $40,000

4. Even though some time may have passed since you began dealing with your situation/loss, you may still be coping with some ongoing issues and reactions. Please read the following statements and indicate if this is true for you. Remember, there are no right or wrong answers.

    (a) I recognize the hole this situation/loss has created in my life.   ☐ True   ☐ False

    (b) I think about the difference this situation/loss has made in my life.   ☐ True   ☐ False

    (c) I experience changes in my life as a result of the situation/loss.   ☐ True   ☐ False

    (d) I feel its effects in bits and pieces.   ☐ True   ☐ False

5. The following are feelings you may have experienced as a result of your situation/loss.
At those times, when you experience these feelings associated with your situation/loss, please indicate how upsetting they are for you. Remember, there are no right or wrong answers.

	Have not experienced	Have experienced but not upsetting	Have experienced, somewhat upsetting	Have experienced, very upsetting
(a) Sad				
(b) Anxious				
(c) Angry				
(d) Overwhelmed				
(e) Heartbroken				
(f) Other (please specify)				

6. The questions below are more about the feelings you may experience related to your situation/loss. Please mark the extent to which each statement below is true for you.
In describing my feelings about my situation/loss, I

    (a) Have ups and downs   ☐ True   ☐ False

    (b) Feel their effects on other parts of my life   ☐ True   ☐ False

    (c) Feel them more strongly now than at first   ☐ True   ☐ False

    (d) Believe they will impact on me the rest of my life   ☐ True   ☐ False

Box 6.1 Burke/Eakes Chronic Sorrow Assessment Tool *(Continued)*

7. There may be certain times when you tend to experience the feelings associated with your situation/loss. Please read the following statements and indicate which is true for you.

   These feelings about my situation/loss come up when I

   (a) Have to seek medical care   ☐ True   ☐ False

   (b) Realize all the responsibilities I have   ☐ True   ☐ False

   (c) Compare where I am now with where others are in their lives   ☐ True   ☐ False

   (d) Think of all I now have to do   ☐ True   ☐ False

   (e) Meet someone else in the same situation   ☐ True   ☐ False

   (f) Experience the anniversary of when this began   ☐ True   ☐ False

   (g) Have a "special day" such as a birthday or holiday   ☐ True   ☐ False

   (h) Other (please specify)

8. The statements below are things you may have found helpful to you in managing the feelings associated with your situation/loss. Please indicate which is true for you.

   It helps me deal with my feelings when I:

	Never tried	Have tried, but not helpful	Have tried, somewhat helpful	Have tried, very helpful
(a) Keep busy				
(b) Take 1 day at a time				
(c) Talk to someone close to me				
(d) Pray				
(e) Exercise				
(f) Count my blessings				
(g) Work on my hobbies				
(h) Go to church, synagogue, or other place of worship				
(i) Talk with others in similar situations				
(j) Take a "can do" attitude				
(k) Talk with a minister, rabbi, or priest				
(l) Talk with a health professional				
(m) Focus on the positive				
(n) Other (please specify)				

(continued)

Box 6.1　Burke/Eakes Chronic Sorrow Assessment Tool *(Continued)*

9. The following questions are to find out how helping professionals can assist people who are dealing with situations/losses such as yours. Please indicate which is true for you. Remember, there are no right or wrong answers.

It helps me deal with my feelings when helping professionals:

	Never tried	Have tried, but not helpful	Have tried, somewhat helpful	Have tried, very helpful
(a) Listen to me				
(b) Recognize my feelings				
(c) Answer my questions honestly				
(d) Allow me to ask questions				
(e) Allow me to ask questions				
(f) Take their time with me				
(g) Provide good care				
(h) Other (please specify)				

10. Friends and family may also be helpful to you as you deal with the feelings associated with your situation/loss. Please read the following and indicate which is true for you.

It helps me deal with my feelings when family and friends:

	Never tried	Have tried, but not helpful	Have tried, somewhat helpful	Have tried, very helpful
(a) Listen to me				
(b) Have a positive outlook				
(c) Accept my feelings				
(d) Provide emotional support				
(e) Offer a helping hand				
(f) Acknowledge my situation/loss				
(g) Other (please specify)				

Thank you for answering these questions. Please return the completed questionnaire at this time.

SUMMARY

Chronic sorrow has gained increased attention in the past three decades, based in large part on the research endeavors of the NCRCS. In addition, increased awareness of the changing nature of grief associated with significant losses, whether ongoing in nature or single loss events, has spurred interest in this phenomenon. The newly established theory of chronic sorrow provides a framework for understanding and working with individuals who have experienced significant loss. Specifically, situations and circumstances that trigger chronic sorrow are identified and management methods deemed helpful to those experiencing chronic sorrow are described. Moreover, the theoretical model of chronic sorrow, along with the recently constructed Burke/Eakes Chronic Sorrow Assessment Tool, will facilitate further expansion of research on chronic sorrow and provide opportunities for testing of the theory. The need for exploration of cultural variations in the experience of chronic sorrow has virtually been ignored and must be addressed in future research. In addition, relevance of the theory of chronic sorrow to types of loss experiences not yet studied (i.e., divorce and abuse) needs to be investigated.

The middle range theory of chronic sorrow has widespread application for nurses and others who strive to better understand individuals' responses to loss and to define effective interventions for those experiencing chronic sorrow. Although chronic sorrow is viewed as a normal response to ongoing disparity resulting from a loss, recognition of the periodic re-grief characteristic of chronic sorrow and provision of supportive interventions can provide an increased level of comfort for those experiencing it.

ANALYSIS OF THEORY

Using the criteria presented in Chapter 2, critique the theory of chronic sorrow. Compare your conclusions about the theory with those found in Appendix A. A nurse who has worked with the theory completed the analysis found in the Appendix.

Internal Criticism

1. Clarity
2. Consistency
3. Adequacy
4. Logical development
5. Level of theory development

External Criticism

1. Reality convergence
2. Utility
3. Significance
4. Discrimination
5. Scope of theory
6. Complexity

CRITICAL THINKING EXERCISES

1. You are a case manager for a family with a young child diagnosed with cerebral palsy. Explain how the theory of chronic sorrow can be used as a framework for planning care and identifying resources for this family.

2. Expand the application of the theory of chronic sorrow to a population not yet studied. Describe the strengths and weaknesses of the theory in relation to the population identified and discuss if the theoretical premises apply.

3. Draft a research study designed to measure outcomes for the external management strategies described in the theory.

WEB RESOURCES

Visit **http://thePoint.lww.com/Peterson3e** for helpful web resources related to this chapter.

REFERENCES

Bettle, A. M. E., & Latimer, M. A. (2009). Maternal coping and adaptation: A case study examination of chronic sorrow in caring for an adolescent with a progressive neurodegenerative disease. *Canadian Journal of Neuroscience Nursing, 31*(4), 15–21.

Bowes, S., Lowes, L., Warner, J., & Gregory, J. W. (2009). Chronic sorrow in parents of children with type 1 diabetes. *Journal of Advanced Nursing, 65*(5), 992–1000.

Burke, M. L. (1989). Chronic sorrow in mothers of school-age children with a myelomeningocele disability. (Doctoral dissertation, Boston University, 1989). *Dissertation Abstracts International, 50*, 233B–234B.

Burke, M. L., Eakes, G. G., & Hainsworth, M. A. (1999). Milestones of chronic sorrow: Perspectives of affected individuals and family caregivers. *Journal of Family Nursing, 5*(4), 374–387.

Burke, M. L., Hainsworth, M. A., Eakes, G. G., & Lindgren, C. L. (1992). Current knowledge and research on chronic sorrow: A foundation for inquiry. *Death Studies, 16*, 231–245.

Clubb, R. L. (1991). Chronic sorrow: Adaptation patterns of parents with chronically ill children. *Pediatric Nursing, 17*, 462–466.

Copley, M. F., & Bodensteiner, J. B. (1987). Chronic sorrow in families of disabled children. *Journal of Child Neurology, 2*, 67–70.

Damrosch, S. P., & Perry, L. A. (1989). Self-reported adjustment, chronic sorrow, and coping of parents of children with Down syndrome. *Nursing Research, 38*, 25–30.

Doornbos, M. M. (1997). The problems and coping methods of caregivers of young adults with mental illness. *Journal of Psychosocial Nursing, 35*(9), 22–26.

Eakes, G. G. (1993). Chronic sorrow: A response to living with cancer. *Oncology Nursing Forum, 20,* 1327–1334.

Eakes, G. G. (1995). Chronic sorrow: The lived experience of parents of chronically mentally ill individuals. *Archives of Psychiatric Nursing, IX,* 77–84.

Eakes, G. G., Burke, M. L., & Hainsworth, M. A. (1998). Middle range theory of chronic sorrow. *Image: Journal of Nursing Scholarship, 30*(2), 179–184.

Eakes, G. G., Burke, M. L., & Hainsworth, M. A. (1999). Chronic sorrow: The lived experience of bereaved individuals. *Illness, Crisis, and Loss, 7*(1), 172–182.

Eakes, G. G., Burke, M. L., Hainsworth, M. A., & Lindgren, C. L. (1993). Chronic sorrow: An examination of nursing roles. In S. G. Funk, E. M. Tornquist, M. T. Champagne, & R. A. Wiese (Eds.), *Key aspects of caring for the chronically ill: Hospital and home* (pp. 231–236). New York: Springer.

Eakes, G. G., Hainsworth, M. E., Lindgren, C. L., & Burke, M. L. (1991). Establishing a long-distance research consortium. *Nursing Connections, 4,* 51–57.

Fraley, A. M. (1986). Chronic sorrow in parents of premature children. *Children's Health Care, 15,* 114–118.

Fraley, A. M. (1990). Chronic sorrow: A parental response. *Journal of Pediatric Nursing, 5,* 268–273.

George, A., & Vickers, M. H. (December 2006–January 2007). Chronic grief: Experiences of working parents of children with chronic illness. *Contemporary Nurse, 23,* 228–242.

Golden, B. (1994). *The presence of chronic sorrow in mothers of children with cerebral palsy.* Unpublished master's thesis, Arizona State University, Tempe.

Gordon, J. (2009). An evidence-based approach for supporting parents experiencing chronic sorrow. *Pediatric Nursing, 35*(2), 115–119.

Hainsworth, M. A. (1994). Living with multiple sclerosis: The experience of chronic sorrow. *Journal of Neuroscience Nursing, 26,* 237–240.

Hainsworth, M. A. (1995). Chronic sorrow in spouse caregivers of individuals with multiple sclerosis: A case study. *Journal of Gerontological Nursing, 21,* 29–33.

Hainsworth, M. A., Busch, P. V., Eakes, G. G., & Burke, M. L. (1995). Chronic sorrow in women with chronically mentally disabled husbands. *Journal of the American Psychiatric Association, 1*(4), 120–124.

Hainsworth, M. A., Eakes, G. G., & Burke, M. L. (1994). Coping with chronic sorrow. *Issues in Mental Health Nursing, 15,* 59–66.

Hobdell, E. F. (2004). Chronic sorrow and depression in parents of children with neural tube defects. *Journal of Neuroscience Nursing, 36*(2), 82–88, 94.

Hobdell, E. F., Grant, M. L.,Valencia, I., Mare, J., Kothare, S. V., Legido, A., et al. (2007). Chronic sorrow and coping in families of children with epilepsy. *Journal of Neuroscience Nursing, 39*(2), 76–82.

Hummel, P. A., & Eastman, D. L. (1991). Do parents of premature infants suffer chronic sorrow? *Neonatal Network, 10,* 59–65.

Isaksson, A., & Ahlstrom, G. (2008). Managing chronic sorrow: Experiences of patients with multiple sclerosis. *Journal of Neuroscience Nursing, 40*(3), 180–191.

Isaksson, A. K., Gunnarsson, L. G., & Ahlstorm, G. (2007). The presence and meaning of chronic sorrow in patients with multiple sclerosis. *Journal of Clinical Nursing, 16*(11c), 315–324.

Johnsonius, J. (1996). Lived experiences that reflect embodied themes of chronic sorrow: A phenomenological pilot study. *Journal of Nursing Science, 1*(5/6), 165–173.

Keamy, P., & Griffin, T. (2001). Between joy and sorrow: Being a parent of a child with a developmental disability. *Journal of Advanced Nursing, 34*(5), 582–592.

Kraft, S. K., & Kraft, L. J. (1998). Chronic sorrow: Parents' lived experience. *Holistic Nursing Practice, 13*(1), 59–67.

Kratochvil, M. S., & Devereaux, S. A. (1988). Counseling needs of parents of handicapped children. *Social Casework, 68,* 420–426.

Lichtenstein, B., Laska, & Clair, J. (2002). Chronic sorrow in the HIV-postive patient: Issues of race, gender and social support. *Aids Patient Care and STDS, 16*(1), 27–38.

Liedstrom, E., Isaksson, A., & Ahlstrom, G. (2008). Chronic sorrow in next of kin of patients with multiple sclerosis. *Journal of Neuroscience Nursing, 40*(5), 304–311.

Lindgren, C. L. (1996). Chronic sorrow in persons with Parkinson's and their spouses. *Scholarly Inquiry for Nursing Practice, 10,* 351–367.

Lowes, L. L., & Lyne, P. (2000). Chronic sorrow in parents of children with newly diagnosed diabetes: A review of the literature and discussion of the implications for nursing practice. *Journal of Advanced Nursing, 32*(1), 41–48.

Lynn, M. (1986). Determination and quantification of content validity. *Nursing Research, 35*(6), 382–385.

Mallow, G. E., & Bechtel, G. A. (1999). Chronic sorrow: The experience of parents with children who are developmentally disabled. *Journal of Psychosocial Nursing, 37*(7), 31–35.

Martin, K., & Elder, S. (1993). Pathways through grief: A model of the process. In J. D. Morgan (Ed.), *Personal care in an impersonal world: A multidimensional look at bereavement* (pp. 73–86). Amityville, NY: Baywood Publishing.

Mayer, M. (2001). Chronic sorrow in caregiving spouses of patients with Alzheimer's disease. *Journal of aging and Identity, 6*(1), 49–60.

Olshansky, S. (1962). Chronic sorrow: A response to having a mentally defective child. *Social Casework, 43,* 191–193.

Patrick-Ott, A., & Ladd, L. D. (2010). The blending of Boss's concept of ambiguous loss and Olshansky's concept of chronic sorrow: A case study of a family who has significant disabilities. *Journal of Creativity in Mental Health, 5*(1), 74–86.

Philips, M. (1991). Chronic sorrow in mothers of chronically ill and disabled children. *Issues in Comprehensive Pediatric Nursing, 14*, 111–120.

Rosenberg, C. J. (1998). Faculty-student mentoring. A father's chronic sorrow: A daughter's perspective. *Journal of Holistic Nursing, 16*(3), 399–404.

Seideman, R. Y., & Kleine, P. F. (1995). A theory of transformed parenting: Parenting a child with developmental delay/mental retardation. *Nursing Research, 44*, 38–44.

Shumaker, D. (1995). *Chronic sorrow in mothers of children with cystic fibrosis.* Unpublished master's thesis, University of Tennessee, Memphis.

Smith, C. S. (2009). Substance abuse, chronic sorrow, and mothering loss: Relapse triggers among female victims of child abuse. *Journal of Pediatric Nursing, 24*(5), 401–412.

Teel, C. S. (1991). Chronic sorrow: Analysis of the concept. *Journal of Advanced Nursing, 16*, 1322–1319.

Warda, M. (1992). The family and chronic sorrow: Role theory approach. *Journal of Pediatric Nursing, 7,* 205–210.

Wikler, L. M., Wasow, M., & Hatfield, E. (1981). Chronic sorrow revisited: Parents vs. professional depiction of the adjustment of parents of mentally retarded children. *American Journal of Orthopsychiatry, 51*, 63–70.

7

Social Support

MARJORIE A. SCHAFFER

DEFINITION OF KEY TERMS

Appraisal support	Affirmation from statements or actions made by another (Kahn & Antonucci, 1980)
Emotional support	Experience of feeling liked, admired, respected, or loved (Norbeck, Lindsey, & Carrieri, 1981)
Formal support	Help from professionals, paraprofessionals, or other service providers from structured community organizations (may be paid or unpaid assistance)
Informal support	Help provided through a person's "lay" social network, such as from family members and friends
Informational support	Knowledge provided to another during a time of stress that assists in problem solving (House, 1981)
Instrumental support	Tangible aid, goods, or services (House, 1981)
Negative support	Interactions that cause stress or are more demanding than helpful (Coyne & DeLongis, 1986)
Perceived support	Generalized appraisal that individuals are cared for and valued, have others available to them, and are satisfied with relationships (Heller, Swindle, & Dusenbury, 1986)
Social network	Structure of the interactive process of persons, who give and receive help and protection (Langford, Bowsher, Maloney, & Lillis, 1997)
Social support	(1) "Aid and assistance exchanged through social relationships and interpersonal transactions" (Fleury, Keller, & Perez, 2009, p. 12); (2) "A well-intentioned action that is given willingly to a person with whom there is a personal relationship and that produces an immediate or delayed positive response in the recipient" (Hupcey, 1998b, p. 313)

INTRODUCTION

Social support is a middle range theory that addresses structure and interaction in relationships. It impacts health status, health behavior, and use of health services (Stewart, 1993). As health professionals, nurses often have access to clients' social networks. Through communication with clients and their family members, nurses can intervene to promote or strengthen social support. The literature identifies many positive consequences of social support, including health-promoting behaviors, personal competence, coping, a sense of well-being, self-worth, and decreased anxiety and depression (Langford et al., 1997). Research on social support interventions can provide nurses with knowledge about the most effective strategies for strengthening social support for clients, which contributes to improved health status.

HISTORICAL BACKGROUND

Cassel (1974), one of the early social support theorists, introduced the term "social support." Based on animal studies, he theorized that strengthening social supports could improve the health of humans. Studies in the early 1970s suggested that social support mediates the negative effects of stress (Roberts, 1984). The "buffer" and attachment theories have been the basis for considerable research on the relationship of social support and health (Callaghan & Morrissey, 1993). The buffer theory suggests that social support protects persons from life stressors (Cassel, 1976; Cobb, 1976). The attachment theory holds that the ability to form socially supportive relationships is related to the secure attachments formed in childhood (Bowlby, 1971). In the mid-1970s to early 1980s, the literature most often described social support in concrete terms, such as an interaction, person, or relationship (Veiel & Baumann, 1992). In recent years, the term has been used more abstractly, to include perceptions, quality and quantity of support, behaviors, and social systems. The analysis and testing of social support theory has gained multidisciplinary interest and is prominent in nursing and social–psychological literature. For nurses, social support can connect family assessment, patient needs, and health outcomes (Hupcey, 1998b).

DEFINITION OF THEORY CONCEPTS

Developers of social support theory have organized definitions of social support by a variety of component labels: aspects, categories, constructs, defining attributes, dimensions, interpersonal transactions, subconcepts, taxonomies, and types (Table 7.1). The variety of definitions of social support provided by theorists illustrates the lack of consensus about the nature of social support. This lack of consensus contributes to complexity in evaluating social support interventions and outcomes, comparing research findings, and developing social support theory.

Although multidimensional definitions predominate, positive interaction or helpful behavior is shared by all social support definitions (Rook & Dooley, 1985). In addition, most social support theories have the assumption that support is given and received by members of a social network, leading to social integration or a feeling of belonging (Diamond, 1985; Norbeck & Tilden, 1988). Recipients perceive that social support facilitates coping with stressors in their lives (Pierce, Sarason, & Sarason, 1990); high levels of stress may be mediated by social support (Chou, Avant, Kuo, & Fetzer, 2008). Social support is defined as "aid and assistance exchanged through social relationships and interpersonal transactions" (Fleury et al., 2009, p. 12). Social support can be structural, focusing on who provides the support, or functional, emphasizing the act of providing social support activities (Callaghan & Morrissey, 1993; Norwood, 1996). In addition, there are many characteristics that influence the quality and adequacy of social support, such as the stability, direction, and source of support (Stewart, 1989a). Social networks can be described by the number and categories of persons who provide social support: family members, close friends, neighbors, coworkers, and professionals (Tardy, 1985). Hupcey (1998a) suggested that a personal relationship is required for social support to take place, defining social support as "a well-intentioned action that is given willingly to a person with whom there is a personal relationship and that produces an immediate or delayed positive response in the recipient" (Hupcey, 1998b, p. 313).

EMOTIONAL, INFORMATIONAL, INSTRUMENTAL, AND APPRAISAL SUPPORTS

The four theoretical constructs or defining attributes of the theory include emotional, informational, instrumental, and appraisal supports (Barrera, 1986; Fleury et al., 2009; House, 1981; Tilden & Weinert, 1987). *Emotional support* involves the experience of feeling liked, admired, respected, or loved. *Instrumental support* is the provision of tangible aid, goods, or services. *Informational support* refers to providing information during a time of stress. *Appraisal support* affirms one's actions or statements (House, 1981; Kahn & Antonucci, 1980; Norbeck, 1981). See Box 7.1 for an application of emotional, instrumental, informational, and appraisal supports to a social support intervention for promoting physical activity among Hispanic women.

TABLE 7.1 Theoretical Multidimensional Definitions of Social Support

Label	Support components
Aspects (Cohen, 1992)	Social networks Perceived support Supportive behaviors
Categories (Hupcey, 1998a)	Types of support provided Recipients' perceptions Intentions/behaviors of provider of support Reciprocal support Social networks
Constructs (Vaux, 1988)	Support network resources Support incidents Support behaviors Support appraisals Support or network orientation
Defining attributes (House, 1981)	Emotional support Informational support Instrumental support Appraisal support
Dimensions (Cutrona, 1990)	Emotional Esteem (appraisal) Tangible (instrumental) Information Social integration
Interpersonal transactions (Kahn, 1979)	Affect—feeling liked or loved Affirmation—of behavior, perceptions, and views Affect—feeling respected or admired Aid—material or symbolic
Subconcepts (Barrera, 1981)	Material aid Physical assistance Intimate interaction Guidance Feedback Social participation
Taxonomies (Laireiter & Baumann, 1992)	Social integration Network resources Supportive climate and environment Received and enacted support Perception of being supported
Types (Wortman, 1984)	Expression of positive affect Expression of agreement Encouragement of open expression of feelings Offer of advice and information Provision of material aid Network of reciprocal help and mutual obligation

NEGATIVE SOCIAL SUPPORT

It is possible for social support to negatively affect one's well-being (Revenson, Schiaffino, Majerovitz, & Gibofsky, 1991). The perception of or the satisfaction with the support one receives (perceived support) is likely to influence the outcome of the support activity (Heller et al., 1986). The support activity could

Box 7.1	Application of Social Support Theory to Practice: Promotion of Physical Activity among Hispanic Women

A culturally relevant program, titled *Mujeres en Accion por Su Salad* (Women in Action for Their Health), used peer counselors to provide social support interventions to promote physical activity among Hispanic women. The peer counselors (*promotoras*) are members of the community. This approach is based on the assumption that individual behavior is influenced by their social network. The peer counselors provided *emotional support* when they shared their ideas and experiences for staying with walking activities, gave encouragement, and developed relationships with women in the community. They provided *instrumental support* by offering pedometers to monitor progress toward reaching specific goals, providing maps of safe walking paths, and organizing walking groups. *Informational support* included offering facts, advice, or reassurance about skills needed for safe walking and problem solving about overcoming barriers. *Appraisal support* occurred through giving feedback about goal achievement and giving positive reinforcement for recording their progress. Social support occurred in personal relationships as well as from supportive resources in the community (Fleury et al., 2009).

actually be unrecognized or perceived negatively by the recipient. Negative social support is perceived as unhelpful and may undermine self-esteem. Characteristics of negative social support include stressful or conflicted social networks, misguided or absent support, inappropriate advice, avoidance, and disagreement (Stewart, 1993). Moreover, costs to the provider of social support such as overload, over commitment, and stressful emotional involvement may occur (Coyne & DeLongis, 1986; La Gaipa, 1990). The balance of rewards and costs is likely to influence both perceptions and effects of social support. Cost, conflict, reciprocity, and equity are sub-dimensions that could be measured to capture the negative aspects of social support (Tilden & Galyen, 1987). Assessing the quality of the social support is important. Research shows that there is a negative relationship between the quality of social support and the caregiver burden (Vrabec, 1997). The amount of conflict in the relationship can result in negative social support that contributes to stress rather than well-being.

VARIATIONS IN THE THEORY OF SOCIAL SUPPORT

A concept analysis of social support, based on an examination of 200 studies published from 1978 to 1996, revealed that most studies did not include a specific reference to a theoretical definition of social support, and that researchers who defined social support often did not use a definition that addressed the interactional nature of social support (Hupcey, 1998b). Although Hupcey suggested that social support exchanges occur in personal relationships, other scholars have discussed the examples of social support provided by professionals or outside the context of personal relationships, such as through communication over the Internet.

Professionals can intervene to strengthen existing social support networks for clients or choose to provide social support when it is lacking by helping individuals and families to access resources in the community that strengthen social support. Schaffer and Lia-Hoagberg (1997) concluded that nurses could provide informational support to partners and others important in the social networks of low-income pregnant women that would enhance the emotional, instrumental, informational, and appraisal support available to the women through their existing social networks. Social support was provided by professionals in a program called the New Mothers Network targeted to single, low-income, African American mothers. Program components included an electronic library, a chat group (asynchronous), and e-mail communication. Advanced practice nurses provided informational, appraisal, and emotional supports through e-mail discussion and offering encouraging messages in the chat group (Hudson, Campbell-Grossman, Keating-Lefler, & Cline, 2008).

Wright and Bell (2003) explained how social support occurs in computer-mediated support groups. Although communication occurs between participants who do not have close personal relationships, the participants experience emotional and informational supports as they communicate about health-related experiences they have in common. Participants may be more open in expressing emotions since there is greater anonymity and protection from stigmatization in comparison to face-to-face interactions. However, the possibility of negative support exists in the case of hostile messages. In addition, there may be greater difficulty in forming long-term relationships and a diminished reliance on family and friends may occur. On the positive side, evidence suggests that electronic social support may decrease the use of health services (Scharer, 2005).

Overlap of other related concepts with social support is also a concern when defining social support. In a study of nurse-provided telephone social support for low-income pregnant women, Finfgeld-Connett (2005) suggested that the telephone-delivered nursing interventions involved something more than the attributes of social support; she reflected that the presence may be a sub-concept of social support and that social support may have become the default variable for nursing research studies because of the unavailability of instruments for measuring nursing presence.

VARIABLES THAT INFLUENCE PERCEPTIONS OF SOCIAL SUPPORT

A number of variables affect the social support that is given and received or experienced. These include perceptions of the need and the availability for support, timing, motivation for providing support, duration, direction, life stage, the source of support, and social network.

The provider of the social support first recognizes another's need for social support before determining the response to the need. If there is a mismatch in the provider's and recipient's perceptions of the need for support or the type of support that is provided, the recipient may not consider the support to be helpful (Dunkel-Schetter & Bennett, 1990; Dunkel-Schetter & Skokan, 1990). Providers of support may assume that the recipient experiencing stress needs support. If this assumption is inaccurate, the act of support could result in feelings of dependency, inadequacy, and lower self-esteem (Dunkel-Schetter, Blasband, Feinstein, & Herbert, 1992). Research data suggest that the perception of the availability of support is more important for health and well-being than the actual receiving of the support (Cohen, Gottlieb, & Underwood, 2001).

Timing is also important, because the support needs of the recipient can change relative to the recipient's appraisal of the situation over time (Jacobson, 1986; Norwood, 1996; Tilden, 1986). Social support is a dynamic process influenced by personal characteristics and situations. Changes that affect both the giving and the receiving of social support include the nature of relationships from a historical perspective, expectations of support from one's network, and personal coping skills (Lackner, Goldenberg, Arrizza, & Tjosvold, 1994).

Motivation for providing social support can affect the quality of the support provided. A sense of obligation on the part of the provider may decrease the recipient's satisfaction with the support (Hupcey, 1998a). Providers of social support are likely to consider the recipient's responsibility and effort relative to the support needed and the costs to the provider that result from the act of support (Jung, 1988). The provider's previous experiences with providing support and previous interactions with the intended recipient will also influence choices of support actions (Hupcey, 1998a).

Duration of the support, referring to length of time or stability of the support, is a consideration for the chronically ill and persons who experience long-term loss (Cohen & Syme, 1985). The long-term effects of stressors on individuals may require ongoing support, as well as support from sources outside the usual social networks. For example, in a longitudinal study of the perceived support and support sources of older women with heart failure, the women identified paid helpers as sources of support at a later time in progression of their illness (Friedman, 1997).

The direction of support may be unidirectional or bidirectional. Bidirectional support is characterized by mutuality and reciprocity (Stewart, 1993). Professional support is usually unidirectional. In family and intimate relationships, the roles of "helper" and "helpee" may alternate (Clark, 1983; Rook & Dooley, 1985). Reciprocity in social support is likely to reduce feelings of burden and strain in providers and inadequacy and lack of control in recipients (Albrecht & Adelman, 1987).

The provision and receiving of social support vary over the life span. Some life stages offer more capability for providing social support, while others require more receiving than giving of social support.

Social support needs are greater during times of change and additional stress, such as during the birth of a child or with the loss of strength and function associated with aging.

Individuals often identify family and friends as sources of support in comparison with professionals (Hupcey & Morse, 1997; Schaffer & Lia-Hoagberg, 1997). However, professionals can intervene to enhance the existing social support resources of clients or can act as surrogates to provide support not currently available in the client's social network (Norbeck, 1988). To enhance informal and formal sources of support, professionals can develop and strengthen relationships with personal support networks, mutual aid groups, neighborhood support systems, volunteer programs, and community resources (Chien & Norman, 2009; Froland, Pancoast, Chapman, & Kimboko, 1981). Formal support is more likely to occur in institutional settings. Newsom, Bookwala, and Schulz (1997) found a high degree of formal support for older adults in nursing homes, residential care facilities, and congregate apartments. The instrumental support available in institutional settings was provided primarily by professional and nonprofessional paid staff. These formal support sources may also provide a sizeable amount of emotional support for older adults who have physical and cognitive challenges, because paid staff are more often available for older adults in group residences (Pearlman & Crown, 1992).

The size of the social network is sometimes considered an indicator of social support. Key sources of support, including immediate family members and close friends, are distinguished from sources viewed as less important—other relatives, coworkers, church and community members, and professional caregivers (Griffith, 1985). However, a large social network does not necessarily guarantee that a large amount of support is present (Kahn & Antonucci, 1980). The quality of the relationships and availability of persons in the social network, as well as the number of persons in the network, contribute to the enacted social support. A variety of network members can better provide the range of needed social support actions. For example, in one study, persons with a cancer diagnosis perceived spouses or partners as helpful for their physical presence, while friends provided practical help (Dakof & Taylor, 1990). In another study with cancer patients, informational support was perceived as helpful from experts but not from friends or families (Dunkel-Schetter, 1984).

THE RELATIONSHIP OF SOCIAL SUPPORT AND HEALTH

Heller et al. (1986) posited that two facets of social support, esteem-enhancing appraisal and stress-related, interpersonal transactions, have an effect on health outcomes. They hypothesized that the appraisal or perception of the social interaction is health protective, rather than the social interaction or support activity itself. Esteem-enhancing appraisal results from an assessment of how one is viewed by others. In stress-related interpersonal transactions, network members provide tangible assistance, which facilitates coping (Fig. 7.1).

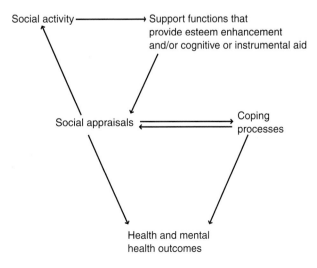

Figure 7.1 Hypothesized relationships between facets of social support, coping, and health outcomes. (From Heller, K., Swindle, R. W., & Dusenbery, L. (1986). Component social support processes: Comments and integration. *Journal of Consulting and Clinical Psychology, 54*[4], 466–470. Copyright © 1986 by the American Psychological Association. Reprinted with permission.)

Cohen et al. (2001) described two models that explain how social support influences health. The stress-buffering model holds that social support contributes to health-promoting behaviors in persons who are experiencing stress. Rather than choosing behaviors that may be harmful to health, the support resources strengthen an individual's perceived ability to cope with a stressful situation (Thoits, 1986). These beliefs lead to a calmer psychological and physiological response to the stressful situation and can decrease negative behavioral responses. In this case, an individual is more likely to have an adaptive response to the stressful situation, thus avoiding a maladaptive response with a greater potential for negative health effects.

The main effect model, the second model described by Cohen et al. (2001), suggests that social support directly impacts psychological and physical health, whether or not an individual is experiencing a stressful situation. Integration into a social network, as contrasted to isolation, can provide social control and peer pressure to engage in health-promoting behaviors and lead to positive psychological states, such as a sense of predictability, stability, purpose, belonging, and security (Cassel, 1976; Hammer, 1981; Thoits, 1983). In addition, social networks can provide multiple sources of information about health care services and may also provide informal health care that prevents progression of illness (Cohen et al., 2001).

Norbeck (1981) proposed a model for using social support as a nursing intervention to improve health outcomes. The social support environment of the client is assessed by determining the need for social support compared with the available social support. An assessment of inadequate social support necessitates developing an intervention plan to increase social support. Possible interventions can focus on strengthening the client's existing social support structure or function, or providing direct support during a crisis. According to this nursing process model, adequate social support will result in a positive health outcome; inadequate social support without intervention will result in a negative health outcome.

Manning-Walsh (2005) offers a research-based model (consistent with the stress-buffering model) in which social support is a mediator that contributes to improved health outcomes. In a study of women with breast cancer, personal support provided by family and close friends mediated the negative effects of common symptoms contributing to distress during the breast cancer treatment and resulted in improved scores on quality of life measures both generally and specific to breast cancer.

Other studies in nursing have resulted in positive relationships between social support and other variables that contribute to improvements in health behavior or positive perceptions about health. In a study of Taiwanese women in early pregnancy, women with higher levels of social support reported less stress; social support along with the additional predictor variables of pregnancy-related nausea and vomiting, perceived stress, and pregnancy planning together explained the variance in maternal psychosocial adaptation (Chou, Avant, Kuo, & Fetzer, 2008). Keller, Allan, and Tinkle (2006) found that social support from friends increased the time postpartum women spent in physical exercise. In a study of nursing home residents in Norway, Drageset et al. (2009) determined that there was positive relationship between social support and health-related quality of life. In a study of older adults who used senior centers in New York, perceived social support was positively associated with autonomy (Matsui & Capezuti, 2008). Latham and Calviollo (2009) explored predictors of successful diabetes management in a sample of 240 low-income Hispanic people. Social support explained 24% of the satisfaction with quality of life and self on the Diabetes Quality of Life measure. Chien and Norman (2009) conducted a literature review to determine the effectiveness of mutual support groups for family caregivers of people with psychotic disorders. Mutual support groups are "informal networks of individuals who share a common experience or issue" (p. 1618). In the review of 25 studies, they found evidence for short-term positive effects on physical and psychosocial health for clients and families. Benefits included more knowledge about the illness and treatment, lower burden and distress, and better coping ability. The researchers suggested that there should be more studies that investigate the long-term effects of mutual support groups.

SOCIAL SUPPORT NURSING ASSESSMENT AND INTERVENTIONS

Beeber and Canuso (2005) suggested five critical assessment questions for nurses to help determine effective emotional, informational, and instrumental social support interventions:

1. Who helps you get the day-to-day things you need in your life?
2. If you had an emergency, who would you call on for help?

3. Who would lend you money to keep or ask to keep your child(ren) if you needed it?
4. Who gives you advice that is useful?
5. Who understands your private worries and feelings? (p. 773).

Logsdon and Koniak-Griffin (2005) developed a clinical pathway for social support of postpartum adolescents, which outlines assessment of social support; assessment of related variables such as depression, risk for harm, and high-risk behaviors; and health care provider interventions. They gave examples of specific assessment questions, suggested relevant instruments for the measurement of social support, and identified professional interventions that strengthen existing social support networks. Identified pathway interventions include counseling and teaching about the reality and demands of the postpartum period, common feelings experienced in the postpartum period, options for social support in their network, and the importance of communication as well as providing social skills training and referral for community services. Such interventions can raise the level of perceived appraisal, emotional, informational, and instrumental supports.

Vandall-Walker, Jensen, and Oberle (2007) used a grounded theory approach to explore the process of nursing support in a sample of 20 family members from 14 families of critically ill adults hospitalized in intensive care. Family members viewed nursing support as "lightening their load." Initially, nurses engaged family members through the following support activities: acknowledging, welcoming, orienting, relating, trusting, and empathizing. The middle phase focused on sustaining family members through nursing actions of being there, communicating, being accountable, sharing responsibility, negotiating, valuing, promoting family member self-care, and connecting family members to other professionals and services. The final stage of disengaging included providing guidance for decisions, helping to find meaning, and preparing family members to say goodbye, which may involve the client's death or the client leaving the unit. The family members identified nursing support activities that helped them to "get through" the situation, which is different than conceptualizations of support as caring (Vandall-Walker et al.). Many of these nursing actions will likely result in the provision of emotional, informational, instrumental, and appraisal supports to families of critically ill adults.

APPLICATIONS OF THE THEORY

CLINICAL APPLICATIONS

Nurses have the knowledge and expertise to assess the interpersonal and social environments of clients, implement health promotion strategies, and facilitate clients in initiating self-care practices (Tilden, 1985). From a prevention perspective, social support can be viewed as "social inoculation" (Pilisuk, 1982). Through "network therapy," nurses can assess social support adequacy, use existing social support measures, determine the roles of professionals and nonprofessional providers of social support to move clients to increasing independence, and organize and evaluate community support groups (Roberts, 1984).

One example of preventive support is comprehensive home visitation for vulnerable young mothers provided by public health nurses (Olds et al., 2007). Nurses provided regular home visits to young mothers beginning during their pregnancy and continuing until their children were two years of age. The purposes of the visits were to improve pregnancy outcomes, to promote children's healthy development, and to improve the financial self-sufficiency of participating families. Nurses both provided formal support and strengthened informal sources of support. Evaluation of the long-term outcomes through a randomized clinical trial demonstrated positive outcomes for mothers (reduced subsequent birth rate, longer interval between first and second birth, and more relationship stability) and children (higher academic achievement and lower mortality from preventable causes).

Additional clinical application examples are described in Table 7.2, which specifies the five social support intervention levels suggested by Stewart (1989b): individual, dyadic, groups, community, and social system. Interventions at these levels include strengthening available social support and providing direct social support with the goal of improving health status. Table 7.2 provides a summary of the level of intervention based on Stewart's framework, social support intervention examples with the relevant social support theoretical constructs (emotional, informational, instrumental, and appraisal supports), and desired health outcomes.

TABLE 7.2 Clinical Application: Social Support Interventions

Intervention level	Situation	Social support interventions	Desired health outcomes
Individual— Modify how individual seeks or per-ceives sup-port provided by others	A pregnant woman is placed on bed rest for a high-risk pregnancy. She has a two-year-old son and her husband works long hours. She views her husband as her primary source of social support and does not know how she will manage get-ting the assistance she needs during her confinement to bed rest. She is receiv-ing care through a hospital-based home care agency that provides nursing care to perinatal clients.	Assess her available components and sources of social support. Educate her about the importance of bed rest for her pregnancy and describe the kind of support she will need (*informational support*). Counsel her about the need to seek social support from other sources during a time of increased stress and need (*appraisal support*). Listen to the client's concerns about her husband's potential reactions asking the client's mother to assist with household tasks and child care (*emotional support*). The client arranges for help with child-care from her mother and several neighborhood families (*instrumental support*).	Reduced family stress Positive coping strategies Healthy infant
Dyadic— Strengthen support from a key network member or introduce outsider to provide sup-port	A 35-year-old woman is having a mastectomy for breast cancer. She states that she has a very close relation-ship with her husband but has not discussed with him about how the surgery will affect their sexual relation-ship.	Assess her available sources of support for talking about her specific concern. Reassure her that this is a common concern that is difficult for couples to discuss (*appraisal support*). Give her information about a program that provides a visitor who has had a breast cancer experience and suggest that referral for couples' counseling is an option (*informational support*). Following a meeting with the visitor from the volunteer program, the client discusses her concerns with her husband and is reassured by his response (*emotional support*).	Maintenance of healthy self-concept Positive couple relationship Reduced complications
*Group—*Enlarge existing infor-mal network, improve skills of natural helpers, refer to or create support groups	A 45-year-old man has MS and recently became wheelchair dependent. His wife has returned to full-time work. The couple has two teenagers. Case management is provided through a home health agency. The wife has become increasingly frustrated with trying to manage her work demands and the needs of her husband.	Assess the family's social support components and sources, extended family, friend, community, and profes-sional support. Suggest that a support group for persons with MS and their families could be helpful in providing them with under-standing and practical ideas for their situation (*informational support*). Because a local support group does not exist, work with a community service agency to develop a support group (*instrumental support*). The family participates in a local sup-port group (*emotional support*). Reevaluate the current nursing services. Provide additional services needed to reduce the wife's workload (*instrumental support*).	Reduced care-giver stress level Effective family functioning Increased commu-nity resources through provision of a support group for clients with MS and their family members

			TABLE 7.2 Clinical Application: Social Support Interventions (*Continued*)

Intervention level	Situation	Social support interventions	Desired health outcomes
Community— Promote social support and social network frequency of interaction in neighborhoods, organizations, and communities	Elderly residents in an urban, ethnically diverse, low-income neighborhood are more isolated in the winter. A Block Nurse program has been recently established to address the health care needs of this population. A high percentage of the clients served by the program have diabetes.	Survey a sample of the neighborhood elderly population to determine health concerns and social support needs. Consult and collaborate with a foot-care nurse to offer a foot-care program in a community clinic, as well as through home visits. During the clinic and home visits, assess the social support needs of the elderly persons. Educate them about foot care and community resources that can offer them assistance with house cleaning and maintenance (*instrumental support and informational support*). Collaborate with a local faith-based organization to extend their visitation ministry to isolated elderly persons in the neighborhood for the purpose of increasing their social interaction (*emotional support and appraisal support*).	Reduction in complications from diabetes in elderly population in neighborhood Elderly residents stay in their own homes for a longer time period Reduction in health care costs for nursing home care
Systems— Promote policy and structural changes to increase social support in environments and/or remove barriers to social support (in schools, municipalities, hospitals)	The percentage of children who are overweight in an elementary school population has increased. The cafeteria serves highly processed food. The school breakfast program includes sugared cereals.	Educate parents and school staff/administrators about the health concern and collaborate with them to develop a plan to respond to the problem (*informational support*). Use social marketing in the school setting (posters, announcements, bulletins) to increase awareness of the problem and provide classroom education about health behaviors that influence body mass (*informational support*). Contribute to the development of policy for more nutritional food choices in the breakfast and lunch program (*instrumental support*). Create a peer support program to encourage positive change in health behavior patterns, such as nutritional food choices and physical activity (*appraisal support*).	Increase in attractive, nutritious food choices and a reduction in the amount of processed food in meals served at the school Increase in knowledge about the contribution of food choices and exercise to body mass index (BMI) among school children Increase in percentage of children with a normal BMI

RESEARCH APPLICATIONS

Researchers have explored a great variety of nursing practice issues from a social support perspective including topics such as chronic illness, persons who are grieving, the relationship of social support to acute chest complaints, new mothers in stressful situations, and administrative support for nurses. Researchers have also investigated how social support interacts with other variables to predict health outcomes. The majority of studies focus on the individual or family level experience of social support. Few researchers have investigated social support from a community or systems perspective.

Social support theory was used to conceptualize a study on the provision of social support to single, low-income, African American mothers through e-mail messages in a program called the New Mothers Network. The authors explained that informational, emotional, and appraisal supports are feasible through an Internet intervention. In addition, negative social support may occur if the interactions are perceived as nonsupportive, even though they may be intended to be positive. Guidelines for nurses' response to e-mail communication included: (1) timely response to the single mothers' messages, (2) use of an informal and caring tone in messages, (3) inclusion of brief questions that addressed earlier interactions to stimulate a reply, (4) presentation of information in brief and simple paragraphs for easy viewing, and (5) messages written at sixth-grade reading level. In addition, links to community resources were often imbedded in the messages. The researchers conducted a qualitative analysis of key themes of the e-mail messages from the mothers to two nurses for a sample of 12 mothers over a six-month time period. Cultural backgrounds of the nurses were similar to the participants. One of the three themes focused on relationships of support. The single mothers discussed both positive and negative supports they received in interactions with family and the infant's father. Data indicated that some mothers were not seeking advice from the nurse (informational support), but rather were discussing a topic in detail. The authors suggested that the mothers may have been seeking emotional and appraisal supports after discussing negative support from the family. Analysis of messages indicated that social support needs of the mothers were greater than the support offered to them by the family and the birth father. Although the mothers generally did not seek informational support, nurses can use the Internet to provide information about topics such as feeding infants and postpartum depression. The authors suggested that nurses can provide emotional support to the young mothers for coping with changes in becoming a mother and appraisal support for new learning about caring for their infant. In addition, nurses can suggest strategies for responding to negative support that mothers may receive from family members, friends, and the infant's father.

Source: Campbell-Grossman, C. K., Hudson, D. B., Keating-Lefler, R., & Heusinvelt, S. (2009). New mothers network: The provision of social support to single, low-income, African American mothers via e-mail messages. *Journal of Family Nursing, 15*(2), 220–236.

See Using Middle Range Theories 7.1 for an example of how social support theory has been used in research. The Bibliography at the end of the chapter lists additional citations on social support research in nursing.

MEASURES OF SOCIAL SUPPORT

Although a great number of social support measures have been developed in several disciplines, many measures do not have adequate reliability and validity testing, and many are situation specific rather than general measures of social support. Available measures address: (a) interconnectedness in a social network; (b) received support, based on a person's report of support that was provided; and (c) perceived support, the support a person believes to be available to them (Sarason, Sarason, & Pierce, 1990). Researchers have primarily developed situation-specific measures of social support for groups who encounter a common stressor event, such as pregnancy or chronic illness (Stewart, 1993). Of 21 social support instruments reviewed by Stewart (1998a), only four were applicable on a general level. Six measures of social support developed by nurse researchers are described in Table 7.3. The selected instruments represent both general and specific measures of social support and have been psychometrically analyzed. None of the instruments are applicable to young children. Additional measures of social support that have been used by but not developed by nurse researchers are listed at the bottom of the table.

Most measures of social support are self-reports. Newsom et al. (1997) discussed the challenge of measuring social support for the cognitively impaired. They suggested that proxy and observational measures of social support may be an alternative strategy for determining the adequacy of social support for persons who cannot provide an accurate self-report. Proxies, such as nursing home staff and primary caregivers, can provide information about social network contacts and interactions. Observational

TABLE 7.3 Selected Social Support Instruments Developed by Nurse Researchers

Instrument	Social support components	Description	Sample item
Interpersonal Relationships Inventory (IPRI) (Tilden, Nelson, & May, 1990)	Social support Reciprocity Conflict	39 items (13 for each subscale) Five-point agree/disagree scale Subscales used separately Internal consistency and test–retest reliability Construct validity for social support and conflict subscales	Someone believes in me (support). I let others know I care (reciprocity). I wish people were more sensitive (conflict).
Norbeck Social Support Questionnaire (NSSQ) (Norbeck et al., 1981, 1983)	Affect Affirmation Aid Loss Duration of relationship Frequency of contact	Identify persons in network Five-point scale on extent of support provided for nine questions Internal consistency and test–retest reliability Construct validity	How much does this person make you feel if liked or loved?
Social Support Questionnaire (SSQ) (Northouse, 1988) Perceived Resource Questionnaire (PRQ-85) (Weinert, 1987, 1988)	Sources of social support Amount of social support Intimacy Social integration Nurturance Worth Assistance	40 items Sources—spouse, family member, friends, nurse, physician Five-point Likert-type agree/disagree scale Internal consistency reliability and concurrent validity Part 1—Identifies resources and satisfaction with help Part 2—25 items on perceived social support; seven-point agree/disagree scale Internal consistency reliability—Part 2 Construct validity—Part 2	If I need advice there is someone who would assist me to work out a plan to deal with the situation.
Support Behaviors Inventory (SBI) (Brown, 1986)	Perceived degree of experiential support during pregnancy—satisfaction with partner support and other support	11 items on shortened version Six-point satisfied/dissatisfied scale Internal consistency reliability for total support score on shortened version	Tolerates my ups and downs and unusual behaviors.
Social Support in Chronic Illness Survey (SSCII) (Hilbert, 1990)	Intimate interaction Guidance Feedback Maternal aid Behavioral assistance Positive social interaction	38 items Six-point satisfied/dissatisfied scale Internal consistency reliability Content validity	Commented favorably when he/she noticed me doing something that the health team recommended.

Note: Additional measures of social support used by Nurse Researchers.

● Family Functioning, Health and Social Support (FAFHES)—social support portion has 37 items for aid, affirmation, and affect subscales (Astedt-Kurki, Tarkaa, Rikala, Lehti, & Paavilainen, 2009)
● Family Support for Exercise Scale (Sallis, Grossman, Pinski, Patterson, & Nader, 1987)
● Friend Support for Exercise Scale (Sallis et al. , 1987)
● Interpersonal Support Evaluation List (ISEL)—15 items include appraisal, belonging, and tangible support (Cohen, 1985; Owen, 2003)
● Multidimensional Scale of Perceived Social Support (MSPSS)—12 items include significant other, family, and friend subscales (Zimet et al., 1988)
● Social Support for Physical Activity Scale—four items measure support from kin, non-kin, and health-care workers (Cousins, 1996)

methods include recording interaction behaviors and videotaping. A coding system can be used to label the source and the type of the support, the recipient response, and other characteristics of the support interaction.

Some researchers have used qualitative approaches for investigating social support, although quantitative measures appear to be predominant. In Finland, nurse researchers asked one open-ended question to explore perceptions of social support after the death of a spouse: "What helped you cope with your grief?" (Kaunonen, Tarkka, Paunonen, & Laippla, 1999). The researchers used content analysis to classify the data by the structure of social relationships and the social support functions of aid, affirmation, and affect in relationships (Kahn, 1979). Lugton (1997) used a strategy called social contact analysis, in addition to interview data, to explore the social support experienced by women treated for breast cancer. Participants drew their social networks, with self at center, using shorter lines for closer relationships and arrows to indicate whether the relationship involved support, strain, or both. The researcher then asked participants to describe how professional and informal persons in the social network had responded to the illness of the participant in supportive and nonsupportive ways. Types of support that facilitated adjustment were emotional support, companionship, practical help, opportunities for confiding, experiential support (from others who had experienced breast cancer), and sexual identity support.

CHALLENGES TO SOCIAL SUPPORT THEORY DEVELOPMENT AND RESEARCH

Future efforts in social support theory development and research need to move from a description of the relationship of social support and health outcomes to the investigation of interactional characteristics, negative aspects, gender and cultural contexts, causal relationships in social support, and effective social support interventions. In particular, multilevel interventions that address both interpersonal support and community-level environmental support could contribute to knowledge about cost-effective social support strategies for improving the health status of populations.

Since researchers have used a variety of definitions of social support and have measured different aspects of social support, it is difficult to compare study results (Heitzmann & Kaplan, 1988; Roberts, 1984). Hupcey (1998b) commented that many other concepts, such as marital status and frequency of contact, have often been included in definitions of social support. A focus on the interactional nature of social support is missing from many studies. To determine effectiveness of social support, an understanding of the perceptions of the providers of social support as well as those of the recipient merits further exploration (Hupcey, 1998b). The reciprocity of social support is an interactional variable that can contribute to understanding effective social support interventions.

Middle range social support theory development could be enhanced by greater exploration of the negative effects of informal social support. Many social support measures do not include negative aspects of relationships (Krishnasamy, 1996; Stewart, 1993). In a review of 50 studies on social support and caregiver burden, Vrabec (1997) recommended further examination of the amount of conflict in the social support network as a predictor of caregiver burden. The Interpersonal Relationships Inventory (IPRI) is one of the few measures that attempts to encompass the full context of relationships through inclusion of reciprocity and conflict subscales (Tilden et al., 1990).

Social support measures also need to be sensitive to the cultural context (Ducharme, Stevens, & Rowat, 1994). Higgins and Dicharry (1991) evaluated the Personal Resources Inventory Part 2 (PRQ) for its applicability to Navajo women. They found that 10 of the 25 items were not applicable to Navajo culture. The 10 items were considered too personal because in the Navajo culture, family problems and feelings are not discussed with others. Different cultural groups may vary in perceptions of the number of persons they consider to be a part of their social network, as well as the relative importance of the different components of social support. Expectations for independence and help may differ. Some types of assistance could be expected and appreciated by one culture and be interpreted as shameful by another culture.

In a study on types of social support in African Americans with cancer, Hamilton and Sandelowski (2004) found that although the broad categories of social support were applicable to the African American sample, strategies for perceived helpful social support differed from Caucasian populations. African Americans perceived presence and distracting activities as emotional support in contrast to verbal expressions of problems. Instrumental support included offers of prayer and other kinds of assistance that were less often identified in other studies of social support.

Martinez-Schallmoser, MacMullen, and Telleen (2005) suggested specific assessment questions that are adapted to the social support needs of the Mexican American pregnant women population. The meaning of social support across cultures needs further exploration. In addition, males are a neglected population in social support research (Langford et al., 1997). Qualitative research approaches could be useful for discovering meanings of social support across cultures.

Causality in social support research needs further exploration. Researchers have conducted many descriptive and correlational studies that link social support to positive health outcomes, but fewer studies substantiate causal links (Callaghan & Morrissey, 1993). The impact of health status on how people seek and receive support has been explored less often than the effects of social support on health status (Stewart, 1993). Changes in health status are likely to influence the amount and components of social support that are needed. With increased stress resulting from threats to health, social support actions can facilitate coping. Moreover, the balance of reciprocity in relationships and the amount of conflict present may change in response to health status changes. One question suggested by Cohen et al. (2001) for future study is whether persons with chronic illness decrease their provision of support, resulting in an imbalance in the social network (reciprocity).

To further develop an understanding of the linkages of social support to health outcomes, theoretically based social support interventions need to be tested in controlled intervention trials across varied settings and age groups (Ducharme et al., 1994). Cohen et al. (2001) suggested that more intervention research should be conducted on promising interventions, such as support groups and support provided in dyads (partner or peer support). In addition, research on interventions that focus on strengthening the social support environments at a community or systems level can develop knowledge about how to use social support to improve the health status of populations. Multilevel interventions may be the most effective. Rook and Dooley (1985) described two categorical approaches to social support interventions—individual and environmental. Individual interventions are used to change how a person perceives or seeks support, while an environmental approach targets the community to improve the social support climate. Social support is likely to be maximized with the implementation of both approaches. Research methods used to test the effectiveness of social support interventions need to be tailored to the intervention level. Measures for any level should include the potential negative aspects of social support in the person's interactions and environment, which, if not considered, can confound the interpretation of study findings. Evaluation of social support interventions at the individual, dyadic, and group levels is likely to focus on the perceptions of social support actions and available support. Evaluation of social support interventions at the community and system levels emphasizes analysis of social support available in networks and the environment.

SUMMARY

Social support theory is important to nurses because it can explain and suggest nursing interventions to improve health outcomes. Although a great variety of social support measures have been developed, many are for specific situations. There is a lack of consensus on the definition of social support. Authors disagree on the dimensionality of social support. A major concern is the omission of considering potential negative aspects of social support. The next step for expanding social support theory is knowledge development about effective multilevel social support interventions.

ANALYSIS OF THEORY

This chapter provides several constructs to view the phenomenon. Using the criteria presented in Chapter 2, critique the body of knowledge presented in this chapter. You will be using each criterion in a manner different from its use when applied to one specific theory. Specific questions related to the use of each criterion in this new context follow. Compare your conclusions about the constructs across theories with those found in Appendix A. A nurse scholar who has worked with this phenomenon completed the analysis found in the Appendix.

Internal Criticism

1. Clarity (Do we have theories of social support that are clear?)
2. Consistency (Is there consistency in approach, that is, terms, interpretations, principles, and methods, across theories?)
3. Adequacy (How adequate is the body of theories in accounting for social support?)
4. Level of theory development (At what level of development are the social support theories?)

External Criticism

1. Reality convergence (Do these theories reflect "real world" nursing experiences of social support?)
2. Utility (How useful are present theories when applied in practice and research?)
3. Significance (Do the theories reflect issues essential to nursing?)
4. Discrimination (Do the theories help distinguish social support from other interpersonal processes?)
5. Scope of theory (What seems to be the scope of the theories?)
6. Complexity (As a group, how would you judge the complexity of social support theories?)

CRITICAL THINKING EXERCISES

Compare two options for providing a social support intervention for parents of children diagnosed with a chronic mental illness: (a) a nurse led monthly face-to-face meeting of parents (with childcare provided) and (b) an asynchronous Internet discussion for the parents.

1. Look at the list of definitions of key terms. Use the key terms to analyze the nature of the social support experience that could be expected from each of the two interventions.

2. Analyze how each of the interventions is consistent or inconsistent with Hupcey's definition of social support.

3. Design evaluation studies, using both quantitative and qualitative approaches, to measure the experience of social support and effectiveness of the intervention for each of the two options. Consider the reliability and validity of suggested measurement strategies.

4. Analyze how the following variables may affect the experience of social support in each of the two options: perceptions of the need for and availability of support, timing, motivation for providing support, duration, direction, life stage, sources of social support, and social network.

5. Analyze the potential effectiveness (improved health outcomes and coping) resulting from professional or nurse-provided social support versus enhancement of social support provided by personal relationships and social networks for parents of children with a chronic mental illness.

WEB RESOURCES

Visit **http://thePoint.lww.com/Peterson3e** for helpful web resources related to this chapter.

REFERENCES

Albrecht, T., & Adelman, M. (1987). Communication networks as structures of social support. In T. Albrecht & M. Adelman (Eds.), *Communicating social support* (pp. 40–61). Newbury Park, CA: Sage.

Astedt-Kurki, P., Tarkka, M. T., Rikala, M. R., Lehti, K., & Paavilainen, E. (2009). Further testing of a family nursing instrument (FAFES). *International Journal of Nursing Studies, 46*, 350–359.

Barrera, M. (1981). Social support in the adjustment of pregnant adolescents: Assessment issues. In B. Gottlieb (Ed.), *Social networks and social support* (pp. 69–96). Beverly Hills, CA: Sage.

Barrera, M., Jr. (1986). Distinctions between social support concepts, measures, and models. *American Journal of Community Psychology, 14*(4), 413–445.

Beeber, L. S., & Canuso, R. (2005). Strengthening social support for the low-income mother: Five critical questions and a guide for intervention. *Journal of Obstetric, Gynecologic & Neonatal Nursing, 34*(6), 769–776.

Bowlby, J. (1971). *Attachment.* London: Pelican.

Brown, M. A. (1986). Social support during pregnancy: A unidimensional or multidimensional concept? *Nursing Research, 35*(1), 4–9.

Callaghan, P., & Morrissey, J. (1993). Social support and health: A review. *Journal of Advanced Nursing, 18*, 203–210.

Cassel, J. (1974). Psychosocial process and "stress": Theoretical perspectives. *International Journal of Health Services, 4*(3), 471–482.

Cassel, J. (1976). The contribution of the social environment to host resistance. *American Journal of Epidemiology, 104*(2), 107–123.

Chien, W., & Norman, I. (2009). The effectiveness and active ingredients of mutual support groups for family caregivers of people with psychotic disorders: A literature review. *International Journal of Nursing Studies 46*, 1604–1623.

Chou, F., Avant, K. C., Kuo, S., & Fetzer, S. J. (2008). Relationships between nausea and vomiting, perceived stress, social support, pregnancy planning, and psychosocial adaptation in a sample of mothers: A questionnaire survey. *International Journal of Nursing Studies, 45*, 1185–1191.

Clark, J. S. (1983). Reactions to aid in communal and exchange relationships. In J. D. Fisher, D. Nadler & B. M. DePaulo (Eds.), *New directions in helping: Vol 1. Recipient reactions to aid* (pp. 281–305). New York: Academic.

Cobb, S. (1976). Social support as a moderator of life stress. *Psychosomatic Medicine, 38*, 300–314.

Cohen, S. (1992). Stress, social support, and disorder. In H. O. Veiel & U. Baumann (Eds.), *The meaning and measurement of social support* (pp.109–204). New York: Hemisphere Publishing.

Cohen, S., Gottlieb, B. H., & Underwood, L. G. (2001). Social relationships and health: Challenges for measurement and intervention. *Advances in Mind–Body Medicine, 17*, 129–141.

Cohen, S., Mermelstein, R., Kmarack, T., & Hoberman, H. M. (1985). Measuring the functional components of social support. In I. G. Sarason & B. R. Sarason (Eds.). *Social support: Theory, research and applications.* Boston, MA: Martinus Nijhoff.

Cohen, S., & Syme, S. L. (1985). Issues in the study and application of social support (pp. 73–94). In S. Cohen & S. L. Syme (Eds.), *Social support and health* (pp. 3–32). New York: Academic.

Cousins, S. O. (1996). Exercise cognition among elderly women. *Journal of Applied Sport Psychology, 8*, 131–145.

Coyne, J. C., & DeLongis, A. (1986). Going beyond social support: The role of social relationships in adaptation. *Journal of Consulting and Clinical Psychology, 54*, 454–460.

Cutrona, C. E. (1990). Stress and social support: In search of optimal matching. *Journal of Social and Clinical Psychology, 9*(1), 3–14.

Dakof, G., & Taylor, S. (1990). Victim's perception of social support: What is helpful from whom? *Journal of Personality and Social Psychology, 58*(1), 80–89.

Diamond, M. (1985). A review and critique of the concepts of social support. In R. A. O'Brien (Ed.), *Social support and health: New directions for theory and research* (pp. 1–32). Rochester, NY: University of Rochester Press.

Drageset, J., Eide, G. E., Nygard, H. A., Bondevik, M., Nortvedt, M. W., & Natvig, G. K. (2009). The impact of social support and sense of coherence on health-related quality of life among nursing home residents—A questionnaire survey in Bergen, Norway. *International Journal of Nursing Studies, 46*, 66–76.

Ducharme, F., Stevens, B., & Rowat, K. (1994). Social support: Conceptual and methodological issues for research in mental health nursing. *Issues in Mental Health Nursing, 15*, 373–392.

Dunkel-Schetter, C. (1984). Social support and cancer: Findings based on patient interviews and their implications. *Journal of Social Issues, 40*(4), 77–98.

Dunkel-Schetter, C., & Bennett, T. L. (1990). Differentiating the cognitive and behavioral aspects of social support. In B. R. Sarason, I. G. Sarason, & G. R. Pierce (Eds.), *Social support: An interactional view* (pp. 267–296). New York: Wiley.

Dunkel-Schetter, C., Blasband, D., Feinstein, L., & Herbert, T. (1992). Elements of supportive interactions.

When are attempts to help effective? In S. Spacapan & S. Oskamp (Eds.), *Helping and being helped* (pp. 83–114). New York: Academic.

Dunkel-Schetter, C., & Skokan, L. A. (1990). Determinants of social support provision in personal relationships. *Journal of Social and Personal Relationships, 7*(4), 437–450.

Finfgeld-Connett, D. (2005). Telephone social support or nursing presence? Analysis of a nursing intervention. *Qualitative Health Research, 15*(1), 19–29.

Fleury, J., Keller, C., & Perez, A. (2009). Social support theoretical perspective. *Geriatric Nursing, 30*(2S), 11–14.

Friedman, M. M. (1997). Social support sources among older women with heart failure: Continuity versus loss over time. *Research in Nursing and Health, 20*, 319–327.

Froland, C., Pancoast, D., Chapman, D., & Kimboko, P. (1981). *Helping networks and human services.* Beverly Hills, CA: Sage.

Griffith, J. (1985). Social support providers: Who are they? Where are they met? And the relationships of network characteristics to psychological distress. *Basic and Applied Social Psychology, 6*(1), 41–60.

Hamilton, J. B., & Sandelowski, M. (2004). Types of social support in African Americans with cancer. *Oncology Nursing Forum, 31*(4), 792–800.

Hammer, M. (1981). "Core" and "extended" social networks in relation to health and illness. *Social Science and Medicine, 17*, 405–411.

Heitzmann, C. A., & Kaplan, R. M. (1988). Assessment of methods for measuring social support. *Health Psychology, 7*(1), 75–109.

Heller, K., Swindle, R. W., & Dusenbury, L. (1986). Component social support processes: Comments and integration. *Journal of Consulting and Clinical Psychology, 54*(4), 466–470.

Hilbert, G. A. (1990). Measuring social support in chronic illness. In O. L. Strickland & C. F. Waltz (Eds.), *Measurement of nursing outcomes* (Vol. 4, pp. 79–95). New York: Springer.

Higgins, P. G., & Dicharry, E. K. (1991). Measurement issues addressing social support with Navajo women. *Western Journal of Nursing Research, 13*(2), 242–255.

House, J. S. (1981). *Work stress and social support.* Englewood Cliffs, NJ: Prentice Hall.

Hudson, D. B., Campbell-Grossman, C., Keating-Lefler, R., & Cline, P. (2008). New mothers network: The development of internet-based social support intervention for African American mothers. *Issues in Comprehensive Pediatric Nursing, 31*, 23–25.

Hupcey, J. E. (1998a). Clarifying the social support theory–research linkage. *Journal of Advanced Nursing, 27*(6), 1231–1241.

Hupcey, J. E. (1998b). Social support: Assessing conceptual coherence. *Qualitative Health Research, 8*(3), 304–318.

Hupcey, J. E., & Morse, J. M. (1997). Can a professional relationship be considered social support? *Nursing Outlook, 45*, 270–276.

Jacobson, D. E. (1986). Types and timing of social support. *Journal of Health and Social Behavior, 27*, 250–264.

Jung, J. (1988). Social support providers: Why do they help? *Basic and Applied Social Psychology, 9*, 231–240.

Kahn, R. L. (1979). Aging and social support. In M. W. Riley (Ed.), *Aging from birth to death: Interdisciplinary perspectives* (pp. 77–91). Boulder, CO: Westview Press.

Kahn, R. L., & Antonucci, T. C. (1980). Convoys over the life course: Attachment, roles, and social support. In P. B. Baltes & G. Brim (Eds.), *Life span development and behavior* (*Vol. 3,* pp. 253–283). New York: Academic.

Kaunonen, M., Tarkka, M., Paunonen, M., & Laippala, P. (1999). Grief and social support after the death of a spouse. *Journal of Advanced Nursing, 30*(6), 1304–1311.

Keller, C., Allan, J., & Tinkle, M. B. (2006). Stages of change, processes of change, and social support for exercise and weight gain in postpartum women. *Journal of Obstetric, Gynecologic, & Neonatal Nursing, 35*(2), 232–240.

Krishnasamy, M. (1996). Social support and the patient with cancer: A consideration of the literature. *Journal of Advanced Nursing, 23*(4), 757–762.

La Gaipa, J. J. (1990). The negative effects of informal support systems. In S. Duck (Ed.), *Personal relationships and social support* (pp. 122–139). London: Sage.

Lackner, S., Goldenberg, S., Arrizza, G., & Tjosvold, I. (1994). The contingency of social support. *Qualitative Health Research, 4*(2), 224–243.

Laireiter, A., & Baumann, U. (1992). Network structures and support functions theoretical and empirical analyses. In H. O. Veiel & U. Baumann (Eds.), *The meaning and measurement of social support* (pp. 33–55). London: Hemisphere Publishing.

Langford, C. P. H., Bowsher, J., Maloney, J. P., & Lillis, P. (1997). Social support: A conceptual analysis. *Journal of Advanced Nursing, 25*(1), 95–100.

Latham, C. L., & Calvillo, E. (2009). Predictors of successful diabetes management in low-income Hispanic people. *Western Journal of Nursing Research, 313*, 364–387.

Logsdon, M. C,, & Koniak-Griffin, D. (2005). Social support in postpartum adolescents: Guidelines for nursing assessments and interventions. *Journal of Obstetric, Gynecologic, and Neonatal Nursing, 34*(6), 761–768.

Lugton, J. (1997). The nature of social support as experienced by women treated for breast cancer. *Journal of Advanced Nursing, 25*(6), 1184–1191.

Manning-Walsh, J. (2005). Social support as a mediator between symptom distress and quality of life in women with breast cancer. *Journal of Obstetric, Gynecologic, and Neonatal Nursing, 34*(4), 482–493.

Martinez-Schallmoser, L., MacMullen, N. J., & Telleen, S. (2005). Social support in Mexican American childbearing women. *Journal of Obstetric, Gynecologic, and Neonatal Nursing, 34*(6), 755–760.

Matsui, M., & Capezuti, E. (2008). Perceived autonomy and self-care resources among senior center users. *Geriatric Nursing, 29*(2), 141–147.

Newsom, J. T., Bookwala, J., & Schulz, R. (1997). Social support measurement in group residences for older adults. *Journal of Mental Health and Aging, 3*(1), 47–66.

Norbeck, J. S. (1981). Social support: A model for clinical research and application. *Advances in Nursing Science, 3*(4), 43–59.

Norbeck, J. S. (1988). Social support. *Annual Review of Nursing Research, 6*, 85–109.

Norbeck, J. S., Lindsey, A. M., & Carrieri, V. L. (1981). The development of an instrument to measure social support. *Nursing Research, 30*(5), 264–269.

Norbeck, J. S., Lindsey, A. M., & Carrieri, V. L. (1983). Further development of the Norbeck social support questionnaire: Normative data and validity testing. *Nursing Research, 32*(1), 4–9.

Norbeck, J. S., & Tilden, V. P. (1988). International research in social support: Theoretical and methodological issues. *Journal of Advanced Nursing, 13*, 173–178.

Northouse, L. (1988). Social support in patients' and husbands' adjustment to breast cancer. *Nursing Research, 37*, 91–95.

Norwood, S. L. (1996). The social support Apgar: Instrument development and testing. *Research in Nursing and Health, 19*, 143–152.

Olds, D. L., Kitzman, H., Hanks, C., Cole, R., Anson, E., Sidora-Arccoleo, K., et al. (2007). Effects of nurse home visiting on maternal and child functioning: Age-9 follow-up of a randomized trial. *Pediatrics, 120*(4), 832–845.

Owen, A. E. (2003). *Evaluation of differences in depression, defensiveness, social support, and coping between acute and chronic CHD patients hospitalized for myocardial infarction and unstable angina.* Unpublished doctoral dissertation, Department of Philosophy College of Arts and Sciences University, South Florida.

Pearlman, D. N., & Crown, W. H. (1992). Alternative sources of social support and their impacts on institutional risk. *The Gerontologist, 32*, 527–535.

Pierce, G. R., Sarason, B. R., & Sarason, I. G. (1990). Integrating social support perspectives: Working models, personal relationships, and situational factors. In S. Duck (Ed.), *Personal relationships and social support* (pp. 173–189). London: Sage.

Pilisuk, M. (1982). Delivery of social support: The social inoculation. *American Journal of Orthopsychiatry, 52*, 20–31.

Revenson, T., Schiaffino, K., Majerovitz, S., & Gibofsky, A. (1991). Social support as a double-edged sword: The relation of positive and problematic support to depression among rheumatoid arthritis patients. *Social Science Medicine, 33*(7), 807–813.

Roberts, S. J. (1984). Social support—meaning, measurement, and relevance to community health nursing practice. *Public Health Nursing, 1*(3), 158–167.

Rook, K. S., & Dooley, D. (1985). Applying social support research: Theoretical problems and future directions. *Journal of Social Issues, 41*(1), 5–28.

Sarason, B. R., Sarason, I. G., & Pierce, G. R. (1990). *Social support: An interactional view.* New York: Wiley.

Sallis, J. F., Grossman, R. M., Pinski, R. B., Patterson, T. L., & Nader, P. R. (1987). The development of scales to measure social support for diet and exercise behaviors. *Preventive Medicine, 16*, 825–836.

Schaffer, M. A., & Lia-Hoagberg, B. (1997). Effects of social support on prenatal care and health behaviors of low-income women. *Journal of Obstetric, Gynecologic, and Neonatal Nursing, 26*(4), 433–440.

Scharer, K. (2005). Internet social support for parents: The state of the science. *Journal of Child and Adolescent Psychiatric Nursing, 18*(1), 26–35.

Stewart, M. J. (1993). *Integrating social support in nursing.* Newbury Park, CA: Sage.

Stewart, M. J. (1989a). Social support instruments created by nurse investigators. *Nursing Research, 38*(5), 268–275.

Stewart, M. J. (1989b). Social support intervention studies: A review and prospectus of nursing contributions. *International Journal of Nursing Studies, 26*(2), 93–114.

Tardy, C. H. (1985). Social support measurement. *American Journal of Community Psychology, 13*(2), 187–202.

Thoits, P. A. (1983). Multiple identities and psychosocial well-being: A reformation and test of the social isolation hypothesis. *American Sociological Review, 48*, 174–187.

Thoits, P. A. (1986). Social support as coping assistance. *Journal of Consulting and Clinical Psychology, 54*(4), 416–423.

Tilden, V. P. (1985). Issues of conceptualization and measurement of social support in construction of nursing theory. *Research in Nursing and Health, 81*, 199–206.

Tilden, V. P. (1986). New perspectives on social support. *The Nurse Practitioner, 11*, 60–61.

Tilden, V. P., & Galyen, R. D. (1987). Cost and conflict: The darker side of social support. *Western Journal of Nursing Research, 9*(1), 9–18.

Tilden, V. P., Nelson, C. A., & May, B. A. (1990). The IPR inventory: Development and psychometric characteristics. *Nursing Research, 39*(6), 337–343.

Tilden, V. P., & Weinert, S. C. (1987). Social support and the chronically ill individual. *Nursing Clinics of North America, 22*(3), 613–620.

Vandall-Walker, V., Jensen, L., & Oberle, K. (2007). Nursing support for family members of critically ill adults. *Qualitative Health Research, 17,* 1207–1218.

Vaux, A. (1988). *Social support—Theory, research, and intervention.* New York: Praeger.

Veiel, H. O., & Baumann, U. (1992). The many meanings of social support. In H. O. Veiel & U. Baumann (Eds.), *The meaning and measurement of social support* (pp. 1–9). New York: Hemisphere Publishing.

Vrabec, N. J. (1997). Literature review of social support and caregiver burden, 1980 to 1985. *Image: Journal of Nursing Scholarship, 29*(4), 383–388.

Wandersman, L., Wandersman, A., & Kahn, S. (1980). Social support in the transition to parenthood. *Journal of Community Psychology, 8,* 332–342.

Weinert, C. (1987). A social support measure: PRQ85. *Nursing Research, 36*(5), 273–277.

Weinert, C. (1988). Measuring social support: Revision and further development of the personal resource questionnaire. In O. L. Strickland & C. F. Waltz (Eds.), *Measurement of nursing outcomes* (*Vol. 1,* pp. 309–327). New York: Springer.

Wortman, C. B. (1984). Social support and the cancer patient: Conceptual and methodologic issues. *Cancer, 53*(10), 2339–2362.

Wright, K. B., & Bell, S. B. (2003). Health-related support groups on the Internet: Linking empirical findings to social support and computer-mediated communication theory. *Journal of Health Psychology, 8*(1), 39–54.

Zimet, G. D., Dahlem, N. W., Zimet, S. G., & Farley, G. K. (1988). The multidimensional scale of perceived social support. *Journal of Personality Assessment, 52,* 30–41.

BIBLIOGRAPHY

Bakan, G., & Akyol A. D. (2007). Theory-guided interventions for adaptation to heart failure. *Journal of Advanced Nursing, 61*(6), 596–608.

Blixen, C., & Kippes, C. (1999). Depression, social support, and quality of life in older adults with osteoarthritis. *Image: Journal of Nursing Scholarship, 31*(3), 221–226.

Bolla, C. D., De Joseph, J., Norbeck, J., & Smith, R. (1996). Social support as road map and vehicle: An analysis of data from focus group interviews with a group of African American women. *Public Health Nursing, 13*(5), 331–336.

Campbell-Grossman, C. K., Hudson, D. B., Keating-Lefler, R., & Heusinvelt, S. (2009). New mothers network: The provision of social support to single, low-income, African American mothers via e-mail messages. *Journal of Family Nursing, 15*(2), 220–236.

Chou, F., Avant, K. C., Kuo, S., & Fetzer, S. J. (2008). Relationships between nausea and vomiting, perceived stress, social support, pregnancy planning, and psychosocial adaptation in a sample of mothers: A questionnaire survey. *International Journal of Nursing Studies, 45,* 1185–1191.

Cossette, S., Levesque, L., & Laurin, L. (1995). Informal and formal support for caregivers of a demented relative: Do gender and kinship make a difference? *Research in Nursing and Health, 18,* 437–451.

Hagerty, B. M., & Williams, R. A. (1999). The effects of sense of belonging, social support, conflict, and loneliness on depression. *Nursing Research, 48*(4), 215–219.

Hubbard, P., Muhlenkamp, A. F., & Brown, N. (1984). The relationship between social support and self-care practices. *Nursing Research, 33*(5), 266–270.

Hudson, A. L., & Morris, R. I. (1994). Perceptions of social support of African Americans with acquired immunodeficiency syndrome. *Journal of National Black Nurses Association, 7*(1), 36–49.

Ihlenfeld, J. T. (1996). Nurses' perceptions of administrative social support. *Issues in Mental Health Nursing, 17,* 469–477.

Kavanaugh, K., Trier, D., & Michelle, K. (2004). Social support following perinatal loss. *Journal of Family Nursing, 19*(1), 70–92.

Logsdon, M. C., Gagne, P., Hughes, T., Patterson, J., & Rakestraw, V. (2005). Social support during adolescent pregnancy: Piecing together a quilt. *Journal of Obstetric, Gynecologic, and Neonatal Nursing, 34*(606–614), 433–440.

Mahon, N. E., Yarcheski, A., & Yarcheski, T. J. (1998). Social support and positive health practices in young adults: Loneliness as a mediating variable. *Clinical Nursing Research, 7*(3), 292–309.

McVeigh, C. A. (2000). Investigating the relationship between satisfaction with social support and functional status after childbirth. *MCN, The American Journal of Maternal/Child Nursing, 25*(1), 25–30.

Meneses, K., McNees, P., Azuero, A., & Jukkala, A. (2010). Development of the fertility and cancer project: An internet approach to help young cancer survivors. *Oncology Nursing Forum, 37*(2), 191–197.

Norbeck, J. S., De Jospeph, J. F., & Smith, R. T. (1996). A randomized trial of an empirically derived social support intervention to prevent low birthweight. *Social Science and Medicine, 43,* 947–954.

Purath, J., Buchholz, S. W., & Kark, D. L. (2009). Physical fitness assessment of older adults in the primary care setting. *Journal of the American Academy of Nurse Practitioners, 21,* 101–107.

Reece, S. M. (1993). Social support and the early maternal experience of primiparas over 35. *Maternal-Child Nursing Journal, 21*(3), 91–98.

Sammaraco, A., & Konecny, L. M. (2010). Quality of life, social support, and uncertainty among Latina and Caucasian breast cancer survivors: A comparative study. *Oncology Nursing Forum, 37*(1), 93–99.

Tarkka, M., & Paunonen, M. (1996). Social support provided by nurses to recent mothers on a maternity ward. *Journal of Advanced Nursing, 23*(6), 1202–1206.

8

Caring

DANUTA M. WOJNAR

DEFINITION OF KEY TERMS

Caring	A nurturing way of relating to a valued other toward whom one feels a personal sense of commitment and responsibility (Swanson, 1991, p. 165).
Knowing	Striving to understand an event as it has meaning in the life of the other. Knowing involves avoiding assumptions about the meaning of an event to the one cared for, centering on the other's needs, conducting in-depth assessment, seeking verbal and nonverbal cues, and engaging the self of both (p. 163).
Being with	Being emotionally present to the other by conveying ongoing availability, sharing feelings, and monitoring that the one providing care does not burden the one cared for (p. 163).
Doing for	Doing for the other what he or she would do for the self if it were at all possible. Doing for the other means providing care that is comforting, protective, and anticipatory, as well as performing duties skillfully and competently while preserving the person's dignity (p. 164).
Enabling	Facilitating the other's passage through life transitions and unfamiliar events by informing, explaining, supporting, focusing on relevant concerns, thinking through issues, and generating alternatives. Enabling promotes the client's personal healing, growth, and self-care (p. 164).
Maintaining belief	Sustaining faith in the other's capacity to get through an event or transition and face a future with meaning. The goal is to enable the other so that within the constraints of his or her life, they are able to find meaning and maintain a hope-filled attitude (p. 165).

INTRODUCTION

Nursing, like other health professions, is based on the ideal of service to humanity. At the core of nursing values lays the ideal of altruistic caring that is guided by theory, research, and a code of ethics. Nursing is focused on creating caring–healing environments that assist individuals, families, and communities attain or maintain a state of optimal wellness in their life experiences from birth, through adulthood, until the end of life (Swanson & Wojnar, 2004). Most individuals choose nursing as a profession because of their desire to care for others. With advances in nursing science, there has been an escalating interest in the concept of caring in nursing. Over the past few decades, philosophical debates, research, and theory development have ensued to define the concept of caring, articulate caring behaviors, and identify outcomes of caring for patients, families, nurses, organizations, and society.

Also of deep concern is detecting and eliminating barriers to caring in clinical practice. Among several prominent frameworks, Swanson's middle range theory of caring has achieved popularity among practitioners because of its simplicity, elegance, relevance, and ease of application in education, research, and clinical practice.

HISTORICAL BACKGROUND

Nursing has a long legacy as a caring–healing profession. In the nineteenth century, Florence Nightingale, the matriarch of modern-day nursing, expressed a belief that caring for the sick is based on the understanding of persons and environment. She saw the uniqueness of nursing in creating optimal environments for restoring the health of individuals, a vision that has now been in operation for over 100 years (Chinn & Kramer, 2004). Nurse theorists, such as Watson (1979, 1988, 1999), Leininger (1981, 1988), Benner (1984), Benner and Wrubel (1989), Boykin (1994), Swanson-Kauffman (1985, 1986, 1988a, b), Swanson-Kauffman and Roberts (1990), and Swanson (1991, 1993, 1998, 1999a, b, c) have reaffirmed the importance of caring for the profession through philosophical debates, theory development, and groundbreaking research. These nursing scholars have led the profession in reminding nurses that caring is essential for delivery of sound nursing care.

THEORY DEVELOPMENT

Swanson's interest in the caring science has been a rapid process. As a novice nurse, she was drawn to working in a hospital that had a clearly articulated vision for professional nursing practice and actively supported primary care nursing (Swanson, 2001). During the theorist's doctoral studies at the University of Colorado, the concept of caring went to the forefront of her professional and scholarly activities and from that point on, caring and miscarriage have become the foci of her scholarship. For her doctoral dissertation, Swanson set out to conduct descriptive phenomenological investigation of 20 women who had recently miscarried and to identify what types of caring behaviors they considered most helpful (Swanson, 1991). Inductive data analysis led Swanson to the development of a Caring Model with five distinct caring processes: *knowing, being with, doing for, enabling,* and *maintaining belief* (Swanson-Kauffman, 1985, 1986, 1988a; Swanson, 1991, 1993). Later, these caring process provided foundation for the development of her middle range theory of caring.

In a subsequent investigation, Swanson focused on exploring caring from the perspective of 19 professional caregivers and 7 parents of infants hospitalized in the Neonatal Intensive Care Unit (NICU) (Swanson, 1990). She discovered that the caring processes she had identified through her dissertation research were also applicable to parents and professionals who were responsible for taking care of babies in the NICU. Swanson was not only able to retain and refine the definitions describing the acts of caring, but was also able to propose that clinical care in a complex environment requires balance of caring for self and others, attaching to others as well as one's role, managing responsibilities, and avoiding bad outcomes for self, others, and society (Swanson, 1990). The next phase in the development of Swanson's caring theory was the "Caring and the Clinical Nursing Models Project" in which Swanson explored how a group of young mothers who received a long-term public health nursing intervention recalled and described nurse caring (NC) (Swanson-Kauffman, 1988b). Based on the findings of this study, Swanson defined caring as a concept and refined the definitions of caring processes (Swanson, 1993).

Subsequently, Swanson's scholarship has shifted to conducting a meta-analysis of data-based publications on caring (Swanson, 1999a) and instrument development. Swanson established psychometric properties of two instruments to measure caring: Caring Mate/Caring Other Scale (see Table 8.1) and Caring Professional Scale. Among other measures, she used the above instruments to determine the level of support women (Swanson, 1999b, c, 2000; Swanson, Connor, Jolley, Pentinato, & Wang, 2007; Swanson, Karmali, Powell, & Pulvermakher, 2003) and couples (Swanson, Chen, Graham, Wojnar, & Petras, 2009) received after miscarriage.

TABLE 8.1 Caring Mate/Caring Other Scale

	As of late, to what extent does your mate:	Not at all	Occasionally	About half the time	Often	All of the time
1.	Strive to understand what miscarriage means to you?	1	2	3	4	5
2.	Share in your feelings about miscarriage?	1	2	3	4	5
3.	Do extra things to help you out?	1	2	3	4	5
4.	Just be with you?	1	2	3	4	5
5.	Provide you with opportunities to discuss the miscarriage if you want to or need to?	1	2	3	4	5
6.	Keep you informed about how she is feeling about the miscarriage?	1	2	3	4	5
7.	Support you emotionally?	1	2	3	4	5
8.	Believe in you and your ability to get through tough times?	1	2	3	4	5
9.	Maintain hope that your plans to have children will all work out as you desire?	1	2	3	4	5
10.	Do little things to show she cares?	1	2	3	4	5

DEFINITIONS OF THEORY CONCEPTS

In 1993, Swanson refined her theory by making explicit her beliefs about the four phenomena of concern to the discipline of nursing: Nursing, Person/Client, Health, and Environment. The concept of caring, central to the theory, as well as caring processes (knowing, being with, doing for, enabling, and maintaining belief) are clearly defined and arranged in a logical sequence (see Fig. 8.1, which depicts how caring is delivered). Swanson also made explicit her beliefs about what it means for nurses to practice in a caring manner to promote health and healing of others. Chinn and Kramer (2004) and McNair, Lorr, and Droppleman (1981) maintain that the simplicity and clarity of a theory refers to a theory with a minimal number of concepts. Simplicity and clarity of language used to define the concepts allow practitioners to understand and apply Swanson's theory in practice.

NURSING

Swanson (1991, 1993) defines nursing as informed caring for the well-being of others. She posits that the discipline is informed by scientific knowledge from nursing and related fields, and by knowledge derived from the humanities, clinical practice, and cultural values and beliefs (Swanson, 1993).

PERSON

Persons are defined as "unique beings who are in the midst of becoming and whose wholeness is made manifest in thoughts, feelings, and behaviors" (Swanson, 1993, p. 352). Swanson asserts that life experiences

The Structure of Caring

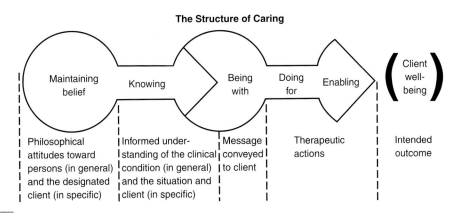

Figure 8.1 The structure of caring as linked to the nurse's philosophical attitude, informed understandings, message conveyed, therapeutic actions, and intended outcome. (From Swanson, K. M. (1993). Nursing as informed caring for the well-being of others. *Image: The Journal of Nursing Scholarship, 25*[4], 352–357.)

of each individual are influenced by a complex interplay of genetics, spiritual endowment, and the person's capacity to exercise free will. Therefore, persons both shape and are shaped by the environment in which they live.

Persons are viewed as dynamic, growing, self-reflecting, yearning to be connected with others, and spiritual beings. Swanson posits that spiritual endowment connects each human being to an eternal and universal source of goodness, mystery, life, creativity, and serenity. The spiritual endowment may be a soul, higher power/Holy Spirit, positive energy, or, simply grace; free will equates with choice and the capacity to decide how to act when confronted with a range of possibilities (p. 352). Yet, she also maintains that limitations set by race, class, gender, socio-political system, or access to care might prevent individuals from exercising free will. Hence, acknowledging free will mandate nursing discipline to honor individuality and consideration of a whole range of possibilities that might be acceptable or desirable to the patients, families, and communities for whom nurses care.

According to Swanson, the "other," whose personhood nursing discipline serves, refers to individuals, families, groups, and societies. With this understanding of personhood, nurses are mandated to take on leadership roles in advocating for human rights, equal access to health care, and other humanitarian causes. Lastly, when nurses think about the "other" to whom they direct their caring, they also need to think of self, other, nurses, and the practice of nursing as the designated "other/recipient" of their caring.

HEALTH

Swanson (1993) asserts that to experience health and well-being is to have a subjective, meaning-filled experience of wholeness that involves a sense of integration and becoming wherein all levels of being are free to be expressed including human spirituality, thoughts, feelings, intelligence, creativity, relatedness, femininity, masculinity, and sexuality, to name just a few. Therefore, reestablishing wholeness involves a complex process of curing and healing at the physical, mental, psychosocial, and spiritual levels.

ENVIRONMENT

Swanson (1993) defines environment as situational rather than physical and views environment as any situation that influences or is influenced by the designated client. Environment is ever changing at the cultural, social, biophysical, political, and economic realms, and by any context that influences or is influenced by the designated client. She suggests that the terms "environment" and "person/client" in nursing can be viewed interchangeably. The environment may be specified to the intra-individual level of a specified client, whereby the "client" may be the cellular level and the environment may be the tissues or body of which the cell is a component. Alternatively, the client may be an entire community and the environment may include cultural, social, and political aspects (p. 353). Therefore, when Swanson's theory is used in research or clinical practice, one must remember that what is considered an environment in one situation may be considered a client in another.

CARING

Swanson believes that NC is grounded on a belief in people and their capacities. Therefore, caring is defined as a nurturing way of relating to a valued other toward whom one feels a personal sense of commitment and responsibility. Swanson maintains that caring involves five processes: (a) knowing, (b) being with, (c) doing for, (d) enabling, and (e) maintaining belief. For detailed definition of the caring processes, refer to section on "Definition of Key Terms."

DESCRIPTION OF THE THEORY OF CARING

PHILOSOPHICAL FOUNDATION

Swanson has drawn on various philosophical and theoretical sources while developing her theory of caring. In the chapter, Swanson (2001) recalled that early in her career, knowledge obtained from formal nursing education and clinical practice made her acutely aware of the centrality of caring to preserving human dignity and promoting healing. She also acknowledged several nurse scholars for influencing her beliefs about nursing and caring. She credits Dr. Jacqueline Fawcett for helping her understand the unique role of nursing in caring for others and importance of altruistic caring for the persons' well-being. Swanson also acknowledges Dr. Jean Watson for encouraging her to inductively study caring. While Drs. Swanson and Watson sustain a deep friendship and respect for each other's scholarship, they both view their scholarship as complementary. They view their programs of research as unique and believe the congruency of their findings add credibility to each other's work. Yet, both scholars see their theories of caring and their programs of research on caring as unique and the congruency of their findings as adding credibility to their individual work (Swanson, 2001). Lastly, Swanson credits Dr. Kathryn M. Barnard for encouraging her to test and apply her theory of caring through randomized clinical trials.

Swanson's theory was developed empirically, using inductive methodology. According to Chinn and Kramer (2004), inductive reasoning involves inducing of hypotheses and relationships by observing or living through phenomena and before reaching definite conclusions. Swanson's theory of caring was inductively developed through descriptive phenomenological inquiry with women who had miscarried (Swanson-Kauffman, 1985, 1986, 1988a, b), with the caregivers of vulnerable infants in the NICU (Swanson, 1990), and with socially at-risk mothers who had received long-term care from master's prepared public health nurses (1991).

THEORETICAL ASSUMPTIONS

Swanson purports that caring, which she defines as "a nurturing way of relating to a valued other toward whom a nurse feels a sense of commitment and responsibility" (1991, p. 162), is not unique to the domain of perinatal nursing. Instead, she posits that caring is an essential component of nurse–client relationship in any setting. She also purports that caring occurs in every nurse–client relationship that involves skillful application of caring processes (knowing, being with, doing for, enabling, and maintaining belief). She also posits that regardless of the amount of nursing experience, caring is influenced by the nurse's attitude (maintaining belief), understanding of client's experience (knowing), verbal and nonverbal interactions with the client (being with), enabling (believing in the client's capacity to live through difficult transitions), and outcomes of caring (intended outcomes of nursing process). Swanson purports that caring processes coexist and overlap, and cannot be delivered in a linear way or in separation from one another. Lastly, Swanson claims that if she had truly identified and defined the universal aspects of caring, then her caring processes should ring true in any situation where caring is a part of an interpersonal relationship. Swanson (1993) depicted the caring processes and the relationships between them in the structure of caring (Fig. 8.1).

EXAMPLES OF THE THEORY APPLICATION IN RESEARCH

Reynolds (1971) suggests that a functional theory is one that can be applied in clinical practice and research. Swanson has persevered in the development of her theory from the point of defining the concept of caring and proposing her Caring Model to the development of middle range theory of caring. She subsequently conducted descriptive prospective studies guided by the theory of caring to determine human responses to miscarriage, and intervention research with women and couples who miscarried using randomized controlled trial (RCT) design.

In her dissertation research, the theorist analyzed data obtained from in-depth interviews with 20 women who have recently miscarried. She proposed two theoretical models as a result of this phenomenological investigation: (1) The Human Experience of Miscarriage Model and (2) The Caring Model. Based on the dissertation findings pertaining to miscarriage, Swanson developed Meaning of Miscarriage Scale (Swanson, Kieckhefer, Powers, & Carr, 1990). In the Caring Model, Swanson proposed that the processes of knowing, being with, doing for, enabling, and maintaining belief give meaning to nursing acts labeled as caring (Swanson-Kauffman, 1985, 1986, 1988a, b). Findings of this investigation provided the foundation for the development of middle range theory of caring.

As part of her postdoctoral studies, Swanson conducted another phenomenological investigation, in which she explored "what was it like to be a provider of care to vulnerable infants in the NICU?" Swanson (1990) found that the caring processes she identified with women who miscarried were also applicable to parents, physicians, and nursing staff responsible for taking care of infants in the NICU. Hence, she decided to retain the wording describing the acts of caring and propose that holistic care in a complex environment like NICU, embraces balance of *caring* (for self and the one cared for), *attaching* (to others and roles), *managing responsibilities* (assigned by self, others, and society), and *avoiding bad outcomes* (Swanson, 1990).

In a later investigation, Swanson (1991) explored what it had been like for socially at-risk mothers to receive supportive, long-term nursing interventions. As a result of this study, she was finally able to define caring and further refine the definitions of caring processes. Collectively, findings of Swanson's research with women who have miscarried, caregivers in the NICU, and socially at-risk mothers provided the foundation for expanding the Caring Model into the middle range theory of caring (Swanson, 1991, 1993).

Subsequently, Swanson tested her theory of caring with women who miscarried in several investigations funded by the National Institutes of Health (NIH), National Institute of Nursing Research (NINR), and other funding sources. Swanson's (1999a, b) intervention study with 242 women who miscarried focused on examining the effects of caring-based counseling sessions on the women's processing of loss and their emotional wellness in the first year after loss. Additional aims of the study were to examine the effects of the passage of time on healing and to design strategies to monitor caring interventions. The main findings of this investigation were that caring was effective in decreasing the participants' overall disturbed mood, depression, and anger. Moreover, all study participants (treated or not) assigned less personal significance to miscarrying, had higher levels of self-esteem and less anxiety, anger, and confusion. In other words, the findings of the study demonstrated that while passing of time had positive effects on women's healing after miscarriage, caring interventions had a positive impact on decreasing the overall disturbed mood, anger, and level of depression. The second aim of this investigation was to monitor the caring variable and identify whether caring was delivered as intended. Swanson monitored caring in three different ways: (a) she transcribed approximately 10% of counseling sessions and analyzed data using inductive and deductive content analysis; (b) she required that before each caring session, the counselor completes McNair, Lorr, and Droppelman's (1981) Profile of Mood States to monitor whether their own mood was associated with women's ratings of caring after each session; and (c) after each session, the counselor completed an investigator developed Counselor Rating Scale and took narrative notes about the counseling session. The most noteworthy finding of monitoring caring was that the majority of participants were highly satisfied with caring received during counseling sessions, suggesting that caring was delivered as intended.

In 2009, Swanson and her research team published results from NIH, NINR funded intervention study "Couples Miscarriage Healing Project" conducted with ($N = 341$) heterosexual couples over a period of 1 year after loss (Swanson et al., 2009). The purpose of this investigation was to determine the effects of miscarriage on couples in committed heterosexual relationships, and to identify effective ways of assisting

In 2009, Swanson and her research team published results of a RCT conducted to examine the effects of three couple-focused interventions and a control condition on women and their partners' resolution of depression and grief during the first year after miscarriage.

A total of 341 couples participated in the study. They were enrolled within the first 12 weeks after pregnancy loss. Subsequently, couples who met the inclusion criteria were randomly assigned to NC intervention that entailed three counseling sessions, SC that consisted of three video and workbook modules, CC that included one counseling session and three SC modules, or controlled condition in which no treatment was offered. Interventions were based on Swanson's caring theory and Meaning of Miscarriage Model. They were offered 1, 5, and 11 weeks after enrollment. Outcomes included depression (CES-D) and grief, pure grief (PG), and grief-related emotions (GRE). Couples' perceptions of Caring Professional and Caring Mate/Caring Other Scales in the aftermath

USING MIDDLE RANGE THEORIES

8.1

of loss were also administered to all participants. Differences in rates of recovery were estimated via multilevel modeling conducted in a Bayesian framework.

Swanson et al. (2009) found that Bayesian odds (BO), ranging from 3.0 to 7.9, favored NC over all other conditions for accelerating women's resolution of depression. BO of 3.2–6.6 favored NC and no treatment over SC and CC for resolving men's depression. BO of 3.1–7.0 favored all three interventions over no treatment for accelerating women's PG resolution, and BO of 18.7–22.6 favored NC and CC over SC or no treatment for resolving men's PG. BO ranging from 2.4 to 6.1 favored NC and SC over CC or no treatment for hastening women's resolution of GRE. BO from 3.5 to 17.9 favored NC, CC, and control over SC for resolving men's GRE.

Swanson et al. (2009) concluded that NC had the overall broadest positive impact on couples' resolution of grief and depression. In addition, grief resolution (PG and GRE) was accelerated by SC for women and CC for men.

Source: Swanson, K. M., Chen, H., Graham, J. C., Wojnar, D. M., & Petras, A. (2009). Resolution of depression and grief during the first year after miscarriage: A randomized controlled trial of couples-focused interventions. *Journal of Women's Health, 18*(8), 1245–1257.

the couples in their healing process. Study participants (couples) were randomly assigned to a control group (no intervention) or one of the three treatment groups: (a) NC (three counseling sessions with a nurse), (b) self-caring (SC) (three videos and workbook modules), (c) combined caring (CC) (one NC session and three videos and workbook modules). Interventions, based on Swanson's caring theory and Meaning of Miscarriage Model, were offered 1, 5, and 11 weeks after enrollment. Differences in rates of recovery were estimated via multilevel modeling conducted in a Bayesian framework. Swanson et al. found that caring-based interventions delivered by Registered Nurse had the overall broadest positive impact on couples' resolution of grief and depression. In addition, grief resolution was accelerated by SC intervention for women, and combined nurse and SC intervention for men. Findings demonstrated that Swanson's theory is an effective framework to facilitate healing of individuals and couples in clinical practice. Using Middle Range Theories 8.1 provides additional information about this study.

APPLICATIONS OF THE THEORY IN RESEARCH BY OTHERS, EDUCATION, AND CLINICAL PRACTICE

Reynolds (1971) asserts that a useful theory provides a sense of understanding and applicability in research, education, and practice. The caring theory has been the theoretical foundation for numerous research studies, master theses and doctoral dissertations, and scholarly projects of undergraduate and graduate nursing students. Literature review of computerized databases (MEDLINE, CINAHL, and Digital Dissertations) indicate that Swanson's theory and research has been cited or otherwise utilized in over 160 data-based publications, while the article "Nursing as Informed Caring for the Well Being of Others" (Swanson, 1993) has been cited over 50 times.

Authors have utilized Swanson's caring theory as a theoretical framework, or a guide for the discussion of their research findings. Kish and Holder (1996) used it to explore clinical scholarship in practice. Yorkston, Klasner, and Swanson (2001) used it to develop guidelines for practitioners working with patients who have multiple sclerosis. Quinn, Smith, Ritenbaugh, and Swanson (2003) developed guidelines for assessing impact of healing relationships in nursing. Sikma (2006) studied caring with elderly population. Kavanaugh, Moro, Savage, and Mehendale (2006) used Swanson's theory to guide their research with teen fathers. Sandblom (2006) utilized caring theory to guide her analysis of grief and depression after miscarriage among couples with history of infertility. Wojnar (2007) used the principles of caring theory to explore the experiences of lesbian couples who miscarried.

Chinn and Kramer (2004) assert that the situations in which the theories may be effectively applied should not be limited. Consistent with Chin and Kramer's view, Swanson's theory has been successfully adapted as a framework for professional nursing practice by various Universities and practice settings across the United States, Canada, and Sweden. Box 8.1 identifies two specific applications.

Swanson's theory of caring may be used effectively to establish therapeutic relationships with diverse populations. Recent examples of the theory application suggest that it may be applied to any nurse–client relationship and any clinical setting offering a framework for enhancing contemporary nursing practice while bringing the discipline to its traditional caring–healing roots.

SUMMARY

The usefulness of Swanson's theory of caring has been demonstrated in research, education, and clinical practice. The belief that caring has a pivotal role in the practice of professional nursing had its beginning in the theorist's clinical practice, the influence of her mentors, and in the findings from her phenomenological investigations. Her later works, including meta-analysis of research on caring (Swanson, 1999c) have demonstrated generalizability and applicability of the theory of caring in education, clinical nursing practice, and research beyond perinatal context.

NC, as demonstrated by Swanson in research with women and couples after miscarriage, caregivers in the NICU, and socially at-risk mothers, recognizes the importance of attending to the wholeness of human experiences and needs.

ANALYSIS OF THEORY

Using the criteria presented in Chapter 2, critique the theory of Caring. Compare your conclusions about the theory with those found in Appendix A. A researcher who has worked with the theory completed the analysis found in the Appendix.

Internal Criticism	External Criticism
1. Clarity	1. Reality convergence
2. Consistency	2. Utility
3. Adequacy	3. Significance
4. Logical development	4. Discrimination
5. Level of theory development	5. Scope of theory
	6. Complexity

CRITICAL THINKING EXERCISES

1. Think about a time when you felt that you or someone close to you experienced caring in the health care environment. What was it like to experience caring? What did the practitioner say or do? How consistent were his or her actions with caring processes identified by Swanson? Alternatively, think about a situation when caring was not delivered. What was missing in your interaction with that practitioner?

2. Think about a situation in your clinical practice when your interaction with the client did not go smoothly. Consider key definitions identified in Swanson's theory and reflect on what caring processes were missing from that interaction. In what ways could that interaction be improved?

3. Consider Swanson's theory of caring as a theoretical framework for a research study relevant to your clinical practice. In what ways would it be applicable?

REFERENCES

Benner, P. (1984). *From novice to expert.* Menlo Park, CA: Addison-Wesley.

Benner, P., & Wrubel, J. (1989). *The primacy of caring.* Menlo Park, CA: Addison-Wesley.

Boykin, A. (1994). *Living a caring-based curriculum.* New York: National League for Nursing.

Chinn, P. L., & Kramer, M. K. (2004). *Integrated knowledge development in nursing* (6th ed.). St. Louis, MO: Mosby.

Kavanaugh, K., Moro, T. T., Savage, T., & Mehendale, R. (2006). Enacting a theory of caring to recruit and retain vulnerable participants for sensitive research. *Research in Nursing and Health, 29*(3), 244–252.

Kish, C. P., & Holder, L. M. (1996). Helping to say goodbye: Merging clinical scholarship with community service. *Holistic Nursing Practice, 10*(3), 74–82.

Leininger, M. M. (1981). The phenomenon of caring: Importance of research and theoretical considerations. In M. M. Leininger (Ed.), *Caring: An essential human need.* Thorofare, NJ: Slak.

Leininger, M. M. (1988). Leininger's theory of nursing: Cultural care diversity and universality. *Nursing Science Quarterly, 1*(4), 152–160.

McNair, P. M., Lorr, M., & Droppleman, L. F. (1981). *Profile of mood states manual* (2nd ed.). San Diego: Educational & Industrial Testing Service.

McNair, D. M., Lorr, M., Droppleman, L. F., & Reynolds, P. D. (1981). *A primer of theory construction.* Indianapolis, IN: Bobs-Merrill.

Quinn, J., Smith, M., Ritenbaugh, C., & Swanson, K. M. (2003). Research guidelines for assessing the impact of the healing relationship in clinical nursing. *Alternative Therapies, 9*(31), 69–79.

Raynolds, P. D. (1971). *A primer of theory construction.* Indianapolis, IN: Bobbs-Merril.

Sandblom, S. (2006). *Does a history of infertility affect the grief and depression response in couples experiencing a spontaneous miscarriage?* Unpublished master's thesis, University of Washington School of Nursing, Washington, DC.

Sikma, S. (2006). Staff perceptions of caring: The importance of a supportive environment. *Journal of Gerontological Nursing, 32*(6), 22–29.

Swanson, K. M. (1990). Providing care in the NICU: Sometimes an act of love. *Advances in Nursing Science, 13*(1), 60–73.

Swanson, K. M. (1991). Empirical development of a middle range theory of caring. *Nursing Research, 40*(3), 161–166.

Swanson, K. M. (1993). Nursing as informed caring for the well-being of others. *Image: Journal of Nursing Scholarship, 25*(4), 352–357.

Swanson K. M. (1998). Caring made visible. *Creative Nursing Journal, 4*(4), 8–11, 16.

Swanson, K. M. (1999a). Research-based practice with women who have had miscarriages. *Image: Journal of Nursing Scholarship, 31*(4), 339–345.

Swanson, K. M. (1999b). The effects of caring, measurement, and time on miscarriage impact and women's well-being in the first year subsequent to loss. *Nursing Research, 48*(6), 288–298.

Swanson, K. M. (1999c). What's known about caring in nursing: A literary meta-analysis. In A. S. Hinshaw, J. Shaver & S. Feetham (Eds.), *Handbook of clinical nursing research,* (pp. 31–60). Thousand Oaks, CA: Sage.

Swanson, K. M. (2000). Predicting depressive symptoms after miscarriage: A path analysis based on Lazarus' paradigm. *Journal of Women's Health and Gender-based Medicine, 9*(2), 191–206.

Swanson, K. M. (2001). A program of research on caring. In M. E. Parker (Ed.), *Nursing theories and nursing practice* (pp. 411–420). Philadelphia, PA: Davis.

Swanson, K. M. (2002) Caring professional scale. In Watson, J. (Ed.), *Assessing and measuring caring in nursing and health science.* New York: Springer.

Swanson, K. M. Chen, H., Graham, J. C., Wojnar, D. M., & Petras, A. (2009). Resolution of depression and grief during the first year after miscarriage: A randomized controlled trial of couples-focused interventions. *Journal of Women's Health, 18*(8), 1245–1257.

Swanson, K. M., Jolley, S. N., Pettinato, M., Wang, T., & Connor, S. (2007). The context and evolution of women's responses to miscarriage over the first year after loss. *Research in Nursing & Health, 30*(1), 2–16.

Swanson, K. M., Karmali, Z., Powell, S., & Pulvermahker, F. (2003). Miscarriage effects on interpersonal and sexual relationships during the first year after loss: Women's perceptions. *Journal of Psychosomatic Medicine, 65*(5), 902–910.

Swanson, K. M., Kieckhefer, G., Powers, P., & Carr, K. (1990). Meaning of miscarriage scale: Establishment of psychometric properties (Abstract). *Communicating Nursing Research, 25*, 365.

Swanson, K. M., & Wojnar, D. (2004). Optimal healing environments in Nursing. *Alternative Therapies in Health and Medicine, 10*(1), 43–51.

Swanson-Kauffman, K. M. (1985). Miscarriage: A new understanding of the mother's experience. *Proceedings of the 50th anniversary celebration of the University of Pennsylvania School of Nursing*, 63–78.

Swanson-Kauffman, K. M. (1986). Caring in the instance of unexpected early pregnancy loss. *Topics in Clinical Nursing, 8*(2), 37–46.

Swanson-Kauffman, K. M. (1988a). The caring needs of women who miscarry. In M. M. Leininger (Ed.), *Care, discovery and uses in clinical and community nursing* (pp. 55–71). Detroit, MI: Wayne State University Press.

Swanson-Kauffman, K. M. (1988b). There should have been two: Nursing care of parents experiencing the perinatal death of a twin. *Journal of Perinatal and Neonatal Nursing, 2*(2), 78–86.

Swanson-Kauffman, K. M., & Roberts, J. (1990). Caring in parent and child nursing. *Knowledge about care and caring: State of the art and future development.* Washington, DC: American Academy of Nursing.

Watson, J. (1979). *Nursing: The philosophy and science of caring.* Boston, MA: Little & Brown.

Watson, J. (1988). New dimensions of human caring theory. *Nursing Science Quarterly, 1*, 175–181.

Watson, J. (1999). *Nursing: Human science and human care: A theory of nursing.* Sudbury, MA: Jones & Barlett.

Wojnar, D. (2007). Miscarriage experiences of lesbian birth and social mothers: Couples' perspective. *Journal of Midwifery and Women's Health, 52*(5), 479–485.

Yorkston, K. M., Klasner, E. R., & Swanson, K. M. (2001). Communication in multiple sclerosis: Understanding the insider's perspective. *American Journal of Speech Language Pathology, 10*, 126–137.

9

Interpersonal Relations

SANDRA J. PETERSON

DEFINITION OF KEY TERMS

Communication	A skill necessary to understand the nurse–patient relationship; composed of "spoken language, rational and nonrational expressions of wishes, needs, and desires, and the body gesture" (Peplau, 1991, p. 289).
Interpersonal relations	Any process that occurs between two people. The interpersonal processes between nurse and patient are identified as the core of nursing (Forchuk, 1993).
Nursing situation	What occurs between the nurse and the patient, thus the interaction of the individual thoughts, feelings, and actions of both.
Observation	A skill necessary to understand the nurse–patient relationship. Its aim, "as an interpersonal process, is the identification, clarification, and verification of impressions about the interactive drama, of the pushes and pulls in the relationship between nurse and patient as they occur" (Peplau, 1991, p. 263).
Personality	"… Pattern that is relatively stable and that characterizes persisting situations in the life of an individual … total assets and liabilities that determine an individual action" (Peplau, 1991, pp. 164, 165). Nurses attempt to provide experiences for patients that promote personality development.
Phases of nurse–patient relationship	Four overlapping but generally sequential aspects of the relationship identified as orientation, identification, exploitation, and resolution.
Psychobiological experiences	Factors that influence the functioning of personalities, providing energy that is converted into constructive or destructive behavior. The primary source of this energy is anxiety.
Psychological tasks	"Tasks encountered in the process of learning to live with people as an aspect of formation and development of personality and as an aspect of the tasks demanded of nurses in their relations with patients" (Peplau, 1991, p. 159), for example, counting on others, delaying satisfaction, identifying self, and participating with others.
Recording	Methods used to create documents of nurse–patient interactions, primarily for the purpose of student learning.
Roles in nursing	Set of functions that nurses use in the context of nurse–patient situations as a means of helping the patient, identified as stranger, resource person, teacher, leader, surrogate, and counselor.

INTRODUCTION

"When the history of nursing theory comes to be written few names will be seen to have been more influential than that of Hildegard Peplau" (Welch, 1995, p. 53). Peplau, who developed the theory of interpersonal relations, is identified as the first contemporary nurse theorist (McKenna, 1997). Sills (1978) credits Peplau with clarifying the relationships between nursing theory, practice, and research. "Theory was used to guide nursing practice. Theory was tested in the real world of practice" (Sills, 1978, p. 122).

Although Peplau entitled her work a conceptual frame of reference, she often referred to it as a theory (Peplau, 1992, p. 13). Peplau produced a testable theory, identifying her work as a "source of hypotheses that may be examined with profit in all nursing situations" (Peplau, 1991, p. ix). The theory of interpersonal relations is currently labeled as a middle range theory (Armstrong & Kelly, 1995; Fawcett, 2000; O'Toole & Welt, 1989). Peplau, herself, defined the scope of her theory as in the middle range. She referred to it as "a partial theory for the practice of nursing as an interpersonal process" (Peplau, 1991, p. 261).

Initially developed with a focus on phenomena of most concern to psychiatric nurses, the theory of interpersonal relations is applicable to all nurses (Peplau, 1964, 1992). Peplau (1997) claimed that "the nurse–patient relationship is the primary human contact that is central in a fundamental way to providing nursing care" (p. 163). The stated purpose of her theory is the improvement of nurses' relations with patients. This is achieved through the nurse's understanding of his or her own behavior, helping others identify personally experienced difficulties, and applying principles of human relations to the problems that arise in the context of relationships (Peplau, 1991, p. xi). This process results in a nursing situation in which both the patient and the nurse learn and grow. A growth-producing relationship with others is a goal that transcends any particular nursing specialty and in her description of the theory, Peplau (1952, 1991) used examples of patients with a variety of health issues, for example, a woman diagnosed with lymphosarcoma, a child having surgery on his hand to correct a congenital problem, a woman in labor, and a man with a coronary occlusion.

HISTORICAL BACKGROUND

What makes Peplau's theory of interpersonal relations so remarkable is that it was conceived during a period in nursing's history when nurses had little or no independent role and little or no investment in the development of nursing theory. Peplau was educated and began her nursing practice, as described in her own words, at a time when "we were absolutely not allowed to talk to a patient, because if we did we might say the wrong thing" (Welch, 1995, p. 54). It was not until the late 1930s while working as a staff nurse at Mount Sinai Hospital, New York, that she discovered "there was more to nursing than just this doing activity, because there we were allowed to talk to the patients" (Welch, 1995, p. 54). In the 1940s Peplau found psychiatric nursing still focused on activities, for example, helping patients with tasks of daily living, which included cleaning patients' rooms and doing patients' laundry (Peplau, 1985, p. 31). It was out of her desire to be more useful to patients that the idea of interpersonal relations theory was developed.

Peplau used both deductive and inductive methods in her theory development work (Reed, 1995). Deductively, she integrated ideas from a number of theories into her theory of interpersonal relations. She was influenced by the work of Sigmund Freud, particularly his interest in unconscious motivation. Harry S. Sullivan's theory of interpersonal relations also contributed to her thinking about interpersonal processes in nursing. For example, she refers to his concepts of anxiety, self-system, and modes of experiencing. Also incorporated into her theory are elements from developmental psychology and learning theory (Armstrong & Kelly, 1995; Lego, 1980) and the ideas of the humanistic psychologists, Abraham Maslow, Rollo May, and Carl Rogers (Gastmans, 1998).

Peplau defined her inductive approach in both general and specific terms. The inductive approach for concept naming that she described included several steps:

1. Observing behaviors for which no explanatory concepts are available
2. Seeking to repeat those observations in others, under similar conditions
3. Noting regularities concerning the nature of the data being observed
4. Naming the phenomena (Peplau, 1989, p. 28)

These steps would be followed by further observation, resulting in the phenomenon becoming more clearly defined, which then allowed for testing with additional patients. "Eventually, useful interventions would be derived from the explanation of the phenomenon and the effects of these interventions upon it also tested" (Peplau, 1969, p. 28).

Peplau's specific inductive process of theory development involved using data from student–patient interactions. "I just happened to hit upon the notion of sitting students down with one patient for a long time and then study what they did with patients" (Peplau, 1985, p. 31). It was from these observations that psychotherapy by nurses in the context of the interpersonal relationship emerged.

Her theory of interpersonal relations, first appearing in 1952 in the book *Interpersonal Relations in Nursing,* has been published unchanged several times. During the 1950s and 1960s, her theory was used and tested in the challenging environment of state psychiatric hospitals. Some of this work is reported in *Basic Principles of Patient Counseling* published in 1964 by Smith, Kline, and French (Sills, 1978, p. 124). In four decades since its inception, interpersonal theory has been expanded by Peplau and other nurse scientists (Peplau, 1991, p. vi). For example, work on therapeutic milieu, crisis, and family therapy has been based on Peplau's theory. Sills (1978) conducted a review of three major nursing journals from 1972 to 1977 (one published for the first time in 1963). She identified 93 citations of Peplau's work and concluded that "it [is] remarkable that twenty-five years after the publication of *Interpersonal Relations in Nursing* that it, with no revisions, is still found useful. And . . . that utilization increases" (Sills, 1978, p. 125).

DEFINITIONS OF THEORY CONCEPTS

Although not specified at the time of the development of the theory in 1952, each domain of the traditional metaparadigm of nursing is addressed by Peplau. Her definitions of these major domain concepts are useful in understanding the rather complex theory of interpersonal relations.

NURSING

The foundation of her theory is her definition of nursing. Perhaps what is unique, but not unexpectedly so, is the primacy of the nurse–patient relationship in her definition. She defines nursing as an interpersonal process, intended to be therapeutic. It "is a human relationship between an individual who is sick or in need of health services" (Peplau, 1991, pp. 5, 6) and a nurse who has appropriate preparation to respond to the need. The use of technical procedures in nursing is acknowledged but relegated to a secondary role. Her most frequently quoted definition is:

> Nursing is a significant, therapeutic, interpersonal process. It functions co-operatively with other human processes that make health possible for individuals in communities....Nursing is an educative instrument, a maturing force, that aims to promote forward movement of personality in the direction of creative, constructive, productive, personal, and community living. (Peplau, 1952, p. 16)

PERSONS

In her theory, Peplau includes two persons as components: the nurse and the client, or more often, the patient (O'Toole & Welt, 1989; Peplau, 1992). Peplau (1952) initially defined man as:

> An organism that lives in an unstable equilibrium (i.e., physiological, psychological, and social fluidity) and life is the process of striving in the direction of stable equilibrium, i.e. a fixed pattern that is never reached except in death. (p. 82)

Forchuk (1991) revised that definition, omitting the terms "organism" and "equilibrium" because they represent a more "mechanical, closed-system perspective" (p. 55) that is inconsistent with Peplau's view of humans as growth seeking. A person is a relational being experiencing "interacting expectations, conceptions, wishes, and desires, as well as feelings when ... in situations with other persons" (O'Toole & Welt, 1989, p. 5). This perspective on persons as relational beings is fundamental to the theory.

NURSE

The nurse is identified as a professional with definable expertise (Peplau, 1992). This expertise should include the ability to "identify human problems that confront patients, the degrees of skill used to meet situations, and be able to develop with patients the kind of relationships that will be conducive to improvement in skill" (Peplau, 1991, p. xiii). The nurse also possesses "a unique blend of ideals, values, integrity, and commitment to the well-being of others" (Peplau, 1988, p. 10).

PATIENT

The patient is defined first as a person, deserving of "all of the humane considerations: respect, dignity, privacy, confidentiality, and ethical care" (Peplau, 1992, p. 14), but a person who has problems that now require the services of a nurse. Ideally, the patient participates actively in the nurse–patient relationship (O'Toole & Welt, 1989, p. 57).

HEALTH

Peplau (1952) provided a definition of health in her initial description of the theory. "It [health] is a word symbol that implies forward movement of personality and other human processes in the direction of creative, constructive, productive, personal, and community living" (p. 12). In addition, she identified two processes that are necessary for health: (a) biological, for example, absorption and elimination and (b) social, which promotes physical, emotional, and social well-being (pp. 12–13).

ENVIRONMENT

Peplau focused on the issue of environment as milieu, using the term to describe a therapeutic environment (O'Toole & Welt, 1989, p. 78). The milieu is composed of structured (e.g., ward government) and unstructured components. The unstructured components consist of the complex relationships between patients, staff, visitors, and other patients, which is often neglected and yet has a significant impact on patient outcomes. Milieu ideally involves the creation of an atmosphere conducive to recovery.

DESCRIPTION OF THEORY OF INTERPERSONAL RELATIONS

Peplau implied a philosophical foundation to her theory of interpersonal relations and provided two basic assumptions, which have been expanded by others, using the initial publication of the theory as the primary source. Peplau did not label the propositional statements in her theory as such; instead, they are integrated into her discussion of the components of the theory.

PHILOSOPHICAL FOUNDATIONS

There are some different perspectives on the nature of the philosophical underpinnings of Peplau's theory of interpersonal relations in Nursing. Sellers (1991) labels the theory:

> ... a mechanistic, deterministic, persistence ontological view; an epistemology that is consistent with the totality paradigm, with its emphasis on a received view of knowledge and logical positivism; and an axiology that values stability, traditionalism, and nursing's close alignment with medicine. (p. 158)

Sellers did not support these conclusions with examples from the theory. Since the complexity of Peplau's theory makes it difficult to categorize, it is not surprising that others have considered it from a different philosophical perspective.

More recently, existential phenomenology has been identified as the philosophical foundation of Peplau's theory (Gastmans, 1998). Consistent with phenomenology, observation of patients as a fundamental task of nursing is seen as contextual and value-laden. It requires openness to and involvement with patients' existential situations. "Nursing has a human interpretive character" (Gastmans, 1998, Phenomenology and Nursing Science, para. 5) with the nurse–patient relationship at its core. Interpretations are meaning-seeking activities that arise as the nurse participates with the patient. This participation with the patient is described as respectful, communicating positive interest, and nonjudgmental regard (Peplau, 1991). Peplau uses the term "professional closeness" (Peplau, 1969) to summarize these characteristics that allow the nurse to communicate care when participating with patients.

Although most of Peplau's philosophy is imbedded in her writings, she does delineate six "beliefs about patients" (Peplau, 1964). She identifies these as her "philosophy about patients and their care" (p. 30), attributed primarily to psychiatric nurses but applicable to all patients:

1. All behavior is purposeful, has meaning, and can be understood.
2. The nurse must observe what is going on; she must interpret what is observed, and then she must decide action on the basis of her interpretations.
3. The nurse meets the needs of the patient.
4. The nurse–patient interaction—the verbal and nonverbal exchanges in the nursing situation—can influence recovery.
5. The personality of the patient is somehow involved in his illness.
6. There are some ideas about nursing care that relate to the word *anxiety* (pp. 30–35).

ASSUMPTIONS

In the initial publication of her theory, Peplau (1952) listed two guiding assumptions, emphasizing the importance of the nurse's own growth and development in establishing helpful interpersonal relationships with patients. Others have expanded that list through personal correspondence with Peplau and review of her writings. Table 9.1 provides a list of the assumptions of the theory of interpersonal relations.

These 13 assumptions serve to illustrate the complexity of Peplau's theory of interpersonal relations.

THEORY DESCRIPTION WITH PROPOSITIONAL STATEMENTS

The core of the theory, the relationship between nurse and patient, is composed of phases, fulfilled through roles, influenced by psychobiological experiences, and requires attending to certain psychological tasks. Peplau also identified methods that can assist the nurse to develop understanding of the nurse–patient relationship. The description of the theory is presented using the same sequence as Peplau (1952, 1991) did in her seminal work, *Interpersonal Relations in Nursing*.

COMPOSED OF PHASES

Peplau (1991) initially defined four phases of the nurse–patient relationship: orientation, identification, exploitation, and resolution. Forchuk (1991) later reconceptualized these phases into three, with the working phase replacing the identification and exploitation phases. These phases are considered overlapping and interlocking, with each phase possessing characteristic functions. They are experienced in every nursing situation.

Phase of Orientation. There are four functions that nurses use during orientation: (a) *provide the resources* of specific, needed information to help the patient understand the problem and the health care situation; (b) *serve as a counselor* to encourage the patient to express thoughts and feelings related to the problem situation; (c) *act as surrogate* to family members so that the patient can reenact and examine relevant issues from prior relationships; and (d) *use technical expertise* to attend to concerns or issues that require the use of professional devices. These nursing functions assist the patient to address the needs experienced during the phase of orientation.

TABLE 9.1 Assumptions of the Theory of Interpersonal Relations

Source	Assumptions
Identified by Peplau (1952)	1. "The kind of person each nurse becomes makes a substantial difference in what each patient will learn as he is nursed throughout his experience with illness" (p. xii). 2. "Fostering personality development in the direction of maturity is a function of nursing and nursing education; it requires the use of principles and methods that permit and guide the process of grappling with everyday interpersonal problems or difficulties" (p. xii).
Based on correspondence with Peplau (Forchuk, 1993)	3. Nursing can claim as its uniqueness, the responses of clients to the circumstances of their illnesses or health problems (1989, p. 28). 4. Because illness provides an opportunity for learning and growth, nurses can assist clients to further develop their intellectual and interpersonal competencies, during the illness experience, by gearing nursing practices to evolving such competencies through nurse–client interactions (1989, p. 28). Peplau references Gregg (1954) and Mereness (1966) in the development of this fourth assumption (Forchuk, 1993, p. 6).
Inferred from Peplau's writings (Forchuk, 1993)	5. Psychodynamic nursing crosses all specialty areas of nursing. It is not synonymous with psychiatric nursing because every nurse–client relationship is an interpersonal situation in which recurring difficulties of everyday life arise (summarized from Peplau (1952), introduction). 6. Difficulties in interpersonal relations recur in varying intensities throughout the life of everyone (Peplau, 1952, p. xiv). 7. The need to harness energy that derives from tension and anxiety connected to felt needs to positive means for defining, understanding, and meeting productively the problem at hand is a universal need (Peplau, 1952, p. 26). 8. All human behavior is purposeful and goal seeking in terms of feelings of satisfaction and/or security (Peplau, 1952, p. 26). 9. The interaction of nurse and client is fruitful when a method of communication that identifies and uses common meanings is at work in the situation (Peplau, 1952, p. 284). 10. The meaning of behavior to the client is the only relevant basis on which nurses can determine needs to be met (Peplau, 1952, p. 226). 11. Each client will behave, during crisis, in a way that has worked in relation to crises faced in the past (Peplau, 1952, p. 255).
Inferred from Peplau's writings (Sellers, 1991)	12. The function of personality is to grow and to develop. Nursing is a process that seeks to facilitate development of personality by aiding individuals to use those compelling forces and experiences that influence personality in ways that ensure maximum productivity (p. 73). 13. Because illness is an event that is experienced along with feelings that derive from older experiences but are reenacted in the relationship of nurse to patient, the nurse–patient relationship is an opportunity for nurses to help patients to complete the unfinished psychological tasks of childhood to some degree (p. 59).

The patient needs to recognize and understand the extent of the difficulty and the help that is needed to address it. Orienting the patient to the nature of the problem is a complex task. It requires that the nurse acts as both a resource person and a counselor. As a resource person, the nurse provides specific information about the problem confronting the patient and helps the patient see the personal relevance of the information. As a counselor, the nurse encourages the patient to be actively involved in identifying and assessing the problem.

The patient also needs to recognize and use the professional services offered. The nurse serves as a resource person to help the patient identify the range and limitations of services provided. It is important for the patient to know what can be expected from the nurse. It is equally important that the patient understands the limitations in the health care environment, both situational (i.e., related to the routines) and cultural (i.e., related to the standards of conduct).

In order for the patient to move successfully to the next phase in the nurse–patient relationship, he or she must harness the energy from the tension and anxiety created by felt needs in a constructive fashion to define, understand, and resolve the problem. The counseling role of the nurse is vital in dealing with the patient's anxiety. The nurse must understand the meaning of the situation to the patient and be alert to evidence of anxiety manifested by apathy, dependency, or overaggressiveness, or terror and panic if the patient fails to deal with it. As a resource person, the nurse helps the patient understand the meaning of the anxiety-promoting events he is experiencing in the health care environment. In the counseling role, the nurse encourages the expression of expectations and feelings by responding unconditionally to the patient. This response communicates to the patient that the focus of the relationship is on his needs, not those of the nurse. Through nondirective listening, the nurse encourages the patient to focus on the problem and express related feelings, without offering advice, reassurance, suggestions, or persuasions. This establishes the foundation for the work of the next phase of the relationship.

Phase of Identification. This phase begins after the patient has, to a degree, clarified first impressions and arrived at some understanding of what the situation has to offer. At this time, the patient can selectively begin to identify with some of the individuals who are offering help in one of the three ways: with interdependence/participation, independence/isolation, or dependence/helplessness. This identification is based on the degree to which the patient believes the nurse will be helpful and on the nature of his past relationships.

The patient who responds interdependently feels less powerless and identifies with and expresses the attitudes of cheerfulness, optimism, and problem solving that he perceives in the nurse. Under these conditions, the patient may express feelings that are not normally considered acceptable (e.g., helplessness or self-centeredness). These expressions are seen as potentially growth producing if the nurse accepts the feelings and continues to meet the needs of the patient.

Not all patients can identify with the nurse offering help because of the influence of earlier negative relationships with others. This experience often leads to a response that is independent or isolative. At this time, the nurse in the surrogate family member role may provide the patient with the opportunity to have new and more positive relational experiences.

Other patients may identify with the nurse too quickly, which can result in an overly dependent response to the nurse. These patients want all their needs to be met by others with no expectations placed on them. This not uncommon response limits the possibility of growth through the experience.

It is important for the nurse to consider the phenomenon of leadership during the identification phase. The nurse attempts to provide opportunities for the patient to assume responsibility in the situation that promotes more constructive rather than imitative learning. The patient is encouraged to develop the skills to perceive, focus, and interpret cues in the situation, and then respond appropriately, independent of the nurse.

Phase of Exploitation. During this phase the patient feels comfortable enough to take full advantage of the services being offered and experience full value from the relationship with the nurse. Varying degrees of dependence and self-directedness are manifested with vacillation between the states. Ideally, the patient begins to identify and orient self to new goals besides solving the immediate problem, for example, in the case of a hospitalized patient, the goal of functioning at home.

Phase of Resolution. As old needs are met, they are replaced by new goals that began to be formulated while the patient engaged in (i.e., exploited) the use of the services provided by the nurse. It is hoped that the patient will experience a sense of security and release that occurs because he or she received help in the time of need. This security is accompanied by less reliance on and decreasing identification with helping persons and increasing reliance on self to deal with the problem. This is the result of a nurse–patient relationship that is characterized during all phases by: (a) an unconditional, patient-focused, and ongoing relationship that provides for the patient's needs; (b) a recognition of and appropriate response to cues that indicate the patient's desire and readiness to grow; and (c) a shift of power from nurse to patient as patient assumes responsibility for achieving new goals (Peplau, 1991, pp. 40, 41).

FULFILLED THROUGH ROLES

The roles of nursing are defined by nurses, endorsed by patients, influenced by society, and promoted by the professional literature. Peplau identified the roles that she considered most relevant to nurse–patient situations and delineated principles for the successful fulfilling of those roles. The roles she identified were as follows:

1. Stranger: The nurse approaches the patient with respect and positive interest.
2. Resource person: The nurse answers questions using level of functioning, psychological readiness, psychological atmosphere, and relevance of the questions to formulate the response.
3. Teacher: The nurse considers what patients already know and level of interest to develop learning situations that enable patients to learn through experience.
4. Leader: The nurse engages patients as active participants in planning their care.
5. Surrogate: The nurse recognizes that patients often respond to him or her as they would to a person from their past and uses that recognition to help patients deal constructively with their feelings and learn new ways or relating to others.
6. Counselor: The nurse observes and listens to patients in a way that helps patients develop fully understanding of themselves, their feelings and actions.

INFLUENCED BY PSYCHOBIOLOGICAL EXPERIENCES

The psychobiological experiences of needs, frustration, conflict, and anxiety influence the functioning of personalities. These experiences are also sources of energy that can result in both constructive and destructive actions. It is through understanding these experiences that individuals can learn to become more productive human beings (Peplau, 1991).

Needs. Although Peplau identifies needs as both physiological and psychological, her emphasis is on those that are psychological in nature. Security, new experiences, affection, recognition, and mastery are identified as psychological needs.

Needs create tension, which individuals strive to reduce through the expenditure of energy (behavior). Behavior is directed at meeting the uppermost need, which may leave other needs unrecognized. Underactivity and overactivity are ineffective ways of meeting unrecognized needs. Unmet needs, if persistent, can lead to ever-increasing tension or anxiety. When immediate needs are met, others emerge, some of which may be more consistent with promoting health (e.g., recovery and personality development).

Frustration. Frustration occurs when fulfillment of a need or pursuit of a goal is blocked. The primary goal identified by Peplau (1991) is the need for a "feeling of satisfaction and/or security" (p. 86). Frustration can be manifested as aggression and/or anxiety. Direct expression of aggression occurs when the source is identified and is the recipient of its expression; indirect expression of aggression occurs when the recipient only resembles the original source. Anxiety is a result of repeated frustrations that are perceived as failure to accomplish goals. Since the experience of anxiety is difficult to tolerate, the individual defends self from it by: (a) modifying the goal to one for which success is more likely, (2) giving up on the goal with the possibility of dissociation of feelings occurring, and/or (3) adopting fixed responses (e.g., stereotyping and delusions). It is important for the nurse and patient to communicate to clarify goals and arrive at some mutually acceptable ones.

Conflict. Another issue that the nurse and patient deal with in their interpersonal relationship is conflicting goals. Conflicting goals are often unrecognized and are expressed in the behavioral responses of hesitation, tension, vacillation, or complete blocking.

Blocking occurs when approaching a goal is completely incompatible with avoiding another one (approach–avoidance conflict). The most common example is the desire to go home (approaching goal) that coexists with the desire to not leave the perceived safety of the hospital (avoiding goal). Fear results and intensifies when approaching a goal for which there is a conflicting goal of avoiding. This fear can express itself as withdrawal or avoidance. If that which is feared can be identified, the nurse can act as a resource person by providing information and experiences that can reduce the strength of avoidance. If the source of the fear cannot be identified, it is referred to as anxiety and is likely an internal conflict that is more difficult to resolve.

Individuals often are required to make choices between two desirable goals (approach–approach conflict). This is manifested with slightly different behavioral responses, for example, ignoring the feelings about the desired goals or keeping them from conscious awareness. The nurse is most helpful by fulfilling the counselor role in this situation. Listening in a way that encourages the expression of feelings allows the individual to recognize the factors that influence the choice to be made.

Unexplained Discomfort/Anxiety. As previously noted, anxiety or unexplained discomfort, as Peplau sometimes referred to it, can occur when there are unmet needs, obstacles to goals, or conflicting goals. Anxiety is often associated with guilt, doubt, fears, and obsessions. Both patients and nurses experience this feeling state that influences behavior productively or destructively through the energy it produces.

Peplau (1991) identifies two principles that nurses can use to assist patients to use anxiety productively:

1. "When anxiety is held within tolerable limits it can be a 'functionally' effective element in interpersonal relations" (p. 127).
2. As anxiety increases in severity, there is a narrowing of perceptual awareness. Mild anxiety can manifest itself as restlessness, sleeplessness, hostility, misunderstanding, repeated questioning, seeking attention or reassurance, and so on. This level of anxiety creates a felt need that can serve as a source of motivation for personality growth. In contrast to mild anxiety, severe anxiety can be crippling and incapacitating. The patient cannot collaborate with the nurse and useful learning cannot take place.

The nurse helps reduce the anxiety to a more manageable and useful level by his or her presence as someone who will listen and provide for the patient's physical needs. The ability of the nurse to be helpful to the patient during the experiences of anxiety is predicated on his or her self-understanding. "If a nurse has developed ability to undergo tension and stress, in order to identify a difficulty that she feels and to take steps that lead to a course of action based on evidence of what is involved, she will be able to help patients to do likewise" (Peplau, 1991, p. 135).

REQUIRES ATTENDING TO CERTAIN PSYCHOLOGICAL TASKS

Psychological tasks are those related to learning to live with others. Peplau addresses the tasks of (a) learning to count on others, (b) learning to delay satisfaction, (c) identifying oneself, and (d) developing skills in participation. These tasks occur not only as an aspect of the development of personality, but also as features of nurse–patient relationships. During this relationship, the nurse has the opportunity to help patients develop in areas of task deficit. In order to provide this assistance, the nurse uses the previously discussed roles and understanding of the previously examined psychobiological experiences. In addition, in order to understand his or her own personality and the patient's, the nurse needs to appreciate the psychological tasks of infants and children as identified by Sigmund Freud and Richard Havighurst (Peplau, 1991, p. 166) and the acculturation processes that enable those tasks to be successfully completed.

Counting on Others. This is the first psychological task of the infant. Initially, comfort and discomfort are the only feeling states experienced. If the caregiver (mother) appreciates the feelings of discomfort being communicated and responds unconditionally and in a way consistent with the infant's biological make-up, the infant learns to rely on the mother for help. Thus, a healthy dependence is learned. If there is maternal rejection and/or overprotection, an ongoing need for dependency may develop. An individual's longing for dependency thus operates as a persistent need that is based on a denial that help is needed or would be useful, or it is based on a belief that others will be able to identify and meet needs without his or her attempts to communicate them.

The nurse encounters varying degrees of both healthy dependency and dependency longings in nursing situations. In response to those situations, nurses help patients learn that they are trustworthy and then assist patients to become more aware of their needs and to express those needs more effectively (Peplau, 1991, p. 181). There are a number of positive consequences of having needs met. The patient experiences a feeling of self-worth and as a result begins to collaborate with the nurse in his or her growth. In addition, as needs are met, new, more mature ones can emerge.

Delaying Satisfaction. The socialization of a child includes the lesson of deferring to the wishes of others and delaying gratification of his own wishes, a lesson that is dependent on having already learned that those being deferred to are also those that can also be counted upon. According to Peplau (1991), this lesson takes place primarily during the process of toilet training. A rigorous and rigid form of training may inhibit the child's natural desire to explore this newly developing skill (i.e., producing feces) and can result in a sense of powerlessness. By contrast, if mother's acceptance is not used as an emotional tool to manipulate the child into what the mother finds acceptable behavior, the child can learn to accept interference with immediate gratification of needs as inevitable, usually reasonable, and possibly a useful life experience (Peplau, 1991, pp. 193, 194).

During the toilet training experience, the child has three possible responses: (a) adapt his needs to those of family and gradually learn to behave in a way consistent with family members with whom he identifies, (b) give up feelings of power and comply with other's demands, or (c) refuse to give up power, becoming defiant and resistant. The latter two responses result in distorted relations with others and unresolved personality issues that persist into adulthood. The nurse may note these issues manifested in patients who are exploitive and manipulative; who hoard and withhold, being unable to share (including the inability to share feelings); and who alter their responses to others in a way that indicates a lack of stability and consistency in personality structure.

Peplau (1991) identified principles that are consistent with healthy toilet training and general socialization activities that help the nurse establish rapport with patients and assist them in developing the ability to delay gratification of needs:

1. Show unconditional interest and acceptance.
2. Encourage expression of needs and feelings.
3. Provide times in which demands are met and they are not met.
4. Promote participation in decision making so that patients can become more self-directing.
5. Allow for some "hoarding," which reinforces feelings of security.
6. Encourage sharing, which can only occur when there is freedom from coercion.

Hopefully, patients learn that delaying gratification can be experienced without an overwhelming sense of anxiety.

Identifying Oneself. Self-identity or concept of self enhances or distorts relationships with others, a fact that is true for both the patient and the nurse. This sense of self develops initially through a child's interactions with adults as he learns to rely on others and delay gratification in relation to needs. The way the child is appraised during these interactions results in three possible views of self: (a) *a sense of competency* to identify wants and needs, communicate them to others, and receive needed assistance; (b) *a sense of helplessness and dependence* on others to provide what is needed and a belief that this helplessness will produce a sense of safety (since making no demands will result in not being deserted); and (c) *a sense of distrust* in others as a source of assistance that results in independently taking what is needed. If a child has to work to get or sustain approval from others or to avoid anxiety of the experience of disapproval, a healthy development of self concept is difficult to achieve.

Concepts of self are established in childhood but can be reinforced or modified by experiences with others throughout life. The nurse can provide experiences that help the patient develop a concept of self that facilitates the establishment of interdependent relationships with others. In order to provide the appropriate experiences, the nurse needs to understand the patient's self-perception. Peplau (1992) suggests a number of activities that help the nurse understand a patient's self concept:

1. Consider own response to patient as a source of information about the patient's perceptions of self and situation confronting him.
2. Develop self-awareness of own habits (e.g., regarding cleanliness) and how they are expressed in the nursing situation.
3. Identify patient's patterns of feeling expressions and other behavioral responses as he encounters situational challenges.
4. Consider patient's specific responses to the nursing situation as indicators of needs to be met.

In addition, the nurse can be helpful to the patient by the following:

1. Being value neutral, "… providing merely conditions and acting as a sounding board against which the patient may air his views and give full expression to his feelings in a nonjudgmental relationship" (Peplau, 1991, p. 226)
2. Communicating hope and acceptance
3. Avoiding the problematic responses of praise, blame, and indifference

The nurse who exhibits these characteristics can enhance the patient's whole concept of self and ability to experience interdependent relationships with others.

Participating with Others. When individuals participate in making decisions that affect them, they are more likely to understand the decisions, be involved in implementing them, and appreciate the contributions of others to the ultimate decision. This task of participating with others is composed of the abilities to (a) *compromise,* arbitrate, and make personal concessions; (b) *compete,* express rivalry, and struggle with peers; and (c) *cooperate,* subordinate individual wishes to achieve mutually beneficial goals. The process of developing these skills is influenced by the appraisals of parents and peers.

The abilities to participate with others are consolidated in a process referred to as consensual validation. The view of self becomes more consistent with the views of peers and a more realistic perspective of life and one's role in it develops. At this time, a child also begins to be able to care for and accept others. This occurs to the degree that the child cares for and accepts self.

The nurse attempts to encourage participation with others through collaboration with the patient in addressing problems. This participatory approach serves to improve the patient's skills in meeting problems. Peplau (1991) describes a three-step process:

1. Assist the patient to identify the problem.
2. Collaborate to "achieve a decision on what is possible, what can be done, and then move into other items that have been mentioned and other *possible courses of action* that can be taken in behalf of and with the co-operation of the patient" (Peplau, 1991, p. 248).
3. Encourage the patient to try out what has been proposed.

As part of the process of identifying the problem, the nurse will need to assess the patient's attitude, since attitude will affect the way the patient will attempt to solve the problem. The two most common attitudes are overconcern or underconcern. If overconcerned, the patient may attempt to arrive at a solution too quickly and the solution will be inadequate. If underconcerned, the patient may not invest sufficient energy in its solution and the solution will be superficial.

In formulating a possible solution to the problem, the nurse needs to allow the patient to determine the pace for working through it. Time pressures are often communicated by the nurse in the form of suggestions about what is wrong and advice as to what needs to be done, leading to premature and ineffective solutions. Nurses can help patients to experience the process of problem solving and to develop the skills needed to actively participate in its solution.

Nursing Methods Used to Understand Interpersonal Processes

Observation, communication, and recording are three basic skills that are "valuable to the use of nursing as an interpersonal process that is therapeutic and educative for patients" (Peplau, 1991, p. 309). Peplau considered these three operations as integral to the nursing process.

Observation. "The aim of observation in nursing, when it is viewed as an interpersonal process, is the identification, clarification, and verification of impressions about the interactive drama, of the pushes and pulls in the relationship between nurse and patient, as they occur" (Peplau, 1991, p. 263). Observation as described by Peplau is composed of four components: (a) intuitive impressions, (b) hypothesis statements, (c) organized observations, and (d) judgment formations.

Intuitive impressions are hunches or generalizations about what is occurring in an experience. They are an important component of understanding the problems of patients. Impressions are the foundation for the development of hypotheses, and it is hypotheses that provide a means of reducing the risk of concentrating prematurely on details of the situation. When the impressions or generalizations are formulated as a hypothesis, they serve to provide a useful focus to the observations. The nurse proceeds to gather evidence related to the hypotheses (units of experience) that provide both elaboration of the whole impression and differentiation of the details.

Peplau (1991) provides a classification of types of observer–observed relationships that the nurse can use to gather evidence:

1. **Spectator:** The patient is unaware of being observed. The nurse is generally engaged in another activity while observing the patient.
2. **Interviewer:** The patient is aware of being observed as he responds to the situation or to the directive or nondirective questioning of the nurse. The nurse frequently takes notes while observing as an interviewer.
3. **Collector:** The nurse uses records and reports created by others as a way of determining what has happened in a particular situation. Observations made using this approach can help form partial impressions.
4. **Participant:** "The nurse engages in ordinary activities connected with nursing a patient and at the same time observes the relationship between the patient and herself" (Peplau, 1991, p. 274). The patient is aware that nursing care is being given, but is unaware that his/her responses are being observed. During participant observation, the nurse must pay attention to his/her behavior in order to evaluate its usefulness in the relationship and modify behavior as needed.

The observations need to be organized. Organization helps provide focus to the multiplicity and complexity of the observations of human behavior in interpersonal relationships. Peplau (1991) suggests hypotheses and the phases of the nurse–patient relationship as two approaches to organizing observations. This organization of observations made through participant observation is the basis of all nursing judgments in practice (p. 283). "Observation and understanding of what is observed are essential operations for making judgments and for designing experiences with patients that aid them in the solution of their problems" (Peplau, 1991, p. 289).

Communication. One of the basic tools of nursing is communication, which requires "awareness of means of communication; spoken language, rational and nonrational expressions of wishes, needs, and desires, and the body gesture" (Peplau, 1991, p. 289). Use of words or verbal communication can convey facts, focus on everyday events, and provide interpretations. Spoken language can reveal personal realities or express hidden meanings, but it can also avoid conveying anything meaningful.

There are two main principles for effective verbal communication: clarity and continuity. Clarity occurs when there is a common frame of reference or when specific efforts are made to arrive at mutual understanding. "Clarity is promoted when the meaning to the patient is expressed and talked over and a new view is expanded in awareness" (Peplau, 1991, p. 291). Continuity occurs when the connections between ideas and the related feelings, events, or themes expressed through the ideas are made evident. "Continuity is promoted when the nurse is able to pick up threads of conversation [that occur over time] … and when she aids the patient to focus and to expand these threads" (Peplau, 1991, p. 293). Following up on what patients say communicates that what they said is important and that as individuals they are worthwhile.

In the process of promoting clarity and continuity in communication, the nurse must also be able to interpret symbols to arrive at the hidden meanings of patients' indirect communications. Self-awareness is one of the primary conditions for achieving understanding. For a nurse, this awareness enables her to express congruence in the use of words, their relevance, and related actions.

Awareness provides the primary distinction between rational and nonrational communications. Rational expressions more likely occur when individuals see themselves rather than others as a source of personal security and when they are oriented toward the future in the context of the present rather than oriented to the past. Nonrational expressions communicate in more ambiguous and indirect ways than do rational expressions. Longings, hopes, and fears are often conveyed in a disguised form. It is the nurse's responsibility to interpret the meaning of the communication by considering the symbols being used to express the underlying emotions.

In addition to the spoken word, gestures can be considered either rational or nonrational expressions. "The body as a whole, as well as parts of it, act as expressional instruments that communicate to others the feelings, wishes, and aspirations of an individual" (Peplau, 1991, p. 304). Underactivity and overactivity are examples of whole-body gestures. Hand gestures (e.g., clenched fist) and facial grimaces (e.g., biting a lip) are examples of more specific gestures. The nurse's responsibility is to observe gestures and attempt to understand both what she and the patient are communicating to each other. Arriving at understanding or meaning is a complicated and ongoing process of observation and communication.

Recording. Peplau focuses primarily on recording for the purpose of student learning. In addition to charting in medical records, students need additional forms for recording what has occurred between student and patient. These additional recordings provide a means of examining the relationship in order to achieve insight into the student nurse's own behavior and the ways the patients responded. How useful the recording is to the student's development of interpersonal skills is dependent in part on the exactness of the wording of the recording. The ultimate goal of recordings, as well as observation and communication, is nurse–patient relationships that result in improved health outcomes for the patient. In nursing education, students still create and analyze "verbatims" to promote learning about themselves and the nature of their relationships.

Applications of the Theory: Research. Peplau's theory of interpersonal relations remains relevant as a foundation for scientific inquiry and nursing practice. A review of the literature, 2000–2010, revealed over 120 publications in which Peplau's work was cited. Theory of interpersonal relations is of interest internationally, with publications by nurse scientists from Australia, Brazil, Canada, China, Denmark, Ethiopia, France, Great Britain, New Zealand, Norway, Slovenia, South Africa, Spain, Sweden, and Turkey. Among the citations to Peplau's work in the last decade are her biography (Callaway, 2002); book chapters on her theory (George, 2005; Reed, Shearer, & Nicoll, 2004), editorials and tributes (Wills, 2010, Zauszniewski, 2009); doctoral dissertations (Mariani, 2007), and numerous articles using her theory as a framework for research or a basis for nursing care practices. In addition, there are articles that describe her theory (McCarthy & Aquino-Russell, 2009) and present her contributions from historical perspectives (Boling, 2003; Silverstein, 2008).

The theory has served as a framework for studying a variety of research questions, using both qualitative and quantitative methods. Although originally a theory designed to describe therapeutic relationships between nurses and psychiatric patients (Forchuk & Reynolds, 2001; Forchuk et al., 2000; Tofthagen, 2004), it is currently used to examine the nature of relationships with other populations. For instance, in qualitative research, the theory has provided the framework to study: (a) helping roles in working with survivors of sexual violence (Courey, Martsolf, Drauker, & Strickland, 2008), (b) home-visiting programs for vulnerable prenatal families (McNaughton, 2005), (c) behaviors used by hospitalized patients to engage nurses in interactions (Shatell, 2005), and (d) promoting wellness in young adults experiencing early stages of psychosis (McCann & Baker, 2001). In addition, a case study that was qualitative in nature, examined the nurse–patient relationship in counseling male patients with acquired immune deficiency syndrome (AIDS) (Gauthier, 2000).

The quantitative studies focus on both nursing practice and nursing education. New to the body of research are several randomized control studies. Table 9.2 provides examples of nursing research using quantitative methods published in English from 2000 to 2010.

TABLE 9.2 Examples of Research Using Theory of Interpersonal Relations

Citation	Focus
Anderson, K. H., Ford, S., Robson, D., Cassis, J., Rodriques, C., & Gray, R. (2010). An exploratory, randomized controlled trial of adherence therapy for people with schizophrenia. *International Journal of Mental Health Nursing, 19,* 340–349. Retrieved from www.wiley.com/bw/journal.asp?ref=1445-8330.	Use of adherence therapy to improve compliance with antipsychotic medication regime in people with psychosis.
Beeber, L. S., Holditch-davis, D., Perreira, K., Schwartz, T. A., Lewis, V., Blanchard, H., et al. (2010). Short-term in-home intervention reduces depressive symptoms in Early Head Start Latina mothers of infants and toddlers. *Research in Nursing & Health, 33*(1), 60–76. doi:10.1002/nur.20363	Use of in-home culturally appropriate psychotherapy intervention to reduce symptoms of depression in Latina mothers of toddlers and infants.
Erci, B., Sezgin, S., Kacmaz, Z. (2008). The impact of therapeutic relationship on preoperative and postoperative patient anxiety. *Australian Journal of Advanced Nursing, 26,* 59–66. Retrieved from www.ajan.com.au	Effect of the Interpersonal Relations Model based on phases of therapeutic relationship on perioperative anxiety.
Oflaz, F., Hatipoglu, S., & Aydin, H. (2008). Effectiveness of psychoeducation intervention on post-traumatic stress disorder and coping styles of earthquake survivors. *Journal of Clinical Nursing, 17,* 677–687. doi:10.1111/j.1365-2702.2007.02047.x	Comparison of psychoeducation (based on phases of therapeutic relationship) alone, medication alone, with combined approach to reduce anxiety and improve coping of survivors of earthquake in Turkey.
Mariani, B. S. (2007). *The effect of mentoring on career satisfaction of registered nurses and intent to stay in the nursing profession.* Unpublished doctoral dissertation, Widener University School of Nursing, Chester, PA.	Effect of mentoring as a representation of an interpersonal relationship on career satisfaction of nurses and their intent to stay in the profession.
McNaughton, D. B. (2005). A naturalistic test of Peplau's theory in home visiting. *Public Health Nursing, 22,* 429–438. Retrieved from www.wiley.com/bw/journal.asp?ref=0737–1209	Phases of the nurse–patient relationship identified in home visits to prenatal clients by public health nurses.
Beebe, L. H., & Tian, L. (2004). TIPS: Telephone intervention—problem solving for persons with schizophrenia. *Issues in Mental Health Nursing, 25,* 317–329. doi:10.108/0161280490274804	Significance of face-to-face meetings in the efficacy of telephone intervention with schizophrenic individuals.
Mahon, N. E., Yarcheski, A., & Yarcheski, T. J. (2004). Social support and positive health practices in early adolescents: A test of mediating variables. *Clinical Nursing Research, 13*(3), 216–236. doi:10.1177/1054773803262407	Relationship between social support and positive health practices of young adolescents.
Carroll, S. M. (2004). Nonvocal ventilated patients' perceptions of being understood. *Western Journal of Nursing Research, 26,* 85–112. doi:10.1177/0193945903259462	Characteristics of nonvocal ventilated patients' communication and the kind of nursing care they desire.

(continued)

TABLE 9.2 Examples of Research Using Theory of Interpersonal Relations (*Continued*)

Citation	Focus
Sorenson, D. S. (2003). Healing traumatizing provider interactions among women through short-term group therapy. *Archives of Psychiatric Nursing, 17,* 259–269. doi:10.1053j.apnu.2003.10.002	Use of cognitive group intervention to resolve trauma of women traumatized by health providers' interactions during childbirth.
Douglass, J. L., Sowell, R. L., & Phillips, K. D. (2003). Using Peplau's theory to examine the psychosocial factors associated with HIV-infected women's difficulty in taking their medications. *The Journal of Theory Construction & Testing, 7,* 10–17. Retrieved from http://tuckerpub.com/jtct.htm	Relationship between the patient and the primary health care provider as it relates to medication adherence of HIV positive women.
Kim, K. H. (2003). Baccalaureate nursing students' experiences of anxiety producing situations in the clinical setting. *A Journal of the Australian Nursing Profession, 14,* 145–155. Retrieved from www.highbeam.com/Australian+Nursing+Journal/publications.aspx?	Relationship between trait anxiety and type of clinical education experiences of student nurses.
Kai, J., & Crosland, A. (2002). People with enduring mental health problems described the importance of communication, continuity of care, and stigma. *Evidence-Based Nursing, 5*(3), 93. Retrieved from http://ebn.bmj.com	Significance of therapeutic relationships in maintaining contacts with primary care and mental health services for individuals with chronic mental illness.
Washington, E. A. (2001). Installation of 3% hydrogen peroxide or distilled vinegar in urethral catheter drainage bag to decrease catheter-associated bacteriuria. *Biological Research for Nursing, 3,* 78–87. doi:10.1177/109980040200300203	Comparison of use of 3% hydrogen peroxide and distilled vinegar to decrease incidence of catheter-associated bacteriuria using Peplau's theory to guide advanced practice nurses' interactions.
Durkin, A. E. (2000). *Comfort levels of nursing students and faculty regarding clinical assignment to an AIDS patient.* University of Connecticut, Storrs, CT.	Relationship of age, education, and prior experience with comfort levels of faculty and students when students care for AIDS patients.
Forchuk, C., Westfall, J., Martin, M., Bamber-Azzapardi, W., Kosterewa-Tolman, D., & Hux, M. (2000). The developing nurse–client relationship: Nurses' perceptions. *Journal of American Nurses Association, 6,* 3–10. doi:10.1177/107839030000600102	Perspectives of nurses in a tertiary care hospital on the nature and progression of the nurse–client relationship and the factors that facilitate or interfere with the development of the relationship.

As noted in the table, nurse scientists have begun to explore the usefulness of Peplau's theory in cross-cultural contexts. Using Middle Range Theories 9.1 describes one such study.

Although instrument development to study the nature of nurse–patient relationships began in the 1960s and continues in a limited fashion, the numbers developed are few. This may be explained in part by the phenomenological nature of the theory (Haber, 2000) and in part by its complexity. Table 9.3 provides an overview of those instruments.

Peplau has contributed to both the processes used to develop nursing's body of knowledge and the content of that knowledge base. "Optimistically, legitimatization of practice-derived theory in the 1990s will make theory-testing and hypothesis-generating qualitative research related to Peplau's model a priority for nurse researchers in the new millennium" (Haber, 2000, pp. 59, 60). Peplau and others have suggested research needs or questions for this new millennium. Peplau (1964) identified the following questions for nurses in general hospital settings:

1. How do nurses distinguish between a demand and a need of a patient?
2. What is the language behavior during the nurse–patient exchange in the general hospital?

This experimental (pretest/posttest) study tested the effect of an intervention based on Peplau's theory of interpersonal relations on depressive symptoms of Latina mothers of infants and toddlers. Hypothesis 1 stated: "mothers who received the intervention would demonstrate significantly less depressive symptom severity, report less child behavioral aggression and fewer concerns about child social-emotional functioning, and demonstrate greater maternal responsiveness midway through the intervention (T2:14 weeks), at the conclusion of the intervention (T3: 22 weeks), and 1 month following completion of the intervention (T4: 26 weeks) compared to mothers who received usual care" (p. 62).

The sample was comprised of 80 newly immigrated, Latina mothers with depressive symptoms who had infants or toddlers. They were recruited for Early Head Start programs located in southeastern United States. The mothers spoke only Spanish or had limited English proficiency. Peplau's theory provided the structure for the intervention that consisted of 16 in-home contacts made by teams of English-speaking master's prepared psychiatric nurses and trained Spanish language interpreters. The focuses of the intervention were: (a) reduction of depressive symptoms and their interpersonal sources,

USING MIDDLE RANGE THEORIES

9.1

(b) choice and use of social support, (c) management of stressful life issues and interpersonal disputes, and (d) development of strategies to increase responsiveness to the child. The CES-D, Spanish version, was used to determine depressive symptoms; child aggression was measured by the Child Behavior Checklist (CBCL), Spanish version, and the Ages and Stages Questionnaire-Social Emotional (ASQ-SE); and responsiveness to child was assessed using the Maternal-Child Observation (MCO) and the Home Observation for Measurement of the Environment (HOME).

The findings were supportive of Peplau's theory:

1. There was a statistically significant greater decrease in depressive symptoms for the mothers receiving the intervention than those who received usual care, T2: $P = 0.02$, T3: $P = 0.01$, and T4: $P = 0.02$.

2. Reports of aggression decreased in the intervention group from T1 to T4 ($P = 0.03$), whereas they increased in the usual care group during the same timeframe.

3. There were no statistically significant differences between the two groups related to maternal interactions and responsiveness.

Source: Beeber, L. S., Holditch-Davis, D., Perreria, K., Schwartz, T. A., Lewis, V., Blanchard, H., et al. (2010). Short-term in-home intervention reduces depressive symptoms in early Head Start Latina mothers of infants and toddlers. *Research in Nursing and Health, 33*(1), 60–76. doi:10.1002/nur.20363

3. How do patients develop sufficient flexibility to incorporate body image changes into views of self after major surgery or major life experiences? What nursing interventions are most helpful to patients during this process?

4. How does the one-to-one relationship fit into the present and the future health care delivery system? (pp. 81, 82).

Perhaps the most fundamental and pervasive question that researchers of the nurse–patient relationship can ask and attempt to answer is, What aspects of the nurse–patient relationship contribute to the welfare and well-being of patients? (Caris-Verhallen, Kerkstra, & Bensing, 1997). The promotion of the welfare of patients is core to all nursing theories, but for Peplau, the means of achieving that goal focuses on the attributes and behaviors of both the nurse and the patient and in the dynamic interaction that occurs between them.

Applications of the Theory: Practice. Peplau's theory of interpersonal relations has remained popular with nurses, in earlier years particularly those practicing psychiatric–mental health nursing. Surveys of psychiatric nurses in Canada and the United States found over half of them claiming to use Peplau's theory in their practices (Forchuk, 1993, p. 28). Most recently in the field of mental health, the theory has been used to (a) conceptualize the role of mental health consultant liaison (Merritt & Procter, 2010), (b) prepare nurse therapists (Vandemark, 2006), (c) promote therapeutic relationships (Stockman, 2005), (d) care for depressed and potentially suicidal elderly (Campbell, 2001), and (e) prioritize in community mental health settings (Bonner, 2001).

The theory has also been used to consider practice issues of general concern to nurses, for instance (a) presence (Zblock, 2010), (b) shared decision making (Wills, 2010), (c) quality of life (McCarthy &

TABLE 9.3 Instruments Used to Test Theory of Interpersonal Relations

Instrument	Reference	Description
Social Interaction Inventory	Methven, D., & Schlotfeldt, R. (1962). The social interaction inventory. *Nursing Research, 11*(2), 83–88.	Inventory comprised of 30 common nurse–patient situations in which the stress faced by the patient and his or her family is identified. For each situation, responses representing five different types are given (i.e., expression of concern that encourages verbalization; expression of sympathy and giving reassurance; inquiry into tangential aspects of the situation; explanations, justifications, or defense of nurse's point of view; rejection or denunciation of patient's need). Validity described.
Therapeutic Behavior Scale	Spring, R., & Turk, H. (1962). A therapeutic behavior scale. *Nursing Research, 11*(4), 214–218.	Tool to rate nurses' responses to patients as therapeutic or nontherapeutic in relation to approach, level, topic, focus, and consistency. Validity and reliability data included.
Facilitative Level of a Therapeutic Relationship	Aiken, L., & Aiken, J. (1973). A systematic approach to the evaluation of interpersonal relationships. *American Journal of Nursing, 73,* 863–867.	Tool to evaluate the implementation of the five core dimensions (empathetic understanding, positive regard, genuineness, concreteness, and self-exploration) using a five-point scale of descriptors of nurse's or patient's behaviors. No data on validity or reliability included.
Working Alliance Inventory (WAI)	Horvath, A. O., & Greenberg, L. (1986). The development of the Working Alliance Inventory. In L. Greenberg & W. Pinsof (Eds.), *Psychotherapeutic process: A research handbook* (pp. 529–556). New York: Guilford Press.	36-item instrument, with parallel forms for client and therapist to self-report sense of bonding and tasks and goals of the developing therapeutic relationship. Validity and reliability data included.
Relationship Form	Forchuk, C., & Brown, B. (1989). Establishing a nurse–client relationship. *Journal of Psychosocial Nursing, 27*(2), 30–34.	Seven-point analog scale of the stages of the nurse–patient relationship, using brief descriptions of both the nurse's and the client's roles at each stage. Validity and reliability data provided.
Engagement with Health Care Provider		13-item scale on which clients rate the nature of their interactions with health care provider using a four-point scale with 1 = always true and 4 = never true. Focuses on issues such as, listening, caring, mutuality in decision making, and respect. Reliability data provided.

Aquino-Russell, 2009), (d) altered body image (Wiest, 2006), patient autonomy (Moser, Houtepen, & Widdershoven, 2007), (e) power struggles (Kozub & Kozub, 2004), (f) process of aging (Wadensten & Carlson, 2003), (g) intentionality (Ugarriza, 2002), (h) stress reduction using reminiscence (Puentes, 2002), and (i) explanation of symptoms (Mahoney & Engebretson, 2000).

Examples of application to practice in the last 10 years demonstrate how useful the theory is in a broad range of nursing situations. The theory has been used to (a) care for patients in end-stage kidney disease (Graham, 2006), (b) promote computer-mediated communication (Hrabe, 2005), (c) serve as a foundation for assessing needs in a patient with heart failure (Davidson, Cockburn, Daly, & Fisher, 2004), (d) work with younger residents in long-term care setting (Schafer & Middleton, 2001), (e) improve

Peplau's theory of interpersonal relations was used to guide the education of patients undergoing urinary diversion. Prior to surgery, patients can experience anger, grief, fear, and anxiety related to their diagnosis, testing experiences, and the surgical procedure. Postoperatively, these patients are at risk for multiple complications, for instance, infections, ileus, thrombophlebitis, altered body image, incontinence, and changes in sexual functioning. Needed life style changes occur that require learning about diet and exercise and the management of an altered urinary system. They may also need to help addressing their psychosocial needs as they return home and reengage with their communities.

The educational strategy was formulated to parallel Peplau's phases of the interpersonal process. In the orientation phase, the nurse and the patient meet with the goal of the patient accepting the nurse and his/her level of expertise so that the nurse can assess the learning needs of the patient and the patient's readiness to learn. Patients' acceptance of their knowledge deficits serves as motivation to learn. Nurse and patient clarify their expectations for future meetings, establishing mutually agreed upon goals. Nurses engage in (a) assessment of patients' prior knowledge and readiness to learn, (b) determination of mutually determined learning goals, (c) presentation of educational materials, and (d) discussion of surgical options and procedures.

USING MIDDLE RANGE THEORIES

9.2

During the identification phase, the focus is on addressing the gaps in the patient's knowledge of the disease, treatment choice, and self-care issues, and establishing goals for the preoperative and immediate postoperative periods and for discharge. During this phase, the patient may exhibit independence, overdependence, or isolation/rejection. In this phase, the nurse teaches neo-bladder care and healthy nutritional practices and works to develop an appropriate activity plan. Successful completion of this stage occurs when the patient recognizes the need for new skills and knowledge to achieve the established goals.

Exploitation is the next stage, characterized by comfort and trust in the relationship between nurse and patient. The patient can identify new learning goals but demonstrates independence and the ability to engage in self-care. In this phase, the nurse reaffirms patient's accomplishments, promotes independence, and helps patient identify community resources. In the final phase, resolution may take place months after discharge from the hospital. The patient experiences security and a sense of independence and self-reliance. The focus during this phase is on quality of life and integration of a changed health status. The nurse encourages participation in support groups and explores quality of life issues with the patient.

The article outlines each phase with related teaching activities and applies the implementation in case study.

Source: Marchese, K. (2006). Using Peplau's theory of interpersonal relations to guide the education of patients undergoing urinary diversion. *Urologic Nursing, 26,* 363–371. Retrieved from http://www.suna.org/cgi-bin/WebObjects/SUNAMain.woa/wa/viewSection?s_id=1073743840&ss_id=536872962

palliative care (Wallace, 2001), and (f) support parents of children with severe meningococcal disease (Haines, 2000). Peplau's theory has also served as a foundation to educate (a) faculty and students on telehealth through distance learning methods (Gallagher-Lepack, Scheibel & Gibson, 2009), (b) patients undergoing urinary diversion to promote their recovery (Marchese, 2006), (c) antepartal patients on prevention of prematurity (Tjedie, 2004), and (d) emigrants on cross-cultural health promotion practices (Kater, 2000). Using Middle Range Theories 9.2 provides an example of the theory applied to a specific practice issue.

Applications of the Theory: Theory and Model Development. Peplau's theory of interpersonal relations has served as a foundation for the development of other middle range theories and models applicable to practice. Examples include: (a) the Model of Simple Reminiscence (Puentes, 2002), (b) Cultural Competence (Warren, 2002), (c) Client–Nurse Interaction Phase of Symptom Management model (Haworth & Dhuly, 2001), and (d) Interface of Anthropology and Nursing Model (Mahoney & Engebretson, 2000). But Peplau's contributions to nursing are not limited to the content of her theory. She is credited with promoting the "scholarship of nursing practice" (Reed, 1996), integrating nursing practice with a process for ongoing development of nursing's knowledge base.

SUMMARY

Peplau is acknowledged as the first theorist of the modern era of nursing. Her theory of interpersonal relations in nursing focuses on the stages experienced, the nursing roles used, and the issues addressed in the context of the nurse–patient relationship. In the nursing profession, the primacy of the nurse–patient relationship is still recognized and Peplau's phenomenological approach to theory development is still valued. "Peplau's work has been influential, particularly (though not exclusively) in mental health nursing and 'her ideas have provided an architectural design for the practice of a discipline'" (Pearson, 2008, p. 80). Peplau was able to pull together "loose, ambiguous data and put them into systematic terms that could be tested, applied, and integrated into the practice of psychiatric nursing" (Lego, 1980, p. 68). Although because of its complexity, research on the theory of interpersonal relations is not a simple undertaking, further testing of Peplau's theory could make significant contributions to nursing's body of knowledge.

ANALYSIS OF THEORY

Using the criteria presented in Chapter 2, critique the theory of Interpersonal Relations. Compare your conclusions about the theory with those found in Appendix A. A nurse scholar who has worked with the theory completed the analysis found in the Appendix.

Internal Criticism	External Criticism
1. Clarity	1. Reality convergence
2. Consistency	2. Utility
3. Adequacy	3. Significance
4. Logical development	4. Discrimination
5. Level of theory development	5. Scope of theory
	6. Complexity

CRITICAL THINKING EXERCISES

1. In what ways might Peplau's theory of interpersonal relations need to be revised to be most useful to nurses in a health care environment in which contact time between nurse and client is limited?

2. The surrogate role is not one that is frequently mentioned in recent nursing practice literature. Is that role as defined by Peplau relevant to nursing practice as currently experienced? If so, in what way? If not, why?

3. Peplau's theory focuses on the one-to-one therapeutic relationship between a nurse and a patient. Are the phases of relationships, roles of the nurse, psychobiological experiences encountered in the relationship, and psychological tasks described by Peplau relevant in other nursing contexts, for example, in relationships between nurses? If so, what are some examples of these contexts? If not, why?

WEB RESOURCES

Visit **http://thePoint.lww.com/Peterson3e** for helpful web resources related to this chapter.

REFERENCES

Armstrong, M. E., & Kelly, A. E. (1995). More than the sum of their parts: Martha Rogers and Hildegard Peplau. *Archives of Psychiatric Nursing, 9*(1), 40–44.

Boling, A. (2003). The professionalization of psychiatric nursing: From doctors' handmaidens to empowered professionals. *Journal of Psychosocial Nursing & Mental Health Services, 41*, 26–40. Retrieved from www.jpnonline.com

Callaway, B. J. (2002). *Hildegard Peplau: Psychiatric nurse of the century.* New York, NY: Springer.

Caris-Verhallen, W., Kerkstra, A., & Bensing, J. (1997). The role of communication in nursing care for elderly people: A review of the literature. *Journal of Advanced Nursing, 25*, 915–933.

Courey, T. J., Martsolf, D. S., Draucker, C. B., & Strickland, K. B. (2008). Hildegard Peplau's theory and the health care encounters of survivors of sexual violence. *Journal of the American Psychiatric Nurses Association, 14*, 136–143. doi:10.1177/1078390308315613

Davidson, P., Cockburn, J., Daly, J., & Fisher, R. S. (2004). Patient-centered needs assessment: Rational for a psychometric measure for assessing needs in heart failure. *Journal of Cardiovascular Nursing, 19*(3), 164–171.

Fawcett, J. (2000). *Analysis and evaluation of contemporary nursing knowledge: Nursing models and theories.* Philadelphia, PA: F. A. Davis.

Forchuk, C. (1991). Peplau's theory: Concepts and their relations. *Nursing Science Quarterly, 4*(2), 54–60.

Forchuk, C. (1993). *Hildegarde E. Peplau: Interpersonal nursing theory.* Park, CA: Sage.

Forchuk, C., & Reynolds, W. (2001). Clients' reflections on relationships with nurses: Comparisons form Canada and Scotland. *Journal of Psychiatric & Mental Health Nursing, 8*, 45–51. Retrieved from onlinelibrary.wiley.com

Forchuk, C., Westwell, J., Martin, M., Bamber-Azzapardi, W., Kosterewa-Tolman, D., & Hux, M. (2000). The developing nurse–client relationship: nurses' perspectives. *Journal of the American Psychiatric Nurses Association, 6*, 3–10. doi:10.1177/107839030000600102

Gallagher-Lepack, S., Scheibel, P., & Gibson, C. C. (2009). Integrating telehealth in nursing curricula: Can you hear me now? *Online Journal of Nursing Informatics, 13*, 1089–9758. Retrieved from http://ojni.org/

Gastmans, C. (1998). Interpersonal relations in nursing: A philosophical-ethical analysis of the work of Hildegard E. Peplau. *Journal of Advanced Nursing, 28*, 1312–1319. Retrieved August 1, 2002, from http://gateway1.ovid.com/ovidweb.cgi.

Gautier, P. (2000). Use of Peplau's Interpersonal Relations Model to counsel people with AIDS. *Journal of American Psychiatric Nurses Association, 6*, 119–125. doi: 10.167/mpn.2000.108534

Graham, J. (2006). Nursing theory and clinical practice: How three nursing models can be incorporated into the care of patients with end stage kidney disease. *Canadian Association of Nephrology Nurses (CANNT) Journal, 16*(4), 28–31.

George, J. B. (2005). *Nursing theories: The base for professional practice.* Boston, MA: Pearson.

Haber, J. (2000). Hildegard E. Peplau: The psychiatric nursing legacy of a legend. *Journal of the American Psychiatric Nurses, 6*(2), 56–62.

Haines, C. (2000). Use of a theoretical framework in pediatric intensive care to provide support for parents of children with severe meningococcal disease. *Nursing in Critical Care, 5*, 87–97. Retrieved from http://www.wiley.com/bw/journal.asp?ref=1362-1017

Haworth, S. K., & Dluhy, N. M. (2001). Holistic symptom management: Modeling the interaction phase. *Journal of Advanced Nursing, 36*, 302–310. Retrieved from www.journalofadvancednursing.com

Hrabe, D. P. (2005). Peplau in cyberspace: An analysis of Peplau's interpersonal relations theory and computer-mediated communication. *Issues in Mental Health Nursing, 26*(4), 397–414.

Kater, V. (2000). A tale of teaching in two cities. *International Nursing Review, 47*, 121–125. Retrieved from http://onlinelibrary.wiley.com/journal/10.1111/(ISSN)1466-7657

Kozub, M. L., & Kozub, F. M. (2004). Dealing with power struggles in clinical and educational settings. *Journal of Psychosocial Nursing & Mental Health Services, 42*(2), 22–31.

Lego, S. (1980). The one-to-one nurse–patient relationship. *Perspectives in Psychiatric Care, 18*(2), 67–89.

Mahoney, J. S., & Engebretson, J. (2000). The interface of anthropology and nursing guiding culturally competent care in psychiatric nursing. *Archives of Psychiatric Nursing, 14*, 183–190. doi:10.1053/apnu.2000.8657

Marchese, K. (2006). Using Peplau's theory of interpersonal relations to guide the education of patients undergoing urinary diversion. *Urologic Nursing, 26*(5), 363–371. Retrieved from http://www.suna.org/cgi-bin/WebObjects/SUNAMain.woa/wa/viewSection?s_id=1073743840&ss_id=536872962

Mariani, B. S. (2007). *The effect of mentoring on career satisfaction of registered nurses and intent to stay in the nursing profession.* Unpublished doctoral dissertation, Widener University School of Nursing, Chester, PA.

Merritt, M. K., & Procter, N. (2010). Conceptualizing the functional role of mental health consultation-liaison nurse in multi-morbidity using Peplau's nursing theory. *Contemporary Nurse: A Journal for the Australian Nursing Profession, 34*, 158–166. Retrieved from http://www.contemporarynurse.com/

McCann, T., & Baker, H. (2001). Mutual relating: Developing interpersonal relationships in the community. *Journal of Advanced Nursing, 34*, 530–537. Retrieved from www.journalofadvancednursing.com/

McCarthy, C. T., & Aquino-Russell, C. (2009). A comparison of two nursing theories in practice: Peplau and Parse. *Nursing Science Quarterly, 22*, 34–40. doi:10.1177/0894318408329339

McKenna, H. (1997). *Nursing theories and models.* London: Routledge.

McNaughton, D. B. (2005). A naturalistic test of Peplau's theory in home visiting. *Public Health Nursing, 22*, 429–438. Retrieved from http://www.blackwellpublishing.com/journal.asp?ref=0737-1209

Moser, A., Houtepen, R., & Widdershoven, G. (2007). Patient autonomy in nurse-led shared care: A review of theoretical and empirical literature. *Journal of Advanced Nursing, 57*(4), 357–365.

O'Toole, A. W., & Welt, S. R. (1989). *Interpersonal theory in nursing practice: Selected works of Hildegard E. Peplau.* New York: Springer.

Pearson, A. (2008). Dead poets, nursing and contemporary nursing practice (4). *International Journal of Nursing Practice. 14*, 79–80. doi:10.1111/j.1440-172X.2008.00682.x

Peplau, H. E. (1952). *Interpersonal relations in nursing.* New York: G.P. Putnam's Sons.

Peplau, H. E. (1964). Psychiatric nursing skills and the general hospital patient. *Nursing Forum, 3*(2), 28–37.

Peplau, H. E. (1969). Professional closeness … as a special kind of involvement with a patient, client or family group. *Nursing Forum, 8*, 343–360.

Peplau, H. E. (1985). Help the public maintain mental health. *Nursing Success Today, 2*(5), 30–34.

Peplau, H. E. (1988). The art and science of nursing: Similarities, differences and relations. *Nursing Science Quarterly, 1*, 8–15.

Peplau, H. E. (1989). Theory: The professional dimension. In A. W. O'Toole & S. R. Welt (Eds.), *Interpersonal theory in nursing practice: Selected works of Hildegard E. Peplau* (pp. 21–30). New York: Springer.

Peplau, H. E. (1991). *Interpersonal relations in nursing: A conceptual frame of reference for psychodynamic nursing.* New York: Springer.

Peplau, H. E. (1992). Interpersonal relations: A theoretical framework for application in nursing practice. *Nursing Science Quarterly, 5*(1), 13–18.

Peplau, H. E. (1997). Peplau's theory of interpersonal relations. *Nursing Science Quarterly, 10*(4), 162–167.

Puentes, W. J. (2002). Simple reminiscence: A stress-adaptation model of the phenomenon. *Issues in Mental Health Nursing, 23*(5), 497–511.

Reed, P. G. (1995). A treatise on nursing knowledge development for the 21st century: Beyond postmodernism [Electronic version]. *Advances in Nursing Science, 17*(3), 70–84.

Reed, P. G. (1996). Transforming practice knowledge into nursing knowledge—A revisionist analysis of Peplau. *Image: The Journal of Nursing Scholarship, 28*, 29–33. Retrieved September 19, 2002, from http://gateway1.ovid. com/ovidweb.cgi

Reed, P. G., Shearer, N. B. C., & Nicoll, L. H. (2004). *Perspectives on nursing theory* (4th ed.). Philadelphia, PA: Lippincott Williams & Wilkins.

Schafer, P., & Middleton, J. (2001). Examining Peplau's pattern integrations in long-term care. *Rehabilitation Nursing, 26*, 192–197. Retrieved from http://www.researchgate.net/journal/0278-4807_Rehabilitation_nursing_the_official_journal_of_the_Association_of_Rehabilitation_Nurses

Sellers, S. C. (1991). *A philosophical analysis of conceptual models of nursing.* Unpublished doctoral dissertation, Iowa State University, Ames, IA.

Shatell, M. (2005). Nurse bait: Strategies hospitalized patients us to entice nurses within the context of interpersonal relationship. *Issues in Mental Health Nursing, 26*, 205–223. doi: 10.1080/01612840590901662

Sills, G. M. (1978). Hildegard E. Peplau: Leader, practitioner, academician, scholar, and theorist. *Perspectives in Psychiatric Care, 16*(3), 122–128.

Silversten, C. M. (2008). From the front lines to the home front: A history of the development of psychi-

atric nursing in the U.S. during the World War II era. *Issues in Mental health Nursing, 29*, 719–737. doi: 10.1080/01612840802129087

Stockman, C. (2005). A literature review of the progress of the psychiatric nurse–patient relationship as described by Peplau. *Issues in Mental Health Nursing, 26*, 911–919. doi:10.1080/01612840500248197

Tiedje, L. B. (2004). Teaching is more than telling: Education about prematurity in a prenatal clinic waiting room. *The American Journal of Maternal Child Nursing, 29*(6), 373–379.

Tofthagen, R. (2004). An encounter between two realities: What experiences do psychiatric nurses gain from their efforts to create a helping relationship with psychotic patients? *Nordic Journal of Nursing Research & Clinical Studies, 24*(2), 4–9.

Ugarriza, D. N. (2002). Intentionality: Applications within selected theories of nursing. *Holistic Nursing Practice, 16*(4), 41–50. Retrieved from http://journals.lww.com/hnpjournal/pages/default.aspx

Vandermark, L. M. (2006). Awareness of self and expanding consciousness: Using nursing theories to prepare nurse-therapists. *Issues in Mental Health Nursing, 363*–371. doi:10.1080/01612840600642885

Wadensten, B., & Carlsson, M. (2003). Nursing theory views on how to support the process of ageing. *Journal of Advanced Nursing, 42*, 118–124. Retrieved from http://www.journalofadvancednursing.com/

Wallace, P. R. (2001). Improving palliative care through effective communication. *International Journal of Palliative Nursing, 7*, 86–90. Retrieved from www.ijpn.co.uk/

Warren, B. J. (2002). The interlocking paradigm of cultural competence: A best practice approach. *Journal of American Psychiatric Nurses Association, 8*(6), 209–213.

Welch, M. (1995). Hildegard Peplau in a conversation with Mark Welch. Part I. *Nursing Inquiry, 2*(1), 53–56.

Wiest, D. A. (2006). Impact of conceptual nursing models in a professional environment. *Topics in Emergency Medicine, 28*(2), 161–166.

Wills, D. E. (2010). Sharing decisions with patients: Moving beyond patient-centered-care. *Journal of Psychosocial Nursing and Mental Health Services, 48*(3), 1–5.

Zauszniewski, J. A. (2009). Mentoring our next generation: Time to dance. *Journal of Child & Adolescent Psychiatric Nursing, 22*(3), 113–114.

BIBLIOGRAPHY

SELECTED WORKS BY PEPLAU

Peplau, H. E. (1984). Help the public maintain mental health (Interview). *Nursing Success, 2*(5), 30–34.

Peplau, H. E. (1986). The nurse as counselor. *Journal of American College Health, 35*(11), 11–14.

Peplau, H. E. (1987). Interpersonal constructs for nursing practice. *Nurse Education Today, 7*(5), 201–208.

Peplau, H. E. (1989). Future directions in psychiatric nursing from the perspective of history. *Journal of Psychosocial Nursing, 27*(2), 18–21, 25–28, 39, 40.

Peplau, H. E. (1994). Quality of life: An interpersonal perspective. *Nursing Science Quarterly, 7*(1), 10–15.

Peplau, H. E. (1995). Some unresolved issues in era of biopsychosocial nursing. *Journal of American Psychiatric Nurses Association, 1*(3), 92–96.

Peplau, H. E. (1996). Fundamental and special—The dilemma of psychiatric mental nursing—commentary. *Archives of Psychiatric Nursing, 10*(4), 162–167.

SELECTED WORKS ON PEPLAU'S THEORY

Beeber, L. S. (1998). Treating depression through the therapeutic nurse–patient relationship. *Nursing Clinics of North American, 33*(1), 153–157.

Beeber, L., Anderson, C. A., & Sills, G. M. (1990). Peplau's theory in practice. *Nursing Science, 3*(1), 6–8.

Bonner, G. (2001). Mental health. The concept of priority as it relates to a community mental health team. *British Journal of Community Nursing, 6*, 86–93. Retrieved from www.bjcn.co.uk/

Campbell, D. M. (2001). Learning to care. *Assignment, 7*, 25–38.

Comley, A. L. (1994). A comparative analysis of Orem's self-care model and Peplau's interpersonal theory. *Journal of Advanced Nursing, 20*(4), 755–760.

Feely, M. (1997). Using Peplau's theory in nurse-client relations. *International Nursing Review, 44*(4), 115–120.

Forchuk, C. (1991a). A comparison of the works of Peplau and Orlando. *Archives of Psychiatric Nursing, 5*(1), 38–45.

Forchuk, C. (1991b). Conceptualizing the environment of the individual with chronic mental illness. *Issues in Mental Health Nursing, 12*, 159–170.

Forchuk, C. (1994). Preconceptions in the nurse–client relationship. *Journal of Psychiatric & Mental Health Nursing, 1*(3), 145–149.

Fowler, J. (1994). A welcome focus on a key relationship: Using Peplau's model in palliative care. *Professional Nurse, 10*(3), 194–197.

Fowler, J. (1995). Taking theory into practice: Using Peplau's model in the care of a patient. *Professional Nurse, 10*(4), 226–230.

Greg, D. E. (1978). Hildegard E. Peplau: Her contributions. *Perspectives in Psychiatric Care, 16*(3), 118–121.

Martin, M. L., Forchuk, C., Santopinto, M., & Butcher, H. K. (1992). Alternatives approaches to nursing practice: Application of Peplau, Rogers, and Parse. *Nursing Science Quarterly, 5*(2) 80–85.

Samhammer, J., & Myers, H. B. (1964). Learning in the nurse–patient relationship. *Perspectives in Psychiatric Care, 2*(3), 20–29.

Schroder, P. J. (1979). Nursing intervention with patients with thought disorders. *Perspectives in Psychiatric Care, 17*(1), 32–39.

Zauszniewski, J. A. (2010). Mentoring our next generation: Time to dance. *Journal of child & Adolescent Psychiatric Nursing, 22*, 113–114. doi:10.1111/j1744-6171.2009.00191x

Zblock, D. M. (2010). Nursing presence in contemporary nursing practice. *Nursing Forum, 45*, 120–124. Retrieved from http://onlinelibrary.wiley.com/journal/10.1111/(ISSN)1744-6198

10

Attachment

TRINE KLETTE

DEFINITION OF KEY TERMS

Attachment	An innate psychobiological urge to form lasting bonds with a primary caregiver
Early interaction	Dyadic activities performed by a child and its caregiver
Patterns of attachment	The distinct ways an individual tends to behave when feeling distressed
Internal working model	Basic assumptions about oneself, others, and the interaction with others
Sensitivity	The ability to perceive and understand signals from others
Affective empathy	An individual's congenital tendency to identify with the emotions of others
Cognitive empathy	A developmentally conditioned ability to understand and take the perspective of others
Comfort	Activities based on an individual's capacity for sensitivity and empathy whose goal is to relieve distress
Health	Composite process and phenomenon including experience of physical well-being, sense of logical coherence, meaningful social functioning, and feeling of security
Care	Watchful and gentle ways of attending to the needs of others
Nursing care	Theoretical and training-based knowledge and skills in ways of attending to the basic needs of individuals or groups of individuals, independent of age, sex, ethnic background, or beliefs, with regard to context and the given environments

HISTORICAL BACKGROUND

Attachment theory was first presented by John Bowlby in 1957 in the form of three lectures for the British psychoanalytic society. In the first lecture, "The nature of the child's tie to its mother," Bowlby claimed that the human child is ready to enter into interaction and relations from the moment it is born. By proposing this, he opposed two of the dominant theories on child development at that time: the theory of secondary drive and the theory of object relations (Klette, 2007). Building on Freud's work on the subconscious and transference but opposing his theories of psychosexual phases and aggression as basic developmental forces, Bowlby proposed that it is the real-life interactions and experiences that are most important for an individual's psychological health. The actual satisfaction or denial of basic needs during the upbringing years (not fantasies or phases) is the basis for an individual's capacity to enter into and maintain social relations. The latter is seen as fundamental to psychological health. By claiming

160

this, Bowlby moved attention on human development and functioning from intrapersonal conflicts to interpersonal relations.

DESCRIPTION OF ATTACHMENT THEORY

Integrating knowledge from medicine, ethology, learning theories, developmental biology, and psychology, John Bowlby presented the theory on human attachment. Observations of animal behaviors had been of great importance when he stated that all primates are conditioned to seek proximity to a caregiver for the purpose of protection and survival (Harlow, 1958). Having an inborn, specific repertoire of communicative expressions and functions, human infants are normally able to exhibit specific behaviors to establish and maintain proximity to caregivers (Simpson & Belsky, 2008). These are smiling and vocalizing (signaling behaviors), crying and screaming (aversive behaviors), and sucking and clinging (active behaviors). During childhood and adolescence these behaviors mature and integrate and will vary in strength until they are *referred to the backseat* as Bowlby put it (Bowlby, 1958). But all the attachment-related behaviors are maintained at different levels of activity and will be used in new combinations throughout life. When danger or threats occur, they may be demonstrated just as strongly as in childhood, especially crying and clinging.

Initially, it was the observations of children's responses to separations from their primary caregivers that had caught Bowlby's attention. These observations led among others to the description of three phases of reactions to such separations: protest, grief, and denial. The longer the separations had lasted and the younger the child had been when the separation had occurred, the more serious the psychological disturbances were observed to be (Bowlby, 1960). Attachment theory describes how and why an infant organizes and integrates behavior focused on a specific mother figure during the first year of life. Because the first attachment relationship is of vital importance to the child, separation from the primary caregiver is experienced as utterly threatening. According to the theory, attachment relationships are the products of a behavior-response system, which "supervise" the physical presence, and the psychological availability of the mother figure and activates/regulates attachment behavior directed at her (Ainsworth & Bowlby, 1989; George & Solomon, 1996). From a biological point of view, such behavior enhances the infant's probability of survival and later reproduction. As long as the infant feels safe, the attachment figure functions as a secure base for exploration, play, and other social activities. But when the child feels distressed, the goals of exploration are normally overruled by the need for protection from the caregiver. Between 8 and 18 months separations from the primary caregiver cause particularly intense distress in a child. Even though the attachment system never locks down, it becomes increasingly invisible over the years (Bowlby, 1958).

DEFINITION OF KEY CONCEPTS

ATTACHMENT

Bowlby described the core of attachment to be a child's preferred wish for contact with its primary caregiver when feelings of threats occur (Bowlby, 1958). The establishment of attachment relationships develops through phases. The first three take place between birth and the age of three. From seven months to three years of age, the three primary functions of attachment are most noticeable:

1. *Proximity maintenance:* staying close to and resisting separations from the attachment figure
2. *Safe haven behavior:* turning to the attachment figure for support and comfort
3. *Secure base behavior:* using the attachment figure as a base for exploration and other nonattachment activities

The fourth phase, which begins about three years of age, normally implies a child's increased ability to take the caregiver's perspective and develop a "goal-corrected partnership" with the caregiver (Posada et al., 1995; Simpson & Belsky, 2008).

INTERNAL WORKING MODELS

On the basis of the child's needs and demands and the caregiver's responses, basic beliefs, expectations, and attitudes about relationships develop. Such mental representations were termed *internal working models* by Bowlby (1988). The development and integration of the internal working model includes and affects the psychological, physiological, social development, and functioning of the child (Hofer, 1994; Luecken, 2000; Roisman et al., 2009; Schore, 1994). The core in a child's working model of the world is the comprehension of who the attachment figure is, where it can be found, and how it can be expected to respond when called upon. The perception of how acceptable the child is in the eyes of the caregiver is seen as the core in the child's inner working model of the self. A child growing up with available, predictable, and supportive parents tends to construct an internal working model of itself as capable and worthy of help and support. Children experiencing little or unpredictable response and support or have caregivers who threaten, harm, or abandon them tend to develop internal working models of themselves as unworthy, unloved, or ineffective. Some of these children might, however, develop positive internal working models of their caregivers to be able to live in and tolerate the relationship. Regardless of the upbringing, as an internal working model matures and integrates, it becomes gradually subconscious and automatic.

PATTERNS OF ATTACHMENT

Bowlby's collaboration with psychologist Mary Ainsworth represented a breakthrough with regard to further research and application of attachment theory. Based on a study of attachment-related behavior among families with small children in Baltimore, Ainsworth was able to describe certain distinct patterns of attachment behavior (Ainsworth et al., 1978). These patterns were respectively termed *secure, anxious avoidant,* and *anxious ambivalent* (see below). Ainsworth also constructed the classic observational method for studying attachment behavior in children between 8 and 18 months: "The Strange Situation Procedure" (Ainsworth & Bell, 1970). The procedure, lasting for about 20 minutes, consists of seven episodes including two short separations between the child and the caregiver. In the first separation episode, the child is left with a stranger and in the second it is left alone. Since the attachment system is open and visible at this age, trained coders will be able to ascribe the children to either of the following categories:

Secure attachment: A securely attached child is generally described as emotionally open and straightforward, claiming comfort and protection from the caregiver when distressed and able to settle down and eventually exhibit creative playfulness when they feel secure. The secure pattern is associated with available, predictable, and sensitive caregiving (see below). Ainsworth described four sub-patterns of the secure pattern.

Anxious avoidance: A child who has developed an anxious-avoidant pattern of attachment generally tries to suppress or hide open manifestations of negative emotions and reactions when distressed, avoiding eye-contact with the caregiver and often using toys as a distraction. This pattern is associated with relatively consistent distant, reserved, rejecting, or punitive caregiving. Maltreated children with this pattern are most likely to have been victims of physical and emotional abuse (Weinfeld, 2008). Ainsworth described two sub-patterns of anxious avoidance.

Anxious ambivalence: Children who develop an anxious ambivalent pattern of attachment show mixed emotions toward their caregiver when distressed. Conspicuous helplessness and passivity alternate with outbursts of aggression or fear. A child with an anxious ambivalent pattern of attachment tends not to explore the surroundings very much but concentrates its attention on the caregiver's whereabouts. The pattern of anxious ambivalence is associated with unpredictable caregiving, where the caregiver tends to follow his/her own impulses rather than consistently responding to the signals and needs of the child. Maltreated children displaying this pattern of attachment are most likely to have been victims of neglect (Weinfeld, 2008). Ainsworth described two sub-patterns of anxious ambivalence.

Disorganized attachment: By describing the pattern of attachment and developing a procedure for observing attachment behavior in small children, attachment research developed rapidly (Cassidy & Shaver, 2008). It soon became clear, however, that some children could not be ascribed to any of

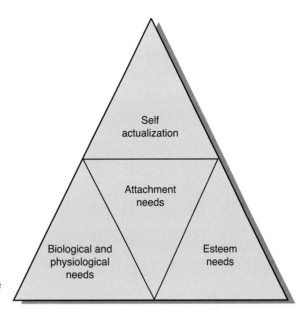

Figure 10.1 Maslows' pyramid modified to integrate attachment needs.

the original patterns described by Ainsworth. These children, who exhibited a confusing mixture of behavioral responses, often combined with tics and other bodily oddities were eventually described as disorganized with regard to attachment (Main & Hesse, 1990; Main & Solomon, 1990). Disorganized attachment is particularly associated with fearful and/or frightening parenting that makes it impossible for the child to develop a coherent attachment pattern. Prolonged isolation, neurological problems, and pharmacological interventions have later been added to the precursors for disorganized attachment. It has been speculated that the seemingly meaningless body movements seen in many children with disorganized attachment, corresponds to what is described as conflict behavior in animals. That is, the movements are expressions of the impossible in the child's situation, caught as it is between the drive and the need to seek closeness to and protection from the caregiver and the impulse to fight or flee from the very same person.

Earned secure: Adults have been observed who, despite strong evidence of unloving parents and a harsh upbringing, appear coherent and balanced with regard to attachment in the Adult Attachment Interview.* These individuals were described as "earned secure" (Hesse, 2008; Pearson, Cohn, Cowan, & Cowan, 1994). Studies indicate that attachment-related behavior is as stable and robust with earned security as with natural secure. Alternative secure attachment and psychological treatment seem to account for such positive changes of an attachment strategy.

ATTACHMENT AS A BASIC NEED

By describing the basic human needs, Abraham Maslow (1970) made a great contribution to the works of a variety of disciplines, including nursing. Although the need for attachment is not explicitly addressed in Maslow's pyramid, it is touched upon through (the needs for) shelter, protection, security, family, relationships, and so on. It is, however, strongly indicated by research that the need for attachment not only is a need in its own right, but also in fact is a central one. With great respect to Maslows' invaluable work, a pyramid that is modified to integrate attachment needs is suggested in Figure 10.1.

---

*The Adult Attachment Interview is a semi-structured interview about attachment-related episodes from the childhood to the present (George, Kaplan, & Main, 1985, 1996). Theories on memory (Schacter & Tulving, 1994; Schacter, 2001) are integrated and utilized in the interview, and Grice's maxims for reliability and validity in conversations (1975) are used in the codings.

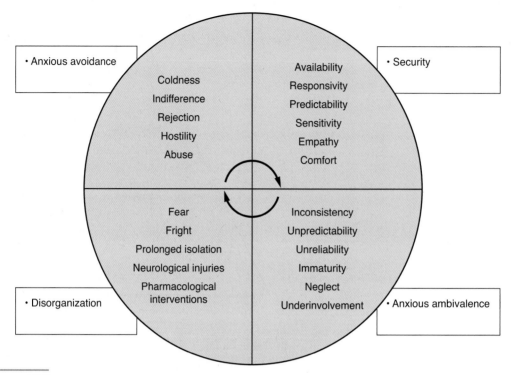

Figure 10.2 Factors underlying the patterns of attachment.

ATTACHMENT AND CARE

Attachment theory gives strong evidence to the importance of meeting a child's need for contact and closeness with understanding, respect, and warmth. It also gives evidence on the importance of care in general and in cases of disease, illness, and loss in particular (see also Chapter 12). Individual care factors known to promote attachment security are availability, predictability, and sensitivity. Socially contributing factors are extended networks, education, stable incomes, preventive health care, and a general social stability (Cassidy & Shaver, 2008; Killén, Klette, & Arenevik, 2006; Solomon & George, 1996).

Individuals who have received adequate care during childhood tend to be open and trusting toward others and also exhibit empathy and caring behavior toward needs of others. Individuals who have experienced rejection, abuse, and little comfort and protection during childhood tend to withdraw, trivialize, or dismiss care needs. Individuals who have been exposed to unpredictable and neglectful care seem to alternate between passivity and intrusive behavior (Klette, 2007).

Attachment relationships will be formed throughout life and when first formed, such relationships tend to be strong and important, for better or worse. Attachment theory offers an opportunity to understand, observe, and change some apparently fixed premises for human behavior. Instead of assigning behaviors merely to genetic conditions and individual dispositions, attachment theory and research has shown that crucial social behavior is *learnt* through interaction and care (see Fig. 10.2).

ATTACHMENT AND HEALTH

Health is understood as a process and phenomenon that includes experience of physical well-being, sense of logical coherence, meaningful social functioning and the feeling of security (see Chapter 14). Seen in this light, secure attachment accounts for many positive health-related conditions and functions. Among other things, a marked lack of securely attached individuals is found in various clinical psychiatric samples (van IJzendoorn, Goldberg, Koonenberg, & Frenkel, 1992). As mentioned earlier, basic beliefs/expectations/attitudes and patterns of self-protective behavior tend to re-emerge in times of threats, illness, or loss (Bretherton & Munholland, 2008). Bowlby described the early behaviors (crying, clinging, etc.) as *old soldiers* who are put to rest, but who will rise again when needed. How and to which extent the old soldiers will fight will vary according to the attachment strategy of the individual. Signs of secure attachment are, among other things, trust and ability to ask for and make use of help and care. Securely attached individuals also tend to be more balanced and flexible than individuals with other attachment experiences, and they are better able to regulate and adjust their feelings and reactions to a stressful situation. Evidence of connections between child abuse and neglect, various diseases, and anxious and disorganized attachment is significant (Klette, 2008). A pioneering study by McWilliams and Bailey (2010) shows strong association between adult attachment ratings and a number of health conditions. The study findings support that insecure (i.e., anxious) attachment is a risk factor for disease and chronic illness, particularly conditions involving the cardiovascular system. See also Donovan et al. (1985), Reite and Field (1985), Spangler (1994) and Hofer (2003) for studies of associations between attachment and psychobiology.

Epigenetic is a new research area that offers significant insights into the interaction between genes and environment. Among others, studies show that the quality of care received in early age inflicts upon the development of the brain and behaviors by altering processes that control the expression of the DNA. Enzymes that block, repair, and switch functions of the genes on and off are described. The findings indicate that psychiatric diseases are related to stress in relation to primary caregivers or significant others in childhood (Donovan, 1985; Fosse, 2009; Heim et al., 2003; Luecken, 2000; Szyf, McGowan, & Meaney, 2008).

DEVELOPMENT AND CHANGE

If the upbringing conditions of a child remain unaltered, the basic attitudes, expectations, and behavioral strategies also tend to remain unchanged. If the conditions change for the better, the internal working model and the pattern of attachment may change in a more secure direction. If the conditions change for the worse, they may change in an anxious or even disorganized direction. Earned security (see above) indicates that attachment status can be altered throughout life, but it appears to become increasingly resistant to change. The problem with changing status of attachment is probably not least due to the subconscious and automatic character of the internal working model. But also the common tendency to believe that an attachment pattern is the product of individual dispositions probably accounts for this. The first years and the puberty period seem to be most susceptible to attachment-related influence and change, but the attachment system also tends to open up for adaption during pregnancy and in the postpartum period as well as in cases of loss, illness, or disease. According to Bowlby, the ability to change is reduced with age, but changes occur throughout life, which means that an individual is always open to positive influence.

APPLICATIONS OF ATTACHMENT THEORY: RESEARCH

Attachment theory and research highlights the importance of preventive health care directed at families with small children. Guidance, practical help, and emotional support with regard to behaviors that facilitates secure attachments appear to be among the best ways to promote health and prevent disease. Obtaining knowledge about attachment may help many parents to improve their interactive behaviors. Others will need much supervision and close follow-up to be able to change destructive patterns. Some parents, independent of the investments made, will still not be able to change, and therefore alternative care should be found. Virginia Henderson's concepts of strength, will, and knowledge may prove very useful in assessing and addressing attachment-related health behaviors. They can be seen as corresponding to the phenomena of the internal working model: expectations, attitudes, and assumptions.

Although it is known to be of great importance for health care behaviors, the phenomenon of will is still quite elusive and unclear. Henderson equaled will to "love of life," and psychologist Rollo May (1969) describes will not as an independent ability or special personality trait, but as a product of care. Will and wish cannot be the basis of care, but rather the opposite, they are found on and manifest themselves as liberated and activated care. By describing the internal working model and the patterns of attachment,

Bowlby and Ainsworth provided new insights into the phenomenon of will. Some patients do apparently not, despite huge investments, want to change their self-destructive behaviors or engage in health-preventive activities. Taking the patient's attachment experiences into account may prove valuable when planning interventions. A definition of will as *the ability to be or do something, rooted in attachment experiences,* is suggested.

A number of measurements and programs for intervention have been developed since Ainsworth's strange situation, and great advances have been made in measuring attachment in early childhood, later adolescence, and adulthood. The use of separation-reunion situations, Q-sort assessments, and the Adult Attachment Interview (van IJzendoorn, 1995) has led to significant findings regarding the importance of attachment throughout life (Hesse, 2008). The Circle of Security Project is one of the many promising intervention programs (Marvin, 2002). The study described in Research Application 10.1 identifies comfort behaviors and their relationship to maternal attachment. The research described in Research Application 10.2 provides an example of an instrument used in the study of attachment.

Research Application   10.1

Mary Ainsworth considered sensitivity to be the most important aspect of caring for the infant (Ainsworth, 1969), and she defined sensitivity as consisting of *awareness, empathy,* and *the ability to adjust reactions and responses to the child's needs.* Among other things, she exemplified sensitivity by the importance of the caregiver's ability to give sufficient comfort to the child. Later studies have shown that motherly sensitivity, as Ainsworth described it, is a necessary but not a sufficient condition for the development of secure attachment (De Wolff and Van IJzendoorn, 1997). One of the problems arising when observing sensitivity in early mother–child interactions is that it is quite difficult to test and measure under normal conditions. Redefining Ainsworth's concepts, the meaning of comfort in early interaction was addressed (Klette, 2007). In the study, sensitivity was simply described as the ability to sense (see, hear, feel, etc.). Empathy was defined as consisting of both an inborn disposition to identify and connect to the feelings of others (affective empathy) and a developmentally conditioned ability to take the perspective of others (cognitive empathy). Sensitivity and empathy were viewed as interconnected and necessary premises for an individual's ability to give comfort, possibly being products of care and comfort themselves. Different from sensitivity and empathy, which being inner states, comfort is the distinct behaviors aimed at calming and relieving distress. Comforting behaviors, which are purposeful actions, are open to observation and measurement.

Seventeen mothers were interviewed using the Adult Attachment Interview and coded according to the experiences of comfort in childhood. The women were recruited from a prospective study described below (Killén et al., 2006). The mothers were then observed in the Ainsworth's strange situation with their children at one year of age with special attention paid to their comforting behavior after the separations. Lastly, the attachment status of the children, which had been coded independently by trained coders, was included. Strong association between the mothers' memories and experiences of comfort, their ability to give comfort to their child and the child's attachment status at one year was registered (Klette, 2007). The study indicated that comfort is an important aspect of childcare and attachment development. The most efficient comforting behavior was holding and stroking the child until the distress was eased. Children, who were comforted in this way during the reunions, would normally want to reengage in explorative behavior after a relatively short while. The children, who were comforted only until the mother thought it was sufficient, normally kept sobbing and trying to get more from her throughout the procedure. Distractions did not work as comfort in any of the observed cases and was not included as comforting behavior. Needs for comfort arise normally in situations perceived as dangerous or painful, and help and support in dealing with negative emotions like fear, pain, and anger is of great importance throughout life. The study seems to indicate that if a child experiences acceptance and reconciliation when distressed, this contributes both to attachment security and also strengthens their ability to give comfort to their own children later. Being observable actions, comforting behaviors may be particularly useful indicators of individual caregiving capacity as it often also involves stress for the caregiver, especially when related to their own children (Klette, 2007).

APPLICATIONS OF THEORY: PRACTICE

Attachment theory has been most frequently applied to work with children. The federal program in the United States, Early Head Start, is the most visible example of a practice application of this theory (Boris & Zeanah, 2011). The theory has also been used with children who have been mistreated (Allen, 2011) and children with disabilities (Howe, 2006; Wilkins, 2010). It has also been found useful in situations where child custody was an issue (Garber, 2009; Marvin & Schultz, 2009), as well with children being adopted or in foster care (Walker, 2008). Using Middle Range Theories 10.1 discusses the use of the theory by health care workers involved in adoption or foster care evaluations.

Research Application 10.2

Measuring Parent–Child Interactions

The aim of the longitudinal prospective study "Attachment and children's development" (see Research Application 10.1) was to investigate relations between early mother–child interaction and the development of attachment (Killén, Klette, & Arenevik, 2006). 293 mother-child dyads were observed from the children were three months until they were four and a half years. The findings presented here are taken from a sub-study of mother–child interaction during the first year, and from a sub-study of children's attachment at one year of age. The sample encompassed dyads from different socioeconomic districts in Norway, and also included dyads from mother–child institutions. The procedures used in the study were the Care Index (see below), Ainsworth's strange situation, and a short questionnaire concerning education, income, social network support, drug abuse, and medical diagnoses.

Care Index

Care Index is a scoring system for observing parent–child interaction under nonthreatening conditions on the basis of short videotapes (Crittenden, 2000). Sensitivity to the child's signals is the central concept that the Care Index coding system is built around. Crittenden defines adult sensitivity as a behavior pattern that pleases the child most, increases its wellbeing, and reduces its distress, and it is seen as a dyadic concept. According to the definition, it also incorporates the child's temperament and mother's empathy. The mothers' behavior is scored by a two-point scoring system on the three dimensions: sensitive, passive, or controlling (open or hidden). The child's behavior is scored on four dimensions: cooperative, difficult, passive, or compulsive compliant. The behaviors scored include seven elements: (1) facial expression, (2) vocal expression, (3) position and body contact, (4) expression of affection,

(5) turn-taking contingent, (6) control, and (7) choice of activity. The first four of these aspects are assessment of affect within the dyad. The final three refer to temporal contingencies. The two points could both be placed on one dimension (for instance sensitive) or they might be split (for instance, between sensitive and controlling). The sum of the score should always be 14 points. Obtaining between 11 and 14 points on the sensitive and cooperative scales can, according to Crittenden, be considered sufficient for the "sensitive" and "cooperative" categories. Scores between 7 and 10 points are classified as "adequate (for adults) and mixed cooperative (for infants)." Less than six sensitive or cooperative items should yield classifications of "inept" (5–6) and "at risk" (0–4), which can be "controlling" and/or "unresponsive" (for adults) and "difficult" and/or "passive" (for infants). Care Index is considered useful in applied settings to screen for risk, guide intervention, and assess some outcomes of treatment. When used diagnostically it is emphasized that the data provided by the Care Index would constitute only one part of information, which could be useful in conjunction with other information.

Strong correlations were found between education, social network, social stress factors, and the mothers' sensitivity at the first two observations. At 6–7 months, but not at 3–4 months there were observed significant differences in sensitivity between mothers exposed to respectively low and high socioeconomic stress. At both points of observation, significantly lower sensitivity was seen in the mothers from the mother–child institutions. The Care Index categories were, however, found to be too detailed for clinical use. It was, therefore, suggested that they should be divided into three: "Good enough" interactions (more than eight points), "At risk" interactions (7–5 points), and "Maltreatment" interactions (4–0 points).

(continued)

Research Application (*Continued*)   `10.2`

Crittenden's sensitivity scale (Crittenden, 2000)		Proposed sensitivity scale	
13–14 points	Mutual delight, joy in one another; a dance	8–14 points	"Good enough" mother–child interaction
11–12 points	Smooth, pleasing interaction; playful shared positive affect		
9–10 points	Quite satisfactory play; no problems, but no dance		
7–8 points	Adequate play, but noticeable periods of dyssynchrony (either controlling or unresponsive)		
5–6 points	Clear, unresolved problems; limited playfulness, but no evidence of hostility or lack of empathy (unresponsiveness)	5–7 points	Mother–child interaction at "Risk"
3–4 points	Clear lack of empathy, nevertheless, some feeble (insufficient or unsuccessful) attempts is made to respond to infant; lack of playful quality	0–4 points	"Maltreatment" interaction between mother and child
0–2 points	Total failure to perceive or attempt to sooth infant's distressed state; no play		

As mentioned earlier, attachment patterns at one year were assessed using Ainsworth's strange situation, and it was expected that the Care Index categories would predict attachment categories. The main finding was that the use of the three classification categories could predict infant attachment at one year and therefore might be used to serve as a basis for selective and indicated prevention as well as early intervention (Killén et al., 2006).

The use of attachment theory is not limited to involvement with children. It has been found useful by counselors and psychotherapists working with individuals with personality disorders (Van den Berg & Oei, 2009; Fogany & Bateman, 2007), depressed adolescents (Bowlby, 1979; Shaw, Dallos, & Shoebridge, 2009), and those suffering from addiction (Flores, 2006). The theory has also been applied to involvement with adult cancer patients and their partners (Burwell, Brucker, & Shields, 2006) and more recently as it relates to spiritual coping in older adults (Munnichs, Bowlby, & Miesen, 1986; Pickard & Nelson-Becker, 2011).

USING MIDDLE RANGE THEORIES

`10.1`

Attachment theory is identified as useful in the selection of substitute caregivers and matching a child with a caregiver for children who are being adopted or placed in foster care. The theory provides a framework for assessing the qualities of potential caregivers. Three attributes are considered most important: (a) the ability to manage a wide range of feelings of self and others, (b) the resolution of past personal losses or traumas, and (c) the ability to engage in reflection. The assessment of the child is also a critical consideration in placement decisions. A trained social worker can assess a child's attachment pattern during times of distress or fear. Of particular concern in placement is manifestation of disorganized attachment, in which children view caregivers as a source of danger and therefore must be controlled in some fashion. The involved adults' attachment pattern is also important and needs to be assessed, as does the dynamics of the couple relationship. A complementary attachment pattern in couples is considered most resilient. With these assessment data, decisions about appropriate placement of children can be more informed and hopefully result in a growth-producing environment for children.

FURTHER RESEARCH

There is a vast area of attachment-research challenges and possibilities relevant to nursing. There are, for instance, strong warrants for further research regarding the role of attachment in the development of specific health conditions (McWilliams & Bailey, 2010). The study of attachment and comfort (Klette, 2007) also calls for further investigations. Other areas of importance are trans-generational continuities and discontinuities of attachment, and the development of the earned secure status. Even though continuity seems to be a rule, there is much evidence of variety and change regarding the internal working models and patterns of attachment in adult attachment relationships. According to Bowlby, it is the quality of interpersonal communication that is the major factor in deciding whether a child or adult is in a secure, anxious, or distressed state (Kobac & Madsen, 2008). Further development of reliable measurements and programs for clinical intervention is also called for, especially with regard to school-age children and the very old.

SUMMARY

John Bowlby had to search multidisciplinary knowledge to explain children's reactions to separations from their primary caregivers. Since then, a number of disciplines have included the theory of attachment in their body of knowledge and contributed to exciting new knowledge (Cassidy & Shaver, 2008). It is time that the discipline of nursing also pays serious regard to the meaning and development of attachment behavior. From a nursing point of view, there are many reasons for this application as attachment theory and research among other things contribute to the clarification of many concepts/phenomena central to nursing, such as empathy, comfort, care, and health. By taking a patient's attachment experiences and status into account, the nurse will be able to improve the understanding of individual possibilities and limitations, possibly in particular with regard to the phenomenon of will. Reflecting upon own attachment history with regard to attitudes, expectations, and patterns of self-protective behavior might also help the individual nurse to be a more conscientious in her work. Attachment theory highlights the importance of prevention, a traditionally central field of nursing. The importance of preventing child abuse and neglect can probably not be underestimated. While attachment theory and research is yielding an increasing amount of knowledge about the development of health and disease in humans, it is strongly recommended that the discipline of nursing starts making use of and contributing to this multidisciplinary and cross-cultural effort to improve human conditions. Attachment theory is a theory about human development and needs from the cradle to the grave, according to Bowlby. It is based on and integrates well-documented knowledge and will probably prove to be of great value in clinical and theoretical nursing.

ANALYSIS OF THEORY

Using the criteria presented in Chapter 2, critique the theory of Attachment. Compare your conclusions about the theory with those found in Appendix A. A researcher who has worked with the theory completed the analysis found in the Appendix.

Internal Criticism

1. Clarity
2. Consistency
3. Adequacy
4. Logical development
5. Level of theory development

External Criticism

1. Reality convergence
2. Utility
3. Significance
4. Discrimination
5. Scope of theory
6. Complexity

CRITICAL THINKING EXERCISES

1. One of the patterns of attachment is referred to as "earned secure." This pattern, characterized by coherence and balance, is achieved by adults who experienced unloving or harsh parenting. What individual characteristics or life experiences might contribute to achievement of this pattern?

2. Based on this theory, what behaviors would a nurse attempt to engender when working with parents to promote healthy attachment?

3. At times of threat, illness, or loss, self-protective behaviors in adults can emerge. How would adults manifest self-protective behaviors?

4. What is a research question that would provide validation of this theory?

WEB RESOURCES

Visit **http://thePoint.lww.com/Peterson3e** for helpful web resources related to this chapter.

REFERENCES

Ainsworth, M. D. S. (1969). *Maternal sensitivity scales.* Baltimore, MD: Johns Hopkins University Press. Retrieved 2004, from www.psychologie.sunysb.edu/ewaters/552/senscoop.htm

Ainsworth, M. D. S., & Bell, S. M. (1970). Attachment, exploration and separation: Illustrated by the behaviour of one-year-olds in a strange situation. *Child Development, 41,* 49–65.

Ainsworth, M. D. S., Blehar, M. C., Waters, E., & Wall, E. (1978). *Patterns of attachment. A psychological study of the strange situation.* Hillsdale, NJ: Erlbaum.

Ainsworth, M. S., & Bowlby. J. (1989). An ethological approach to personality development. *American Psychologist 46*(4), 333–341.

Allen, B. (2011). The use and abuse of attachment theory in clinical practice with maltreated children, Part II: Treatment. *Trauma, Violence & Abuse, 12*(1), 3–12.

Boris, N. W., & Zeanah, C. H. (2011). Attachment research and Early Head Start: From data to practice. *Attachment & Human Development, 13*(1), 99–104.

Bowlby, J. (1958). "The nature of the child's tie to his mother." *International Journal of Psycho-Analysis 39,* 350–373.

Bowlby, J. (1960). Separation anxiety. *The International Journal of Psycho-analysis. XLI,* 89–113.

Bowlby, J. (1979). *The making & breaking of affectional bonds.* London: Tavistock.

Bowlby, J. (1988). *A secure base: Clinical applications of attachment theory.* London: Routledge.

Bretherton, I., & Munholland., K. A. (2008). Internal working models in attachment relationships: Elaborating a central construct in attachment theory. In J. Cassidy & P. R. Shaver (Eds.), *Handbook of attachment* (2nd ed., pp. 102–127). New York: Guilford Press.

Burwell, S. R., Brucker, P. S., & Shields, C. G. (2006). Attachment behaviors and proximity-seeking in cancer patients and their partners. *Journal of Couple & Relationship Therapy, 5*(3), 1–16

Cassidy, J., & Shaver, P. R., Ed. (2008). *Handbook of attachment: Theory, research, and clinical applications* (2nd ed.). New York: Guilford Press.

Crittenden, P. M. (2000). *CARE-Index manual.* Miami, FL: Family Relations Institute.

De Wolff, M., & van IJzendoorn, M. H. (1997). Sensitivity and attachment: A meta-analysis on parental antecedents of infant attachment. *Child Development, 68*(4), 571–591.

Donovan, W. L., & Leavitt, L. A. (Eds.). (1985). Cardiac responses of mothers and infants in Ainsworth's Strange situation. *The psychobiology of attachment and separation.* Orlando, FL: Academic.

Flores, P. J. (2006). Conflict and repair in addiction treatment: An attachment disorder perspective. *Journal of Groups in Addiction & Recovery, 1*(1), 5–26.

Fogany, P., & Bateman, A. W. (2007). Mentalizing and borderline personality disorder. *Journal of Mental Health, 16*(1), 83–101.

Fosse, R. (2009). Ingen gener for psykiske lidelser (No genes for psychiatric diseases). *Tidsskrift for Norsk Psykologforening, 46*(6), 596–600.

Garber, B. D. (2009). Attachment methodology in custody evaluation: Four hurdles standing between developmental theory and forensic application. *Journal of Child Custody, 6*(1–2), 38–61.

George, C., & Solomon, J. (1996). Representational models of relationships: Links between caregiving and attachment. *Infant Mental Health Journal, 17*(3), 198–216.

Grice, H. P. (1975). Logic and conversation. In P. Cole & J. L. Morgan (Eds.), *Syntax and semantics: Speech acts* (3rd ed.). New York: Academic.

Harlow, H. (1958). The nature of love. In J. M. Notterman (Eds.), *The evolution of psychology; Fifty years of the American psychologist* (pp. 41–64). Washington, DC: American Psychological Association.

Heim, C., Newport, D. J., Bonsall, R., Miller, A. H., & Nemeroff, C. B. (2003). Altered pituitary-adrenal axis responses to provocative challenge tests in adult survivors of childhood abuse. *American Journal of Psychiatry, 158*, 575–581.

Hesse, E. (2008). The adult attachment interview. Historical and current perspectives. In J. Cassidy & P. R. Shaver (Eds.), *Handbook of attachment* (pp. 552–598). New York: Guilford Press.

Hofer, M. A. (1994). Hidden regulators in attachment, separation, and loss. *Monographs of the society for research in child development, 59*, 192–207.

Hofer, M. A. (2003). The emerging neurobiology of attachment and separation. In S. W. Coates, J. L. Rosenthal & Schechter, D. S. (Eds.), *September 11: Trauma and human bonds* (pp. 191–209). Hillsdale, NJ: Analytic Press.

Howe, D. (2006). Disabled children, parent–child interaction and attachment. *Child & Family Social Work, 11*(2), 95–106.

Killén, K., Klette, T., & Arenevik, E. (2006). Tidlig mor-barn samspill i norske familier (Early mother–child interaction in Norwegian families). *Tidskift for Norsk Psykologforening, 43*, 694–701.

Killén, K., Arenevik, E., & Klette, T. (2007). Early mother–child interaction and children's attachment at 1 year in Norway. Unpublished manuscript

Klette, T. (2007). *Tid for trøst. En undersøkelse av sammenenger mellom trøst og trygghet over to generajsoner (Time for comfort. A study of connections between comfort and security across two generations)*, In *Nova Rapport 17/07*. Oslo: Nova.

Klette, T. (2008). Omsorgssvikt og personlighetsforstyrrelser (Child maltreatment and personality disorders), *Tidskrift for norsk legeforening, 128*, 1538–1540.

Kobac, R., & Madsen, S. (2008). Disruptions in attachment bonds: Implications for theory, research and clinical intervention. In J. Cassidy & P. R. Shaver (Eds.), *Handbook of attachment* (pp. 23–37). New York: Guilford Press.

Luecken, L. J. (2000). Parental caring and loss during childhood and adult cortisol responses to stress. *Psychology and Health, 15*, 841–851.

Main, M., & Hesse, E. (1990). Parent's unresolved traumatic experiences are related to infant disorganized attachment status: Is frightened and/or frightening parental behaviour the linking mechanism? In M. T. Greenberg, D. Cicchetti & E. M. Cummings (Eds.), *Attachment in the preschool years* (pp. 273–310). Chicago, IL: University of Chicago Press.

Main, M., & Solomon, J. (1990). Procedures for identifying infants as disorganized/disoriented during the Ainsworth strange situation. In M. Greenberg, D. Cicchetti & E. M. Cummings (Eds.), *Attachment in the preschool years*. Chicago, IL: University of Chicago Press.

Marvin, R. (2002). The circle of security project: Attachment-based intervention with caregiver–preschool child dyads. *Attachment and Human Development 4*(1), 107–124.

Marvin, R. S., & Schutz, B. M. (2009). One component of an evidence-based approach to the use of attachment research in child custody evaluations. *Journal of Child Custody, 6*(1–2), 1537–9418.

May, R. (1969). *Love and will*. New York: Norton.

McWilliams, J. A., & Bailey, S. J. (2010). Associations between adult attachment ratings and health conditions: Evidence from the National Comorbidity Survey Replication. *Health Psychology American Psychological Association, 29*(4), 446–453.

Munnichs, J., Bowlby, J., & Miesen, B. (1986). *Attachment, life-span and old-age*. Deventer: Van Loghum Slaterus.

Pearson, J. L., Cohn, D. A., Cowan, P. H., & Cowan, C. P. (1994). Earned and continuous-security in adult attachment: Relation to depressive symptomatology and parenting style. *Development and Psychopathology, 6*(2), 359–373.

Pickard, J. G., & Nelson-Becker, H. (2011). Attachment and spiritual coping: Theory and practice with older adults. *Journal of Spirituality in Mental Health,13*(2), 138–155.

Posada, G., Gao, Y., Wu, F., Posada, R., Tascon, M., Schöelmerich, A., et al. (1995). The secure-base phenomenon across cultures: Children's behaviour, mother's preferences and experts concepts. In E. Waters (Ed.), *Monographs of the society for research in child development* (pp. 27–48). Chicago, IL: University of Chicago Press.

Reite, M., & Field, T. (Eds.). (1985). *The psychobiology of attachment and separation. Behavioral biology*. Orlando, FL: Academic.

Roisman, G. I., Susman, E., Barnett-Walker, K., Booth-LaForce, C., Owen, M. T., Belsky, J., et al. (2009). Early family and child-care antecedents of awakening cortisol levels in adolescence. *Child Development, 80*(3), 907–992.

Schacter, D. L. (2001). *The seven sins of memory: How the mind forgets and remembers*. Boston, MA: Houghton Mifflin.

Schacter, D. L., & Tulving, E. (Eds.). (1994). *Memory systems 1994*. Cambridge, MA: MIT Press.

Schore, A. N. (1994). *Affect regulation and the origin of the self, the neurobiology of emotional development*. Hillsdale, NJ: Erlbaum.

Shaw, S. K., Dallos, R., & Shoebridge, P. (2009). Depression in female adolescents: An IP analysis. *Clinical Child Psychology & Psychiatry, 14*(2), 167–181.

Simpson, J. A., & Belsky. J. (2008) Attachment theory within a modern evolutionary framework. In J. Cassidy & P. R. Shaver (Eds.), *Handbook of attachment* (pp. 131–157). New York: Guilford Press

Solomon, J., & George, C. (1996). Defining the caregiving system: Toward a theory of care-giving. *Infant Mental Health Journal, 17*(3), 183–197.

Spangler, G. Schieche, M., Ilg, U., Maier, U., & Ackerman, C. (1994). Maternal sensitivity as an external organizer for bio-behavioural regulation in infancy. *Developmental Psychology, 27*(7), 425–437.

Szyf, M., McGowan, P., & Meaney, M. J. (2008). The social environment and the epigenome. *Environmental and Molecular Mutagenesis, 49*, 46–60.

Van den Berg, A., & Oei, K. T. I. (2009). Attachment and psychotherapy in forensic patients. *Mental Health Review Journal, 14*(3), 40–51.

van IJzendoorn, M. H. (1995). Adult attachment representation, parental responsiveness and infant attachment: A meta analysis on the predictive validity of the adult attachment interview. *Psychological Bulletin, 117*, 387–403.

van IJzendoorn, M. H., Goldberg, S., Koonenberg, P. M., & Frenkel, O. J. (1992). The relative effects of maternal and child problems on the quality of attach-ment: A meta-analysis of attachment in clinical samples. *Child Development, 63*, 840–858.

Walker, J. (2008). The use of attachment theory in adoption and fostering. *Adoption and Fostering, 32*(1), 49–57.

Weinfeld, N. S., Sroufe, L. A., Egeland, B., & Carlson, E. (2008). Individual differences in infant-caregiver attachment: Conceptual and empirical aspect of security. In J. Cassidy & P. R. Shaver (Eds.), *Handbook of attachment* (pp. 880–905). New York : Guilford Press.

Wilkins, D. (2010). I'm not sure what I want (and I don't know how to get it): How do social care workers perceive the parental relationships of children with autism spectrum conditions? *Journal of Social Work Practice, 24*(1), 89–101.

11

Modeling and Role-Modeling

ELLEN D. SCHULTZ

DEFINITION OF KEY TERMS

Adaptation	Adaptation is the "process by which an individual responds to external and internal stressors in a health and growth-directed manner" (Erickson, Tomlin, & Swain, 1983, p. 252).
Affiliated-individuation	Affiliated-individuation is an inherent need to be dependent on support systems while maintaining a sense of autonomy and separateness from those systems.
Environment	The client's environment includes internal and external stressors as well as internal and external resources (Erickson, 1989). The theorists see environment in the "social subsystems as the interaction between self and other both cultural and individual" (Erickson, 2002a, p. 452).
Facilitation	Through the interactive process of facilitation, the nurse assists the client to "identify, mobilize, and develop" personal strengths. The nurse does not affect the outcomes for the client, but rather helps in the process of moving toward holistic health.
Health	Health is a state of equilibrium among the subsystems of the holistic person. It is not defined by the absence of disease, but rather the client's perception of mental, physical, and social well-being.
Holism	"The interaction of the multiple subsystems and the inherent bases creates holism. Holism implies that the whole is greater than the sum of the parts" (Erickson et al., 1983, p. 45). There is a blending of conscious and unconscious.
Inherent endowment	Inherent endowment includes both the genetic makeup of the person and the inherent characteristics resulting from disease and/or birth that may influence the person's health status.
Lifetime growth and development	Persons change throughout the lifetime, responding to an inherent desire to fulfill their potential in the areas of basic needs and psychological and cognitive stages.
Modeling	Modeling is "the process the nurse uses as she develops an image and understanding of the client's world—an image and understanding developed within the client's framework and from the client's perspective" (Erickson et al., 1983, p. 95).

(*Definition of Key Terms continued on next page*)

DEFINITION OF KEY TERMS CONTINUED

Nursing	"Nursing is the holistic helping of persons with their self-care activities in relation to their health. This is an interactive, interpersonal process that nurtures strengths to enable development, release, and channeling of resources for coping with one's circumstances and environment. The goal is to achieve a state of the perceived optimum health and contentment" (Erickson et al., 1983, p. 49). This requires that the nurse unconditionally accepts the client.
Nurturance	"Nurturance fuses and integrates cognitive, physiological and affective processes with the aim of assisting a client to move toward holistic health" (Erickson et al., 1983, p. 48). In order to nurture, the nurse must understand the client's model of the world.
Person	"Human beings are holistic persons who have multiple interacting subsystems" (Erickson et al., 1983, p. 44). These dynamic subsystems are the biophysical, cognitive, psychological, and social subsystems. Intersecting and permeating these subsystems are the genetic base and spiritual drive.
Role-modeling	In role-modeling, the nurse uses purposeful interventions, based on nursing science, that are unique to the client, to assist the client toward holistic health.
Self-care knowledge	Self-care knowledge is one's personal understanding of what interferes with or what promotes his or her own health and development.
Self-care resources	Self-care resources are internal and external resources that serve as a foundation for growth and can be mobilized to promote holistic health.
Self-care action	Clients demonstrate self-care action when they develop and use self-care knowledge and self-care resources. "Through self-care action the individual mobilizes internal resources and acquires additional resources that will help the individual gain, maintain and promote optimal level of holistic health" (Erickson et al., 1983, p. 48).
Stressor	A stressor is a stimulus experienced by the individual as a challenge that mounts an adaptive response.
Unconditional acceptance	The individual is accepted as a unique and worthwhile human being.

INTRODUCTION

Modeling and Role-Modeling (MRM) is a theory and paradigm for nursing and serves as a foundation for nursing research, education, and practice. It is among the theories "most commonly used by holistic nurses" (Frisch, 2009, p. 116). As a theory that is strongly tied to nursing practice, it is a positive response to the criticism cited by Fawcett that many models and theories are "invented by scholars and academics" and therefore may have little relevance for nursing practice (1995, p. 519).

Chapter 1 describes the hierarchy of nursing knowledge and the classification of nursing theories as grand, middle range, or practice theories. While MRM is included here among the middle range theories, consensus has not been established on this classification. Tomey and Alligood (1998) originally classified MRM as a middle range theory but later stated that MRM theory could serve as a guide for nursing practice due to its specificity, yet it is abstract enough that middle range theories could be derived from it (Tomey & Alligood, 2002). McEwin and Wills (2002) consider MRM to be a grand theory and categorized it as one of the interactive process theories, while Parker and Smith (2010) list MRM in the category of grand theory in the interactive/integrative paradigm.

One system for classifying theory is to consider the scope of the theory. A grand theory includes the nursing metaparadigm concepts of nursing, health, environment, and person, all of which are addressed in

MRM. This chapter is appropriately included in this text because it presents, as components of the grand theory, a number of middle range concepts that have developed from MRM theory. These concepts are best understood within the context of the grand theory.

MRM is a client-centered nursing theory that places the client's perceptions, or model of the world, at the center of the nurse–client interaction. The theory integrates concepts from several interdisciplinary theories including psychosocial development (Erikson, 1968), cognitive development (Piaget, 1952), basic human needs (Maslow, 1968), and stress adaptation (Engel, 1962; Selye, 1976). The expanded description of the theory included energy-based concepts (Brekke & Schultz, 2006). These concepts are linked to those unique to MRM theory. Through the processes of MRM, the nurse facilitates and nurtures the client to achieve high-level, holistic wellness.

HISTORICAL BACKGROUND

MRM is a theory "born in practice," as described by Dickoff, James, and Weidenback (1968). "… Using nursing practice as a basis for theory development promotes not only a broader view of reality but also an increased relevance of theory to practice" (McClosky & Grace, 1994, p. 78). Through observations made in clinical practice in a variety of nursing settings, Helen Erickson became consciously aware of the nurse's role as a healer. Based on a combination of insights gleaned through personal experience, clinical practice, and discussions with her father-in-law, renowned psychotherapist, Milton Erickson, Helen Erickson began, in the mid-1970s, to formulate the ideals that later became MRM theory (Keegan & Dossey, 1998). As a graduate student, Erickson began testing components of the theory, beginning with research on the Adaptive Potential Assessment Model (APAM) (M. E. Erickson, 2002b; Erickson & Swain, 1982), followed by additional testing of this concept (Barnfather, Swain, & Erickson, 1989a) and the concept of self-care resources (Erickson & Swain, 1990).

The process of articulating and researching MRM concepts and the effects of MRM interventions led the way to the publication of *Modeling and Role-Modeling: A Theory and Paradigm for Nursing* (Erickson et al., 1983). This text made the theory more accessible to nurses, thus promoting the use of MRM in practice, education, and research. The publication of *Modeling and Role-Modeling: A View from the Client's World* (Erickson, 2006) offered a deeper understanding of the basic concepts of the theory, an articulation of beliefs that were implied but not specifically described in the first text on MRM theory, as well as additional ways to apply the theory in practice. Erickson discusses beliefs that are central to her model of the world. She thoughtfully articulates her reason for being in this way. "Reflection … has led me to conclude that my Life Purpose is to nurture growth in others.… Looking back at my life … attaching meaning to significant experiences and memories, I've concluded that nurturing growth is tantamount to facilitating self-actualization of finding-of-Self in others.… I am satisfied that this is my Life Purpose" (p. 28).

The link between knowledge and practice, the basis for Erikson's work, continues to be articulated in *Exploring the Interface Between the Philosophy and Discipline and Holistic Nursing: Modeling and Role-Modeling at Work* (Erickson, 2010a). This text is a rich blend of the philosophy of MRM and holistic nursing with the practical application of the theory in both nursing education and practice.

UTILIZATION OF MRM THEORY IN NURSING EDUCATION AND PRACTICE

MRM theory serves as a foundation for nursing education in several nursing programs. Table 11.1 lists the programs using MRM ranging from integration in specific courses to the serving as the foundation for the curriculum. Nurses in many settings who have been exposed to MRM either through the literature or as students have introduced the concepts into their practice environments formally or informally. For example, nurses on a surgical unit at the University of Michigan developed and implemented an assessment tool that is based on MRM (Campbell, Finch, Allport, Erickson, & Swain, 1985; Finch, 1990; Walsh, VandenBosch, & Boehm, 1989); the nurses in the vascular surgery unit use MRM as their practice framework (University of Michigan, 2002). Health care facilities across the country that are currently using MRM theory as the foundation for nursing practice are listed in Table 11.2.

TABLE 11.1 Nursing Programs Utilizing Modeling and Role-Modeling Theory

Academic Program	Utilization of MRM Theory
Century College White Bear Lake Minnesota	Currently integrating MRM theory into the curriculum in the Associate Degree Nursing Program
East Carolina University Greenville, North Carolina	Theoretical foundation for the transition from RN to graduate student
Harding University School of Nursing Search, Arkansas	Theoretical foundation for clinical course in pediatric nursing
Humboldt State University School of Nursing Eureka, California	Theoretical foundation for the BSN and RN-BSN programs
Inver Hills Community College Inver Grove, Minnesota	Currently integrating MRM theory into the curriculum in the Associate Degree Nursing Program
Lamar University Dishman Department of Nursing Beaumont, TX	Framework for high-fidelity simulation experiences and integrated into medical-surgical nursing course
Metropolitan State University Department of Nursing St. Paul, Minnesota	Theoretical foundation for RN-BSN, LPN-BSN, Entry-Level MSN programs, and currently being integrated in the development of BSN-DNP program
The College of St. Catherine School of Nursing St. Paul, Minnesota	Integrated into the foundation courses in the Associate of Science in Nursing degree
The University of Texas at Austin School of Nursing Austin, Texas	Theoretical foundation for the Alternate Entry Program
Washtenaw Community College School of Nursing Ypsilanti, Michigan	Theoretical foundation for Associate Degree Program

Source: Chisholm, Deges, and Hale (2010), Erickson (2010b), Gryczman (personal communication, 2010), mrmnursingtheory.org.

TABLE 11.2 Health Care Facilities Implementing MRM Theory in Nursing Practice

Health care facility	Location
Contemporary Health Care	Austin, TX
Homestead Assisted Living Volunteers of America	Maplewood, MN
Oregon Health and Science University Hospital	Portland, OR
Salina Regional Health Center	Salina, KS
The University of Texas Health System	San Antonio, TX
The University of Tennessee Medical Center	Knoxville, TN

Source: Erickson (2010b), Johnson (personal communication, 2010), mrmnursingtheory.org.

The Society for the Advancement of Modeling and Role-Modeling was established to advance the development and application of the theory by promoting the study and integration of the theoretical propositions and philosophical underpinnings, developing a support network, disseminating knowledge and information, and promoting the improvement of holistic health (Bylaws, 2010). The society has sponsored biennial conferences since 1986 and provides grants to support the testing, development, or implementation of MRM theory or concepts.

EXPANDED DEFINITIONS OF MODELING AND ROLE-MODELING CONCEPTS

MRM theory is described in terms of its theoretical bases, including how people are alike and how they are different, a philosophy of nursing and a paradigm for the practice of nursing. For the purpose of defining the major concepts of the theory, they can be categorized into concepts that relate to nursing and those that relate to persons.

CONCEPTS RELATED TO NURSING

Erickson has identified and described several concepts that related to the discipline of nursing. They include nursing, facilitation, nurturance, unconditional acceptance, modeling, and role-modeling.

MODELING

Modeling is a central concept in the theory because understanding the client's viewpoint is the foundation for implementing the nursing process. Modeling is defined as "the process the nurse uses as she develops an image and understanding of the client's world—an image and understanding developed within the client's framework and from the client's perspective" (Erickson et al., 1983, p. 95). Modeling begins with the initiation of the relationship with the client as the nurse seeks to determine the person's world view. Modeling is a central concept because "this worldview helps us to understand what that person perceives to be important, what has caused his problems, what will help him, and how he wants to relate to others" (Erickson, 2010a, p. 205).

Both the art and the science of nursing are reflected in modeling. The art is demonstrated through the use of therapeutic communication to develop an accurate picture of the client's situation. The science is demonstrated in the data aggregation and analysis based on scientific principles and the concepts from the theory.

ROLE-MODELING

"Role-modeling is the facilitation of the individual in attaining, maintaining, or promoting health through purposeful interventions" (Erickson et al., 1983, p. 95). Role-modeling can occur only after the nurse accurately understands the client's worldview. The art of role-modeling is demonstrated by planning and implementing nursing interventions that are based on the client's model of the world and are, therefore, unique. The science of role-modeling is demonstrated through planning theory-based interventions. Data are analyzed using the theory propositions and linkages, discussed elsewhere in this chapter.

NURSING

MRM emphasizes the holistic, interpersonal nature of nursing. Nursing is described as an interactive process that nurtures client strengths to "enable development, release and channeling of resources for coping with one's circumstances and environment. The goal is to achieve a state of perceived optimal health and contentment" (Erickson et al., 1983, p. 49). In the process of assisting clients to achieve holistic health, the nurse must nurture the client; facilitate, not effect, the process; and accept the client unconditionally.

FACILITATION

Through the interactive process of facilitation, the nurse assists the client to identify, mobilize, and develop personal strengths as he or she moves toward health. The nurse does not produce the outcomes for the client, but rather "aids the client in meeting his or her own needs so that he or she may have the necessary resources" for coping with stressors, growth, development, and self-actualization (Erickson, 1990, p. 13).

NURTURANCE

In the process of nurturance, the nurse promotes the integration of the client's affective, cognitive, and physiological processes as the client moves toward holistic health. For nurturance to occur, the nurse must seek to understand and support the client's model of the world and appreciate the value of the client's self-care knowledge. This understanding can be used to develop nursing interventions that are unique to the client.

UNCONDITIONAL ACCEPTANCE

The nurse accepts the client as a "unique, worthwhile, important individual with no strings attached" (Erickson et al., 1983, p. 255). Empathy is used to communicate nonjudgmental respect with the client. The experience of receiving unconditional acceptance leads to sense of dignity and worth and "trust in the provider" (Erickson, 2006, p. 342).

CONCEPTS THAT RELATE TO PERSONS

In describing the concepts that relate to person, Erickson has included concepts formulated for the theory and others that rely on borrowed theories from other disciplines. While nursing seeks to develop "distinctive knowledge" related to the discipline of nursing, the linking of borrowed theory with nursing theory is appropriate if there is congruence between the worldviews of the two (Villarruel, Bishop, Simpson, Jemmott & Fawcett, 2001). Concepts that relate to persons that have been described in MRM theory include person, health, environment, ways the people are alike, and ways in which they differ.

PERSON

The individual is viewed as holistic, having multiple interacting subsystems. These dynamic subsystems are the biological, cognitive, psychological, and social subsystems. The person's genetic makeup and spiritual drive permeate and intersect the subsystems. When caring for the person, the nurse does not focus on one subsystem but on the integrated, dynamic relationships among the subsystems of the person. The spiritual drive draws energy from the universe, unifies the subsystems, and gives energy back to the universal energy afield through continual energy exchange. When caring for the person, the nurse does not focus on one subsystem but on the integrated, dynamic relationships among the subsystems of the person. His or her internal model of the world determines the person's perceptions and interpretations of the environment.

HEALTH

Health is a holistic sense of well-being. Health is not defined by an absence of disease but rather a state of equilibrium among the subsystems of the holistic person. Included in health are the person's beliefs about the quality of his or her life, ability to find meaning in life, and to have a positive future orientation (Erickson, 2010a). The sense of well-being may be experienced in the presence of illness. A goal of nursing is to facilitate the client's achievement of perceived optimal health.

ENVIRONMENT

The concept of environment was not defined in Erickson's original work but has been described in later publications. The concept includes the client's internal and external stressors as well as internal and external resources. "The theorists see environment in the social subsystems as the interaction between self and others both cultural and individual" (Erickson, 2002, p. 452). The importance of the interpersonal environment is emphasized in the theory.

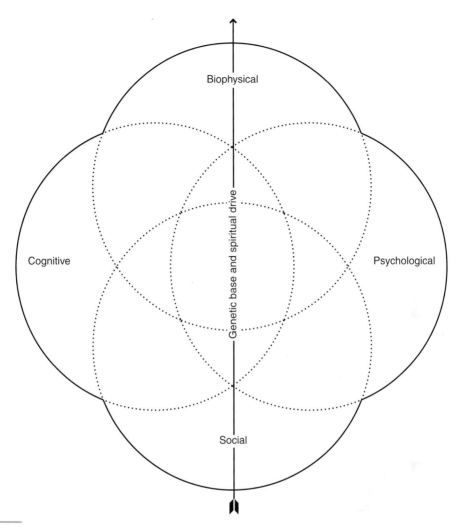

Figure 11.1 Model of the holistic person. (From Erickson, H. C., Tomlin, E. M., & Swain, M. A. (1983). *Modeling and role-modeling: A theory and paradigm for nursing* (p. 45). Englewood Cliffs, NJ: Prentice-Hall. Used with permission.)

How People Are Alike

While recognizing the uniqueness of persons, MRM identifies ways in which people are alike: They are holistic, they experience lifetime growth and development, and they have a need for affiliated-individuation. In understanding how people are alike and how they are different, Erickson synthesizes a number of interdisciplinary theories identified below.

Holism. Dynamic relationships exist among mind, body, emotion, and spirit. Figure 11.1 shows the holistic model of the person. This figure demonstrates the integration of biophysical, psychosocial, cognitive, and social aspects of the person. While identified as separate parts, the figure shows that the multiple subsystems are interconnected and permeated by the genetic base and spiritual drive. Spiritual energy permeates and influences the subsystems while unifying the dimensions of the holistic person. The subsystems interact and function as a total unit.

Lifetime Growth: Basic Needs. People are alike in that they all have basic needs. MRM theory incorporates Maslow's (1968) hierarchy of needs as the framework for understanding basic need satisfaction. Individuals have an inherent desire to fulfill one's potential. Holistic growth is impeded when basic needs are unmet. Consistent with the concept of modeling, the theory supports the view that "all human beings have basic needs that can be satisfied, but only from within the framework of the individual" (Erickson et al., 1983, p. 58).

Lifetime Development. People are also alike because they mature and develop over the lifetimes. The theoretical support for psychosocial development comes from the work of Erik Erikson (1968). As an individual moves through the eight developmental stages, he or she resolves the tasks or crisis of that stage. Resolution of the developmental stage results in the acquisition of lasting strengths and virtues.

Piaget's (1952) theory provides the framework for understanding how people are alike in their cognitive development. Individuals progress through a series of stages in which the ability to think and reason becomes more complex.

Affiliated-Individuation. "Individuals have an instinctual need for affiliated-individuation. They need to be able to be dependent on support systems while simultaneously maintaining independence from these support systems" (Erickson et al., 1983, p. 47). The need for affiliation motivates individuals to seek support. As the need for affiliation is met through supportive contacts, an "affiliative resource" is developed. A healthy sense of individuation is developed as individuals make independent choices, feel good about themselves, and feel esteem from others (Acton, 1997).

How People Are Different

Although people are alike in that they are holistic and share a common process of growth and development, each person is unique. MRM theory identifies these unique aspects of people as the inherent endowment, the ability to adapt, and one's personal model of the world.

Inherent Endowment. A person's inherent endowment is comprised of both the genetic base and the inherent characteristics. The genetic base determines, to some extent, how a person progresses through the developmental processes and responds to stressors. The inherent characteristics also influence health and growth and development. These characteristics include "malformation, brain damage, or other physiological states secondary to birth, prenatal disease, sicknesses, or other factors" (Erickson et al., 1983, p. 75).

Adaptation. People differ in the ability to adapt. Individuals are confronted with stressors, both internal and external on a continuous basis. When the response to these stressors is growth directed, adaptation results. Within MRM theory, adaptation is approached from an integrated perspective. Theoretical support for the physiological response to stressors comes from the work of Selye (1976), particularly the general adaptation syndrome. The psychosocial perspective is supported by Engel's (1962) research on the human response to stressors.

Erickson conceptualized a biophysical-psychosocial model, the APAM that identified states of coping that "reflect an individual's potential to mobilize self-care resources," the individual's adaptive potential. When a stimulus is experienced as a challenge, it is a stressor; when experienced as threatening, it is a distressor and leads to a maladaptive response (Barnfather et al., 1989b; Erickson & Swain, 1982; Erickson et al., 1983).

Three categories are identified in the APAM: arousal, equilibrium, and impoverishment. As shown in Figure 11.2 the experience of a stressor leads to a state of arousal. Arousal may be experienced by feelings of tenseness and anxiousness, accompanied by elevations in blood pressure, pulse rate, respirations, and motor-sensory behavior. From arousal, the person may move to a state of equilibrium or impoverishment. In a state of impoverishment, the individual experiences marked feelings of tension and anxiety with feelings of fatigue, sadness, or depression. In addition to elevated pulse, respiration, blood pressure, and motor-sensory behavior,

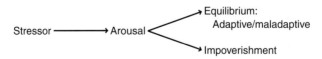

Figure 11.2 Adaptive potential assessment model. (From Erickson, H. C., Tomlin, E. M., & Swain, M. A. (1983). *Modeling and role-modeling: A theory and paradigm for nursing* (p. 81). Englewood Cliffs, NJ: Prentice-Hall. Used with permission.)

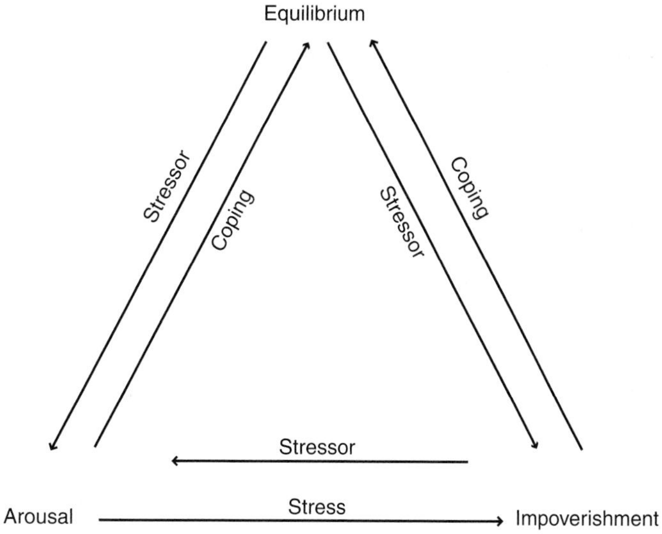

Equilibrium

Stressor

Coping

Stressor

Coping

Stressor

Figure 11.3 Dynamic relationships among states of the adaptive potential assessment model. (From Erickson, H. C., Tomlin, E. M., & Swain, M. A. (1983). *Modeling and role-modeling: A theory and paradigm for nursing* (p. 82). Englewood Cliffs, NJ: Prentice-Hall. Used with permission.)

Arousal ——————— **Stress** ———————→ Impoverishment

there is an elevation in verbal anxiety. Equilibrium may be adaptive or maladaptive. In adaptive equilibrium, the individual has normal vital signs and sensory-motor behavior, expresses hope, has low or absent feelings of tenseness, fatigue, sadness, and depression. In a state of maladaptive equilibrium, one may appear to be coping with stressors but at the expense of draining energy from another subsystem (Erickson et al., 1983).

Each state is associated with different coping potentials or different abilities to mobilize coping resources. Movement among the states, either to equilibrium or impoverishment, depends on the ability to mobilize resources and the presence of new stressors. Figure 11.3 shows the relationship among the APAM states. Assessment of the person's adaptive potential provides important information for the nurse as it is an indication of the resources available, the degree to which the person can mobilize the resources independently, and the level at which the nurse needs to intervene to facilitate adaptation. Nursing interventions are directed toward assisting the client to identify, secure, and mobilize resources (Erickson et al., 1983).

Person's Model of the World—Self-care Knowledge, Resources, and Action. Each person has a unique world view. Nurses use the process of modeling to develop an understanding of how the person perceives the world from her own perspective. One aspect of this "model of the world" that relates to health is self-care knowledge. Each person knows, at some level, what interferes with and what promotes his or her own health and development. This self-care knowledge makes the client the primary source of information in nurse–client interactions. There are two additional self-care concepts related to self-care knowledge. Self-care resources include both internal and external resources that can be mobilized to promote holistic health. Finally, self-care action is the "development and utilization" of self-care knowledge and self-care resources. Activities include both the acquisition of additional resources and the mobilization of self-care resources toward the goal of achieving optimal holistic health. Nursing intervention can assist the client in acquiring and mobilizing resources (Erickson et al., 1983). Figure 11.4 shows the relationship among MRM self-care concepts.

Figure 11.4 MRM self-care concepts. (From Hertz, J. E., & Baas, L. (2006). Self-care: Knowledge, resources, and actions. In H. Erickson (Ed.), *Modeling and role-modeling: A view from the client's world* (p. 98). Cedar Park, TX: Unicorns Unlimited. Used with permission.)

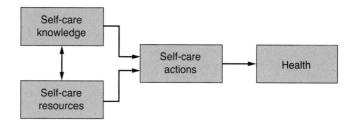

DESCRIPTION OF THE THEORY OF MODELING AND ROLE-MODELING

THEORETICAL LINKAGES

MRM theory draws on concepts from several theorists. Each theorist places emphasis on one aspect of the person. However, Erickson's creation of a holistic nursing theory explains the dynamic relationships among basic need satisfaction, growth, developmental processes, loss, grief, and adaptation. The functional relationships among these concepts lead to theoretical linkages. Relationships exist between/among:

- Need satisfaction and developmental task resolution
- Need satisfaction and adaptive potential
- Need satisfaction, object attachment, and loss, grief, growth, and development
- Developmental residue and self-care resources (H. C. Erickson, 1990; M. E. Erickson, 2002)

Figure 11.5 shows the relationships among the MRM concepts of basic need satisfaction, resolution of developmental tasks, and adaptive potential. For example, the figure demonstrates possible outcomes in adaptive potential when basic needs are met or unmet. When needs are met, the individual is able to mobilize self-care resources and then contend with new stressors that may occur. Satisfaction of basic needs also supports the resolution of developmental tasks, which then result in the individual acquiring positive developmental residual that facilitates the person in demonstrating behaviors that sustain and promote holistic health. However, when the individual fails to have basic needs met, the ability to mobilize self-care resources is compromised leading to difficulty in contending with new stressors. When needs are not met, the person has difficulty in resolving developmental tasks, leading to negative developmental residual and to behaviors that impede holistic health.

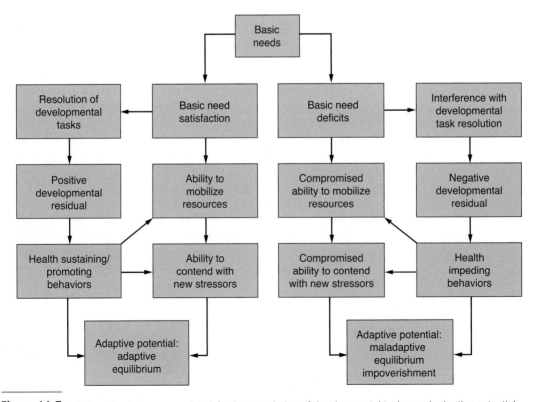

Figure 11.5 Relationships between need satisfaction, resolution of developmental tasks, and adaptive potential.

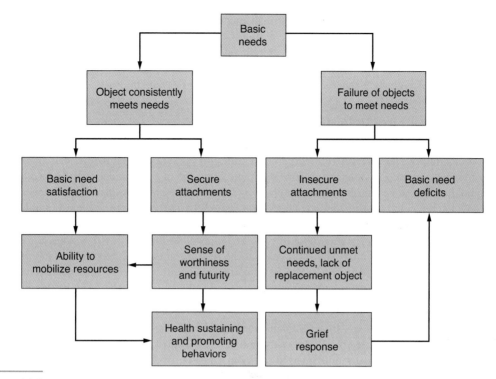

Figure 11.6 Relationships between basic needs and attachment.

The relationship between the MRM concepts of need satisfaction and object attachment is shown in Figure 11.6. When objects consistently meet one's needs, secure attachments form, leading to a sense of worthiness and futurity and the ability to mobilize self-care resources. In contrast, when objects fail to consistently meet individual's needs, insecure attachments form. In the case of loss, replacement objects are necessary to help resolve the grief associated with the loss. Lack of a secure replacement object results in a grief response, which is associated with basic need deficits.

Although the concepts presented in the theory, when viewed individually, may seem simple, the interactions among the factors demonstrate the complexity of the theory. When providing holistic care, the nurse is challenged to view the client not only from interactions of multiple subsystems, but also from the interacting dynamics of basic needs, developmental processes, attachments, mobilization of resources, and others, to achieve holistic health.

From these theoretical linkages, Erickson identified 13 propositions that can be used to predict outcomes, direct the planning of nursing care, and evaluate care.

1. Individuals' ability to contend with new stressors is directly related to the ability to mobilize resources needed.
2. Individuals' ability to mobilize resources is directly related to their need deficits and assets.
3. Distressors are related to unmet basic needs; stressors are related to unmet growth needs.
4. Objects that repeatedly facilitate the individual in need satisfaction take on significance for the individual. When this occurs, attachment to the object results.
5. Secure attachment produces feelings of worthiness.
6. Feelings of worthiness result in a sense of futurity.
7. Real, threatened, or perceived loss of the attachment object results in the grief process.
8. Basic need deficits coexist with the grief process.
9. An adequate alternative object must be perceived available in order for the individual to resolve the grief process.

10. Prolonged grief due to an unavailable or inadequate object results in morbid grief.
11. Unmet basic and growth needs interfere with growth processes.
12. Repeated satisfaction of basic needs is prerequisite to working through developmental tasks and resolution of related developmental crises.
13. Morbid grief is always related to need deficits (Erickson, 1990, p. 28).

PARADIGM FOR NURSING PRACTICE

The practice paradigm of MRM is presented within the framework of the nursing process, emphasizing the importance of both the interactive, interpersonal nature of nursing and the theoretical and scientific bases of nursing practice. Nursing care begins by determining the client's model of the world and then focusing on the most immediate concerns expressed by the client. The practice paradigm directs data collection, data aggregation, analysis, and synthesis, and provides a framework for planning nursing interventions. Critical thinking is required to implement these activities.

Consistent with the concept of modeling, the client is viewed as the primary data source. The nurse and family members are secondary data sources and the rest of the health care team are the third data source. The nurse looks for congruence between data received from the client and that received from significant others and health care professionals. Data are collected and organized in the following categories:

- Description of the situation—to develop an overview of the client's perspective of the situation
- Expectations—to determine the client's expectations for the future
- Resource potential—to determine internal and external resources available to the client
- Goals and life tasks—to determine developmental status and personal model of the world (Erickson et al., 1983)

Erickson (2010b) has described strategies, done within the context of unconditional acceptance, that facilitate a trusting relationship with the client. This relationship is the basis for implementation of interventions. The first strategy is "establishing a mind-set" (p. 216). This involves centering in the present moment and setting the intent to nurture and facilitate the client's healing. The second strategy involves "creating a nurturing space" or creating a healing environment. "It is important to remember that you are entering the client's space and to respect it" (p. 217). The third strategy is "facilitating the story." Active listening is used to understand the client's self-care knowledge.

The use of standardized nursing interventions is not consistent with MRM beliefs. The theory does provide general aims of interventions that are associated with the principles of the theory and facili-

TABLE 11.3 Relationship Between Aims of Intervention and MRM Principles

Aim	Principle
Build trust	The nursing process requires that a trusting and functional relationship exist between nurse and client.
Promote client's positive orientation	Affiliated-individuation is dependent on the individual's perceiving that he or she is an acceptable, respectable, and worthwhile human being.
Promote client's control	Human development is dependent on the individual's perceiving that he or she has some control over his or her life, while concurrently sensing a state of affiliation.
Affirm and promote client's strengths	There is an innate drive toward holistic health that is facilitated by consistent and systematic nurturance.
Set mutual goals that are health directed	Human growth is dependent on satisfaction of basic needs and facilitated by growth-need satisfaction.

Source: Erickson et al. (1983, p. 170).

TABLE 11.4 Selected Practice Studies Related to Modeling and Role-Modeling Theory

Reference	Focus of study
Baldwin, C. M. (2004). Interstitial cystitis and self-care: Bearing the burden. *Urologic Nursing, 24*(2), 111–113.	Application of self-care concepts to the treatment of interstitial cystitis
Barnfather, J. S. (1991). Restructuring the role of school nursing in health promotion. *Public Health Nursing, 8*(4), 234–238.	Modeling and role-modeling (MRM) theory applied to the role of the school nurse
Erickson, H., & Swain, M. (1982). A model for assessing potential adaptation to stress. *Research in Nursing and Health, 5,* 93–101.	Relationship between MRM and well-being
Erickson, H., & Swain, M. (1990). Mobilizing self-care resources: A nursing intervention for hypertension. *Issues in Mental Health Nursing, 11,* 217–235.	Utilizing MRM as an intervention for hypertension
Hagglund, L. A. (2009). Challenges in the treatment of factitious disorder: A case study. *Archives of Psychiatric Nursing, 23*(1), 58–64.	Application of MRM in the treatment of a client with factitious disorder
Haylock, P. J. (2010). Advanced cancer: A mind-body-spirit approach to life and living. *Seminars in Oncology Nursing, 26*(3), 183–194.	MRM theory is applied to the unique care of individuals living with advanced cancer
Irvin, B. L., & Acton, G. J. (1997). Stress, hope, and well-being of women caring for family members with Alzheimer's disease. *Holistic Nursing Practice, 11*(2), 69–79.	Stressor of care givers for people with Alzheimer's disease was studied within the context of MRM
Lombardo, S. L. (2005). Clinician's forum. *Home Healthcare Nurse, 23*(7), 425.	Application of MRM theory to morbid obesity
Scheela, R. (1999). A nurse's experience working with sex offenders. *Journal of Psychosocial Nursing and Mental Health Services, 37*(9), 25–31.	MRM theory is the basis for the concept of "remodeling" with sex offenders

tate the planning of systematic interventions. These are to build trust, promote client's positive orientation, promote client's control, affirm and promote client's strengths, and set mutual goals that are health directed. Table 11.3 shows the aims of intervention and the MRM principle associated with each intervention. *Modeling and Role-Modeling: A Theory and Paradigm for Nursing* (Erickson et al., 1983) provides specific examples of how the aims of interventions can be linked to basic need satisfaction. In the implementation of nursing interventions, the goal is to carry out one intervention that reflects each aim during every contact with the client. A single intervention can meet more than one of the general aims of intervention. Selected publications that demonstrate the application of MRM theory in practice are presented in Table 11.4.

APPLICATIONS OF THE THEORY

MRM has been the theoretical foundation for numerous published research studies, master's theses, and doctoral dissertations. Many of the studies test the middle range concepts found in MRM theory or explore the relationships between or among concepts.

AFFILIATED-INDIVIDUATION

Acton (1997) tested the concept of affiliated-individuation to determine its ability to be a mediator between stress and burden of caregivers and caregiver satisfaction with family caregivers of adults with dementia. Acton and Miller (1996) investigated the effects of a theory-based support group intervention on affiliated-individuation with a group of caregivers of adults with dementia.

ADAPTIVE POTENTIAL ASSESSMENT MODEL

The APAM was first tested by Erickson (1976).

Erickson and Swain (1982) studied the model to statistically validate the three categories of the APAM, arousal, equilibrium, and impoverishment, and to determine whether a relationship existed between the categories and the length of hospital stay. Further testing of the validity of the model was conducted by Barnfather et al. (1989a) to determine if subjects could be classified into the three adaptive states, as a measure of ability to mobilize coping resources. Barnfather (1987) applied the APAM to healthy subjects to test the relationship between basic need satisfaction and the ability to mobilize coping resources. In another study, Barnfather (1993) conducted additional testing of the model and the relationship between basic need status and adaptive potential with male students experiencing stress.

HEALTH/WELL-BEING

Research conducted by Irvin and Acton (1996) tested a model of caregiver stress mediation to determine if perceived support and self-worth had a mediating effect on well-being. Acton and Malathum (2000) studied the relationship between basic need satisfaction and health-promoting behavior and determined the best predictors of health-promoting self-care behavior. The relationship between basic need satisfaction and emotional eating was studied by Timmerman and Acton (2001). They found that a lower level of needs satisfaction was associated with increased emotional eating. "The findings of this study support the proposition from the conceptual framework [MRM] the individuals with higher levels of basic need satisfaction will be better able to deal with stress and thus, engage in healthier behaviors" (p. 699).

SELF-CARE RESOURCES/ACTIONS

Erickson and Swain (1990) conducted a nursing intervention study with hypertensive clients to determine the efficacy of MRM-based interventions directed toward mobilizing self-care resources. Irvin (1993), identifying social support, self-worth, and hope as self-care resources, studied the relationships among these resources and caregiver stress. Using hope as a self-care resource, Irvin and Acton (1997) studied stress mediation in women caregivers, testing ways that stress and well-being were affected by self-care resources. The purpose of Rosehow's (1992) research was to identify self-care actions perceived as significant for persons six months after myocardial infarction. Preferences and rankings of self-care actions were also identified. Baldwin, Hibben, Herr, Lohmer, and Core (2002) investigated the perception of self-care in an Amish community.

Research by Baas (1992) identified the predictor variables related to self-care resources on life satisfaction in persons following myocardial infarction. The concept of self-care resources was also studied in its relationship to quality of life (Bass, Fontana, & Bhat, 1997). The researchers conducted an exploratory pilot study with individuals diagnosed with heart failure to determine potential differences among the groups in measures of self-care needs, resources, and quality of life.

A new concept, perceived enactment of autonomy (PEA), was developed based on the concept of self-care (Baas, Curl, Hertz, & Robinson, 1994; Hertz, 1991). PEA is conceptually defined as "a state of sensing and recognizing the ability to freely choose behaviors and courses of action on one's own behalf and in accordance with one's own needs and goals" (Hertz, 1995, p. 269).

The results of two studies of older adults living in the community "supported a theoretical relationship between PEA and selected self-care health indicators" (Hertz & Anshultz, 2002, p. 179). PEA was shown to be significantly related to self-care knowledge, concepts of life satisfaction, and perceived control.

The investigation of MRM self-care concepts with children has been the focus of three dissertations. Baldwin (1998) studied the effects of a self-care health curriculum on third-grade students' overall health care characteristics and self-care actions. In this study, self-care subconcepts were identified as hope, control, satisfaction with daily life, support, and physical health. The research demonstrated that the group that received the self-care curriculum had higher mean scores of hope and satisfaction with daily living. Nash (2003) studied the impact of the Empowerment Program on self-care resources of middle-school-aged children. In another study of middle-school-aged children, Bray (2005) investigated the two theoretical propositions of MRM: the relationship between resolution of developmental tasks and need satisfaction and the relationship of need satisfaction to coping ability. Self-care resources identified in the study included motivation, engagement, and interpersonal relationships. The study supported the relationship between measures of health and self-care resources as well as the significance of self-care resources in explaining variances in health.

OTHER STUDIES

Additional studies, not related to the categories of concepts included above-employed MRM as the theoretical foundation. Examples of the concepts researched are comfort (Kennedy, 1991), compassionate visiting (Holl, 1992), psychophysiological processes of stress (Kline, 1988), uncertainty, spiritual well-being and psychological adjustment to illness (Landis, 1991), unmet needs of persons with chronic mental illness (Perese, 1997), psychological development and coping ability (Miller, 1986), and nurse–patient interactions (Rogers, 2002). Using Middle Range Theories 11.1–11.3 provide examples of research examining the effectiveness of MRM with individuals in assisted living situations, with community-living older adults, and with women diagnosed with factitious disorder.

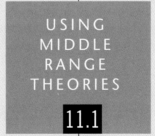

MRM theory served as the theoretical foundation for this Doctor of Nursing Practice project. The focus of this project was to determine the effect of a culture change intervention that utilized nursing-directed activities, person-centered care plans, and integrative interventions on perceived quality of life from the perspective of elders, families, and nursing staff in an assisted-living facility. MRM theory was clinically applied through the use of the "I" care plan, based on a personal relationship with the client, the client's model of the world, and unique interventions designed to meet the needs of the client. In addition to the individualized care plans, a Plan-Do-Study-Act cycle was utilized to plan meaningful, growth-promoting activities for residents. Integrative therapies were included as part of the services offered to residents.

Culture change was measured through the use of the Artifacts of Culture Change instrument. An observational tool, the Observable Indicators of Nursing Home Care Quality Indicators, was used to evaluate the health promotion program. Finally, Quality-of-Life surveys (adapted from Ohio KePRO) were administered. Post-project review of the residents' Culture Change tool and Quality-of-Life indicated a "marked increase" in measures of quality of life. The Artifacts of Culture Change organizational tool showed an increase of 18% on the domain of care practices and a 22% increase in the domain of outcomes.

The project highlighted the importance of person-centered care in assisted living, an area often neglected. In addition, the project focused on combining evidence-based approach to change with a solid foundation in nursing theory. This project won a national "Promoting Excellence in Assisted-Living Person-Centered Care Award" from the Center for Excellence in Assisted Living and first place in the Evidence-Based Practice category at the Midwest Nursing Research Society Annual Conference.

USING MIDDLE RANGE THEORIES 11.1

Source: Staus, R. (2010, April). Culture Change in an Assisted-Living Facility: A MRM Approach, Presentation at Facilitating Spiritual Well-Being: The Society for the Advancement of Modeling and Role-Modeling Biennial Conference, San Antonio, TX.

The purpose of this descriptive, correlational study was to examine the relationship of PEA with internal and external self-care resources (MRM-based concepts) of community-based older adults. Participants (*n* = 120), recruited from six senior centers, completed three instruments that measured study concepts of autonomy, social support, and functional status. The instruments used in the study were the Hertz Perceived Enactment of Autonomy Scale (HPEAS), the Multidimensional Scale of Perceived Social Support (MPPSS), and the Barthel Index (BI).

Researchers found that participants had high scores on the HPEAS, indicating positive perceived autonomy. Functionality scores, measured by the BI, indicated that as a group the participants were highly independent. Function was highly correlated with perceived autonomy. External self-care resources, satisfaction with services, and social support were significantly connected to perceived autonomy as were internal self-care resources. When discussing the implications of the findings for practice, the researchers caution against nurses' use of actions or language that may discourage self-care. They suggest that nurses engage in activities that increase the client's perception of control such as providing information that supports informed decision making and independent action.

USING MIDDLE RANGE THEORIES

11.2

Source: Matsui, M., & Capezuti, E. (2008). Perceived autonomy and self-care resources among senior center users. *Geriatric Nursing, 29*(2), 141–147.

INSTRUMENTS USED IN EMPIRICAL TESTING

Several instruments have been developed to test MRM theory. Table 11.5 lists instruments that have been used in MRM research.

SUMMARY

MRM is a nursing theory and paradigm for nursing practice. MRM synthesizes theories of development, basic needs, stress, and loss, and explains interrelationships among these concepts. These concepts are liked to several concepts specific to MRM theory, such as holism, adaptation, affiliated-individuation, nurturance, facilitation, self-care, and unconditional acceptance. At the heart of the theory is modeling,

In this article, MRM theory is applied to the treatment of a woman with factitious disorder, a complex diagnosis characterized by intentionally feigning psychological or physical symptoms that is motivated by assuming the sick role. Hagglund (2009) describes the multiple symptoms presented by the client over a number of years including, but limited to, sprained limbs, asthma, dizziness, blackouts, nausea, panic attacks, depression, anorexia, fevers, irritable bowel syndrome, and visual disturbances. MRM theory was utilized by the advanced practice psychiatric nurse (APPN) to understand the client's world view (modeling) and to interpret the client's situation and design nursing interventions (role-modeling).

The client was assessed as being in a state of maladaptation, lacking self-care knowledge. Interventions that were implemented based on MRM theory were as follows: establish trust through empathy and validation, accept the client unconditionally, implement therapeutic communication techniques, promote the client's control in asking for help when needed, empower the development of self-care knowledge, and promote strengths in using available self-care resources. "MRM provides a meaningful framework in which the APPN is able to apply the concepts of nurturance and acceptance, which ultimately leads to cohesion among the health team and facilitates the client's behavior in a growth-directed manner" (Hagglund, 2009, para 25).

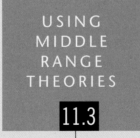
USING MIDDLE RANGE THEORIES

11.3

Source: Hagglund, L. A. (2009). Challenges in the treatment of factitious disorder: A case study. *Archives of Psychiatric Nursing, 23*(1), 58–64 doi:10.1016/j.

TABLE 11.5 Instruments Commonly Used in MRM Research

Instrument	Variable(s) measured	Source
Basic Need Satisfaction Inventory	Basic need satisfaction tool based on Maslow's five basic needs, operationalizes the construct of need satisfaction	Leidy (1994)
Erickson Maternal Bonding-Attachment Tool	Assessment of maternal bonding-attachment process within the context of need satisfaction	Erickson (1996)
Health-Promoting Lifestyle Profile II	Health-promoting, self-care behavior	Walker, Sechrist, & Pender (1995)
Modified Erikson Psychosocial Stage Inventory	Erikson's eight stages of the life cycle in adults	Darling-Fisher & Leidy (1988)
Perceived Enactment of Autonomy (PEA) Scale	Potential for self-care action, links self-care knowledge, resources and actions; PEA and its attributes: individuality, self-direction, and voluntariness	Hertz (1991)
Patient Assessment Form	Form used to collect assessment data on client based on MRM	Campbell, Finch, Allport, Erickson, & Swain (1985)
Robinson Self-appraisal Inventory	Self-reported denial	Robinson (1991)
Self-care Resource Inventory	Self-care resources, including resources available, resources needed, and differences in resources	Baas (1992)

the process of "stepping into" and understanding the client's thoughts, feelings, and needs. The nurse uses role-modeling to design scientifically based nursing interventions that are developed within the understanding of the client's model of the world that assist clients to move toward perceived optimal health. MRM serves as a framework for nursing research, education, and practice.

ANALYSIS OF THEORY

Using the criteria presented in Chapter 2, critique the MRM theory. Compare your conclusions about the theory with those found in Appendix A.

Internal Criticism	External Criticism
1. Clarity	1. Reality convergence
2. Consistency	2. Utility
3. Adequacy	3. Significance
4. Logical development	4. Discrimination
5. Level of theory development	5. Scope of theory
	6. Complexity

CRITICAL THINKING EXERCISES

1. The APAM identifies states of coping as arousal, equilibrium, and impoverishment. Consider a client for whom you are caring. Given a specific nursing diagnosis, how would your nursing interventions differ depending on the adaptive state of the client?

2. The client's model of the world is a primary concept in MRM. Using the assessment data that you have compiled about a client, write a description of the client's model of the world in the "first person."

3. MRM was developed for application to an individual client. Can MRM be applied to the family? Does a family have a model of the world, an adaptive state, and developmental stages, for example?

WEB RESOURCES

Visit **http://thePoint.lww.com/Peterson3e** for helpful web resources related to this chapter.

REFERENCES

Acton, G. J. (1997). Affiliated-individuation as a mediator of stress and burden in caregivers of adults with dementia. *Journal of Holistic Nursing, 15*(4), 336–357.

Acton, G. J., & Malathum, P. (2000). Basic need status and health-promoting self-care behavior in adults. *Western Journal of Nursing Research, 22*(7), 796–811.

Acton, G. J., & Miller, E. W. (1996). Affiliated-individuation in caregivers of adults with dementia. *Issues in Mental Health Nursing, 17*, 245–260.

Baas, L. S. (1992). The relationship among self-care knowledge, self-care resources, activity level and life satisfaction in persons three to six months after myocardial infarction. *Dissertation Abstracts International, 53*, 04B.

Baas, L. S., Curl, E. D., Hertz, J. E., & Robinson, K. R. (1994). Innovative approaches to theory-based measurement: Modeling and role-modeling research. In Chinn (Ed.). *Advanced methods of inquiry in nursing*. Gaithersburg, MD: Aspen.

Bass, L. S., Fontana, J. A., & Bhat, G. (1997). Relationships between self-care resources and quality of life of persons with heart failure: A comparison of treatment groups. *Progress in Cardiovascular Nursing, 12*(1), 25–38.

Baldwin, C. M. (1998). An investigation of health outcomes for urban elementary children utilizing an innovative self-care health curriculum model as compared to the traditional health curriculum. Unpublished doctoral dissertation, Bowling Green State University.

Baldwin, C. M., Hibbein, J., Herr, S., Lohner, L., & Core, D. (2002). Self-care as defined by members of an Amish community utilizing the theory of modeling and role-modeling. *Journal of Multicultural Nursing & Health, 8*(3), 60–64.

Barnfather, J. S. (1987). Mobilizing coping resources related to basic need status in healthy, young adults. *Dissertation Abstracts International, 49*, 02B.

Barnfather, J. S. (1991). Restructuring the role of school nursing in health promotion. *Public Health Nursing, 8*(4), 234–238.

Barnfather, J. S. (1993). Testing a theoretical proposition for modeling and role-modeling: Basic need and adaptive potential status. *Issues in Mental Health Nursing, 14*, 1–18.

Barnfather, J. S., Swain, M. A., & Erickson, H. C. (1989a). Construct validity of an aspect of the coping process: Potential adaptation to stress. *Issues in Mental Health Nursing, 10*, 23–40.

Barnfather, J. S., Swain, M. A., & Erickson, H. C. (1989b). Evaluation of two assessment techniques for adaptation to stress. *Nursing Science Quarterly, 2*(4), 172–182.

Bray, C. O. (2005). The relationship between psychosocial attributes, self-care resources, basic need satisfaction and measures of cognitive and psychological health of adolescents: A test of the modeling and role-modeling theory. *Dissertation Abstracts International, 66*, 03B.

Brekke, M., & Schultz, E. D. (2006). Energy theories: Modeling and role-modeling. In H. Erickson (Ed.), *Modeling and role-modeling: A view from the client's world*. Cedar Park, TX: Unicorns Unlimited.

Bylaws. (2010). Society for the Advancement of Modeling and Role-Modeling. Retrieved October 21, 2010, from www.mrmnursingtheory.org/bylaws/htm

Campbell, J., Finch, D., Allport, C., Erickson, H., & Swain, M. A. (1985). A theoretical approach to nursing assessment. *Journal of Advanced Nursing, 10*, 111–115.

Darling-Fisher, C. S., & Leidy, N. K. (1988). Measuring Eriksonian development in the adult: The modified Erikson psychosocial stage inventory. *Psychological reports, 62*, 747–754.

Dickoff, J., James, P., & Weidenback, E. (1968). Theory in a practice discipline: Practice oriented theory. *Nursing Research, 5*, 415–435.

Engel, G. S. (1962). *Psychological development in health and disease*. Philadelphia, PA: WB Saunders.

Erickson, H. C. (1976). Identification of state of coping utilizing physiological and psychological data. Unpublished master's thesis, University of Michigan, Ann Arbor, MI.

Erickson, H. C. (1989). *Looking at patient's needs through new eyes: Modeling and role-modeling*. Unpublished manuscript.

Erickson, H. C. (1990). Theory based practice. *Modeling and Role-Modeling: Theory, Practice and Research, 1*(1), 1–27.

Erickson, H. C. (Ed.) (2006). *Modeling and role-modeling: A view from the client's world.* Cedar Park, TX: Unicorns Unlimited.

Erickson, H. C. (2010a). *Exploring the interface between the philosophy and discipline of holistic nursing: Modeling and role-modeling at work.* Cedar Park, TX: Unicorns Unlimited.

Erickson, H. C. (2010b). Helen Erickson, Eveyln Tomlin and Mary Ann Swain's theory of modeling and role-modeling. In M. E. Parker & M. C. Smight (Eds.), *Nursing theories and nursing practice* (3rd ed.). Philadelphia, PA: Davis.

Erickson, H. C., & Swain, M. A. (1982). A model for assessing potential adaptation to stress. *Research in Nursing and Health, 5*(2), 93–101.

Erickson, H. C., & Swain, M. A. (1990). Mobilizing self-care resources: A nursing intervention for hypertension. *Issues in Mental Health Nursing, 11,* 217–235.

Erickson, H. C., Tomlin, E. M., & Swain, M. A. (1983). *Modeling and role-modeling: A theory and paradigm for nursing.* Englewood Cliffs, NJ: Prentice-Hall.

Erickson, M. E. (1996). *Relationships among support, needs satisfaction and maternal attachment in adolescent mothers.* Unpublished doctoral dissertation, University of Texas, Austin.

Erickson, M. E. (2002a). Modeling and role-modeling. In A. M. Tomey & M. R. Alligood (Eds.), *Nursing theorists and their work.* St. Louis, MO: Mosby.

Erickson. M. E. (2002b). Modeling and role-modeling theory in nursing practice. In M. R. Alligood & A. M. Tomey (Eds.), *Nursing theory utilization & application* (2nd ed.). St. Louis, MO: Mosby.

Erikson, E. (1968). *Identity, youth and crisis.* New York: Norton.

Fawcett, J. (1995). *Analysis and evaluation of conceptual models of nursing* (3rd ed.). Philadelphia, PA: Davis.

Finch, D. A. (1990). Testing a theoretically based nursing assessment. *Modeling and Role-Modeling: Theory, Practice and Research, 1*(1), 203–213.

Frisch, N. C. (2009). Nursing theory in holistic nursing practice. In M. B. Dossey & L. Keegan (Eds.), *Holistic nursing a handbook for practice* (5th ed., pp. 113–123). Boston, MA: Jones & Bartlett.

Hagglund, L. A. (2009). Challenges in the treatment of factitious disorder: a case study. *Archives of Psychiatric Nursing, 23*(1), 58–64 doi:10.1016/j.apnu.2008.03.002.

Hertz, J. E. (1991). The perceived enactment of autonomy scale: Measuring the potential for self-care action in the elderly. *Dissertation Abstracts International, 52,* 04B.

Hertz, J. E. (1995). Conceptualization of perceived enactment of autonomy in the elderly. *Issues in Mental Health Nursing, 17,* 261–273.

Hertz, J. E., & Anshultz, C. A. (2002). Relationships among perceived enactment of autonomy, self-care, and holistic health in community-dwelling older adults. *Journal of Holistic Nursing, 20*(2), 166–186.

Holl, R. M. (1992). The effects of role-modeled visiting in comparison to restricted visiting on the well-being of clients who had open heart surgery and their significant family members in the critical care unit. *Dissertation Abstracts International, 53,* 08B.

Irvin, B. L. (1993). Social support, self-worth, and hope as self-care resources for coping with caregiver stress. *Dissertation Abstracts International, 53,* 06B.

Irvin, B. L., & Acton, G. J. (1996). Stress mediation in caregivers of cognitively impaired adults: Theoretical model testing. *Nursing Research, 45*(3), 160–166.

Irvin, B. L., & Acton, G. J. (1997). Stress, hope, and well-being of women caring for family members with Alzheimer's disease. *Holistic Nursing Practice, 11*(2), 69–79.

Keegan, L., & Dossey, B. M. (1998). *Profile of nurse healers.* Albany, NY: Delmar.

Kennedy, G. T. (1991). A nursing investigation of comfort and comforting care of the acutely ill patient. *Dissertation Abstracts International, 52,* 12B.

Kline, N. W. (1988). Psychophysiological processes of stress in people with a chronic physical illness. *Dissertation Abstracts International, 49,* 06B.

Landis, B. J. (1991). Uncertainty, spiritual well-being, and psychosocial adjustment to chronic illness. *Dissertation Abstracts International, 52,* 08B.

Leidy, N. K. (1994). Operationalizing Maslow's theory: Development and testing of the basic need satisfaction inventory. *Issues in Mental Health Nursing, 15,* 277–295.

Maslow, A. H. (1968). *Toward a psychology of being.* New York: Van Nostrand Reinhold.

Matsui, M., & Capezuti, E. (2008). Perceived autonomy and self-care resources among senior center users. *Geriatric Nursing, 29*(2), 141–147.

McClosky, J., & Grace, H. (1994). *Current issues in nursing* (4th ed.). St. Louis, MO: Mosby.

McEwin, M., & Wills, E. (2002). *Theoretical basis for nursing.* Philadelphia, PA: Lippincott.

Miller, S. H. (1986). The relationships between psychosocial development and coping ability among disabled teenagers. *Dissertation Abstracts International, 47,* 10B.

Nash, K. (2003). *Evaluation of a holistic peer support and education program aimed at facilitating self-care resources in adolescents.* Unpublished doctoral dissertation, University of Texas Graduate School of Biomedical Sciences, Galveston, TX.

Parker, M. E., & Smith, M. C. (Eds.). (2010). *Nursing theories & nursing practice* (3rd ed.). Philadelphia, PA: Davis.

Perese, E. F. (1997). Unmet need of persons with chronic mental illnesses: Relationship to their adaptation to community living. *Issues in Mental Health Nursing, 18,* 19–34.

Piaget, J. (1952). *The origins of intelligence in children.* New York: International Universities Press.

Robinson, K. R. (1992). Developing a scale to measure responses of clients with actual or potential myocardial infarctions. *Dissertation Abstracts International, 53,* 12B.

Rogers, S. R. (2002). *Nurse–patient interactions: What do patients have to say?* Unpublished doctoral dissertation, University of Texas at Austin, Austin, TX.

Rosehow, D. J. (1992). Multidimensional scaling analysis of self-care actions for reintegrating holistic health after myocardial infarction. *Dissertation Abstracts International, 53,* 04B.

Scheela, R. (1999). A nurse's experience working with sex offenders. *Journal of Psychosocial Nursing and Mental Health Services, 37*(9), 25–31.

Selye, H. (1976). *The stress of life.* New York: McGraw-Hill.

Staus, R. (2010, April). *Culture change in an assisted-living facility: A MRM approach.* Presentation at Facilitating Spiritual Well-Being: The Society for the Advancement of Modeling and Role-Modeling Biennial Conference, San Antonio, TX.

Timmerman, G., & Action, G. (2001). The relationship between basic need satisfaction and emotional eating. *Issues in Mental Health Nursing, 22,* 691–701.

Tomey, A. M., & Alligood, M. R. (1998). *Nursing theorists and their work* (4th ed.). St. Louis, MO: C. V. Mosby Company.

Tomey, A. M., & Alligood, M. R. (2002). *Nursing theorists and their work* (5th ed.). Philadelphia, PA: Davis.

University of Michigan. (2002). *5B vascular surgery unit.* Retrieved July 1, 2002, from http://www.med.umich.edu/nursing/5b.htm

Villarruel, A. M., Bishop, T. L., Simpson, E. M., Jemmott, L. S., & Fawcett, J. (2001). Borrowed theories, shared theories, and the advancement of nursing knowledge. *Nursing Science Quarterly, 14*(2), 158–163.

Walker, S. N., Sechrist, K., & Pender, N. (1995). *The health-promoting lifestyle profile II.* Omaha, NE: University of Nebraska Medical Center, College of Nursing.

Walsh, K. K., VandenBosch, T. M., & Boehm, S. (1989). Modeling and role-modeling: Integrating theory into practice. *Journal of Advanced Nursing, 14,* 755–761.

BIBLIOGRAPHY

Acton, G. J., Irvin, B. L., Jensen, B. A., Hopkins, B. A., & Miller, E. W. (1997). Explicating middle-range theory through methodological diversity. *Advances in Nursing Science, 19*(3), 78–86.

Baker, C. (1999). From chaos to order: A nursing-based psycho-educational program for parents of children with attention-deficit hyperactivity disorder. *Canadian Journal of Nursing Research, 31*(2), 7–15.

Baldwin, C. M. (1996). Perceptions of hope: Loved experiences of elementary school children in an urban setting. *Journal of Multicultural Nursing and Health, 2*(3), 41–45.

Barnfather, J. S., & Ronis, D. L. (2000). Test of a model of psychosocial resources, stress, and health among undereducated adults. *Research in Nursing and Health, 23,* 55–66.

Erickson, M. E. (1996). Factors that influence the mother-infant dyad relationships and infant well-being. *Issues in Mental Health Nursing, 18,* 185–200.

Kinney, C. K. (1990). Facilitating growth and development: A paradigm case for modeling and role-modeling. *Issues in Mental Health Nursing, 11,* 375–395.

Rogers, S. (1996). Facilitative affiliation: Nurse–client interactions that enhance healing. *Issues in Mental Health Nursing, 17,* 171–184.

Schultz. E. D. (1998). Academic advising from a nursing theory perspective. *Nurse Educator, 23*(2), 22–25.

12

Comfort

KATHARINE KOLCABA

INTRODUCTION

The concept of comfort has had an historic and consistent association with nursing. Nurses traditionally provide comfort to patients and their families through actions that, in this theory, are called comfort interventions. The theory of comfort, as applied in a *ComfortPlace™*, explicates a philosophy of care whereby

193

holistic comfort needs of patients, families, and nurses are identified and addressed. Intervening variables are accounted for in planning and assessment. The desired and immediate outcome of this type of care is enhanced comfort, an altruistic and patient-centered goal. Later, Kolcaba expanded this desired outcome to apply to nurses and other members of health care teams. This application is useful when institutions are applying for national designations, such as Magnet Status from the American Association of Certification for Nurses, the American Association of Critical Care Nurses Beacon Award, or the Gold Seal of Approval from the Joint Commission Association for Health care Organizations. In addition, enhanced comfort is related to subsequent desirable outcomes such as higher patient or nurse function, quicker discharge, fewer readmissions, increased satisfaction with care, longevity of employment, and stronger cost–benefit ratios for the institution. These subsequent outcomes provide additional rationale for health care leaders and teams to adopt a model of comfort as a unifying framework for care delivery.

HISTORICAL BACKGROUND

Nightingale was perhaps the first health care worker to recognize that comfort was essential for patients. She said, "It must never be lost sight of what observation is for. It is not for the sake of piling up miscellaneous information or curious facts, but for the sake of saving life and increasing health and comfort" (Nightingale, 1859, p. 70). In this quote, Nightingale implied that the relationship between health and comfort is strong, direct, and that both are equally important.

At the beginning of the twentieth century, the term *comfort* was used in a general sense, much as Nightingale had used it, and comfort was highly valued in nursing. Moreover, the ability to provide comfort determined, to a large degree, the nurse's skill and character.

At this time, nurses believed that the provision of comfort was their unique mission. Comfort was especially important because curative medical strategies were not yet developed. Enhancing patient comfort was seen as a positive nursing goal that also was strengthening, and, in most cases, should entail an improvement from a previous state or condition. Comfort resulted from physical, emotional, and environmental interventions, but orders for specific comfort measures were under the physician's authority. Some common "comfort orders" in this period were for poultices, heat, and positioning of the patient in bed (McIlveen & Morse, 1995).

Although emotional care was not one of the specified roles of nurses, physical comfort interventions were intended to bring about mental comfort of patients, indicating that physical and mental comfort were closely related. In early nursing texts, the meaning of comfort was implicit, hidden in context, complex, and general. Many semantic variations, such as comforting, to comfort, in comfort, and comfortable, were used and the term could be in the form of a verb, noun, adjective, or adverb. Comfort also referred to the process of comforting ("The nurse comforted the patient") or the outcome of comfort ("The patient was comforted by the nurse").

From its general meaning and significant worth in nursing at the beginning of the twentieth century, comfort evolved to a less important nursing goal with a connotation more specific to the physical sense. In the 1950s, as analgesics became popular for pain control, few additional treatments for comfort were described (McIlveen & Morse, 1995). At this time, nurses took responsibility for patients' feelings, although nurses were told to refrain from discussing patients' medical conditions with them.

In the 1950s and 1960s, the term remained undefined for nursing, and it was narrowly interpreted, written about rarely, and of course, not measured or documented. These conditions rendered comfort interventions by nurses, and the results on comfort of patients, invisible.

The 1980s saw many advances in medicine and cures often resulted from surgery, antibiotics, radiation therapy (RT), and chemotherapy. Narcotics were used for treating severe pain. The importance of family comfort began to emerge at this time and families were considered legitimate recipients of care and comfort interventions (McIlveen & Morse, 1995). Correlation between the comfort of patients and the comfort of their families was implied.

Also, during the 1980s, nurses promoted self-care for patients whenever possible. Comfort was the main goal of nursing only when patients were terminally ill, an observation that supported Glaser and

Strauss' earlier suggestion that the goal of nursing reverted to comfort when there were no available cures (1965). Where health care settings were less influenced by technology, such as hospice and long-term care, comfort was more important as a nursing goal. McIlveen and Morse (1995) suggested that this trend had broad implications for nursing in the twenty-first century, as demographics would shift to large numbers of elders who may wish for less technology and more comfort in their last years of life.

DEFINITIONS OF THEORY CONCEPTS

When a concept is germane to a discipline, as comfort is, but it has not yet been specifically defined, a concept analysis is necessary. Thus, in 1988, this task was undertaken by Kolcaba. It began with a study of several contemporary dictionaries, each of which contained six or eight definitions of comfort. Those meanings were compared to usages found in an extensive literature search in the journals and textbooks of several disciplines (nursing, medicine, theology, ergonomics, psychology, and psychiatry). From ergonomics came the insight that comfort of persons, for example, in their work place or their cars, was important for optimum function or productivity (Kolcaba & Kolcaba, 1991). Kolcaba extended this insight to patients and their families.

Also consulted for the concept analysis were nursing history books and the Oxford English Dictionary (OED), which traces the origins and evolution of English words. In 1988, the nursing diagnosis (NANDA) for altered comfort was limited to specific physical discomforts such as pain, nausea, and itching. In nursing textbooks, comfort was discussed in terms of pain management. But the origins of comfort supported a significant association with strengthening, because the concept itself came from the Latin word *confortare,* which means "to strengthen greatly." That obsolete meaning of comfort, not included in modern dictionaries, was still very appropriate for nursing! From the OED, the following definitions of comfort were explicated: (a) strengthening; encouragement, incitement, aid, succor, support and (b) physical refreshment or sustenance; refreshing or invigorating influence (Kolcaba & Kolcaba, 1991). These meanings, and the link to optimum function in the ergonomic literature, provide theoretical significance for comfort in nursing.

From this process, which took two years, three technical types of comfort were derived and labeled: relief, ease, and transcendence. *Relief* was defined as the experience of a patient who has had a specific comfort need addressed; its theoretical background was consistent with Orlando's need-based philosophy of nursing (1961/1990). *Ease* was defined as a state of calm or contentment; its theoretical background was enriched by the writings of Henderson (1978) about 13 essential human requirements. *Transcendence* was defined as the state in which one rises above problems or pain. Transcendence was a term previously used in the nursing literature by two psychiatric nurses to denote "more-being" achieved through relationships with nurses (Paterson & Zderad, 1976/1988). More being was deemed important for "rising above" or "working through" difficult situations or symptoms.

Author's Note: Publishing this concept analysis (Kolcaba & Kolcaba, 1991) took one year, as the language was complicated. The analysis was comprehensive but not particularly welcomed by American journals. Hence, this first article actually was published at the same time as Kolcaba's second article (1991), described below.

After presenting these three types of comfort at a research conference, audience feedback was so stimulating that, in the middle of the night, Kolcaba awoke with the idea that the types of comfort (relief, ease, and transcendence) occurred physically and mentally. She sketched out a preliminary grid with the three types of comfort across the top and *physical* and *mental* down the side. Thus, there were six cells in this first grid. After presenting this preliminary grid to colleagues and professors at Case Western Reserve University (where she was a doctoral student), Kolcaba was advised that her "physical" and "mental" categories were not holistic, and to go back to the nursing literature to discover how holism was conceptualized. Doing so took another year. Four contexts of holistic experience were subsequently derived from the literature, which were labeled physical, psychospiritual, social, and environmental (Kolcaba, 1991). *Physical comfort* pertained to bodily sensations and homeostatic mechanisms. *Psychospiritual comfort* pertained to the internal awareness of self, including esteem, sexuality, and meaning in one's life; it also encompassed one's relationship to a higher order or being. *Social comfort* pertained to interpersonal, family, and

	Relief	Ease	Transcendence
Physical			
Psychospiritual			
Environmental			
Sociocultural			

Figure 12.1 Taxonomic structure of comfort.

societal relationships (later, this term was changed to *sociocultural comfort* and family/cultural traditions and financial circumstances were added to the definition). *Environmental comfort* pertained to the external background of human experience; it encompassed light, noise, ambience, color, temperature, and natural versus synthetic elements. Environmental comfort did not include energy fields at this time.

When the three types of comfort were juxtaposed with the four contexts of experience, a 12-cell grid or taxonomic structure (TS) was created (Fig. 12.1) (Kolcaba, 1991). The grid depicted the defining attributes of comfort, and was helpful for deriving the technical definition of comfort (provided at the beginning of this chapter): *the immediate experience of being strengthened by having needs for relief, ease, and transcendence met in four contexts (physical, psychospiritual, sociocultural, and environmental)* (Kolcaba, 1992). This grid has been useful for assessing comfort needs of patients, families, and nurses, planning interventions to address those needs, informally evaluating the effectiveness of those interventions to enhance comfort, and measuring the desired outcome of enhanced comfort for research and practice.

DESCRIPTION OF THEORY: MAJOR COMPONENTS AND THEIR RELATIONSHIPS

ASSUMPTIONS

Assumptions are a theorist's point of view about reality, stated clearly so that future readers know where the theorist is "coming from." Kolcaba's (1994) assumptions are as follows:

- Human beings have holistic responses to complex stimuli.
- Comfort is an immediate and desirable holistic state of human beings that is germane to the discipline of nursing.
- Human beings strive to meet, or to have met, their basic comfort needs. It is an active endeavor.

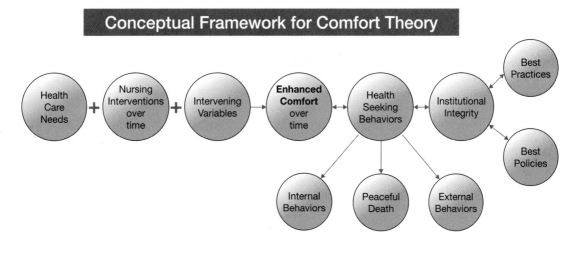

© Kolcaba (2007)

Figure 12.2 Theoretical framework for comfort theory. (*Source:* Kolcaba, K. (2002). *Conceptual framework for comfort theory.* Retrieved November 11, 2007, from http://thecomfortline.com/conceptualframework.html)

CONCEPTS

Concepts are ideas that make up the building blocks of specific theories. The concepts for the middle range theory of comfort are those listed and defined at the beginning of this chapter: comfort needs, comfort interventions, intervening variables, enhanced comfort, health-seeking behaviors (HSBs), and institutional integrity (InI). Consistent with middle range theories, these concepts are at a low level of abstraction (easily defined and measured) and are limited in number. All of these above concepts are relative to patients, families, and nurses; the term *family* encompasses significant others as determined by the patient (Kolcaba, 2003; Kolcaba, Tilton, & Drouin, 2006).

Figure 12.2 is a diagram that shows three levels of abstraction from highest (at the top of the diagram) to lowest (at the bottom of the diagram)—a depiction called a substruction. This particular diagram served as the organizing framework for Kolcaba's dissertation study with women going through RT, discussed later in this chapter. Such diagrams are helpful for planning research studies; they are used in many of Kolcaba's articles and on her web site (Kolcaba, 1997).

PROPOSITIONS

Propositions are relational statements that link concepts together. At the middle range level (Fig. 12.2, Line 1), the following propositions link those respective variables (Kolcaba, 2001):

1. Nurses and other members of the health care team identify comfort needs of patients and their family members, especially those needs that have not been met by existing support systems. Nurses also identify their own comfort needs in their work places, and work constructively for the fulfillment of these needs.
2. Comfort interventions are designed and coordinated to address those unmet comfort needs.
3. Intervening variables are taken into account in designing interventions and determining their probability for success.
4. When interventions are effective, and delivered in a caring manner, the immediate outcome of enhanced comfort is attained.
5. Patients, nurses, and other members of the health care team agree upon desirable and realistic HSBs.
6. If enhanced comfort is achieved, patients, family members, and/or nurses are strengthened to engage in HSBs, which further enhances their comfort.

7. When patients and their family members engage in HSBs as result of being strengthened by comfort interventions, patients, families, and nurses are more satisfied with health care and demonstrate better health-related and institutional outcomes.

8. When patients, families, and nurses are satisfied with health care delivery in a specific institution, improved outcomes and public acknowledgement about the institutions' contributions to health will contribute to those institutions remaining successful.

Comfort Theory (CT) can be adapted to any health care setting, health care discipline, or age group, whether in the home, hospital, or community. For research or practice, the concepts can be further defined, at a lower level of abstraction, in terms of specific populations.

PRACTICE APPLICATIONS

CT has been used to assess the comfort needs of patients and their families, to develop interventions to address those needs, and to evaluate their effectiveness for increasing recipients' comfort (Kolcaba, 1997). It also provides an ethical perspective for decision making in difficult health care situations. For example, when families are faced with difficult choices for their dying loved ones, it is helpful to consider what will make the *patient* more comfortable (Kolcaba, 2003).

CT can be adopted throughout an agency, health care system, private practice, or college of nursing to establish criteria for innovations in orientation for new employees, unified research programs, compassionate and value-based care, needs assessment for patients or personnel, actions to take to improve quality, electronic documentation, evaluation of progress toward goals, and/or performance review. Research Application 12.1 provides an example of a hospital systemwide use of CT.

Specifically, CT has been used by nurse educators as a framework to enhance learning environments for student nurses (Goodwin, Sener, & Steiner 2007). The theory also has been used by nurse leaders to enhance working environments, especially for nurses, and for working toward national institutional recognitions (Kolcaba et al., 2006). As a quality improvement initiative, CT has been utilized as a framework for raising patient satisfaction scores as developed by the Hospital Consumer Assessment of Healthcare Providers Service (HCAHPS). These scores are federally mandated from every hospital for the purpose of comparison on an open web site. Unpublished data have been provided to Kolcaba by her participating agencies that show a correlation between implementation of CT increased HCAHPS scores (see Using Middle Range Theories 12.1).

March and McCormack (2009) determined that slight modifications of CT could render it suitable for the thinking and work of other health care disciplines. Recommended modifications were primarily those of vocabulary inclusiveness, such as changing the words from "theory for nursing" to "theory for health care." Such changes were made on Kolcaba's web site to facilitate coordinated usage of CT for interdisciplinary communication, assessment, planning, and evaluation throughout a given hospital, health system, or agency.

RESEARCH APPLICATIONS FOR THE THEORY OF COMFORT

Generally, in an experimental design, patients meeting inclusion criteria are randomly assigned to levels of intervention such as a usual care group, an intervention group, and/or an enhanced intervention group. Researchers use the General Comfort Questionnaire (GCQ) as a starting point, removing items that are not relevant to their research setting or population, and adding items that are relevant. They plot all items on the TS, making sure that the content domain of comfort is evenly represented. Similar numbers of positive and negative items are utilized, unless patients are very frail cognitively. In that case, mostly positive items are used (Cohen & Mount, 1992). Kolcaba usually uses three measurement points, the first being baseline measures of the selected outcome(s). Power analysis is computed using a medium effect size, 0.80 power, and alpha of 0.10 for most interventions or protocols where known side effects are nonexistent, such as guided imagery (GI) or music therapy. The preferred test statistic is Repeated Measures Multivariate Analysis of Variance (RM-MANOVA) (or if using a covariate, MANCOVA). These are appropriate statistics for comfort research because they capture holistically the interaction between time and intervention(s) (group assignment) and they have strong power (less subjects needed). Accounting for the impact of the

Research Application   12.1

Jim, 75 years old, is apprehensive about his upcoming knee surgery. He is afraid of a general anesthetic, pain, blood loss, loss of mobility, and loss of dignity and independence during the procedure and in the postoperative period. All of these separate fears seem rather minor when considered objectively and separately. However, when Jim experiences them simultaneously (holistically), sitting in the waiting room, they create panic. "This is MY body, MY surgery, MY unknowns. I'm going under the knife!" Jim's whole-person response is greater or stronger than if he thought only about immobility one time, blood loss at another time, and so on.

A study could be designed where the intake nurse asks Jim to rate his comfort from zero to 10, zero being no comfort and 10 being the highest overall comfort possible. From the description of his fears, we are not surprised that Jim has "two" at Time 1. The nurse explores with Jim his detractors from comfort while taking Jim's vital signs (blood pressure, pulse, and respirations are high!). Jim is demonstrating a fight or flight response and really would just like to leave.

The nurse talks with Jim about alternatives to general anesthesia and about patient-controlled analgesia after surgery. The nurse talks about exercises to strengthen his knee and about minimal blood loss usually associated with his surgery. The nurse assures Jim that the surgeon will carefully drape him and that the anesthetist will maintain constant supervision over Jim during the entire procedure. Most reassuring, perhaps, is the fact that Jim's nurse will accompany him into the operating room and will stay with him. The nurse fully understands how he feels about his personal dignity and will be his advocate. This type of coaching is called "usual care" in a research study.

The nurse can see that Jim is calming down. Jim now rates his comfort as "five" (Time 2, after usual care) and vital signs are improved. Then, the nurse begins a GI exercise with Jim. Jim is asked to close his eyes, picture himself in a favorite place, relax his body incrementally, and then imagine the surgery in the most positive ways as suggested by the nurse. "You will feel no pain upon awaking, you will barely have any bleeding," and so on. Kolcaba calls this type of extra interventions "comfort food for the soul." When Jim completes the GI, he is fully relaxed and confident and now rates his comfort at "nine" (Time 3), and his vital signs are even better. The nurse documents the GI intervention and Jim's response to it. This is a test of part I of CT.

The nurse quickly looks at Jim's three comfort scores at each time point and notices that his comfort scores improved considerably at each time point. "Well, coaching improved Jim's comfort but not as much as the guided imagery. And it is interesting that his vital signs improved with each time point although there was a bigger change between Time 2 and Time 3 . . . could increased comfort be related to improved vital signs?" The second part of CT proposes that the immediate outcome of comfort is related to the subsequent outcome of improved vital signs. Other subsequent outcomes of interest might be postoperative bleeding or pain. All of these are HSBs. Institutional outcomes of interest could also be related to Jim's immediate and subsequent outcomes to test the third part of CT. Suggestions for institutional outcomes are patient satisfaction or length of stay in outpatient surgery.

In this way, concepts such as comfort gain importance when they are related to other concepts. Nurses and other members of the health team have rationale taking extra time to enhance patient comfort, in addition to the altruistic reason from which nurses usually are motivated. And nurses can demonstrate that GI improves patient outcomes—a quality improvement issue. (Of course, the design of this study would be much stronger with an experimental group [receives GI] and comparison group [usual care], each consisting of a large number of patients undergoing a similar surgery.)

interaction between time and intervention(s) (in other words, do any of the interventions increase comfort over time?) is congruent with CT. Although comfort is not a stable state from one moment to another, a trend for increased comfort over time can be demonstrated given effective comfort interventions.

All or parts of CT can be tested for research. The *first part* of the theory, Propositions 1–4, is the most frequently tested portion to date. An example from 2006 was the test of a new patient-controlled heated gown, as requested by the manufacturer. The gown was designed to be used pre- and postoperatively to enhance patients' comfort, satisfaction with care, and reduce anxiety. The manufacturer consulted with Kolcaba to adapt the Thermal Comfort Questionnaire from the GCQ. Findings of the study, which

Nurse Smith RN, DNP, worked for Brightside Hospital (fictional names), a large metropolitan teaching hospital and reported directly to the President and CEO. Two years ago, Nurse Smith was called upon to raise patient satisfaction scores on three hospital units with the lowest average scores. Since 2010, HCHAPS have been publically available and used to compare quality of care across different health care systems. The scores quickly became competitive incentives for health care dollars and contracts spread thinly across individual units, agencies, or hospitals.

The CEO was concerned that Brightside's scores were lower compared to the other area hospital of similar size and mission. Smith looked closely at the data that the President had and together they discussed strategies to reach their benchmarks. Smith then conducted a meeting with the nurse leaders on the three lowest units, also including nurses from other units with higher HCHAPS scores. Chris, a leader on a higher scoring unit, 3 west, shared that those nurses had been utilizing CT as a framework for organizing their practice. This initiative grew out of Chris' successfully completed DNP capstone project. In Chris' capstone, the nurses on 3 west were introduced to the value-added potentials of theory-based practice and applications of her favorite type of theory, mid-range. The nurses decided to try applying this mid-range theory (CT) because it was one they could relate to, it was concrete and easy to understand, it reflected specifically what they wanted to do for patients, and it entailed a direct measure of success as perceived by the patient. They also noticed that of the 10 HCHAPS items, seven were entailed in Kolcaba's TS of comfort and were also "nurse-sensitive." For raising HCHAPS scores, CT seemed a logical choice.

USING MIDDLE RANGE THEORIES

12.1

According to CT, the patients' perception of their own comfort was measured before and after nursing care. As a way to document increased patient comfort in the medical records and for later data analysis, Chris suggested including a question about comfort that was parallel to the one about pain; that is, patients were asked to rate their total comfort from 0 to 10 every shift and/or with each comforting intervention. Patients' ratings of their comfort would be used to demonstrate the effectiveness of specific nursing activities. Lower comfort scores (less comfort) would also initiate conversations about detractors from comfort, which would be addressed on an individual basis. Examples of unit-wide and individual comforting interventions that were implemented were quiet time, comfort rounds, hand massage, and efficiently administered complementary therapies.

After discussing CT with other nurses in the meeting, methods for increasing comfort on 3 west were then implemented in the units with weak HCHAPS scores. As nurses became more familiar with CT, they also began designing their additional comforting interventions, such as Welcome Books, Transfer Instructions, Suggestions for Coping with End of Life, better signage for the comfort of visitors, and reduction of environmental noise.

After the year was over, Nurse Smith examined many Inl variables on the weaker units and discovered that their scores more than met benchmarks for Nurse-Sensitive Standards, nurse satisfaction, retention of nurses, and HCHAPS. Scores for Brightside were above national averages after one year (proprietary data) and these effects were sustained every year after adoption of CT. Documentation of patient comfort, and when appropriate, family comfort continued to be included in the patients' records to enable ongoing data analysis about correlations of patient comfort with specific HSBs and institutional outcomes.

supported the manufacturer's claims, were published in a preeminent nursing journal for operating room nurses (Wanger, Byrne, & Kolcaba, 2006).

The *second part* of the theory is represented by Propositions 5 and 6, relating comfort to selected HSBs. This part provides rationale for why nurses and other health care providers should focus on patient, family, and/or nurse comfort, beyond altruistic reasons. Because HSBs include internal and external behaviors, almost any health-related outcome that is deemed important by the patient or family in a given research setting can be classified as an HSB. The task for the investigator is to justify the choice of HSBs and discuss reasons that recipients would want to engage in those HSBs, whether consciously or unconsciously. Kolcaba and colleagues tested Propositions 5 and 6 in their studies with persons who have urinary incontinence (UI) (Dowd, Kolcaba, & Steiner, 2000, 2002, 2003). They found that people with higher comfort were more likely to engage in HSBs and be successful in increasing bladder function and management of UI. That is, comfort was a good predictor of the extent of engagement in HSBs.

The *third part* of CT is represented by Propositions 7 and 8, relating patients' comfort and their engagement in HSBs to InI. The concept of InI was added to the theory in order to provide direction for outcomes research that would support the disciplines of nursing and other health professions. Comfort, patient satisfaction, and nurse satisfaction, currently, are among the few *positive* outcomes being utilized for this type of research. In addition, because institutions are driven by market competition to produce high patient satisfaction scores, those same institutions will be interested to know that patient and/or nurse comfort are strong predictors of patient satisfaction as well as other positive outcomes such as shorter lengths of stay, fewer hospital readmissions, and lower turnover of health care employees, especially nurses. Achieving sought-after national recognitions is another measure of InI.

The research examples in Using Middle Range Theories 12.2 and 12.3 show how all two or three parts of CT were tested simultaneously. Effects of hand massage on patient comfort (immediate outcome) and satisfaction with care (institutional outcome) were measured in a population of long-term nursing home residents (Kolcaba, Schirm, & Steniner, 2006). In a two-group design, those who received hand

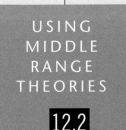

For her dissertation study, Kolcaba tested part 1 of CT. She developed a GI audiotape for women with breast cancer going through conservative treatment. Breast conserving therapy consisted of lumpectomy and RT. The research question was: Will women who receive GI while going through RT for early stage breast cancer have greater comfort over time compared to a usual care group? (see Fig. 12.2).

The audiotape facilitated the delivery of the same holistic message every day to all women in the treatment group. In the script for GI, positive statements were directed to every cell in the TS of comfort known to be important for this population. Input for construction of the audiotape and design of the study was received from the RT nurses, technicians, and physicians.

The instruments used in this study were the Radiation Therapy Comfort Questionnaire (RTCQ), adapted from the GCQ, and four visual analog scales (one each for total comfort, relief, ease, and transcendence). During the pilot test for the methods, the women were asked specifically if there was anything left out of the questionnaire, anything that was forgotten or awkward in the audiotape, and if the instruments were easy to use. When everyone was satisfied with the protocol, the study began.

Nurses told the women who met the inclusion criteria about the study during their first appointment in the RT department. When the patients first heard about the study, about half the women burst into tears; the other half wanted to enroll. The nurses faxed to the data collectors the names and phone numbers of those who wanted to enroll, and the intake visit took place prior to the women's simulation visit. The women in the treatment group were asked to listen to the tape every day, in their own homes, with tape players that

the study provided. They indicated in journals and during interviews that they complied with this request diligently for the first three weeks of RT, after which some were tired of the audiotape. When this occurred, they were encouraged to continue listening to the music side of the tape that would reinforce recall of the GI script. In this way, the script could be internalized.

Three complete data sets were collected (three visits for each woman) on 53 women, which took one year after IRB approvals were obtained. RM MANOVA was used to test the hypotheses. Alpha was set at 0.10 because the intervention had no risks and the higher alpha reduced Type II error (Lipsey, 1990).

Results. This study was a test of the new CT, a test of the effectiveness of the GI intervention, and a test of the ability to show quantitative differences in the complex phenomenon of patient comfort before and after this comfort intervention. Analysis of group differences at baseline on demographic data and comfort revealed that the groups were similar for all baseline variables. This was the desired result for Time 1 data. The result of the MANOVA, which analyzed data from all three time points simultaneously, was that the groups were significantly different on comfort at Times 2 and 3 ($P = 0.07$), a second desired result. Then, two posttests were conducted. The first was to determine which group had higher comfort (the treatment group did) and the second was to perform a trend analysis, looking at the "slopes" of the comfort data for both groups. This analysis revealed a linear slope over time, meaning that differences between the groups increased steadily over time. A simplified picture of the trend analysis for this study is in Figure 12.3. All of these results confirmed the efficacy of GI and supported the theory of comfort.

USING MIDDLE RANGE THEORIES 12.2

Source: Kolcaba, K., & Fox, C. (1999). The effects of guided imagery on comfort of women with early stage breast cancer undergoing radiation therapy. *Oncology Nursing Forum, 26*(1), 67–72.

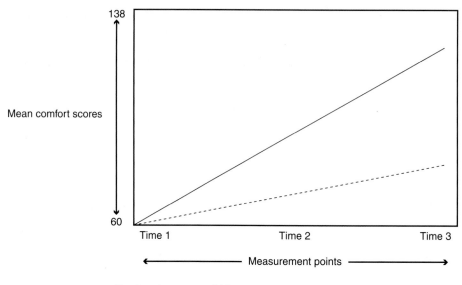

Treatment group = solid line
Comparison group = dotted line

Figure 12.3 Trend analysis for breast cancer study. (*Source:* Kolcaba, K., & Fox, C. (1999). The effects of guided imagery on comfort of women with early stage breast cancer undergoing radiation therapy. *Oncology Nursing Forum,* *26*[1], 67–72.)

The purpose of this study was to test the effectiveness of audiotaped cognitive strategies for improving comfort with innovative bladder management strategies and the HSB of actual bladder function, operationalized by incontinence and/or frequency. The research question was: Will the group practicing cognitive strategies have higher comfort and better bladder function compared to the usual care group over time?

A substructed diagram similar to the RT diagram was used to organize the study. Following this diagram, the known comfort needs of this population were targeted with cognitive strategies recorded on a new audiotape. The TS was used as a guide to cover the domain of comfort with the recorded statements. Possible covariates (intervening variables) were age, gender, and particulars of bladder health history. To measure comfort in this population, the UIFCQ was adapted from the GCQ and was pilot tested before using it in this study. The HSB was improved bladder function operationalized by the Bladder Function Questionnaire (researcher developed).

Most of the methods from the breast cancer study, described previously, were replicated because

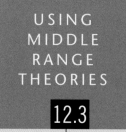

USING
MIDDLE
RANGE
THEORIES

12.3

of their success, including having persons in the treatment group listen to the tape daily, having three data collection points, and using the same method of data analysis.

Results indicated that the treatment group had more comfort and improved bladder function over time compared with the usual care group. In addition, a crossover component was added when those in the original comparison group listened to the audiotape for three weeks, after which data were collected again from both groups. A significant improvement on bladder function was found in the crossover group and their comfort had increased to the level of the treatment group after three weeks of the intervention.

Another interesting finding was that the UIFCQ predicted which participants ($N = 17$, or 90% of the treatment group) would demonstrate improvement in incontinence. Because comfort was a strong predictor of benefit from treatment for incontinence and frequency, these findings also supported the strengthening component of the theory of comfort (Dowd et al., 2000).

Source: Dowd, T., Kolcaba, K., & Steiner, R. (2000). Using cognitive strategies to enhance bladder control and comfort. *Holistic Nursing,* 14(2), 91–103.

massage by their nursing assistants (NAs) as a part of their hygienic care were compared to residents who received usual care (no hand massage). The intervention was incorporated easily into the (NAs) routine, but lack of administrative encouragement led to a decrease in interest in the study and performance of the intervention. Therefore, unlike other comfort studies, a trend toward gradually increasing comfort in a linear direction was not demonstrated. A systematic program of recognition of the NAs work and contribution to science by the administrators might have resulted in positive findings.

In a three-group design, a modified GCQ was utilized to measure differences in comfort and stress between groups of college students, ages 18–24, randomly assigned either to healing touch (HT), coaching, or a combined intervention of HT and coaching. Repeated measures revealed that HT had better immediate results on both outcomes, while coaching had better carryover effects. Findings for the combined treatment group were inconsistent, probably due to methodological issues (Dowd, Kolcaba, Steiner, & Fashinpaur, 2007).

The TS of comfort was utilized to create a Portuguese instrument for hospitalized psychiatric patients to test the effectiveness of GI for increasing comfort (immediate outcome) and decreasing depression, anxiety, and stress (subsequent outcomes). Repeated measures revealed that the treatment group had significantly improved comfort and decreased depression, anxiety, and stress over time (Apostolo & Kolcaba, 2009).

For health care research, patient comfort can be correlated with institutional factors such as nurse–patient ratios, levels of nursing education, new hospital policies or protocols, strategies for nurse retention, and/or specific nursing interventions (especially those considered to be holistic or adjunctive to medical strategies). A full taxonomy of comfort measures is now available in the electronic NANDA data base as nursing diagnoses, interventions, and outcome measures. The patient outcome of comfort can be added to other electronic data bases or paper records as well. Identifying and tracking value-added nursing outcomes by staff nurses on their units and nursing leaders for the entire division, agency, or hospital is important for (a) earning recognition for ones' sphere of influence, (b) elevating the specific contribution of nursing to health care of patients, and (c) counteracting the negative and dangerous reputations that have been created regarding hospital stays.

In addition, in a pay-for-performance (futuristic) reimbursement environment, comfort is a value-added and nursing-sensitive outcome; that is, when patients' and their families' experience increased comfort, a benefit that they desire and need, through the direct actions and behaviors of a nurse, those actions and behaviors could be reimbursed separately. The credibility and validity of the GCQ and its modifications is ideally suited for this purpose. In 2003, the complete instrument was registered as a multidisciplinary outcome indicator by the National Quality Measures Clearinghouse (NQMC). This type of positive (value-added) patient/family measure is unusual because it is a *direct* indicator of quality, rather than an indirect indicator. Indirect indicators are actually indicators of *poor* quality such as "death among surgical patients," "prevalence of pressure ulcers," and "incidence of inpatient falls with injuries" as listed in the current version of the National Quality Forum nursing-related outcome indicators (Dunton, Gonnerman, Montalvo, & Schumann, 2011).

INSTRUMENTS USED IN EMPIRICAL TESTING

GENERAL COMFORT QUESTIONNAIRE

If you want to do a comfort study yourself, and a comfort instrument needs to be constructed for your unique population, you can start with the GCQ and adapt it using your knowledge of the population. Detailed instructions for doing so are on the web (Kolcaba, 1997) and a full discussion of how the GCQ was developed is in Kolcaba (1992) and Kolcaba (2003).

As with the other comfort questionnaires available, the GCQ began with the TS. The GCQ contains two positive and two negative items for each of the 12 cells in the TS, resulting in 48 items. A four-response Likert-type scale was used for the pilot test, although subsequent questionnaires have six responses, which increase sensitivity of the instrument. An even number of responses also forces the responder to choose one side of the comfort fence or the other.

The GCQ was pilot tested in the community ($N = 30$) and several types of hospital units ($N = 226$). Results of this first instrumentation study were encouraging, as the Cronbach's alpha was 0.88, very high for a new instrument. (Perhaps, working from a theoretically driven map of the content domain helped!) Factor analysis, using principal components analysis extracted 13 factors with eigenvalues above 1.0. The 13th factor had only one item and was collapsed into one of the other factors that was semantically similar, producing 12 factors consistent with the TS. In addition, factors clumped together in three subscales on the screen plot and semantically were similar to the types of comfort (relief, ease, and transcendence). This factor structure accounted for 63.4% of the variance in the 48 items (Kolcaba, 1992).

Reliabilities for the subscales (factors) ranged from 0.66 to 0.80, which were lower than for the whole GCQ (0.88). This is because lower numbers of items generally decrease reliability scores. The GCQ revealed significant sensitivity in expected directions between several groups (construct validity). Findings were that: (a) the community group had higher comfort than the hospital group, and (b) people with higher comfort demonstrated a higher correlation with their own estimates of progress in rehabilitation.

When researchers adapt the GCQ to fit their population, they can use the psychometric properties and description of the instrumentation study (above) to support their choice of a comfort instrument. If appropriate, the number of items can be shortened or whole subscales that are not relevant can be removed. However, with each of those strategies, reliability scores may decrease. It is important, therefore, to pilot test adapted instruments with at least 15 subjects who are characteristic of those in the proposed study. A Cronbach's alpha of at least 0.70 is desirable for a new instrument. Kolcaba appreciates submission of your new instruments to her web site (Kolcaba, 1997), so future researchers do not have to "reinvent the wheel" and the preliminary psychometric statistics that support use of comfort instruments.

The credibility and validity of the GCQ and its modifications is ideally suited for this purpose. In 2003, the complete instrument was registered as a multidisciplinary outcome indicator by the National Quality Measures Clearinghouse (NQMC, 2002). This type of positive (value-added) patient/family measure is unusual because it is a *direct* indicator of quality, rather than an indirect indicator. Indirect indicators are actually indicators of *poor* quality such as "death among surgical patients," "prevalence of pressure ulcers," and "incidence of inpatient falls with injuries" as listed in the current version of the National Quality Forum nursing-related outcome indicators (Dunton et al. 2011). In addition, in a pay-for-performance (futuristic?) reimbursement environment, comfort is a value-added and nursing-sensitive outcome; that is, when patients' and their families' experience increased comfort, a benefit that they desire and need, through the direct actions and behaviors of a nurse, those actions and behaviors could be reimbursed separately.

VERBAL RATING SCALES

For clinical research, patient comfort can be assessed with verbal ratings similar to those now conducted for pain. When a patient is asked to rate his/her comfort from 0 to 10, meaningful conversations can be initiated about detractors from comfort in the clinical setting and possible solutions. Findings from the use of verbal rating of either total comfort or discomfort can easily be added to documentation forms in health care settings. In a test of their reliability, verbal ratings of total comfort provided statistically significant data when comparing the effects of two comfort interventions, coaching and HT, for the goal of increasing comfort and decreasing stress of college students (Dowd et al., 2007).

Verbal ratings can be correlated with institutional factors such as nurse–patient ratios, levels of nursing education, new hospital policies or protocols, strategies for nurse retention, and specific nursing interventions (especially those considered to be holistic or adjunctive to medical strategies). A full taxonomy of comfort measures is now available in the electronic NANDA data base as nursing diagnoses, interventions, and outcome measures. Identifying and tracking value-added nursing outcomes by nursing leaders is important for (a) earning recognition for ones unit, agency, or hospital, (b) elevating the contribution of nursing to health care in general, and (c) counteracting the negative and dangerous reputations that have been created regarding hospital stays.

RADIATION THERAPY COMFORT QUESTIONNAIRE

To adapt the GCQ to women with breast cancer, items that were not relevant for RT were deleted. The literature identified critical comfort needs specific to this population. From this list of needs, positive and negative items were developed to complete and balance the questionnaire for this population.

A consideration when developing the Radiation Therapy Comfort Questionnaire (RTCQ) was the length of time it would take for the women to answer it. The nurses thought, and it was later confirmed, that many research participants would choose to complete the questionnaires in the RT department rather than in their homes. In addition, the design of the study was to administer all questionnaires immediately prior to RT. A 48-item questionnaire was deemed too long by the RT staff, and probably too stressful for the women. So, for this study, a 26-item RTCQ was pilot tested. The instrument performed fairly well in the final study with a Cronbach's alpha of 0.76 ($N = 53$, 26 items).

URINARY INCONTINENCE AND FREQUENCY COMFORT QUESTIONNAIRE

For the comfort study with persons with UI, the Urinary Incontinence and Frequency Comfort Questionnaire (UIFCQ) was adapted from the GCQ and contained 23 positive and negative items specific to the experience of living with UI. A six-response Likert-type format, ranging from strongly agree to strongly disagree, was used. After reverse coding negative items, higher scores indicated higher comfort. In this study, 31 women and 9 men participated. The Cronbach's alpha averaged 0.82 across the four measurement points indicating good reliability. The instrument was sensitive to changes in comfort over time ($P = 0.01$) (Dowd et al., 2000).

HOSPICE COMFORT QUESTIONNAIRE (FAMILY AND PATIENT)

For this population, the GCQ was adapted again to create a 49-item Hospice Comfort Questionnaire (HCQ). Family members were asked to rate their own comfort, not that of their patient. The adapted instruments were tested in two phases (Novak, Kolcaba, Steiner, & Dowd, 2001). In phase I, patient and FM questionnaires had a six-item Likert scale response set, ranging from "strongly agree" to "strongly disagree," and higher scores indicated higher comfort. Each questionnaire took about 12 minutes for patients to complete and usually less time for FMs. Approximately equal numbers of positive and negative items were created for the FMs' EOL questionnaire, items were worded more simply and with less alternating between positive and negative orientations. This adaptation was necessary because of decreased mental agility in dying patients (Cohen & Mount, 1992).

In phase II, patient and caregiver questionnaires were reduced to a four-item Likert response set, because of concerns of the data collectors that six responses were too confusing. However, results showed that the instrument in phase I (six responses) had the strongest psychometric properties for both FMs and patients. Cronbach's alpha for the FM questionnaire was 0.89 ($N = 38$) and for the patient questionnaire was 0.83 ($N = 48$) (Novak et al., 2001).

In spite of these high reliability scores, nurse researchers working with this population a few years later thought that 49 items were too many, and they asked a panel of experts to prioritize the items that were most important. From that list of priority items, 24 of the highest items were plotted on the TS and balanced over the content domain. The result is a 24-item HCQ. This instrument was used in an experiment with hospice patients in which a hand massage protocol was tested with 31 patients over a three-week period. Despite a lenient alpha of 0.10, the study did not yield significant results overall. However, of clinical significance is that comfort increased somewhat in the treatment group even as patients approached death while, in the usual care group, comfort scores decreased steadily over the three weekly measurement points (Kolcaba, Dowd, Steiner, & Mitzel, 2004).

HEALING TOUCH COMFORT QUESTIONNAIRE

The Healing Touch Comfort Questionnaire (HTCQ) was adapted from the GCQ following the same procedure described previously. Three experts reviewed it for appropriateness of wording and content, eight

HT practitioners distributed the questionnaire to their clients, and 53 persons completed them within several days of the treatment. The questionnaires were returned in self-addressed envelopes provided by the research team. Cronbach's alpha for the HTCQ was 0.94 for total comfort. Those who had received five or more HT treatments had comfort scores of 13.7 points higher than those who had received one to four treatments. Further analysis showed that there was a trend to a curvilinear relationship between number of treatments and comfort. Comfort seems to increase slightly as the number of treatments increases until about 20 treatments; then comfort levels off and possibly decline. More information is needed about this relationship (Dowd et al., 2006).

The HTCQ was utilized in the study with college students described earlier (Dowd et al., 2007) to establish reliability of the findings from the verbals. Cronbach's alpha in this study revealed an average of 0.93 over three measurement points. The HTCQ was highly and positively correlated with verbal ratings for comfort.

COMFORT BEHAVIORS CHECKLIST

Research with patients near end of life and their family members is in its infancy. Comfort is consistently stated as a desired outcome in hospice standards of care, which makes CT particularly cogent for research with patients near end of life. Making it even more applicable for hospice or palliative research is Schlotfeldt's (1975) inclusion of peaceful death as an HSB, another subsequent outcome. Sometimes, a peaceful death is the most realistic outcome in a particular situation and Schlotfeldt's elevating peaceful death to an HSB was an example of how her thinking was "ahead of her time." However, data collection with patients near end of life is fraught with difficulties. For these reasons, Kolcaba developed a Comfort Behaviors Checklist (CBC), which data collectors can use to rate a patient's *apparent* comfort if the patient loses the cognitive ability to rate his or her own comfort (Kolcaba, 1997). While not as desirable as actually asking a patient about his or her comfort, the instrument fills a gap regarding data collection in very frail or cognitively limited patients. This CBC was recently adapted for clinical documentation of babies' apparent comfort by pediatric nurses from a large western health care system (Kolcaba, 1997).

Other patients whose comfort could be indirectly assessed by nurses are those who are mentally disabled, brain injured, heavily sedated, or unconscious. Using the CBC, a nurse or data collector rates the patient's comfort based on observable behaviors. It contains 29 observations with possible responses of Not Applicable, No, Somewhat, Moderate, and Strong (Kolcaba, 1997). The instrument includes positive indicators of comfort in addition to signs that indicate a lack of comfort. Directions for scoring of the CBC are on Kolcaba's web site, where she directs researchers how to calculate results as a percentage instead of adding total points.

Inter-rater comparisons were performed with long-term care residents to test the reliability of the instrument. A deviation of 20 percentage points between raters for each subject was considered clinically and empirically unreliable. Conversely, a deviation between raters of 10 percentage points for each subject was considered to be acceptable, and a deviation of 5 percentage points was a demonstration of very strong inter-rater consistency. Distributions of the differences in ratings in 39 data sets were as follows: (a) 36 data sets revealed a 10-point difference or less between raters 1 and 2 for each subject ($P = 0.92$; alpha 0.95), and (b) 31 data sets revealed a 5-point difference or less between raters 1 and 2 for each subject ($P = 0.80$; alpha 0.95). These findings indicated strong inter-rater consistency. These findings were repeated with a version of the CBC modified for pediatric surgical patients.

However, when scores from the CBC were correlated with residents' responses on the traditional GCQ, low correlations were revealed, averaging a Cronbach's alpha of 0.14 over three distinct time points. These disappointing findings seemed to indicate that the interior life or feelings of human beings cannot be fully appreciated until they are asked. The stoic demeanors of the long-term care residents, which appeared to indicate comfort, masked many complex feelings about their own comfort. However, in the absence of the ability to verbalize or indicate specific feelings about comfort, the CBC is, perhaps, better than no comfort assessment at all and can serve to indicate increases in percentage points associated with comfort interventions or protocols.

All of these instruments, and others under development or in different languages, are available on Kolcaba's web site (Kolcaba, 1997).

SUMMARY

The theory of comfort provides a framework for research in any setting where patients have comfort needs and enhancing their comfort is valued. The theory has been used to test the effectiveness of specific holistic interventions for increasing comfort, to demonstrate the correlation between comfort and subsequent HSBs, and to relate HSBs to desirable institutional outcomes. It is important as a framework for interdisciplinary care and research because the focus is on the unifying and positive outcome of patient comfort. As such, CT has been used in many health care specialties, both nationally and internationally. As a value-added indicator of improved quality, the desired outcome of comfort is used by nursing leaders for practice and research.

ANALYSIS OF THEORY

Using the criteria presented in Chapter 2, critique the theory of Comfort Care. Compare your conclusions about the theory with those found in Appendix A. A researcher who has worked with the theory completed the analysis found in the Appendix.

Internal Criticism

1. Clarity
2. Consistency
3. Adequacy
4. Logical development
5. Level of theory development

External Criticism

1. Reality convergence
2. Utility
3. Significance
4. Discrimination
5. Scope of theory
6. Complexity

CRITICAL THINKING EXERCISES

1. Nurse leaders attempt to advance practice one unit or agency at a time. In order to bring a philosophy of comfort management to your practice setting, rationale must be developed and presented. Compile logical and compelling rationale for implementing comfort management at your site, and a brief proposal for how you would implement this model.

2. In order to practice comfort management, evidence must be collected about patients'/families' comfort needs, comfort interventions to address those needs, and assessment of baseline comfort compared to comfort after the intervention(s). Design appropriate comfort management documentation for your unit.

3. Research evidence suggests that patients do better when their expectations about specific benefits of nursing care are discussed and met. Design a "comfort contract" whereby patients or their surrogates designate an expected level of postsurgical overall comfort, and also where they can specify chronic discomforts and interventions that they use at home for relief.

WEB RESOURCES

Visit **http://thePoint.lww.com/Peterson3e** for helpful web resources related to this chapter.

REFERENCES

Apostolo, J., & Kolcaba K. (2009). The effects of guided imagery on comfort, depression, anxiety, and stress of psychiatric in patients with depressive disorders. *Archives of Psychiatric Nursing, 23*(6), 403–411.

Cohen, S., & Mount, B. (1992). Quality of life in terminal illness: Defining and measuring subjective well-being in the dying. *Journal of Palliative Care, 8*(3), 40–45.

Dowd, T., Kolcaba, K., & Steiner, R. (2000). Using cognitive strategies to enhance bladder control and comfort. *Holistic Nursing Practice, 14*(2), 91–103.

Dowd, T., Kolcaba, K., & Steiner, R. (2002). Correlations among six measures of bladder function. *Journal of Nursing Measurement, 10*(1), 27–38.

Dowd, T., Kolcaba, K., & Steiner, R. (2003). The addition of coaching to cognitive strategies. *Journal of Ostomy and Wound Management, 30*(2), 90–99.

Dowd, T., Kolcaba, K., & Steiner, R. (2006). Development of an instrument to measure holistic client comfort as an outcome of healing touch. *Holistic Nursing Practice, 20*(3), 122–129.

Dowd, T., Kolcaba, K., Steiner, R., & Fashinpaur, D. (2007). Comparison of a healing touch, coaching, and a combined intervention on comfort and stress in younger college students. *Holistic Nursing Practice, 21*(4), 194–202.

Dunton, N., Gonnerman, D., Montalvo, I., & Schumann, M. (2011). Incorporating nursing quality indicators in public reporting and value-based purchasing initiatives. *American Nurse Today, 6*(1), 14–17.

Glaser, C., & Strauss, A. (1965). *Awareness of dying.* Chicago, IL: Aldine.

Goodwin M., Sener I., & Steiner, S. (2007). A novel theory for nursing education: Holistic comfort. *Journal of Holistic Nursing, 25*(4), 278–285.

Henderson, V. (1978). *Principals and practice of nursing.* New York: Macmillan.

Kolcaba, K. (1991). A taxonomic structure for the concept comfort. *Journal of Nursing Scholarship, 23*(4), 237–239.

Kolcaba, K. (1992). Holistic comfort: Operationalizing the construct as a nurse-sensitive outcome. *Advances in Nursing Science, 15*(1), 1–10.

Kolcaba, K. (1994). A theory of holistic comfort for nursing. *Journal of Advanced Nursing, 19,* 1178–1184.

Kolcaba, K. (1997). *The Comfort Line.* Retrieved October 7, 2011, from http://www.thecomfortline.com

Kolcaba, K. (2001). Evolution of the mid range theory of comfort for outcomes research. *Nursing Outlook, 49*(2), 86–92.

Kolcaba, K. (2003). *Comfort theory and practice: A vision for holistic health care and research.* New York: Springer.

Kolcaba, K., Dowd, T., Steiner, R., & Mitzel, A. (2004). Efficacy of hand massage for enhancing comfort of Hospice Patients. *Journal of Hospice and Palliative Care, 6*(2), 91–101.

Kolcaba, K., & Fox, C. (1999). The effects of guided imagery on comfort of women with early stage breast cancer undergoing radiation therapy. *Oncology Nursing Forum, 26*(1), 67–72.

Kolcaba, K., & Kolcaba, R. (1991). An analysis of the concept of comfort. *Journal of Advanced Nursing, 16,* 1301–1310.

Kolcaba, K., Schirm V., & Steiner R. (2006). Effects of hand massage on comfort of nursing home residents. *Geriatric Nursing, 27*(2), 85–91.

Kolcaba, K., Tilton C., & Drouin, C. (2006). Use of comfort theory to enhance the practice environment. *Journal of Nursing Administration, 36*(11), 538–544.

Lipsey, M. (1990). *Design Sensitivity.* New Park, CA: Sage.

March, A., & McCormack D. (2009). Nursing theory-directed healthcare. *Holistic Nursing Practice, 23*(2), 75–80.

McIlveen, K., & Morse, J. (1995). The role of comfort in nursing care: 1900–1980. *Clinical Nursing Research, 4*(2), 127–148.

Nightingale, F. (1859). *Notes on nursing.* London: Harrison.

Novak, B., Kolcaba, K., Steiner, R., & Dowd, T. (2001). Measuring comfort in caregivers and patients during late end-of-life care. *American Journal of Hospice & Palliative Care, 18*(3), 170–180.

NQMC. (2002). *National Quality Measures Clearinghouse.* Accessed January 18, 2011, from http://quality measures.ahrq.gov/comfort.

Oerlemans, M. (1972). Eli. *American Journal of Nursing, 72,* 1440–1441.

Orlando, I. (1961/1990). *The dynamic nurse–patient relationship.* New York: National League for Nursing.

Paterson, J., & Zderad, L. (1976/1988). *Humanistic nursing.* New York: National League for Nursing.

Schlotfeldt, R. (1975). The need for a conceptual framework. In P. Verhonic (Ed.), *Nursing research* (pp. 3–25). Boston, MA: Little & Brown.

Stevens, J. (1992). *Applied multivariate statistics for the social sciences* (2nd ed.). Hillsdale, NJ: Erlbaum.

Van Dijk, M., De Boer, J., Koot, H., Tibboel, D., Passchier, J., & Duivenvoorden, H. (2000). The reliability and validity of the comfort scale as a postoperative pain instrument in 0-3-year-old infants. *Pain, 84*(2–3), 367–377.

Vullo-Navich, K., Smith, S., Andrews, M., Levine, A., Tischler, J., & Veglis, J. (1998). Comfort and incidence of abnormal serum sodium, BUN, creatinine and osmolality in dehydration of terminal illness.

The American Journal of Hospice & Palliative Care, 15(2), 77–84.

Wagner, D., Byrne, M., & Kolcaba, K. (2006). Effect of comfort warming on preoperative patients. *AORN Journal, 84*(3), 1–13.

13

Health-Related Quality of Life

KRISTIN E. SANDAU

TIMOTHY S. BREDOW

SANDRA J. PETERSON

DEFINITION OF KEY TERMS

Health-related quality of life (HRQOL)	Subset of quality of life (QOL) representing satisfaction in areas of life likely to be affected by health status; HRQOL is subjective, multidimensional, and temporal.
Life domains	Basic components of QOL and HRQOL referring to specific aspects of life, most commonly physical, cognitive, socioeconomic, and psychological/spiritual.
Nursing interventions	Although rarely included as a component in formal theoretical models of HRQOL, involve delivering specific care or treatments targeted for an individual or group who have deficits or potential deficits in an identified domain that may impact HRQOL.
Quality of life	Satisfaction in areas of life deemed important to the individual.

INTRODUCTION

Quality of life (QOL) has been a philosophical and sociopolitical phenomenon for hundreds, if not thousands, of years. Because QOL is not clearly identified with one theorist, it is difficult to define and describe. This lack of specificity has not diminished its popularity as an outcome measure among patients tested in hundreds of studies published both nationally and internationally. QOL has been identified as a middle range theory (Meleis, 1997) representing a specific phenomenon, with a limited number of related concepts, that has obvious applications to practice. The more limited construct of health-related QOL in the context of health care (often referred to as HRQOL) may be even more fitted as a middle range theory because HRQOL is somewhat more limited in focus on areas of life most directly influenced by one's health.

HISTORICAL BACKGROUND

The concept of QOL, concerned with an individual's personal satisfaction with life, has its roots in classical Greek thought and religious teachings. Aristotle is credited with the initial conceptualization of QOL, defined as happiness, the good life, or the outcome of a life of virtue (Morgan, 1992). In the New Testament (John 10:10), Jesus stated that he came to give life and give it abundantly (The Lockman Foundation, 1995). The 10 stages of enlightenment in Buddhism start with achieving joy in life (Stryk, 1968).

Pigou has been credited with modern introduction of the term in 1920 in his book on economics and welfare (Wood-Dauphinee, 1999). Politically, use of the concept, QOL, was limited until it was reintroduced in remarks made by Presidents Johnson and Nixon in speeches on environmental and social issues (Campbell, 1981; Dalkey, Rourke, Lewis, & Snyder, 1972). QOL has its academic roots in the disciplines of psychology and sociology (Spranger, 2001). In the 1970s, these disciplines began to consider the issue of QOL. In the 1970s, the business world adopted the term *QOL* to make claims about the ability of a product to enhance a person's life in the milieu of everyday living.

The WHO's more encompassing definition of health as physical, psychological, and social well-being, and not just the absence of illness or infirmity (World Health Organization, 1948), provided early impetus to the consideration of QOL as a relevant human experience for health care professionals. In 1978, the WHO provided a statement on the application of its definition of health, indicating that individuals have the right "to psychosocial care and adequate QOL in addition to physiologic care" (King & Hinds, 1998, p. xi). Nursing's interest in QOL is long-standing. Florence Nightingale's involvement with the British military provided multiple examples of how nurses can promote the QOL for individuals. This interest has intensified and become a focus of research for nurses.

HRQOL, a subcategory of global QOL, is a more recent concept. Health care trends have contributed to the emergence of HRQOL as an important phenomenon. In the past 15–20 years, the concern for patients has become more inclusive, focusing not just on the treatment of disease, but also on the restoration and promotion of health (Read, 1993). With increased client longevity, health care professionals are attending to the lifestyle issues that accompany chronic disease and often affect QOL. The Food and Drug Administration (FDA) is reflecting this changing emphasis. It can require documentation of not only the safety and efficacy of new products, but also their effect on a user's QOL (Spilker, 1996).

QOL has emerged as a concept of interest to many disciplines. This multiplicity of discipline-specific perspectives has led to little consensus on a definition. Philosophers consider the nature of existence and what is meant by the "good life." Ethicists are concerned with social utility. Economists pursue cost-effectiveness in producing the greatest good. Physicians focus on health- and illness-specific issues, while nurses may approach the issue of QOL more holistically (Anderson & Burckhardt, 1999).

DEFINITION OF THEORY CONCEPTS

QOL and the subconstruct HRQOL have suffered from a lack of clarity for both conceptual and operational definitions in research studies. Regrettably, some researchers published results of HRQOL outcome studies without first stating their conceptual definition of HRQOL. Similarly, several researchers have not accurately matched their conceptual definition with their operational definition. For example, researchers have inaccurately stated that they are measuring the broad construct of QOL but have instead operationalized QOL as an objective measure, such as *length of time without return to surgery* (Elkins, Knott-Craig, McCue, & Lane, 1997).

In the 1980s and early 1990s, many researchers reported outcomes as QOL or HRQOL but had only measured one domain, such as physical functional status. However, functional status is not interchangeable with the construct HRQOL and is most appropriately considered only one of several components contributing to overall HRQOL. Functional status has traditionally been defined by degree of disability to perform standard activities in life (Stineman, Lollar, & Ustun, 2005); a more detailed framework of functional status is provided by Leidy (1994). QOL is an even broader construct than HRQOL: inclusive of all life domains important to a person. The construct HRQOL developed as an entity separate from global QOL as a means of specifying health-related domains of particular interest to researchers (Wenger, Naughton, & Furberg, 1996). Its concepts "tend to cross different nursing fields and reflect a wide variety of nursing situations" (Meleis, 1997, p. 18).

Some authors have used the term *subjective health status* interchangeably with HRQOL, considering it a more accurate descriptor of the phenomenon (Staniszewska, 1998). However, Ferrans categorized approaches to HRQOL measurement as *perceived status* or *evaluative* approaches to HRQOL (Ferrans, Zerwic, Wilbur, & Larson, 2005). HRQOL *perceived* status measures ask patients to rate their functional abilities, such as the commonly used SF-36 survey (Ware & Sherbourne, 1992) and the EORTC Quality of Life Questionnaire (Aaronson et al., 1993). Alternatively, HRQOL *evaluation* measures, such as the Ferrans and Powers Quality of Life Index (Ferrans, 1990a) and the Quality of Life Scale for Cancer (Padilla et al., 1983), place less emphasis on the specific functional abilities and more emphasis on the patient's perception of how satisfied he or she is with his or her abilities or life domains. Both status and evaluation measures have a purpose in research. Perceived status may be helpful in testing specific effects of an intervention, while evaluation status may capture more personal judgments of life satisfaction based on internal expectations that are changeable within the individual. Some measures incorporate both status and evaluative approaches. Such is the case with the WHO Quality of Life Assessment, which covers physical, psychological, social, and spiritual domains, and as a result is quite lengthy (World Health Organization, 1995). The McGill Quality of Life Questionnaire uses evaluation approaches for its four domains, with additional status approaches for two of these domains (Cohen, Mount, Strobel, & Bui, 1995).

Despite significant confusion over related terminology, theorists and researchers have increasingly described the constructs of QOL and HRQOL as having three characteristics: HRQOL is *multidimensional, temporal,* and *subjective.* The multidimensional aspect of HRQOL (Aaronson et al., 1993; Faden & Leplege, 1992; Staniszewska, 1998) is reflected by the major life domains, commonly identified as physiological, psychological, and sociological (Padilla & Grant, 1985). Other investigators have stated that a spiritual domain is of importance (Ferrans & Powers, 1985; Cella & Tulsky, 1990). Recent publications have featured physical, psychosocial, spiritual, emotional, and cognitive/mental dimensions. Osoba (1994) has suggested that researchers can appropriately refer to their study as measuring HRQOL if at least three life domains received assessment.

HRQOL is temporal in nature; patients can change their self-perceptions as they experience events in everyday life and process what they feel are quality-of-life priorities (Sprangers & Schwartz, 1999; Peplau, 1994). Some scholars state that HRQOL is primarily subjective in nature but may include objective assessments at times (Oleson, 1990; Zhan, 1991). However, most researchers now consider HRQOL as subjective in nature (Cella, 1992; Cooley, 1998; Harrison, Juniper, & Mitchell-DiCenso, 1996; Murdaugh, 1997). Further investigation is needed for practical considerations related to ethical implications of allowing those other than the patients to make treatment decisions based on assumed HRQOL when the patients are unable to speak for themselves, such as those in vegetative states. Work has been done to test the validity of parallel administration of subjective HRQOL with proxy health status measures completed for patients by health care providers or family members (Addington-Hall & Kalra, 2001). Measures obtained by others would be most accurately referred to as proxy subjective health status or evaluation measures rather than HRQOL.

DESCRIPTION OF THE THEORY OF QUALITY OF LIFE AND HEALTH-RELATED QUALITY OF LIFE

There are many models of QOL or HRQOL (Cowan, Graham, & Cochrane, 1992; Ferrell, Grant, Dean, Funk, & Ly, 1996; Ferrans, 1990b; Oleson, 1990; Padilla & Grant, 1985; Zhan, 1992, as found in King & Hinds, 1998), most of which omit the relationship between specific interventions and the factors that affect HRQOL. Three seminal models of QOL were provided in the 1990s. Spilker (1996) provided an introductory framework for QOL in health care by illustrating QOL as a pyramid of three levels (Fig. 13.1). A model by Ferrans and Powers (1993) also identified QOL as a main outcomes measure, rather than HRQOL (Fig. 13.2). However, HRQOL researchers have sometimes chosen to concentrate on specific parts of the model rather than the entire model. Researchers have adapted models for use according to the specific condition or population they wish to study (Sandau, Lindquist, Treat-Jacobson, & Savik, 2008). While technically a model may be designed to illustrate QOL, clinicians wishing to research the more limited construct of HRQOL have made adaptations. Researchers should provide clarity about how any adapted or abbreviated conceptual definition supports their selected operational measures.

Nurses Ferrans and Powers developed a theory in which they provided the seminal definition of QOL as a person's "sense of well-being that stems from satisfaction or dissatisfaction with the areas of life that

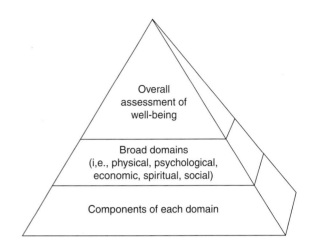

Figure 13.1 Three levels of quality of life. (From Spilker, B. (Ed.). (1996). *Quality of life and pharmacoeconomics in clinical trials* (2nd ed., p. 2). Philadelphia, PA: Lippincott-Raven.)

are important to him/her" (Ferrans & Powers, 1992, p. 29). Since their model encompassed all major life domains, their resulting operational measure, the Ferrans and Powers QOL Index, is a global multidimensional measure designed to represent the comprehensive construct of QOL (Fig. 13.2). The listed domains are health and functioning, socioeconomic, psychological/spiritual, and family.

A commonly cited model in health care disciplines is that of Wilson and Cleary (1995). Although both authors are physicians, the model combines the "social" paradigm with the "medical" paradigm. This model represents the relationships between the basic concepts of QOL (Fig. 13.3). The model identifies five determinants that exist on a "continuum of increasing biological, social, and psychological complexity" (p. 60). These leveled determinants of QOL are referred to as taxonomy and consist of biological factors, symptoms, functioning, general health perceptions, and overall QOL. They are in turn influenced by characteristics of the individual and environment.

Sousa and colleagues tested the Wilson and Cleary model, using multiple linear regression path analysis to evaluate the variables for empirical linkages to overall QOL (Sousa, Holzemer, Henry, & Slaughter, 1999). They reported that data were consistent with the theory, and reported a 32% variance in overall

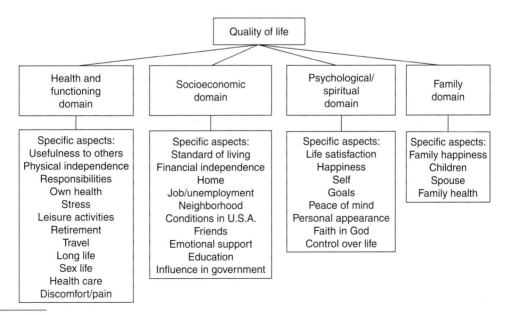

Figure 13.2 Quality of life framework. (From Ferrans, C. E. (1990). Quality of life: Conceptual issues. *Seminars in Oncology Nursing, 6*[4] 248–254.)

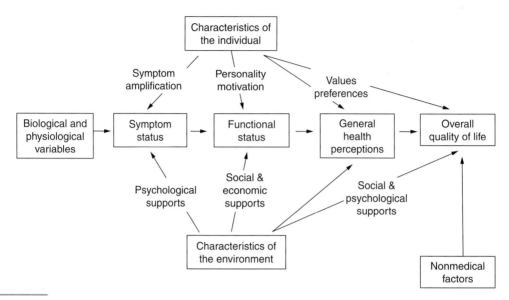

Figure 13.3 HRQOL conceptual model. (From Wilson, I. B., & Cleary, P. D. (1995). Linking clinical variables with health-related quality of life. *JAMA, 273*[1], 60.)

QOL among their sample of persons with human immunodeficiency virus (HIV). However, biological and physiological variables provided the weakest correlations with the other variables, suggesting little influence. The authors indicated that further research was necessary in areas such as other potential influences of personality, motivation, and social and economic supports, as well as the influences of time over the model (Sousa et al., 1999). Sousa and Chen (2002) continued work using structural equation modeling to address conceptual issues of HRQOL. The Wilson and Cleary model encompasses several large constructs as variables, so theory testing the model in its entirety is an intensive feat and is rarely done.

Anderson and Burckhardt (1999) suggest that a major limitation of the Wilson and Cleary model is that the medical factors seem central, rather than the nonmedical factors, to the overall QOL. Similarly, Murdaugh (1997) contends that the Wilson and Cleary model may be more accurately referred to as a taxonomy of patient outcomes due to its continuum of intuitively linked pathways with little empirical support. The majority of variance for overall QOL was unexplained, and many questions remain. Further study of relationships between other variables that can be affected by independent nursing interventions affecting QOL and HRQOL (such as interventions to support resiliency, self-efficacy, and hope) is encouraged.

Wilson and Cleary have described the arrows in the figure to represent the dominant causal relationships without excluding reciprocal connections between either adjacent or nonadjacent components of the model. Ferrans and nursing colleagues offered a revision to the Wilson and Cleary model (Ferrans et al., 2005), in which they made three major changes: (a) added arrows to show that biological function is influenced by characteristics of the environment and individual, (b) deleted nonmedical factors, and (c) deleted labeling on arrows, which tends to restrict relationships.

Work by Padilla and Grant (1985) occurred as early as the above models, but aside from the oncology realm, appears to have been less recognized among health disciplines. Their work deserves discussion because it offered one of the first QOL models to specifically include independent nursing process interventions as a component in the formal model (Fig. 13.4). These include caring attitude, specific nursing interventions, and promotion of self-care. These interventions are perceived by the patient and influence outcome variables that can be categorized by QOL dimensions. For example, the nursing interventions to promote healthy body image in a patient with a new colostomy can influence the patient's overall QOL by contributing to enhanced or maintained body image. Extraneous variables are recognized in the model, such as the individual's prognosis and personal characteristics, and whether the colostomy is temporary or permanent.

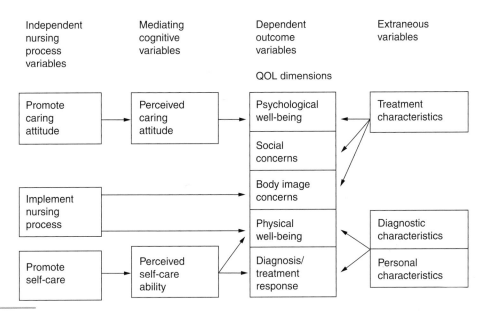

Figure 13.4 A model of the relationship between the nursing process and the dimensions of quality of life. (From Padilla, G. V., & Grant, M. M. (1985). Quality of life as a cancer nursing outcome variable. *Advances in Nursing Science, 8*[1], 45–60.)

Nurse researchers Haase and colleagues (Haase, Heiney, Ruccione, & Stutzer, 1999) used a mixed-method approach to first derive a conceptually valid understanding of what QOL is by interviewing adolescents; they then developed a measurement tool. Qualitative methods of phenomenology, simultaneous concept analysis, focus groups, and thematic analysis were used to generate their Adolescent Resilience Model. The authors defined QOL as a sense of well-being, but measured it based on self-transcendence, mastery, and self-esteem. Testing of the model began by administering existing quantitative instruments and used structural equation modeling. The model consisted of six indirectly measured variables: awareness of condition; ways of coping; relationships with others; spirituality, hope, and spiritual perspective; being courageous; and the outcome variable of QOL. Work continues on this model as the authors study influences of stage of illness and combination of variables into higher-order factors to provide a better fit in the model (Haase et al., 1999).

For their model, nurse researchers Stuifbergen and colleagues (2000) used structural equation modeling to test the selected factors influencing health-promoting behavior or QOL in persons with chronic disabling conditions. QOL was defined as "an individual's overall sense of health, well-being, and satisfaction with life" (2000, p. 124). A complex interaction of contextual factors (severity of illness being most dominant), antecedent variables, and health-promoting behaviors all contributed to QOL in their proposed model. Interventions to enhance mediating factors of social support, acceptance, decreased barriers to self-efficacy, and increased self-efficacy for health behavior can contribute to health-promoting factors and enhanced QOL. The purposeful use of concepts that are currently being tested in nursing makes this model unique to nursing and within the scope of independent nursing interventions. In addition, Leplege and Hunt (1997) commended the authors for acknowledging the interconnectedness of QOL with other aspects of existence such as changes in work, coping strategies, personal relationships, and self-image.

APPLICATIONS OF THE THEORY

Dudgeon (1992) suggested that past conflicts occurring between nurses and physicians over the care of patients with incurable illness might be mitigated by interdisciplinary cooperative efforts to improve

Harrison and colleagues conducted a 12-week, prospective, randomized controlled trial to evaluate the effect of transitional care on HRQOL, rates of readmission, and emergency room use of patients with heart failure ($n = 157$). The nurse-led intervention included education and support for self-management for a period of two weeks after hospital discharge. HRQOL was operationalized by using both a generic health status (SF-36) and a disease-specific QOL measure (Minnesota Living with Heart Failure [MLHFQ] questionnaire). At six weeks after hospital discharge, the overall MLHFQ score was better among the patients randomized to receive the nurse-led intervention than among the usual care patients. However, there was no significant difference in any of the subscales for the SF-36. At 12 weeks after discharge, more of the control group had been readmitted compared to the intervention group (31% vs. 23%); and significantly more of the usual care group visited the emergency department compared with the transitional group (46% vs. 29%). This study provides evidence-based support for nurse-led interventions to successfully improve HRQOL.

The article, like many published in clinical journals, lacked a conceptual definition for HRQOL. However, the authors are to be commended for attempting to address whether or not the statistically significant improvements on the MLHFQ could be considered clinically significant. The authors added a "minimally clinical importance difference" (MCID) analysis, which they defined as a five-point or greater change in the total MLHFQ score. Relative changes in score between baseline and 12 weeks postdischarge were compared for both groups; the most contrast in scores was with the MLHFQ emotional dimension, where improvement was 36% for the transitional group (vs. <1% for the control group). Finally, the fact that the generic SF-36 scores were not improved, while the MLHFQ scores were improved, highlights the importance of knowing one's sample and selecting a measure that will be sensitive to changes expected by a particular intervention in a select population.

USING MIDDLE RANGE THEORIES

13.1

Source: Harrison, M. B., Browne, G. B., Roberts, J., Tugwell, P., Gafni, A., & Graham, A. D. (2002). QOL of individuals with heart failure: A randomized trial of the effectiveness of two models of hospital-to-home transition. *Medical Care, 40*(4), 271–282.

HRQOL. Interdisciplinary efforts based on HRQOL theory provide a bridging between the biomedical and illness models of medicine and nursing.

HRQOL measurement provides an understanding of the patient-perceived outcome experience of chronic illness, evaluation of a procedure, medication, or other intervention between groups, among individuals, or between populations. More recently, HRQOL measures have been used to evaluate efforts of health promotion, including independent nursing interventions such as education and counseling (see Using Middle Range Theories 13.1). Use of formal HRQOL measures has not been routine in clinical practice. The gap between research and clinical practice is fed by the lack of understanding the definition of HRQOL and that HRQOL measures are not "soft" measures but helpful in clinical practice (Rumsfeld, 2002). Rubenstein (1996) provided a table summary of recommendations for incorporating routine and symptom-specific HRQOL screenings into office practice. McClane (2006) recommended three specific HRQOL measures for use by clinical nurse specialists in routine clinical assessment of elderly persons.

INSTRUMENTS USED IN EMPIRICAL TESTING

CATEGORIES OF MEASUREMENT

Measurement tools for HRQOL can be categorized in a variety of ways. For example, one category of measure is based on the number of life domains that are encompassed within the measure. If a tool is designed to examine a full spectrum of life domains, it may be considered *global*. Global tools are important because they may show QOL changes in all domains of life. Heart failure, for example, may have a pervasive effect on patients' ability to generate income, socialize, and be sexually intimate. The Minnesota Living with Heart Failure (Rector, Kubo, & Cohen, 1987) questionnaire attempts to capture a global

TABLE 13.1 Measures Commonly Used to Assess HRQOL

Type	Examples
Generic measures	Ferrans and Powers Quality of Life Index (Ferrans & Powers, 1992) WHOQOL Assessment Tool (World Health Organization, 1995) Nottingham Health Profile (Hunt, McEwan, & McKenna, 1985) SF-36 (Ware & Sherbourne, 1992) EuroQOL (EuroQOL Group, 1990) Sickness Impact Profile (Bergner et al., 1981)
Disease-specific, condition-specific, and treatment-specific measures	Ferrans and Powers Quality of Life Index—Cancer Version (Ferrans, 1990a) Minnesota Living With Heart Failure (Rector et al., 1987) Seattle Angina Questionnaire (Spertus et al., 1995) The Arthritis Impact Measurement Scales (Meenan, 1992) Children's Health Survey for Asthma (Sullivan et al., 1995) Quality of Life Index: Hemodialysis (Ferrans & Powers, 1993) QLQ-C30 Version 3.0 is the generic measure that can be supplemented with disease-specific modules (breast, lung, head & neck, oesophageal, ovarian, gastric, and cervical cancers, and multiple myeloma) (Aaronson et al., 1993)
Symptom-specific measures	McGill Pain Questionnaire (Melzack, 1975) Hospital Anxiety and Depression Scale (Zigmond & Snaith, 1983)
Quality-adjusted life-year (QALY), health utilities, and time trade-off measures	EQ-5D (Agt, Essink-Bot, Krabbe, & Bonsel, 1990) Time Without Symptoms or Toxicity (Q-TWIST) (Gelber et al., 1996)
Qualitative measures	Interviews Focus groups Preference-based with interview script

perspective of the impact of a specific disease on various domains of life. In contrast to global measures, another category is that of measures that target a single domain, such as psychological health, as is offered by the Hospital Anxiety and Depression Scale (Zigmond & Snaith, 1983).

Table 13.1 provides one method of categorizing types of tools used to measure QOL and HRQOL. *Generic* tools, while not specific to disease or treatment, are helpful for making comparisons across studies and between populations (Guyatt, Feeny, & Patrick, 1993). The Nottingham Health Profile has been commonly used in the UK as a generic tool, but is also considered global because of its broad coverage of various life domains (Hunt, McEwen, & McKenna, 1985). The SF-36, which is a generic measure of subjective health status, provides two main summary scores for self-perceived physical and mental functioning, as well as eight more specific health scales (Ware & Sherbourne, 1992).

Recently, researchers have tended toward augmenting generic measures with *disease- or condition-specific measures* in order to capture both overall health status and perceived effects of a certain condition (Bliven, Green, & Spertus, 1998). Disease-, condition-, or symptom-specific tools provide more sensitivity than generic tools for clinicians looking for changes in disease patterns, such as frequency of loose stools or angina. Similarly, use of treatment or therapy-specific tools is helpful to care providers in evaluating specific responses by individual patients to treatments or changes as a result of intervention (see Using Middle Range Theories 13.1).

A quality-adjusted life-year (QALY) instrument is used by some researchers to measure the extent of health improvement due to an intervention combined with the costs associated with the intervention, resulting in a mathematical formula that is used to assess their relative worth of the intervention from an economic perspective (Phillips & Thompson, 2007). For example, a year of perfect health may be worth a score of 1, but a year of less than perfect health life expectancy may be worth −1 point, and death may be worth 0 points. These measures are somewhat controversial and limited in chronic illness, where QOL is more important than survival, and limited by heterogeneity in the samples being measured (Phillips & Thompson, 2007). They are used most often in pharmacoeconomic studies.

Finally, qualitative measures are valuable for development of theoretical definitions and new HRQOL measures, as well as for validity testing of an existing tool in a new or changing population. Qualitative measures may be used to augment a quantitative measure. Typically, qualitative methodologies in HRQOL include personal interviews and focus groups, with possible open-ended questions.

GUIDELINES FOR MEASUREMENT

Investigators selecting measures for HRQOL studies must make sure that they have a clear conceptual definition of HRQOL, and their selection of operational measures should match. Unfortunately, this has not always been the case in the early surge of HRQOL studies. An investigator attempting to measure HRQOL among hospice patients should consider which domains are conceptually important, or have been shown in past research or through clinical experience, to be important in that population. For example, an HRQOL investigator wishing to assess HRQOL among hospice patients would appropriately select a measure that includes the spiritual domain, or augment a generic measure with assessment of subjective spiritual status. Similarly, if an investigator plans to use a generic HRQOL measure among patients undergoing treatment for prostate cancer, this generic measure would most appropriately be augmented by a subjective measure that includes self-evaluation of the social and sexual dimensions.

Gill and Feinstein (1994) provided guidelines for proper measurement of HRQOL, including allowing patients to rate the importance of domains, as in the Ferrans and Powers QOL Index (1992). Gill and Feinstein also recommended allowing patients to supplement standardized measures. Although supplementing quantitative measures with qualitative measures may not be feasible in every study, this practice may provide a test of content validity to the quantitative measure. Study participants may alert investigators of important concerns that were not addressed on the quantitative questionnaire. Similarly, qualitative research in HRQOL, such as interviews, focus groups, and journaling, may provide foundational information for researchers striving to measure HRQOL in a previously understudied population. Although Gill and Feinstein encouraged HRQOL investigators to provide an aggregate score so that study results can be compared with others, some debate the conceptual clarity of mathematically combining several measures to produce an artificially aggregated score. However, obtaining a global satisfaction measure in addition to disease-specific measures may be helpful for comparing results for specific interventions in a discrete population.

Researchers studying HRQOL must be prepared to address challenges in psychometric properties among the vast variety of measures available. Challenges to reliability include aberrancies in data collection (such as one research assistant giving more extensive coaching to some participants than others), the absence of a baseline HRQOL measure, and the use of only pieces of HRQOL measures (unless they have been tested for reliability as a subset). Challenges to validity in HRQOL research include potential concurrent life changes. For example, an investigator wishing to study the effect of an intervention for back pain may have confounding results when a generic HRQOL measure is complicated by a life change in a participant (e.g., loss of spouse) that is unrelated to the treatment for back pain. Practical considerations in use of HRQOL measures include timing of study measures. For example, if one is evaluating how a surgery such as mastectomy may affect HRQOL, it may not be appropriate to obtain measures while the patient is still recovering from postoperative incisional pain, unless the investigator's intention is a purposeful longitudinal assessment. Other practical considerations include subject burden (length of the survey) and clinical relevance (what degree of change in a score will be considered clinically significant). Further discussion of desired psychometric properties of HRQOL measures are provided by DeVon and Ferrans (2003). In summary, selection of a measure includes finding a good match with one's conceptual definition of HRQOL, identifying the life domains and concerns most important to the study population, being clear on the research purpose, investigating past performance of the measure for validity and reliability, and evaluating feasibility of the measure.

Research Application   **13.1**

A nurse researcher was interested in determining whether the inclusion of a nurse-run education and peer-support group improved the outcomes for elementary-school-aged asthmatics. Using a prospective research design, in an asthma clinic, the researcher matched patients by age, nature and severity of symptoms, and treatment regimens. The patients were randomly assigned to either group involvement or no group involvement. Before treatment began, the nurse researcher administered the Pediatric Asthma Quality of Life Questionnaire (AQOLQ-P, see Appendix B) to a new patient, a 10-year-old male. The patient was asked to identify the life domains most affected by the asthma, and he selected "activity limitations" domain, which included riding his bicycle, playing recreational baseball, and playing tag with his friends. The patient also chose the "symptoms" domain, and he identified getting a good night's sleep and being disturbed at school with coughing. The patient then completed the self-administered AQOLQ-P.

The patient, through random selection, was placed in the experimental treatment group. The group met weekly for three months. At the end of the three-month period, the patient returned to the asthma clinic, and the nurse researcher readministered the questionnaire, addressing the same domains that were assessed the first time. Any changes in the ratings fell along a continuum from positive to negative, with positive indicating that a desired outcome relating to HRQOL was achieved. The individual patient data were grouped with other data, and, through statistical analysis, the researcher determined if the group treatment made a statistically significant difference in the QOL outcomes in elementary-school-aged children diagnosed with asthma.

HEALTH-RELATED QUALITY OF LIFE AS AN OUTCOME MEASURE IN NURSING

The goal of nursing interventions in HRQOL research is to have a positive impact on a patient's perceived satisfaction with HRQOL (see Research Application 13.1). This is a central component of HRQOL in that the patient provides a subjective and personal expression of both the level of satisfaction (Staniszewska, 1998) and the degree to which the specific nursing interventions contribute to that level (Robinson, Whyte, & Fidler, 1997). Thus, patient-perceived satisfaction with HRQOL becomes a significant indicator of the success of an intervention. Patient satisfaction is conceptualized as a mediating variable, based on the work of Donabedian (1980), who has consistently regarded patient satisfaction as an outcome. He contended that satisfaction with care represents the patient's judgment of quality of care (Yang, Simms, & Yin, 1999, p. 3).

The Cochrane Database has begun to publish reviews evaluating the effectiveness of specific nursing interventions on QOL or HRQOL. By reviewing results in the Cochrane database for *nursing interventions* and *quality of life,* one can learn, for example, whether breast care nurses can improve QOL for patients (Cruickshank, Kennedy, Lockhart, Dosser, & Dallas, 2008). A more extensive review of Cochrane studies using the terms *nursing* and *quality of life* provides readers with a realistic and somewhat sobering overview of attempts by nurses to improve QOL. The reader is left with a sense that (a) comparatively few nursing interventional studies with QOL as an outcome variable currently exist with randomized or comparison groups, and (b) most nursing interventional studies may be better off avoiding a hypothesis that the outcome of global QOL will be an improved outcome of a single nursing intervention.

What may be a realistic goal for nursing interventions is to make a clinically meaningful improvement in a particular domain, such as the social or mental domain, rather than expect changes to the huge construct of QOL (or even HRQL), which are immense outcome variables potentially affected by a myriad of confounding factors. It may be easier for researchers studying a surgical or pharmaceutical intervention to report improvements to overall QOL, but as nurses, we remember that life continues to present some complex conditions for which there is no simple cure. It is for these conditions (i.e., HIV, end-of-life, heart failure, diabetes, and depression) that we should perhaps most energetically focus our efforts. Our work to identify, and combat alongside our patients, the persistent conditions of depression and anxiety, for example, that occur concomitant with chronic conditions, provide us with challenges for years to come.

Researchers wishing to evaluate the impact of specific nursing interventions on HRQL should consider which specific domain or part of a domain their interventions will most likely impact. For example, though the Cochrane review of interventions by breast care nurses (Cruickshank et al., 2008) was unable to support a significant impact on overall QOL, the review reported early evidence (tempered by lack of large sample sizes) that interventions by breast care nurses significantly improved anxiety and helped early recognition of depressive symptoms (major factors in the psychosocial domain of HRQL). Likewise, though a Cochrane review of structured nursing interventions among patients with lung cancer (Solà, Thompson, Subirana Casacuberta, Lopez, & Pascual) found no improvement in overall QOL, significant results were seen for symptom management of breathlessness as well as some improvements in emotional functioning. These are respectable and important contributions to people living with a complex and potentially isolating disease. Further, researchers have found depression to be an independent predictor for both physical and mental well-being (Mallik et al., 2005); thus, nursing interventions may have an effect difficult to measure but nonetheless contributory toward overall life quality.

Nursing researchers investigating HRQOL often use approaches and interventions from other models and theories, allowing connections to be made between HRQOL and these models or theories. For instance, Stuifbergen, Seraphine, and Roberts (2000) related health-promoting behaviors from Pender's theory with HRQOL as an outcome. HRQOL as a middle range theory allows for concurrent application of theories that support health within illness, a concept thread that runs through the work of Peplau, Rogers, Parse, Newman, and others (Moch, 1989; Newman, 1984; Parse, 1994; Peplau, 1994; Rogers, 1970). As previously discussed, HRQL is subjective, and therefore we must listen to the patient's own summaries. As a theorist and researcher Ferrans concludes, "A disability that makes life not worth living to one person may only be a nuisance to another" (Ferrans, 1990b, p. 252).

SUMMARY

HRQOL is *subjective, multidimensional,* and *temporal.* As an interdisciplinary middle range theory, HRQOL is particularly well matched to nursing because it involves measurement of variables that have traditionally been important to nursing, that is, holistic consideration of the person's responses to real or potential illness. QOL is a concept with a long history, which has, in the last 20 years, become of interest to a number of disciplines. Models of the middle range theory, HRQOL, often comprise three components: (a) *Life domains* refer to the areas of life being affected by a specific condition; (b) *interventions* involve the actions taken to bring about a desired outcome, an improved QOL; and (c) *perceived satisfaction* is the patient's subjective appraisal of well-being. Nurses wishing to understand the impact of a condition on their patients or to judge the effectiveness of an illness treatment can make use of this middle range theory and the instruments designed to measure it.

ANALYSIS OF THEORY

Using the criteria presented in Chapter 2, critique the model of HRQOL suggested by Wilson and Cleary (1995). Compare your conclusions about the theory with those found in Appendix A. A researcher who has worked with the theory completed the analysis found in the Appendix.

Internal Criticism	External Criticism
1. Clarity	1. Reality convergence
2. Consistency	2. Utility
3. Adequacy	3. Significance
4. Logical development	4. Discrimination
5. Level of theory development	5. Scope of theory
	6. Complexity

CRITICAL THINKING EXERCISES

1. Does HRQOL have subjective and objective components?

2. What are the underlying assumptions and potential ramifications of having proxy subjective health status or evaluation measures for children or those unable to speak for themselves?

3. Should further measurement tools only be accepted if based on commonly accepted conceptual definitions?

4. What are appropriate ways for researchers to test validity of HRQOL measures within their population? (Should an HRQOL measure be tested against an objective health status measure?)

WEB RESOURCES

Visit **http://thePoint.lww.com/Peterson3e** for helpful web resources related to this chapter.

REFERENCES

Aaronson, N. K., Ahmedzai, S., Bergman, B., Bullinger, M., Cull, A., & Duez, N., et al. (1993). The European Organization for Research and Treatment of Cancer QLQ-C30: A quality-of-life instrument for use in international clinical trials in oncology. *Journal of the National Cancer Institute, 85*, 365–376.

Addington-Hall, J., & Kalra, J. (2001). Measuring quality of life: Who should measure quality of life? *British Medical Journal, 332*, 1417–1420.

Agt, H. M. V., Essink-Bot, M. L., Krabbe, P. F., & Bonsel, G. J. (1994). Test–retest reliability of health state valuations collected with the EuroQol questionnaire. *Social Science Medicine, 39*(11), 1537–1544.

Anderson, K. L., & Burckhardt, C. S. (1999). Conceptualization and measurement of quality of life as an outcomes variable for health care intervention and research. *Journal of Advanced Nursing, 29*(2), 298–306.

Bergner, M., Bobbitt, R. A., Carter, W. B., & Gilson, B. S. (1981). The Sickness Impact Profile: Development and final revision of a health status measure. *Medical Care, 19*, 787–805.

Bliven, B. D., Green, P., & Spertus, J. A. (1998). Review of available instruments and methods for assessing QOL in anti-anginal trials. *Drugs & Aging, 13*(4), 311–320.

Campbell, A. (1981). *The sense of well being in America.* New York: McGraw-Hill.

Cella, D. F. (1992). Quality of life: The concept. *Journal of Palliative Care, 8*(3), 40–45.

Cella, D. F., & Tulsky, D. S. (1990). Measuring quality of life today: Methodological aspects. *Oncology, 4*(5), 29–38.

Cohen, S. R., Mount, B. M., Strobel, M., & Bui, F. (1995). The McGill Quality of Life Questionnaire: A measure of quality of life appropriate for people with advanced disease. *Palliative Medicine, 9*, 207–291.

Cooley, M. E. (1998). Quality of life in persons with non-small cell lung cancer: A concept analysis. *Cancer Nursing, 21*(3), 151–161.

Cowan, M. J., Young Graham, K., & Cochrane, B. L. (Jan 1992). Comparison of a theory of quality of life between myocardial infarction and malignant Melanoma: A pilot study. *Progress in Cardiovascular Nursing, 7*(1), 18–21.

Cruickshank, S., Kennedy, C., Lockhart, K., Dosser, I., & Dallas, L. (2008). Specialist breast care nurses for supportive care of women with breast cancer. *Cochrane Database of Systematic Reviews,* (1). Art. No., CD005634. doi:10.1002/14651858.CD005634.pub2

Dalkey, N. C., Rourke, D. L., Lewis, R., & Snyder, D. (1972). *Studies in the quality of life, delphi and decision making.* Toronto, ON: Lexington Books, D.C. Heath and Company.

DeVon, H. A., & Ferrans, C. E. (2003). The psychometric properties of four quality of life instruments used in cardiovascular populations. *Journal of Cardiopulmonary Rehabilitation, 23*(2), 122–138.

Donabedian, A. (1980). *The definition of quality and approaches to its assessment.* Ann Arbor, MI: Health Administration Press.

Dudgeon, D. (1992). QOL: A bridge between the biomedical and illness models of medicine and nursing? *Journal of Palliative Care, 8*(3), 14–17.

Elkins, R. C., Knott-Craif, C. J., McCue, C., & Lane, M. M. (1997). Congenital aortic valve disease: Improved survival and quality of life. *Annals of Surgery, 225*(5), 503–511.

EuroQol Group. (1990). EuroQol—A new facility for the measurement of health-related QOL. *Health Policy, 16*, 199–208.

Faden, R., & Leplege, A. (1992). Assessing quality of life, moral implications for clinical practice. *Medical Care, 30*(5, Suppl.), 166–175.

Ferrans, C. E. (1990a). Development of a quality of life index for patients with cancer. *Oncology Nursing Forum, 17*, 15–19.

Ferrans, C. E. (1990b). Quality of life: Conceptual issues. *Seminars in Oncology Nursing, 6*(4), 248–254.

Ferrans, C., & Powers, M. (1985). Quality of Life Index: Development and psychometric properties. *Advances in Nursing Science, 8*, 15–24.

Ferrans, C., & Powers, M. (1992). Psychometric assessment of the Quality of Life Index. *Research in Nursing and Health, 15*, 29–38.

Ferrans, C. E., & Powers, M. J. (1993). QOL of hemodialysis patients. *ANNA Journal, 20*(5), 575–582.

Ferrans, C. E., Zerwic, J. J., Wilbur, J. E., & Larson, J. L. (2005). Conceptual model of health-related QOL. *Journal of Nursing Scholarship, 37*(4), 336–342.

Ferrell, B. R., Grant, M., Dean, G. E., Funk, B., & Ly, J. (1996). "Bone tired": The experience of fatigue and its impact on quality of life. *Oncology Nursing Forum, 23*, 1539–1547.

Gelber, R. D., Goldhirsch, A., Cole, B. F., Wieand, H. S., Schoeder, G., & Krrok, J. E. (1996). A quality-adjusted time without symptoms or toxicity (Q-TWiST) analysis of adjuvant radiation therapy and chemotherapy for resectable rectal cancer. *Journal of the National Cancer Institute, 88*(15), 1039–1045.

Gill, T., & Feistein, A. (1994). A critical appraisal of the quality-of-life measurements. *The Journal of the American Medical Association, 272*, 619–620.

Guyatt, G. H., Feeny, D. H., & Patrick, D. L. (1993). Measuring health-related quality of life. *Annals of Internal Medicine, 118*, 622–628.

Haase, J. E., Heiney, S. P., Ruccione, K. S., & Stutzer, C. (1999). Research triangulation to derive meaning-based quality-of-life theory: Adolescent resilience model and instrument development. *International Journal of Cancer, 12*, 125–131.

Harrison, M. B., Juniper, E. F., & Mitchell-DiCenso, A. (1996). Quality of life as an outcomes measure in nursing research: "May you have a long and healthy life." *Canadian Journal of Nursing Research, 28*(3), 49–68.

Hunt, S. M., McEwen, J., & McKenna, S. P. (1985). Measuring health status: A new tool for clinicians and epidemiologists. *Journal of the Royal College of General Practitioners, 35*, 185–188.

King, C., & Hinds, P. (1998). *Quality of life.* Sudbury, MA: Jones and Bartlett.

Leidy, N. K. (1994). Functional status and the forward progress of merry-go-rounds: Toward a coherent analytic framework. *Nursing Research, 43*, 196–202.

Leplege, A., & Hunt, S. (1997). The problem of quality of life in medicine. *The Journal of the American Medical Association, 278*, 47–50.

The Lockman Foundation (Eds.). (1995). *New American standard bible.* Chicago, IL: Moody Press.

Mallik S., Krumholz H. M., Lin Z. Q., Kasl S., Mattera J. A., & Roumains S. A., et al. (2005). Depression as a risk factor for coronary artery disease: Evidence, mechanisms, and treatment. *Circulation, 111*, 271–277.

McClane, K. S. (2006). Screening instruments for use in a complete geriatric assessment. *Clinical Nurse Specialist, 20*(4), 201–206.

Meenan, R. F., Mason, J. H., Anderson, J. J., Guccione, A. A., & Kazis, L. E. (1992). AIMS2. The content and properties of a revised and expanded Arthritis Impact Measurement Scales Health Status Questionnaire. *Arthritis and Rheumatism, 35*(1), 1–10.

Meleis, A. I. (1997). *Theoretical nursing: Development and progress* (3rd ed.). Philadelphia, PA: Lippincott-Raven.

Melzack, R. (1975). The McGill Pain Questionnaire: Major properties and scoring methods. *Pain, 1*, 277–299.

Moch, S. D. (1989). Health within illness: Conceptual evolution and practice possibilities. *Advances in Nursing Science, 11*(4), 23–31.

Morgan, M. L. (1992). *Classics of moral and political theory.* Indianapolis, IN: Hacket.

Murdaugh, C. R. (1997). Health-related quality of life as an outcome in organizational research. *Medical Care, 35*(11 Suppl.), NS41–NS48.

Newman, M. A. (1984). Nursing diagnosis: looking at the whole. *American Journal of Nursing, 85*, 1496–1499.

Oleson, M. (1990). Subjectively perceived quality of life. *Image: Journal of Nursing Scholarship, 22*(3), 187–190.

Osoba, D. (1994). Lessons learned from measuring health-related quality of life in oncology. *Journal of Clinical Oncology, 12*, 199–220.

Padilla, G. V., & Grant, M. M. (1985). QOL as a cancer nursing outcome variable. *Advances in Nursing Science, 8*(1), 45–60.

Padilla, G. V., Presant, C., Grant, M. M. Metter, G., Lipselt, J., & Heide, F. (1983). Quality of life index for patients with cancer. *Research in Nursing and Health, 6*(3), 117–126.

Parse, R. R. (1994). Quality of life: Sciencing and living the art of human becoming. *Nursing Science Quarterly, 7*(1), 16–20.

Peplau, H. E. (1994). Quality of life: An interpersonal perspective. *Nursing Science Quarterly, 7*(1), 10–15.

Phillips, C., & Thompson, G. (2007). What is a QALY? *Hayward Medical Communications, 1*(6). Retrieved January 22, 2007, from http://www.evidence-based-medicine.co.uk/what_is_series.html

Read, J. L. (1993). The new era of quality of life assessment. In S. R. Walker & R. M. Rosser (Eds.), *Quality of life assessment: Key issues in the 1990s* (pp. 3–10). London: Kluwer.

Rector, T. S., Kubo, S. H., & Cohen, J. N. (1987). Patients' self-assessment of their congestive heart failure. Part 2: Content, reliability and validity of a new measure, the Minnesota Living with Heart Failure questionnaire. *Heart Failure, 3*, 198–209.

Robinson, D., Whyte, L., & Fidler, I (1997). Quality of life measures in a high security environment. *Nursing Standard, 11*(49), 34–37.

Rogers, M. E. (1970). *An introduction to the theoretical basis of nursing.* Philadelphia, PA: Davis.

Rubenstein, L. V. (1996). Using QOL tests for patient diagnosis or screening, or to evaluate treatment. In B. Spilker (Ed.), *QOL and pharmacoeconomics in clinical trials* (2nd ed., pp. 362–372). Philadelphia: Lippincott-Raven.

Rumsfeld, J. S. (2002). Health status and clinical practice: When will they meet? (editorial). *Circulation, 106*(1), 5–7.

Sandau, K. E., Lindquist, R. A., Treat-Jacobson, D., & Savik, K. (2008). Health-related quality of life and subjective neurocognitive function three months after coronary artery bypass graft surgery. *Heart & Lung, 37*(3), 161–172.

Solà, I., Thompson, E., Subirana Casacuberta, M., Lopez, C., & Pascual, A. (2004). Non-invasive interventions for improving well-being and quality of life in patients with lung cancer. *Cochrane Database of Systematic Reviews*, (4). Art. No. CD004282. doi:10.1002/14651858.CD004282.pub2

Sousa, K. H., & Chen, F. F. (2002). A theoretical approach to measuring quality of life. *Journal of Nursing Measurements, 10*(1), 47–58.

Sousa, K. H., Holzemer, W. L., Henry, S. B., & Slaughter, R. (1999). Dimensions of health-related quality of life in persons living with HIV disease. *Journal of Advanced Nursing, 29*(1) 178–187.

Spertus, J. A., Winder, J. A., Dewhurts, T. A., Deyo, R. A., Prodzinski, J., & McDonell, M., et al. (1995). Development and evaluation of the Seattle Angina Questionnaire: A new functional status measure for coronary artery disease. *Journal of the American College of Cardiology, 25*(2), 333–341.

Spilker, B. (1996). *Quality of life and pharmaco economics in clinical trials* (2nd ed.). New York: Lippincott-Raven.

Spranger, M. J. (2001). *International Society of Quality of Life Newsletter 6*(1). Retrieved June 15, 2001, from www.ISOQOL.org

Sprangers, M. A. G., & Schwartz, C. E. (1999). Integrating response shift into health-related quality of life research: A theoretical model. *Social Science and Medicine, 48*(11), 1507–1515.

Staniszewska, S. (1998). Measuring quality of life in the evaluation of health care. *Nursing Standard, 12*(17), 36–39.

Stineman, M. G., Lollar, D. J., & Ustun, T. B. (2005). International classification of functioning, disability, and health: ICF empowering rehabilitation through an operational bio-psycho-social model. In J. A. DeLisa (Ed.), *Physical medicine and rehabilitation principles and practice* (pp. 1099–1108). Philadelphia, PA: Lippincott Williams & Wilkins.

Stryk, L. (1968). *World of Budha: A reader.* Garden City, NY: Doubleday.

Stuifbergen, A. K., Seraphine, A., & Roberts, G. (2000). An explanatory model of health promotion and quality of life in chronic disabling conditions. *Nursing Research, 49*(3), 122–129.

Sullivan, S. A., & Olson, L. M. (1995). Developing condition-specific measures of functional status and well-being for children. *Clinical Performance and Quality Health Care, 3*, 132–138.

Ware, J. E., & Sherbourne, C. D. (1992). The MOS 36-item short-form health survey (SF-36). *Medical Care, 20*, 473–483.

Wenger, N. K., Naughton, M. J., & Furberg, C. D. (1996). Cardiovascular disorders. In B. Spilker (Ed.), *Quality of life and pharmacoeconomics in clinical trials* (2nd ed., pp. 883–891). Philadelphia, PA: Lippincott-Raven.

Wilson, I. B., & Cleary, P. D. (1995). Linking clinical variables with health-related quality of life. *Journal of the American Medical Association, 273*(1), 59–65.

Wood-Dauphinee, S. (1999). Assessing quality of life in clinical research: From where have we come and where are we going? *Journal of Clinical Epidemiology, 55*, 355–363.

World Health Organization. (1948). Constitution of the World Health Organization. *Chronicle of the World Health Organization, 1*(1/2), 13.

World Health Organization. (1995). The World Health Organization Quality of Life Assessment (WHOQOL): Position paper from the World Health Organization. *Social Science and Medicine, 41*, 1403–1409.

Yang, K., Simms, L. M., & Yin, J. (1999). Factors influencing nursing-sensitive outcomes in Taiwanese nursing homes. *Journal of Issues in Nursing, 4*(2). Retrieved June 14, 2001, from www.nursingworld.org

Zhan, L. (1991). Quality of life: Conceptual and measurement issues. *Journal of Advanced Nursing, 17*, 795–800.

Zhan, L. (1992). Quality of life: Conceptual and measurement issues. *Journal of Advanced Nursing, 17*(7), 795–800.

Zigmond, A. S., & Snaith, R. P. (1993). The hospital anxiety and depression scale. *Acta Psychiatrica Scandinavica, 67*, 361–370.

BIBLIOGRAPHY

Ferrans, C. E. (1992). Conceptualizations of QOL in cardiovascular research. *Progress in Cardiovascular Nursing, 2*(7), 2–6.

King, C. R., & Hinds, P. S. (2003). *QOL: From nursing and patient perspective.* Sudbury, MA: Jones & Bartlett.

McDowell, I., & Newell, C. (1996). *Measuring health: A guide to rating scales and questionnaires* (2nd ed.). New York: Oxford University Press.

14

Health Promotion

MARJORIE COOK McCULLAGH

DEFINITIONS OF KEY TERMS

Health Promoting Behavior	Behaviors or actions that people carry out with the intention of improving their health
Prior Related Behavior	Experience with the health-promoting behavior
Personal Factors: Biological, Psychological, Sociocultural	Factors about the person that influence health-promoting behavior. Examples of biologic factors are age, body mass index, and aerobic capacity. Examples of psychologic factors are self-esteem, self-motivation, and perceived health status. Examples of sociocultural factors are race, ethnicity, acculturation, education, and socioeconomic status. The variables may be specific to each health-promoting activity, i.e., factors influencing healthy dietary behaviors may not be the same as those affecting exercise behavior
Perceived Benefits of Action	Beliefs about the positive or reinforcing consequences of a health-promoting behavior
Perceived Barriers to Action	Beliefs about the unavailability, inconvenience, expense, difficulty, or time-consuming nature of a health-promoting behavior
Perceived Self-efficacy	A person's judgment of his or her own abilities to accomplish a health-promoting behavior
Activity-related Affect	Subjective feelings associated with the health-promoting activity
Interpersonal Influences	Beliefs concerning the behaviors, the beliefs, or the attitudes of others regarding a health-promoting behavior. Ideas include social norms, social support, and modeling
Situational Influences	Beliefs about the situation or context of the health-promoting behavior. These ideas may include perceptions of the available options, demand characteristics, and aesthetic features of the environment in which a given behavior is proposed to take place
Commitment to a Plan of Action	A commitment to carry out a health-promoting behavior. The plan should be specific to time, place, and specify whether it will be with specified persons or alone
Immediate Competing Demands	Distracting ideas about other things that must be done (e.g., childcare) immediately prior to their intention to carry out a health-promoting behavior
Immediate competing preferences	Distracting ideas about other attractive activities to engage in (e.g., shopping) immediately before engaging in a health-promoting behavior

INTRODUCTION

During the past century, the major cause of health problems has shifted from infectious diseases to chronic illnesses. Many chronic illnesses are closely related to lifestyle factors such as diet, exercise, and stress management. In order to improve the health of a population experiencing high rates of chronic illness, it is apparent that changes in lifestyle factors are required.

Nurses, as well as many other health professionals, are interested in learning more about how they can help their patients, families, and communities improve their lives. In seeking a way to bring greater longevity and a higher quality of life, some nurses are attracted to interventions that enhance health and quality of living. The Health Promotion Model (Pender, Murdaugh, & Parsons, 2010) has achieved popularity among nurses as a model that serves this purpose.

Health promotion has many benefits. The benefits of living a healthier lifestyle exceed prevention of disease, and include greater vigor and a subjective feeling of wellness. While these benefits can be enjoyed by the individual, society as a whole also profits from health promotion when people create personal and family lifestyles that are consistent with economic prosperity and interpersonal harmony. Health promotion can decrease social problems, such as violence, suicide, and sexually transmitted diseases. Further, health promotion has the potential to significantly decrease health care costs in the years ahead.

Health promotion is a concept well suited to the needs and interests of nurses and their clients. Nurses commonly work in schools, churches, homes, workplaces, and health care agencies. Many of these settings are ideal locations for the promotion of health. Nurses are skilled in many areas that are necessary for health promotion, such as education, counseling, and advocacy. For example, a parish nurse may offer classes to congregational members in a variety of health-related topics such as parenting and caring for aging family members. A school nurse may facilitate self-help group meetings for bereaved children. An occupational health nurse may advocate for inclusion of mental health services in employee health benefit packages. In addition, clients are likely to be receptive to nursing interventions to promote health, because they trust nurses and are accustomed to seeking assistance of these professionals in dealing with their health care needs.

HISTORICAL BACKGROUND

Nola Pender first published her Health Promotion Model in 1982. Some early study results (Garcia et al., 1995) suggested the need for addition of concepts to the model in order to increase its predictive power. Based on the analysis of the empirical support provided by each of the studies based on the model, Pender revised the model, retaining selected model concepts, and deleting others. In addition, three new concepts and associated relationships were added to the model. The added concepts included prior related behavior, immediate competing demands and preferences, and commitment to a plan of action. These revisions to the model, based on both research and theoretical considerations, were made to increase its explanatory power and its potential for use in structuring health-promoting nursing interventions. The revised model was first published in 1996, and most recently in the sixth edition of *Health Promotion in Nursing Practice* (Pender, Murdaugh, & Parsons, 2010).

PENDER'S DEFINITION OF HEALTH

Nurses are accustomed to assessing their patients for evidence of disease or dysfunction. However, the assessment process commonly reflects a focus on illness, rather than health. This approach is limiting in several ways. First, it risks reducing the patient to a sum of his or her parts (e.g., respiratory, neurological, cardiovascular, etc.). Second, it fails to determine the meaning the client attaches to health and illness. This approach is a negative approach to health in that it views health as an absence of disease. Some consider health and illness to be opposite concepts. This way of thinking suggests that persons with disabilities, chronic illness, and those who are near death cannot achieve health. However, many nurses experienced in working with these clients may oppose this view. Negative approaches to health as the absence of illness are inadequate for health professionals at a time that they are increasingly concerned with quality of life and healthy longevity.

Pender's (2010) definition of health is positive, comprehensive, unifying, and humanistic. She believes that health includes a disease component, but does not make disease its principal element. Her definition of health encompasses the whole person and their lifestyle, and includes strengths, resiliencies, resources, potentials, and capabilities. Pender defines health as the actualization of inherent and acquired human potential through goal-directed behavior, competent self-care, and satisfying relationships with others, while adjustments are made as needed to maintain structural integrity and harmony with relevant environments.

A major strength of Pender's definition of health is that it offers an expanded view of health. This expanded view provides for greatly increased opportunities to improve client health, as it is not limited to absence of disease or even limitations in functioning or adaptation. For example, Pender's positive view of health permits the development of nursing interventions that are not limited to decreasing risks for disease, but also aimed at strengthening resources, potentials, and capabilities. This creates broader opportunities for nurses to assist individuals, families, and communities to achieve improved health, enhanced functional ability, and better quality of life.

HEALTH PROMOTION

Health professionals have long recognized the benefits of early detection and treatment of illness, or secondary prevention. However, recently there has been increased appreciation for the role of primary prevention and health promotion in improving health and quality of life. Primary prevention involves activities aimed at the prevention of health problems before they occur and the avoidance of disease. An example of primary prevention is the administration of tetanus immunization to prevent tetanus infection. Health promotion is intended to increase the level of well-being and self-actualization of an individual or group. Examples of health promotion activities include physical activity and healthy nutrition.

While health promotion and primary prevention are distinct theoretical concepts, in practice they often overlap. Many activities directed toward health promotion will also have preventive effects. Indeed, many adults engage in healthy behaviors with the dual intent of increasing wellness and avoiding illness. For example, an adult may adopt a low fat diet with two purposes in mind. One intention may be to lower blood cholesterol and, therefore, prevent future cardiovascular problems (primary prevention, also referred to by Pender as health protection). An accompanying intention may be to gain the benefits of weight loss, such as feeling more energetic (health promotion). Other examples of health behaviors that may have both health promotion and preventive benefits include physical activity, adequate rest, and management of stress.

Health promotion is activity directed toward actualization of human potential through goal-directed behavior, competent self-care, and satisfying relationships with others, while adjustments are made as needed to maintain structural integrity and harmony with relevant environments (Pender et al., 2010). The concept of health promotion is based on Pender's expanded definition of health that focuses on the whole person and promotes the positive aspects of health. This definition applies to all persons, including persons who are well, and those who are experiencing an illness or disability.

Pender advocates the use of health promotion at a variety of levels and settings. Although health promotion is most commonly directed toward the individual, Pender suggests that interventions directed toward the family and community are most likely to be successful in creating a healthy society. Furthermore, Pender discusses health promotion in a variety of settings, including schools, workplaces, homes, and nurse-managed community health centers. In a broad sense, health promotion involves education, food production, housing, employment, and health care. It is multidimensional, encompassing individual, family, community, environmental, and societal health.

DESCRIPTION OF THE HEALTH PROMOTION MODEL

Pender's model is based on theories of human behavior. There is increased recognition of the role of behavior in primary prevention and health promotion, and there is increased attention among health professionals in helping clients adopt healthy behaviors. Motivation for healthy behavior may be based on a desire to prevent illness (primary prevention) or to achieve a higher level of well-being and self-actualization (health promotion). The Pender Health Promotion Model is primarily based on two theories of health behavior: expectancy-value theory and social-cognitive theory. The first, expectancy-value theory, is based on the work by Fishbein and Ajzen (Fishbein, & Ajzen, 1975). The theory explains that people are more likely to work toward goals that are of value to them. This proposition by Fishbein and Ajzen relates to Pender's proposition that people will engage in "behaviors from which they anticipate deriving personally valued benefits" (Pender et al., 2010, p. 55). Expectancy-value theory also explains that people are more likely to invest their effort in goals that they believe are achievable and will result in the desired outcome.

The second parent theory is Bandura's (1986) social-cognitive theory. A major tenet of social-cognitive theory is self-efficacy. Self-efficacy is the confidence a person has in his or her ability to successfully carry out an action. Bandura's theory proposes that the greater a person's self-efficacy for a behavior, the more likely the person will engage in it, even when faced with obstacles. The concept of self-efficacy is one of the behavior-specific cognitions of Pender's model. Pender's belief is that when a person has high perceived competence or self-efficacy in a certain behavior, it results in a greater likelihood that the person will commit to action and actually perform the behavior.

Some have observed that the Health Promotion Model resembles the Health Belief Model. While it is true that the Health Promotion Model shares some concepts with the Health Belief Model, the Health Promotion Model differs from the Health Belief Model in at least one important way. The Health Promotion Model is a competence- or approach-oriented model that focuses on attainment of high level wellness and self-actualization. This is contrasted with the Health Belief Model, which was intended for use in explaining patients' use of medical diagnosis and treatment of disease, such as tuberculosis. Further, the Health Belief Model incorporates fear or threat of disease as a motivation for action. While this perspective may be valid for diseases that have shorter prodromal periods, the Health Promotion Model does not consider fear or threat as a powerful motivation for distant threats to health.

The Health Promotion Model (Pender et al., 2010) consists of two major categories of predictors (individual characteristics and experiences, behavior-specific cognitions and affect), and the behavioral outcome. Pender identifies the behavior-specific cognitions and affect as the major motivational mechanisms for health promotion behavior. These include: perceived benefits of action, perceived barriers to action, perceived self-efficacy, activity-related affect, interpersonal influences, and situational influences. Individual characteristics and experiences included in the model are prior related behavior and personal factors. The model also includes additional concepts influencing the behavioral outcome, such as immediate competing demands and preferences, and commitment to a plan of action. These concepts are briefly described in Definitions of Key Concepts, which appears earlier in this chapter. Relationships of the concepts are described in the model's theoretical propositions (Box 14.1). The schematic representation of the model (Fig. 14.1) shows the relationship of model concepts to the behavioral outcome, health-promoting behavior.

The model includes multiple concepts and relationships, though some concepts and relationships may be more salient than others to a given health behavior. However, the model does not provide assistance in selecting which concepts and relationships are appropriate for specific behaviors. Therefore, the researcher who seeks to use the model should select concepts and relationships based on previous research, theoretical foundations, clinical experience, and practical limitations in regard to a specific behavior. Indeed, extant research using the Health Promotion Model shows the selectivity of researchers in determining which model concepts to include in their study designs.

IMPLICATIONS OF THE MODEL FOR CLINICAL PRACTICE

The Health Promotion Model offers a conceptual framework for the provision of effective nursing care directed at improved health and functional ability. First, the model provides a method for the assessment of client's health-promoting behaviors. The model directs nurses to systematically assess clients for their perceived self-efficacy, perceived barriers, perceived benefits, interpersonal influences, and situational influences that are relevant to the selected health behavior.

Second, the model identifies several additional client characteristics as targets for assessment. These client characteristics include prior behavior, demographic characteristics, and perceived health status. While these characteristics are not amenable to alteration, they offer a basis for tailoring of nursing interventions, as discussed below.

Box 14. 1 Theoretical Propositions of the Health Promotion Model

- Prior behavior has "both direct and indirect effects on the likelihood of engaging in health-promoting behaviors. Prior behavior indirectly influences health-promoting behavior through perceptions of self-efficacy, benefits, barriers, and activity-related affect" (p. 52).
- Personal factors (such as age, self-esteem, and socioeconomic status) may influence cognitions, affect, and health behaviors.
- "Perceived benefits directly motivate behavior as well as indirectly motivate behavior through determining the extent of commitment to a plan of action to engage in the behaviors from which the anticipated benefits will result" (p. 53).
- "Perceived barriers to action affect health-promoting behavior directly by serving as blocks to action as well as indirectly through decreasing commitment to a plan of action"(p. 53).
- "The more positive the affect, the greater the perceptions of efficacy is present. Self-efficacy influences perceived barriers to action, with higher efficacy resulting in lowered perception of barriers. Self-efficacy motivates health-promoting behavior directly by efficacy expectations and indirectly by affecting perceived barriers and level of commitment or persistence in pursuing a plan of action" (p. 54).
- "Activity-related affect influences health behavior directly as well as indirectly through self-efficacy and commitment to a plan of action" (p.54).
- "Interpersonal interaction influences health-promoting behavior directly as well as indirectly through social pressures or encouragement to commit to a plan of action" (p. 55).
- "Situational influences directly influence health behavior, and indirectly influence health behavior through commitment to a plan of action" (p. 56).
- "Commitment to a plan of action propels the individual into and through the behavior unless a competing demand that cannot be avoided or a competing preference that is not resisted occurs" (p, 56).

Source: Pender, N., Murdaugh, C., & Parsons, M. (2006). *Health promotion in nursing practice* (5th ed.). Upper Saddle River, NJ: Prentice Hall.

Third, the model suggests that nursing interventions can be designed to alter clients' perceptions in these areas. Success in these interventions is expected to result in more frequent health behaviors and resultant improved wellness.

Although the model identifies foci for nursing interventions, it does not explicitly describe how nurses can effect changes in client perceptions. While these nursing interventions directed at changing client perceptions are proposed by the Health Promotion Model, few studies that test the effectiveness of these proposed interventions have been completed.

Pender prescribes use of the nursing process as the method of producing behavior change. She emphasizes nursing assessment of health, health beliefs, and health behavior using established frameworks, such as North American Nursing Diagnosis Association (NANDA) and Gordon's functional health patterns. In addition, she recommends the use of model-based assessments such as the Health Promoting Lifestyles Profile II (HPLP-II). Pender emphasizes use of the nursing process in empowering self-care across the life span. She outlines a multi-step process for health planning that includes reinforcing client strengths, developing a plan based on client preferences and Prochaska et al.'s (1994) stages of change, addressing facilitators and barriers, and committing to goals.

Areas of intervention for health promotion include exercise, nutrition, stress management, and social support. Pender (2010) reviews several interventions in each of these areas, many of which are research based, but not model based. These are directed toward increasing the client's capacity for a vigorous and productive life.

USE OF THE HEALTH PROMOTION MODEL IN TAILORING NURSING INTERVENTIONS

Model variables, such as client characteristics, cognitions, and affect may be used to tailor or target nursing interventions to clients. Tailoring of interventions involves shaping of health messages based on

Individual Characteristics   Behavior-specific   Behavioral Outcome
and Experiences   Cognitions and Affect

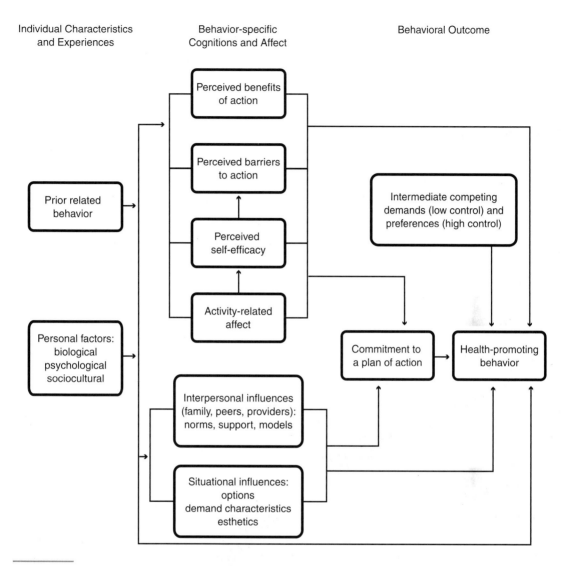

Figure 14.1 Health Promotion Model (*Source:* Pender, N., Murdaugh, C., & Parsons, M. (2010). *Health promotion in nursing practice* (6th ed.). © Reprinted by permission of Pearson Education, Inc., Upper Saddle River, NJ).

characteristics unique to that person. Several comparison studies have found tailoring interventions to increase intervention effectiveness (Kroeze, Werkman, & Brug, 2006; Neville, O'Hara, & Milat, 2009; Velicer, Prochaska, & Redding, 2006). This innovative intervention strategy offers exciting opportunities for designing health promotion interventions that are designed to meet the unique needs of each individual client. Once the nurse assesses the client on each of the relevant factors of the model, this information can be used to custom-design a health promotion program for that individual client. Recent applications of the Health Promotion Model have used computers to quickly and accurately assess the health of the client on model-based variables. With the help of computer technology, nurses have used this information to design a health promotion intervention that is unique to the needs of this individual (Kerr, Savik, Monsen, & Lusk, 2007). This computer-assisted approach offers nurses the opportunity to provide interventions that are more appropriate to the individual, and may, as a result, enhance intervention effectiveness. In a similar manner, model variables may be used to design interventions for groups of clients who share characteristics.

SELECTING THE HEALTH PROMOTION MODEL

Nurses are faced with selecting among a variety of models for use in clinical practice and research. This selection may be based on a variety of factors, including philosophy, research, clarity, and utility.

The Health Promotion Model is appealing to many nurses because it offers a view of health consistent with their motivation for pursuing the profession of nursing. Its holistic and humanistic view is congruent with many nurses' own personal philosophy of health and nursing. The model reflects a belief that persons are capable of introspection and are capable of personal change. In turn, the model proposes that health care is more than treatment and prevention of disease, but involves creating conditions where clients can express their unique human potential. The nurse is presented as an agent for creating behavioral and environmental changes.

The Health Promotion Model has been used successfully in several research studies, as discussed earlier in this chapter. While some models have been tested more extensively, the Health Promotion Model does have a body of extant literature that provides support for its use. A more thorough discussion of studies using the Health Promotion Model is presented in Pender's fifth edition (Pender, Murdaugh, & Parsons, 2006). Examples of research applications of the Health Promotion Model are presented in Research Application 14.1 and Using Middle Range Theories 14.1.

Most nurses will find that the Health Promotion Model is straightforward and easy to understand. It uses terms that are readily comprehended, and its propositional statements are presented clearly. The phenomena addressed by the model are familiar to nurses, and most nurses will require minimal learning of new terms and concepts in order to use and understand the model. The model is clearly presented in graphic form.

Research Application

Noise-induced hearing loss is widespread among construction workers, but only 5% of workers use hearing protection all the time they are exposed to noise. Kerr and colleagues compared the effectiveness of interventions based on the Pender Health Promotion Model to promote use of hearing protection devices among construction workers. A total of 343 noise-exposed construction workers from a large municipal employer and two unions in metropolitan areas of the Midwest were recruited for this random controlled intervention study. Workers in this convenience sample completed pre-test measurements of Health Promotion Model concepts and demographic variables. These concepts included health-related behavior (use of hearing protection), interpersonal influences, situational factors, perceived control of health, perceived self-efficacy, definition of health, perceived health status, perceived benefits, and perceived barriers. Participants were randomly assigned to one of the four experimental conditions: tailored or targeted intervention, each with and without a mailed booster intervention delivered to their home address after six months. Participants in the tailored intervention groups received model-based messages delivered by computer according to their pre-test responses; participants in the targeted intervention groups received similar concepts that were not individually tailored to pre-test responses. Post-tests of hearing protector use were made after one year. Post-tests revealed an increase in use of hearing protective devices (HPD) among all groups; there was no significant difference between groups receiving the tailored and the targeted messages, or between booster and non-booster conditions. These results suggest that the more economical targeted interventions offer a better value in the context of construction workers and promotion of use of hearing protection device use. The authors recommend additional study of the effects of tailored and targeted interventions, and boosters, in influencing health behavior.

Measurement of Model Concepts

Instruments have been developed to measure a variety of concepts related to the Health Promotion Model. Primary of these is the HPLP-II (Susan Walker, personal communication, June 24, 2002). Due to the broad nature of the model, many instruments have been developed to measure behavior-specific attitudes and beliefs. A sample of these is described in Table 14.1.

Kerr et al. (2007).

Marci, age 49, takes daily medication for diabetes, hypertension, and seizures which are not well controlled. Due to seizures, Marci lost her full-time job as a computer data entry technician and stopped driving. She is supported by disability payments, is consequently ineligible for Medicaid, and is waiting for eligibility for Medicare benefits. Members of her church and family provide transportation for medical appointments.

The outpatient clinic nurse assessed Marci for the importance (value) of medication adherence in her life, the extent to which she feels capable of adhering to her medication regimen (self-efficacy), her goals of driving and returning to full-time work (definition of health), her perceived benefits and barriers to medication adherence, access and availability of medications, the presence of other persons in her life who may serve as medication-taking role models, social support for medication adherence, and her use of reminders (cues) for taking medication.

Based on the assessment, the nurse learns that Marci's medication supply is frequently interrupted by her lack of finance (barriers), and that she was sometimes sacrificing her food and other needs in order to purchase her medications (immediate competing demands). In addition, the nurse learns that Marci occasionally forgets medication doses (situational influences), and feels that even if she takes her medications, she will continue to experience seizures, diabetes, and hypertension (self-efficacy).

The nurse initiates several interventions on behalf of Marci based on the assessment. First, the nurse makes a referral to a patient assistance program for assistance with purchasing her seizure and other medications (addressing one barrier to medication administration and her immediate competing demands). Working together, the nurse and Marci develop a plan to place a written reminder to take medications on her refrigerator door, and to use a medication set to organize her daily medications (addressing her situational influences). They also decide to record seizures, blood pressure readings, and HA1c levels on a calendar, for review at the next clinic appointment, as a means of monitoring the success of the plan (addressing her self-efficacy).

The Health Promotion Model has been used in a variety of settings, including schools, workplaces, ambulatory treatment facilities, a rehabilitation center, and a prison. Its use has been with a wide variety of health behaviors, including exercise, nutrition, and use of hearing protection. The studies have involved diverse clients in regard to gender and age. The model has a limited history of application in culturally diverse groups. However, samples of Korean, Taiwanese, Thai, and Japanese individuals have participated in prior studies. It is noteworthy that persons included as study participants have been well or experiencing chronic illness, such as HIV infection.

The Health Promotion Model has been used by nurses working in a variety of community-based settings, such as occupational health and public health. The model is well suited to clients whose health status is stable, and whose basic needs are met. Although Pender's definition of health is broad and encompasses persons who are experiencing illness, application of the Health Promotion Model is untested in acute care settings, and with clients whose health concerns are urgent or living conditions are unstable.

SUMMARY

Pender has proposed a model of health promotion to guide nurses in helping clients achieve improved health, enhanced functional ability, and better quality of life. The need for behavioral and environmental changes to effect improvements in a society where lifestyle factors account for a large proportion of health problems provide justification for the model. The model is based on established theories of human behavior, including expectancy-value theory and social-cognitive theory. The Health Promotion Model claims that a variety of client characteristics and cognitive–affective factors combine with competing demands

TABLE 14.1 Health Promotion Model Instruments

Instrument	First author, date	Description
Health Promoting Lifestyles Profile II (HPLP-II)	Susan Walker, personal communication, June 24, 2002	52-item questionnaire in a 4-point response format measures the frequency of health-promoting behaviors in six domains (health responsibility, physical activity, nutrition, spiritual growth, interpersonal relations, and stress management).
HPLP Spanish Language Version	Walker, Sechrist, & Pender, 1997	This instrument provides a Spanish language version of the HPLP.
HPLP—Japanese Version	Wei et al., 2000	This instrument provides a Japanese language version of the HPLP.
Exercise Benefits/Barriers Scale (EBBS)	Sechrist, Walker, & Pender, 1987	This Likert scale measures the person's "perceived benefits to undertaking preventive behaviors that reduce risk factors in coronary artery disease."
Perceived Self-efficacy of Hearing Protector Use Scale	Lusk, Ronis, & Hogan, 1997	This 10-item scale asks respondents to rate the extent to which they have confidence in their ability to use hearing protection. An example of an item from this scale is, "I am sure I can use my hearing protection so it works effectively."
Perception of Accessibility and Availability of Hearing Protectors Scale	Lusk et al., 1997	This 9-item scale asks respondents to report on this dimension of situational factors influencing this health behavior. A sample item from this scale is, "Ear plugs are available to pick up at my job sites."
Interpersonal Influences on Hearing Protector Use Scale	Lusk et al., 1997	This scale includes three subscales measuring dimensions of this variable: interpersonal norms, interpersonal modeling, and interpersonal support. The Interpersonal Norms Subscale includes four items that query respondents about their beliefs about how much others (family members, friends, supervisor, and co-workers) think they should wear hearing protection. The Interpersonal Support Subscale measures encouragement or praise from family, friends, co-workers, and supervisors about the respondent's use of hearing protection. The Interpersonal Modeling Subscale measures how much they believe others use hearing protection when exposed to noise.

and preferences as well as commitment to a plan of action to explain the likelihood of health-promoting behavior. The model has been tested in several clinical studies using a variety of settings, health behaviors, and client characteristics. It presents exciting possibilities for the creation of interventions that are tailored to the unique characteristics and needs of individual clients.

The model was revised in 1996 following the review and analysis of results of model testing and intervention effectiveness research based on the model. The model authors acknowledge the need for development of measures of model concepts that fit the target population and the design of robust interventions that can change model beliefs and subsequently, health outcomes. Interventions that address not only individuals but families and communities in creating multi-level interventions employing the HPM in combination with community action models are most likely to achieve success.

ANALYSIS OF THEORY

Using the criteria presented in Chapter 2, critique the Health Promotion Model. When you are finished, you can compare your ideas about the model with those of a researcher who has worked with the model (Appendix A).

Internal Criticism

1. Clarity
2. Consistency
3. Adequacy
4. Logical development
5. Level of theory development

External Criticism

1. Reality convergence
2. Utility
3. Significance
4. Discrimination

CRITICAL THINKING EXERCISES

The Pender Health Promotion Model identifies benefits and barriers as factors influencing health behavior. Respond to the following items, considering clients from your own clinical practice.

1. What are the barriers to and the benefits of adopting a selected healthy behavior, such as exercise?

2. Generate several questions designed to elicit specific information about your clients' perceptions of their barriers and benefits?

3. How can you use this information to improve the effectiveness of your efforts to influence your clients' adaptation of healthy behaviors?

WEB RESOURCES

Visit **http://thePoint.lww.com/Peterson3e** for helpful web resources related to this chapter.

ACKNOWLEDGEMENT

The author gratefully acknowledges the critical review of the first edition of this chapter by Dr. Nola Pender.

REFERENCES

Bandura, A. (1986). *Social foundations of thought and action: a social cognitive theory.* Englewood. Cliffs, NJ: Prentice-Hall.

Fishbein M., & Ajzen, I. (1975). *Belief, attitude, intention and behavior: An introduction to theory and research.* Reading, MA: Addison-Wesley.

Garcia, A. W., Broda, M. A., Frenn, M., Coviak, M., Pender, N. J., & Ronis, D. L. (1995). Gender and developmental differences in exercise beliefs among youth and their prediction of their exercise behavior. *Journal of School Health, 65,* 213–219.

Kerr, M. J., Savik, K., Monsen, K. A., & Lusk, S. L. (2007). Effectiveness of computer-based tailoring versus targeting to promote use of hearing protection. *The Canadian Journal of Nursing Research; Revue Canadienne De Recherche En Sciences Infirmieres, 39,* 80–97.

Kroeze, W., Werkman, A., & Brug, J. (2006). A systematic review of randomized trials on the effectiveness of computer-tailored education on physical activity and dietary behaviors. *Annals of Behavioral Medicine: A Publication of the Society of Behavioral Medicine, 31,* 205–223. doi:10.1207/s15324796abm3103_2

Lusk, S. L., Ronis, D. L., & Hogan, M. M. (1997). Test of the health promotion model as a causal model of construction workers' use of hearing protection. *Research in Nursing & Health, 20,* 183–194.

Neville, L. M., O'Hara, B., & Milat, A. J. (2009). Computer-tailored dietary behaviour change interventions: a systematic review. *Health Education Research,* 24:699–720.

Pender, N. (1996). *Health promotion in nursing practice* (3rd ed.). Stamford, CT: Appleton & Lange.

Pender, N., Murdaugh, C., & Parsons, M. (2006). *Health promotion in nursing practice.* Upper Saddle River, NJ: Prentice Hall.

Pender, N. J., Murdaugh, C. L., & Parsons, M. A. (2010). *Health promotion in nursing practice* (6th ed.). Upper Saddle River, NJ: Prentice Hall.

Prochaska, J., Velicer, W., Rossi, J., Goldstein, M., Marcus, B., Rakowski, W., ... Rosenbloom, D. (1994). Stages of change and decisional balance for 12 problem behaviors. *Health Psychology, 13,* 39–46.

Sechrist, K., Walker, W., & Pender, N. (1987). Development and psychometric evaluation of the exercise benefits/barriers scale. *Nursing in Research and Health, 10,* 357–365.

Velicer, W. F., Prochaska, J. O., & Redding, C. A. (2006). Tailored communications for smoking cessations: past successes and future directions. *Drug and Alcohol Review, 25,* 49–57.

Walker, S., Sechrist, K., & Pender, N. (1997). The health-promoting lifestyle profile: Development and psychometric characteristics. *Nursing Research, 39,* 268–273.

Wei, C. N., Yonemitsu, H., Harada, K., Miyakita, T., Omori, S., Miyabayashi, T., … Ueda, A. A. (2000). Japanese language version of the health-promoting lifestyle profile. *Nippon-Eiseigaku-Zasshi, 54,* 597–606.

15

Deliberative Nursing Process

MERTIE L. POTTER

DEFINITION OF KEY TERMS

Automatic nursing process	Actions (visible behaviors) the nurse takes based on reasons other than the patient's immediate needs.
Deliberative nursing process	Means by which the professional nurse purposefully explores with the patient the nurse's perceptions (stimulation of any one of the five senses), thoughts, and/or feelings related to the patient's immediate need for help.
Dynamic nurse–patient relationship	Interactive contact/connection between nurse and patient, when the nurse begins to explore the meaning behind the patient's verbal and nonverbal behaviors.
Immediate need for help	Requirement of the patient in a specific situation. Help for the need relieves or diminishes the patient's immediate distress or improves the patient's immediate sense of adequacy or well-being.
Nursing situation	Circumstance that involves a patient's behavior, the nurse's reaction (perceptions, thoughts, and feelings combined together), and the nurse's action (activity the nurse completes with or for the patient).
Patient distress	Feeling experienced by a patient when the patient cannot meet certain needs and is not helped in meeting such needs.
Patient outcomes/product	Improved verbal and nonverbal patient behaviors that can result from the nurse's deliberative and effective action(s) with the patient.
Validation	Ongoing process of exploring and determining with a patient if the nursing reaction was accurate and if the nursing action was helpful.

INTRODUCTION

The birthing of Deliberative Nursing Process by Ida J. Orlando culminated in 1961, after a number of years laboring to define both the function and the product of professional nursing (Orlando, 1961). The theory began to take shape through Orlando's experiences within nursing practice and nurse education. She reviewed more than 2,000 anecdotal recordings of faculty, students, and nurses related to their interactions with patients and began to see patterns of effective and ineffective nursing process in various nurse–patient situations (Pelletier, 1976). Emerging from these early experiences, Deliberative Nursing Process since has matured into a significant, enduring, and practical nursing theory.

As a middle range theory, Deliberative Nursing Process has a limited number of variables and is limited in scope (McEwan, 2002; Walker & Avant, 1995). However, it is specific and adequate enough to apply and test in research and practice. Although categorized as a grand theory by some (Walker & Avant, 1995; Wills, 2002), Deliberative Nursing Process demonstrates the following middle range theory characteristics: comprehensive yet focused, generalizable, restricted in its concepts, clear in its propositions, and conducive to testable hypotheses (McEwan, 2002).

An unusual paradox within Deliberative Nursing Process is its proclivity toward both simplicity and complexity as a theory. This paradox partially explains the attractiveness of using this theory. Generally, it is straightforward in its presentation, while being multifaceted in its applications. For example, developing a nurse–patient relationship that is dynamic and unique is not complicated. However, the dynamics of the nurse–patient relationship itself may be very complex (Orlando, 1961).

A unique feature related to the development of this theory is the inductive manner in which Orlando defined effective nursing (Schmieding, 2002). Orlando determined effective and ineffective nursing from her observations of "good" and "bad" nursing practice (Orlando, 1961, 1972; Pelletier, 1976; Schmieding, 1993a). From her observations of specific phenomena (nurse–patient interactions), she identified relationships with other phenomena to develop propositions that led to the development of larger concepts and, ultimately, the theory (Johnson & Webber, 2001).

Orlando desired that nurses become educated to assist patients to express what help they actually need (Pelletier, 1967). Another distinctive feature of Deliberative Nursing Process is that patient input is critical. It is the nurse's professional responsibility to involve the patient in the process of identifying and meeting the patient's immediate needs for help (Orlando, 1961, 1972, 1990).

HISTORICAL BACKGROUND

The need for nurses to have a distinct body of knowledge to direct and enhance nursing practice and the movement of nursing toward becoming a profession were beginning to take place at the turn of the twentieth century (Alligood, 2002). Orlando's Deliberative Nursing Process evolved during an era when nurses were attempting to distinguish nursing from other disciplines, and when psychiatric-mental health nurses were determining their place among nurses of other specialties. Deliberative Nursing Process came into being as Orlando realized that nursing needed to address three areas: "nurse–patient relationships, the nurse's professional role and identity, and the development of knowledge which is distinctly nursing" (Orlando, 1961, p. viii).

Orlando first published work related to this theory after she examined what made nursing interventions effective or ineffective. She asserted early on that effective nursing was "good nursing," and ineffective nursing was "bad nursing" (Orlando, 1976; Schmieding, 1993a). Although this terminology might not be acceptable during today's trend of political correctness and relativity, Orlando was bold in her assertion that nursing was either "good" or "bad." She also stressed that nursing needed to define exactly what "nursing" was, and contended that nursing could not be a profession unless it was able to distinguish what nurses did that was unique (Orlando, 1961).

Orlando was asked to determine what mental health principles were needed in a nursing curriculum. However, she became acutely aware during the project that professional nursing did not have a clear function or product. Nursing was at a crossroads. Orlando understood that nurses were unclear in their attempts to define what nursing was (Orlando, 1961). For someone concerned with meeting patients' immediate needs, here was an immediate need for nurses—to define and to distinguish nursing's function and product. She recognized that the patient and the patient's needs were getting lost in nurses' assumptions of what those needs were. During a project funded by the National Institute of Mental Health, Orlando began to examine nurses' interactions with patients.

DEFINING NURSING AND OUTCOME VARIABLES

Resolute in her mission, Orlando set forth in her later work to assist nurses further in defining what nursing is and what it should entail to distinguish it from other disciplines. Key goals became the following: to define the distinct professional function of nurses; to encourage nurses to assume authority to carry out that function; and to educate nurses to use process discipline (deliberative nursing process) to assure that the product of nursing function involves the patient and others who impact the patient's care (Orlando, 1972). She developed a user-friendly theory that was readily understandable and broadly applicable.

Orlando held that "to nurse" and "nursing" were very different from "to doctor" and "doctoring" (Orlando, 1961, 1972; Orlando & Dugan, 1989). She asserted that doctors' orders are designed for patients, not nurses, and that nurses keep themselves on a dependent path when they focus on following doctors' orders rather than assisting patients to meet their needs for help, which may include the patient's needing to comply with doctors' orders (Orlando, 1987). Orlando contended that licensure authorizes nurses to fulfill a professional role, but authority is only implicit until the nurse engages in a process with the patient to meet the function of nursing, namely to help the patient meet immediate needs for help that the patient is unable to meet on his or her own (Orlando, 1972).

Orlando suggested that the concept of "nursing" derives its meaning from the nursing of infants and the need to have someone nurture and assist infants in obtaining what they need from the environment to survive. She postulated that, at times, individuals might need assistance from others to obtain what is needed from the environment to meet their needs when they are unable to nurse themselves (Orlando, 1961, p. 4; Orlando & Dugan, 1989). Orlando (1972, 1987) distinguished the difference between lay and professional nursing by stating that a professional nurse is needed when a lay person cannot assure that the patient's distress will be identified or relieved.

In some of her works, she questioned whether or not expanded roles of nursing should be considered in the realm of nursing or that of doctoring at a lower cost (Orlando & Dugan, 1989). She used straightforward and uncomplicated language. She contemplated and encouraged nurses to discern what the words "to nurse" meant and referred to a dictionary to emphasize her point of what nursing should entail. She accepted Funk and Wagnall's definition of "to nurse" to mean: "to encourage, to look after; to nourish, protect, and nurture; to give curative care to an ailment" (Orlando, 1987, p. 408).

The conceptual framework of nursing proposed by Orlando identified promotion of "comfort," or the relieving of distress, as crucial to the task of nursing. Orlando's work contributed to the evolution of the concept of comfort by subsequent nursing theorists (Tutton & Seers, 2003). In particular, She designated the nursing role as addressing matters prohibiting a client's "mental and physical comfort" (Orlando, 1961, p. 23). In a review of the development of the concept of comfort in nursing, Tutton and Seers (2003) note that while Orlando does not define the "exact nature of comfort," her promotion of Deliberative Nursing Process to enhance patients' perceived needs makes comfort "pivotal" to her definition of nursing, as it relates to both physical and psychological care (p. 691).

Notably, Orlando was ahead of her time in her concern for and measurement of outcome variables. She promoted progressive ideas, such as defining professional nursing, employing critical thinking within the nursing process, involving the patient in the nursing process, and measuring patient outcomes. Orlando was aware that ineffective nursing activities impacted areas, such as nursing care costs, patient progress, material costs, and medication costs. She was concerned that nursing was acquiring too many nonprofessional tasks that would take the nurse away from helping the patient (Orlando, 1961). Always seeking patient involvement in the provision of nursing care, Orlando looked for a "helpful outcome" as validated with the patient to include "change in the behavior of the object indicating either relief from distress or that a solution to a living or work problem had been found" (Orlando, 1972, p. 61). She addressed work problems involving staff members, as well as patient problems in her 1972 reported studies.

ORLANDO'S LEGACY

Work on Deliberative Nursing Process theory has spanned more than a half century. Orlando's initial development on this theory began in the early 1950s, and work on the theory's development continues. Her early works referred to the "deliberative nursing process." Orlando began using the term "nursing process discipline" in 1972 because she asserted that nursing process was a discipline that could be learned (Orlando, 1972, p. 2). The term "deliberative nursing process" will be used throughout this chapter for consistency.

It is obvious in both her published and unpublished writings that Orlando not only was intensely passionate about nursing as an individual, but also was a determined advocate for nursing (Orlando, 1961, 1972, 1976, 1983, 1987). Several basic tenets come through strongly in her work, primarily: (a) the function of nursing is to meet the patient's immediate need for help when the patient is unable to do so without the nurse's help; and (b) that the product of nursing is to relieve the patient's distress caused by the immediate need for help and to be able to observe improvement either verbally or nonverbally (Orlando, 1961, 1972). Furthermore, her theory promotes the uniqueness of nurses and maintains that patients must be involved in the identification and determination of their immediate needs for help (Orlando, 1961). Orlando was not hesitant to express her grave concern with the definition of nursing promoted in the American Nurses Association Social Policy Statement of 1980—she found "no operational meaning" in it and no differentiation between professional and lay nursing (Orlando, 1983, p. 2). Her passion for nursing clearly was evident throughout her life, accompanied by her assertion that the profession needed to define nursing (I. J. Orlando, personal communication, June 24, 2002).

Ida Jean Orlando Pelletier continues as a symbol of nursing leadership and theory development, having taught and implemented her theory at some of the nation's most respected academic institutions; she was formally recognized as a "Nursing Living Legend" by the Massachusetts Registered Nurse Association in 2006—the year prior to her death (Potter, 2008; Tyra, 2008).

DEFINITION OF THEORY CONCEPTS

DELIBERATIVE NURSING PROCESS

Deliberative Nursing Process remains relevant and significant as a nursing theory due to its patient-focused approach, nurse exploration of nurse perceptions, thoughts, and feelings with patients, and effective outcomes that result from its use. Orlando (1961) proposes a practical approach, with a broad application within nursing education, practice, and research. She focuses on the nurse's unique and deliberative response to the patient who has expressed an immediate need for help. This is accomplished by the nurse's exploration and validation of the nurse's perceptions, thoughts, and feelings about the patient's behavior with the patient. Furthermore, it is the nurse's responsibility in deliberative nursing to see to it that the patient's need for immediate help is met either by the nurse's own activity or by eliciting the help of others (Orlando, 1961).

Orlando acknowledges and affirms the nurse's distinctive interpretation and validation of observations made. Furthermore, she stresses the independent function performed during a deliberative nursing interaction. She recognizes that what makes nurse–patient relationships dynamic is nurses' continually sharing their unique perceptions, thoughts, and feelings (i.e., their immediate reaction) about patients' unique behaviors within a deliberative process with patients (Orlando, 1961, 1972).

Orlando asserts that good nursing initially involves a nurse's determining with the patient a number of elements: (a) What does the patient think is occurring? (b) What does the patient define as the immediate distress? (c) Is the patient's distress related to an immediate need for help? (d) Is the nurse's help needed for the patient to obtain relief? She also observed that nurse–patient interactions involving Deliberative Nursing Process resulted in positive outcomes, namely both verbal and nonverbal positive changes within the patient (Pelletier, 1976).

Deliberative Nursing Process was renamed Nursing Process Discipline by Orlando (1972). She also refers to Deliberative Nursing Process as effective nursing (Orlando, 1961, 1972), or good nursing (Orlando, 1976). She analyzed nurse–patient interactions and determined that effective interactions involved open disclosure of the nurse of perceptions, thoughts, and feelings and validation of the same with the patient. After implementing a nursing action, the nurse validates with the patient if the nursing action met the patient's immediate need for help (Fig. 15.1; Orlando, 1961).

Orlando also noted that ineffective interactions often involved a more secretive style. Both patient and nurse were not aware of each other's perceptions, thoughts, and feelings in such interactions (Fig. 15.2).

Orlando (1972, p. 28) developed a Nursing Process Record to assist in learning deliberative nursing process (process discipline) and to be better able to discern nursing process done in secret or using open disclosure (Fig. 15.3). Orlando referred to the nurse's perceptions, thoughts, and feelings as part of the nurse's reaction, and whatever the nurse said and/or did to, with, or for the patient as the nurse's action (see Fig. 15.3; Orlando, 1972, p. 56).

AUTOMATIC NURSING PROCESS

Automatic nursing process refers to any actions or interventions a nurse takes to help a patient that may not be related to the process of helping the patient. Automatic nursing process may be impacted by other influences, such as nursing care costs, patient progress, or additional expenses. Automatic nursing process

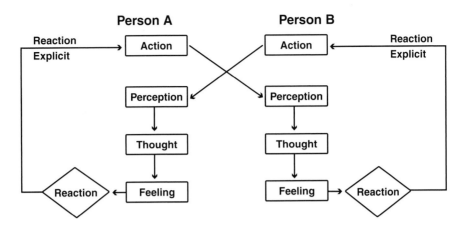

Figure 15.1 The action process in a person-to-person contact functioning by open disclosure. The perceptions, thoughts, and feelings of each individual through the observable action. (Used with permission from Orlando, I. J. (1972). *The discipline and teaching of nursing process* [*An evaluative study*] (p. 26). New York: Putnam.)

also is referred to as Nursing Process Without Discipline (Orlando, 1972), ineffective nursing (Orlando, 1961, 1972), and bad nursing (Orlando, 1976).

Orlando asserted that automatic nursing process activities were ineffective when they: (a) involved nursing action without determining the meaning of the patient's behavior to the patient or the need that caused the behavior, (b) did not assist the patient to inform the nurse how the activity influenced the patient, (c) did not connect the nursing activity to the patient's need, (d) were implemented because of the nurse's inability to explore the nurse's reaction to the patient's behavior, or (e) did not indicate that the nurse was attuned to how the nursing activity influenced the patient (Orlando, 1961, p. 65). Such activities are not necessarily wrong or negative, but they do not determine if the activity is perceived as helpful in relieving the patient's immediate needs. Furthermore, automatic nursing activities indicated to Orlando that nursing care had been given without a disciplined or deliberative professional process (Orlando, 1976).

An example of the difference between use of an automatic nursing process, which involves nurses' assumptions, and a deliberative nursing process, which involves nurses' exploration of the patients' immediate needs for help, is demonstrated in a study by Bochnak, Rhymes, and Leonard (1962). When

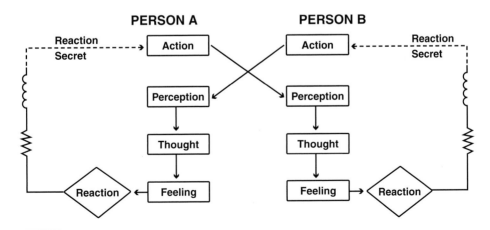

Figure 15.2 The action process in a person-to-person contact functioning in secret. The perceptions, thoughts, and feelings of each individual are not directly available to the perception of the other individual through the observable action. (Used with permission from Orlando, I. J. (1972). *The discipline and teaching of nursing process* [*An evaluative study*] (p. 26). New York: Putnam.)

Nursing Process Record

Perception of or About the Patient	Thought and/or Feeling About the Perception	Said and/or Did to, with, or for the Patient
PROCESS A Mr. G walking back and forth; face red	Looks angry; something must have happened. I'm afraid to ask because he might hit me.	"Good morning, Mr. G."
PROCESS B Mr. G walking back and forth; face red	Looks angry; something must have happened. I'm afraid to ask because he might hit me.	"I'm afraid you will hit me if I ask a question. Should I be afraid?"

Figure 15.3 Process A illustrates the nursing process functioning in secrecy. Process B illustrates the nursing process functioning by open disclosure. (Used with permission from Orlando, I. J. (1972). *The discipline and teaching of nursing process* [*An evaluative study*] (p. 28). New York: Putnam.)

two different types of nursing activities to address patients' complaints of pain were examined, statistically significant results occurred at the 0.05 level. In the control group, it was assumed that any complaint of pain indicated a need for pain-relieving medication, and when patients complained of pain, they were given pain-relieving medication. Relief was variable and slow. However, in the experimental group, nurses who used a deliberative approach to determine more accurately what the patients' complaints of pain were about did not automatically administer pain-relieving medication. Their explorations with the patients led to various interventions that provided more extensive relief and quicker relief for the patients (Bochnak et al., 1962).

DYNAMIC NURSE–PATIENT RELATIONSHIP

According to a recent study, patients are most concerned with personal care issues related to five essential themes: having their needs met, being treated pleasantly, being cared for, having competent nurses, and having care provided promptly (Bolden & Larrabee, 2001). These areas relate to meeting patients' immediate needs for help, which are foundational in Orlando's Theory of Deliberative Nursing

Process. Orlando based her ideas about a dynamic nurse–patient relationship on principles from other theories, such as behavioral theory, which postulates that humans are living and behaving organisms who interact continually with one another and within the environment (Orlando, 1961).

Defining the function and product of nursing is explicit in Orlando's definition of the dynamic nurse–patient relationship. Orlando fervently strove to have nurses define the unique function and product of nursing. She defined nursing function as helping the patient and defined nursing product as the improvement or helpful result in the patient's behavior, observable both verbally and nonverbally (Orlando, 1961, 1972, 1983).

IMMEDIATE NEED FOR HELP

Immediate need for help refers to the patient's inability to fulfill a need for help; the patient may or may not need assistance identifying and/or communicating what the actual need for help is (Orlando, 1961). The observed behavior of the patient is assumed until the meaning behind the behavior is explored (1961, p. 23). Behaviors observed by the nurse may be nonverbal or verbal. Nonverbal behaviors include motor activity, physiological manifestations, and vocalizations. Verbal behaviors take into account complaints, requests, questions, refusals, demands, comments, and statements (1961, pp. 36, 37). Immediate needs for help also are referred to simply as "need" in earlier writings (1961).

Therefore, an immediate need for help is any condition in which patients need to have immediate distress relieved or diminished, or their sense of sufficiency or welfare improved (Orlando, 1961, p. 5). Immediate need for help definitely implies that the patient cannot meet the need without professional help.

PATIENT DISTRESS

Patient distress occurs when a patient's immediate needs are unmet. It is a sense of discomfort that arises when a patient is unable to communicate his or her needs adequately or clearly. Orlando cited physical challenges, unfavorable reactions to the environment, and unfavorable occurrences as examples of circumstances that keep the patient from being able to meet immediate needs (Orlando, 1961, p. 11).

Patient distress is what the patient perceives to be stressful. Orlando holds that behavior has meaning, and that nurses cannot assume what the behavior means without exploring with the patient what the behavior and accompanying distress mean to the patient.

NURSING SITUATION

According to Orlando (1961, p. 36), a nursing situation encompasses three elements and is dependent upon the nurse's use of them: (a) the patient's behavior, (b) the nurse's reaction, and (c) the nurse's actions intended for the patient's benefit. The interaction of these three elements comprises nursing process.

VALIDATION

Validation is an ongoing nursing action within the Deliberative Nursing Process. It involves checking with the patient if the nurse's perceptions, thoughts, and/or feelings were accurate in relation to the patient's behavior, and if the nurse's interventions were "correct, helpful, or appropriate" (Orlando, 1961, p. 56). In addition, Orlando sees the nurse as primarily responsible for initiating the process of exploration and discovery in relation to how the patient is responding to any nursing action (1961). The presence or absence of validation in the nurse–patient relationship and subsequent actions differentiates the deliberative process (with patient validation) from the automatic response (without patient validation), as visualized in Figure 15.4 (Aponte, 2009).

PATIENT OUTCOMES/PRODUCT

The end result of a nursing action is to "bring about improvement" (Orlando, 1961, p. 6). That improvement should be observable both verbally and nonverbally in the patient's behavior (Orlando, 1972,

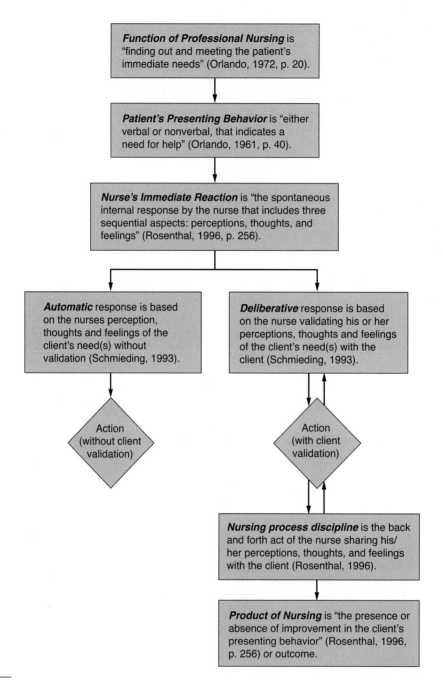

Figure 15.4 Orlando's *Dynamic Nurse–Patient Relationship Nursing Framework.* (From Aponte, J. (2009). Meeting the linguistic needs of urban communities. *Home Healthcare Nurse, 27*[5], 327. Copyright 2009 by Wolters Kluwer Health. Reprinted with permission.)

p. 21). Patient outcomes also should be both "predictable and helpful," and may include such outcomes as "avoidance, relief or diminution of helplessness suffered or anticipated by the individual in an immediate experience" (Orlando, 1972, p. 9). The nurse's activity may result in help, no help, or be unknown (Orlando, 1961, p. 67). If the outcome does not transpire as predicted, then the nurse must continue to explore what else may be needed to meet the patient's immediate need for help.

DESCRIPTION OF THE THEORY OF DELIBERATIVE NURSING PROCESS

SIMPLE YET COMPLEX THEORY

Deliberative Nursing Process is a theory that is readily understood, has a specific focus (i.e., meeting patients' immediate needs for help), addresses patient problems and probable outcomes (felt distress and lowered distress, respectively), and is explicit to nursing. Its concepts and their relationships are testable and they answer questions about nursing, which are indicators of a middle range nursing theory (Marriner-Tomey, 1998). Orlando's work helped refocus nurses on patients rather than on tasks and on an active, rather than passive, role of patients in their own care.

Complexity refers to the "richness" of a theory to elucidate more variables and their interrelationships (Stevens-Barnum, 1990, p. 97). Part of the theory's complexity involves learning how to use it. Becoming proficient in the use of Deliberative Nursing Process necessitates time, practice, and self-reflection, often in the form of a supervisory experience. The use of Nurse Process Recordings (see Fig. 15.3) helps the nurse distinguish between perceptions, thoughts, and feelings—no small task in itself. Learning Deliberative Nursing Process often involves a close supervisory experience in which the learner reconstructs and examines interactions. The process of becoming comfortable in owning one's perceptions, thoughts, and feelings and sharing them with patients is at times difficult and complex.

FUNCTION OF NURSING

Orlando observed patients in distress and asserted that it was professional nursing's role to determine and meet their immediate needs for help by exploring with the patient the nurse's unique thoughts and feelings resulting from perceptions related to the observed patient behaviors (Orlando, 1961, 1972, 1990). When the nurse shares perceptions, thoughts, and/or feelings, it is considered to involve open disclosure; by not sharing, the patient is unaware of the nurse's reaction (Orlando, 1972, p. 26). Nurses must not make assumptions, but must explore their perceptions, thoughts, and feelings about the patient's behavior with patients. Orlando's (1961) incorporation of nurses' exploration of their thoughts with patients as part of a deliberative process indicates how critical thinking is an essential part of the deliberative nursing process (Schmieding, 2002).

MAJOR COMPONENTS AND THEIR RELATIONSHIPS

Nursing is independent, has its own unique professional function, and has its own distinct product (Pelletier, 1976, p. 17). The dynamic nurse–patient relationship involves reciprocity between the nurse and patient; each is influenced by what the other does and says (Marriner-Tomey, 1998). It is dependent upon a nurse-initiated exploration of perceptions, thoughts, and feelings about the patient's behavior, and validation that the nurse's perceptions, thoughts, and feelings are accurate.

The nurse initiates the deliberative process to determine the immediate need for help by helping the patient identify and express the meaning of his or her behavior (Orlando, 1961). Further, the nurse helps the patient explore distress related to the immediate need for help to determine the help needed (p. 29). Within the dynamic nurse–patient relationship, the nurse observes a patient whom the nurse thinks is in distress. This dynamic relationship is dependent upon "what the nurse and patient start with, to the length of their contact and to what they are able to accomplish" (Orlando, 1961, p. 91).

As Schmieding points out, nurses using Deliberative Nursing Process realize "that the patient is the source of the nurse's power" (Schmieding, 2002, p. 327). The nurse uses reflection as part of a critical thinking process to help ascertain the meaning of the patient's behavior according to the patient, and to determine how the behavior relates to the nurse's assumption that an immediate need exists, which is leading to distress for the patient. Nurses obtain information either directly from the patient or indirectly from other sources, such as family, friends, and nursing staff. Orlando considers that nurses have access to a tremendous amount of information about the patient (Orlando, 1961).

The nurse using a deliberative process will check what the meaning of the information is with the patient. In an automatic process, the nurse assumes what the information means. Most likely, the outcomes would be significantly different, depending upon which process the nurse uses. Using the deliberative process, the patient partners with the nurse to identify the need, and a successful outcome is more likely. When an automatic process is used, the patient is not included in the assessment or decision-making processes, making a successful outcome less likely (Orlando, 1961, 1972).

Deliberative Nursing Process is a learned and practiced process (Orlando, 1972). The nurse validates with the patient that the patient has an immediate need for help, and that the immediate need for help cannot be met without a professional nurse's help. The nurse intervenes, after exploring with the patient what meaning the patient ascribes to behaviors related to the situation that resulted in an immediate need for help. The nursing situation involves: (a) the patient's behavior, (b) the nurse's reaction, and (c) the nurse's activity or actions to assist the patient. Nursing process is the interaction of the three elements contained within a nursing situation (Orlando, 1961, p. 36).

The nurse validates that the immediate need for help has been met by asking the patient and evaluating if the anticipated product or patient outcome of the nursing action, namely improvement and relief of distress, have occurred. If the nursing action has resulted in the patient's relief, the nursing action has been effective in achieving the desired and predicted patient outcome or product. As mentioned, Orlando used Nursing Process Recordings to study nursing process and to educate nurses in Deliberative Nursing Process.

Assumptions and propositions will be described, based upon Johnson and Webber's (2001) definitions. Assumptions are assumed truths that are associated with the relationships (p. 15). Patients' becoming distressed when they cannot meet their own needs is an example of an assumption within Deliberative Nursing Process (Orlando, 1961). A more complete listing of assumptions implied within Orlando's Deliberative Nursing Process Theory can be found in Table 15.1.

Propositions direct the relationship between concepts and provide a description of the relationship between concepts (Johnson & Webber, 2001, p. 15). An example that Orlando cited was that "the professional function of nursing is distinct and of central importance to patients in any treatment setting" (Pelletier, 1967, p. 30). Implied propositions within Orlando's Deliberative Nursing Process Theory are listed in Table 15.1.

APPLICATIONS OF THE THEORY

Deliberative Nursing Practice has been applied to a broad range of practice settings, including inpatient and acute nursing settings, residential care facilities, as well as in outpatient or community settings by advanced practice nurses. Deliberative Nursing Process application and outcome measures may be utilized to validate clients' needs and perceived outcomes to improve nursing care. Furthermore, it may lead to professionalization of nursing's role in any of these practice settings, as it demonstrates efficacy and potential impact of nursing. The following examples represent a sampling of contexts in which Deliberative Nursing Practice has been incorporated.

DELIBERATIVE NURSING PROCESS IN THEORY DEVELOPMENT

Deliberative Nursing Process has been linked with recent models of social information processing to develop a new nursing theory. Sheldon and Ellington (2008) applied the Crick and Dodge model of social information processing to interactions within nursing responses to patient behaviors. By evaluating interviews with experienced nurses, nursing scholars identified Deliberative Nursing Process as foundational for understanding nurse–patient relationships. They concluded that social information processing theory was instrumental to further describe how nurses learn to effectively respond to patients' social cues and environmental factors (Sheldon & Ellington, 2008). Their research suggests that the coupling of Deliberative Nursing Process and social information processing may contribute to new nursing theory and curriculum development, in order to enhance nursing training programs and communication skills and improve patient care.

DELIBERATIVE NURSING PROCESS IN A GROUP CONTEXT

The author supervised nurses in 12-week group leadership training. Nurses received contact hours for coleading a weekly patient group session for 12 weeks, completing written assignments and readings,

TABLE 15.1 Assumptions and Propositions Within Orlando's (1961) Deliberative Nursing Process

Assumptions	Propositions
1. Patients require the expertise of professional nurses to meet certain immediate needs for help.	1. Nurses can determine patients' immediate needs for help by using a deliberative nursing process to ascertain with the patient what the immediate need is.
2. Patients experience distress when they cannot meet their own needs.	2. Nurses can help alleviate patients' distress most effectively when implementing actions based upon a deliberative nursing process because the actions will be designed to meet the need causing distress.
3. Nursing can be evaluated as either good or bad.	3. Good nursing involves open disclosure of and validation with the patient of the nurse's perceptions, thoughts, and/or feelings related to the patient's behavior, and validation with the patient that the nursing action taken met the patient's immediate need for help.
4. It is the responsibility of professional nurses to meet patients' immediate needs for help or to assure that those needs are met by someone else.	4. Professional nurses using a deliberative nursing process function differently than lay nurses because they are trained in a process whereby they validate with patients: (a) what the patients' needs are, and (b) if the needs have been met effectively by the nursing actions implemented.
5. Each nursing situation with a patient is unique and dynamic.	5. Patients' individualized needs and nurses' distinctive styles create individually unique nursing situations, and each nursing situation is dynamic because it involves ongoing deliberation by the nurse.
6. The desired outcome of good nursing is that the patient reports or demonstrates: (a) relief from distress, (b) experience of less distress, or (c) improvement in "adequacy or well-being" (p. 5).	6. The nurse can determine with the patient if nursing actions based on the deliberative nursing process alleviated or decreased the distress or helped the patient gain a sense of improved "adequacy or well-being" (p. 5).

and participating actively in supervision throughout the group experience (Potter, Williams, & Costanzo, 2004). Each group focused upon the following:

■ Meeting patients' immediate needs for help
■ Validating that nurse coleaders understood what group members stated was their immediate need for help
■ Sharing nurse coleaders' perceptions with patient group members, thoughts, and/or feelings in response to behaviors (verbal or nonverbal) that group members presented within the group

Group members often commented, either during or at completion of group sessions, how helpful they felt the group had been and frequently commented that they felt better. Group members found that check-ins and check-outs were extremely helpful in addressing patients' immediate needs for help and decreasing patient distress. Positive feedback was given on post-group surveys as well.

Nurses were educated to use deliberative nursing process within a nursing situation (involving the patient's behavior, the nurse's reaction, and the nurse's action) to identify with the patient what the meaning of the patient's behavior is, so that the patient's immediate need for help could be met and distress relieved. Involvement of the patient in discerning the meaning of his or her behavior was found to effectively promote a dynamic nurse–patient relationship. Validation with the patient that the need had been correctly identified and met resulted in positive patient outcomes (Potter et al., 2004).

DELIBERATIVE NURSING PROCESS WITH PROSPECTIVE NURSING STUDENTS

Nursing Camp 2002 was a 2-week camp for 8th-grade students that ran during the summer at Saint Anselm College in Manchester, New Hampshire. Nursing Camp 2002 was a partnership between the Manchester School-to-Careers Partnership, Saint Anselm College, Elliot Hospital, Hanover Hill Health-care, New Hampshire Hospital (NHH), and Visiting Nurses Association Childcare Center. Sylvia Durette, camp director, and this writer introduced 27 students to Orlando's Deliberative Nursing Process as part of their overview of the nursing profession. Students also participated in an interactive experience related to Deliberative Nursing Process.

DELIBERATIVE NURSING PROCESS IN A PRACTICE SETTING

Nursing staff at an extended care facility requested assistance from their nursing supervisor regarding problematic night behaviors of two older adult patients (Faust, 2002). The supervisor incorporated Deliberative Nursing Process to determine apparent unmet needs of the patients. She met with staff and formulated a plan of action. She assigned an additional nursing assistant to that wing, assumed responsibility for the two patients, observed the patients' behaviors, and validated her perceptions with these patients. Both patients demonstrated less distress and increased sleep during the nights.

DELIBERATIVE NURSING PROCESS IN MEASURING NURSING OUTCOMES

The nursing executive leadership at NHH established Orlando's dynamic nursing process theory as a foundation for practice in 1996, and utilized Deliberative Nursing Process as a driving principle in the formation and functioning of a Nursing Practice Enhancement Project (NPEP) (Allen, Bockenhauer, Egan, & Kinnaird, 2006). The NPEP was instituted with the purpose of "redesign[ing] a model" to apply in psychiatric nursing care at NHH. The nursing leadership at NHH identified the interpersonal nurse–client professional relationship as key to healing and psychiatric care. In the process of developing the NPEP, Deliberative Nursing Process was instrumental in helping nurse staff to find a "common approach" to a broad range of clients; furthermore, affirmation of the nursing role as described in the Deliberative Nursing Process became "one of the cornerstones of empowered nursing practice" (Allen et al., 2006, p. 141). A Nursing Practice Outcomes Committee was formed to measure the effectiveness of the redesigned nursing model of psychiatric care at NHH, and found that the revised model of care was effective in reducing the occurrence of seclusion-restraint, improving both patient satisfaction and nurses' job satisfaction (Allen et al., 2006).

DELIBERATIVE NURSING PROCESS IN RESEARCH APPLICATIONS

Deliberative Nursing Process has been categorized as a nursing process theory (Orlando, 1990), a prescriptive theory (Wooldridge, Skipper, & Leonard, 1968), and a reflective practice theory (Schmieding, 2002). The inductive, research-based approach Orlando used to develop Deliberative Nursing Process as a theory was unique. Meleis (1997, p. 348) points out that Orlando used field methodology before it became widely accepted in research use.

Diverse Range of Research Applications

Orlando's theory has been widely used as a framework for numerous studies in a variety of settings. Areas studied encompass nursing theory, practice, education, and administration. Both qualitative and quantitative approaches have been employed.

Deliberative Nursing Process has been applied in theory analysis (Alligood & Choi, 1998; Andrews, 1989; Walker & Avant, 1995). A number of patient outcomes have been studied using Deliberative Nursing Process including, but not limited to pain (Barron, 1966; Bochnak, 1963; Bochnak et al., 1962), postoperative recovery (Eisler, Wolfer, & Diers, 1972), blood pressure and pulse rates (Mertz, 1963), vomiting (Dumas & Leonard, 1963), and levels of distress (Potter & Bockenhauer, 2000). Additional

Research Application   15.1

Nurses at New Hampshire Hospital (NHH), a university-affiliated, state psychiatric facility, were interested in determining if implementation of Safety Agreements would affect patient outcomes and nursing comfort levels when working with patients at risk for self-harm (Potter et al., 2005). Registered nurses (RNs) serving on a Continuous Quality Improvement (CQI) committee had examined the use of safety contracts by nurses at the facility and developed a Safety Agreement tool that they thought would facilitate incorporating Orlando's Deliberative Nursing Process when assessing patients at risk for self-harm.

Validity of safety contracts in general has not been tested. Confusion and controversy exist in relation to the definition and the use of safety contracts with patients who are suicidal (Potter & Dawson, 2001). It is suspected that this confusion and controversy lead to a discomfort and a lack of direction when nurses "contract" with patients for safety.

It has been demonstrated by nurses at NHH that Deliberative Nursing Process can make a difference in patient outcomes (Potter & Bockenhauer, 2000). Hence, these investigators postulated that a more standardized process, using Orlando's Deliberative Nursing Process to enhance communication, might promote patients' agreeing to be safe and, in turn, decrease the rate of self-harm incidents and increase RNs' comfort levels when working with patients at risk for self-harm.

Safety agreements were implemented as the standard of care on all units in Acute Psychiatric Services (APS). Incidents of self-harm were collected via the organizational-wide data collection system pre- and postimplementation. Instruction for RNs in the use of safety agreements occurred the month before implementation of Safety Agreements. Registered Nurses already used Deliberative Nursing Process as a framework for nursing care. The RNs were invited to complete two different surveys on the use of Safety Agreement—first was offered at the end of the first 3-month period and the second was offered at the end of 12 months. There were two convenience sample databases: (a) anonymous lists of self-harm incidents (only chart numbers used, not patient names) and (b) all RNs who performed direct patient care (44 RNs responded to Survey I, and 49 RNs responded to Survey II) in APS.

The investigators used t-tests to detect differences in pre- and postintervention outcomes and Stat Pac Gold computer software to analyze data for statistical differences. The mean rate of self-harming incidents did not change significantly pre- and postimplementation of Safety Agreements. Registered nurses were equally divided in relation to thinking Safety Agreements enhanced or did not enhance nurse–patient interactions. However, RNs did report improvement in the following areas related to use of Safety Agreements: patient responsibility, nurse contact with patients, guidance for safety concerns, discussions with patients related to safety, and time guidelines around issues of safety.

Source: Potter, M. L., Vitale-Nolen, R., & Dawson, A. M. (2005). Implementation of safety agreements in an acute psychiatric facility. *Journal of the American Psychiatric Association, 11*(3), 144–155.

areas explored using Deliberative Nursing Process include spousal grieving (Dracup & Breu, 1978), breastfeeding (Clausen, 1983), and cancer (Reid-Ponte, 1988). Nursing education (Haggerty, 1987; Orlando, 1972) and nursing administration (Schmieding, 1984, 1992) also have been examined using the Deliberative Nursing Process. (For additional studies using Deliberative Nursing Process, refer to the Bibliography.)

Potter, Vitale-Nolen, and Dawson (2005) designed a study to determine if implementation of a Safety Agreement tool made a difference in the rate of patient self-harm incidents and in nurses' feeling more comfortable interacting with patients at risk for self-harm. A Safety Agreement was designed to assist nurses in incorporating Deliberative Nursing Process when interacting with patients at risk for self-harm (see Research Application 15.1).

Bezanson (2002) proposed a theoretical application of Deliberative Nursing Process for an outpatient surgery center of an acute care, community-based hospital. Bezanson asserts that implementation of Deliberative Nursing Process could provide opportunities to improve nursing practice, increase patient satisfaction, and enhance staff satisfaction with their nurse–patient interactions. Bezanson also suggests that mechanisms of evaluation might include patient-focused satisfaction surveys, staff self-reports of satisfaction in practice, and improved patient outcomes.

A quasi-experimental pilot study was undertaken in a large, university-affiliated state psychiatric facility to determine if implementation of Orlando's nursing theory-based practice (Deliberative Nursing Practice) made a difference in patient outcomes when compared with patient outcomes resulting from interventions using nonspecified nursing practice. Two inpatient units were selected that matched most closely in staffing patterns, patient census, and acuity levels. Ten registered nurses (RNs) participated—six in the experimental group and four in the control group. The experimental and control groups of RNs had no significant differences in their demographic composition. Thirty patients were involved in the study—19 in the experimental group and 11 in the control group. Patient experimental and control groups were statistically similar. The RNs were educated in use of the Bockenhauer–Potter Scale of Immediate Distress (BPSID), a five-point Likert-scaled instrument that quantifies the level of patient-demonstrated distress. The BPSID was developed to control for subjectivity when assessing patients'

USING MIDDLE RANGE THEORIES

15.1

levels of distress. The two investigators, a consultant in Orlando's theory, and three hospital RN nurse specialists reviewed and enhanced reference points on the scale. Videotaped simulated interactions helped nurses to learn how to use the BPSID, thus increasing inter-rater reliability. RNs in the experimental group received instruction in Deliberative Nursing Process. Data collection took place over a 12-week time frame. Distress levels of patients were measured before and after RN interventions. A greater reduction ($p = .04$) in patients' levels of distress occurred in the group in which RNs used the Deliberative Nursing Process. Interestingly, RNs who used the Deliberative Nursing Process reported that having a "road map" helped them feel more effective in their nursing interventions. Further research is suggested to control the possible "halo effect" of additional attention provided to the experimental group of RNs via weekly support and education and to obtain verbal feedback from patients who experience nursing interventions that incorporate Deliberative Nursing Process.

Source: Potter, M. L., & Bockenhauer, B. J. (2000). Implementing Orlando's nursing theory: A pilot study. *Journal of Psychosocial Nursing and Mental Health Services, 38*, 14–21.

Deliberative Nursing Process can be used as a framework to design research in various settings and to examine specific patient outcomes. The study illustrated in Using Middle Range Theories 15.1 demonstrates patient outcomes related to reduction in levels of distress when Deliberative Nursing Process was implemented in an acute care psychiatric hospital setting.

Olson and Hanchett (1997) carried out a study examining Orlando's assertion that relationships exist between nurse-expressed empathy and several patient outcomes. They used a descriptive, correlational format, described in Using Middle Range Theories 15.2.

DELIVERING CULTURALLY COMPETENT CARE

Recently, Deliberative Nursing Process was used in the formation and implementation of the Influenza Initiative in New York City—a collaborative nursing effort to meet linguistic needs and provide culturally competent care. This project involved delivering education and immunizations for influenza prevention to an urban population (Aponte, 2009). In this program, bilingual nursing students were paired with nursing providers from a home health care agency to translate for non–English-speaking Spanish, Chinese, Russian, and Ukrainian residents participating in the Influenza Initiative in Fall 2006 and 2007. With Deliberative Nursing Process as a nursing framework for providing care, nursing students were able to confirm and validate clients' needs, ensure accurate understanding of information, confirm consent for treatment, and direct registered nurses (RNs) to administer immunizations in a safe and culturally competent manner (Aponte, 2009).

ETHICAL VALUES IN CARING FOR OLDER ADULTS

In a study by Jonasson (2009), the dynamic nurse–patient relationship is presented as crucial to the process of determining the ethical care of older adults. In her study of nurse–patient interactions between nurses, older adults, and their next of kin, Jonasson points to the processes of validation and evaluation as crucial to providing true benefit to the patient and their family. Through observation and interview data collection, she found that

Relationships between nurse-expressed empathy and two patient outcomes (patient-perceived empathy and patient distress) were explored in a descriptive, correlational study. The hypotheses were: (a) a negative relationship will exist between measures of nurse-expressed empathy and measures of patient distress; (b) a positive relationship will exist between measures of nurse-expressed empathy and patient-perceived empathy, and (c) a negative relationship will exist between patient-perceived empathy and measures of patient distress.

One hundred and forty subjects comprised the sample. Seventy staff registered nurses (RNs) were selected from a pool of 50% of all eligible nurses who were invited. Seventy patients for whom the nurses cared during a day shift were randomly selected to participate.

Nurse participants completed the Staff–Patient Interaction Response Scale (SPIRS) and the Behavioral Test of Interpersonal Skills (BTIS). Both measure

nurse-expressed empathy. Patient participants completed the Empathy Subscale of the Barrett-Lennard Relationship Inventory (BLRI) to determine patient-perceived empathy measures; their patient distress scores were measured using the Profile of Mood States (POMS) and the Multiple Affect Adjective Check List (MAACL).

Testing of hypothesis was as follows: (a) hypothesis one and three were tested together by means of one canonical correlation and (b) hypothesis three was tested by means of multiple regression analysis. All three hypotheses received statistically significant support with the BTIS measurement. A fuller description of methodology and findings are recorded in a report by Olson (1995). This study supported Orlando's (1961, 1972) assertion that relationships exist between accurate perceptions of patients' needs (nurse-expressed empathy and patient-expressed empathy) and patient distress.

USING MIDDLE RANGE THEORIES

15.2

Source: Olson, J., & Hanchett, E. (1997). Nurse-expressed empathy, patient outcomes, and development of a middle-range theory. *Image: Journal of Nursing Scholarship, 29,* 71–76.

body language, elements of respect, and behavior elements of the initial approach of a nurse with an older adult client are crucial in developing a therapeutic nursing relationship. Moreover, the patient and next of kin's perceptions of the nurses' availability and approachability led to improved patient and family feelings of being valued and acknowledged. Jonasson challenges nurses to recognize the extent to which their approach to patients impacts patients' feelings and outcomes, as dependent upon nurse "attitude and actions" (Jonasson, 2009, p. 26).

Nursing Informatics

In a paper regarding Nursing Process Theory and the development of nursing information systems to improve care delivery in the future, Alexander (2007) highlights the role of Orlando's prescribed elements of nursing process: observations, actions, reporting, and recording. In particular, Alexander proposes a nursing informatics model, called the nurse–patient trajectory framework. This trajectory incorporates both patient and provider inputs to coordinate patient care and nursing process elements with human computer interaction to direct the overall plan of care (Alexander, 2007). In comparison to other models of nursing informatics to determine the plan of care, this model would uniquely involve patient input. This would ensure inclusion of validation and evaluation of the client's needs and perceived sources of distress and comfort, rather than promoting an automatic nursing process through technology-guided information processing.

INSTRUMENTS USED IN EMPIRICAL TESTING

There are no set means or tools to measure Deliberative Nursing Process. This is indicative of the nature of the theory because Orlando emphasized that Deliberative Nursing Process involves a nursing situation in which the uniqueness of the nurse is brought to the experience to meet the immediate needs for help, as expressed by the patient, explored by the nurse and the patient, and validated by the nurse with the patient. Each circumstance or nursing situation will be unique and different, because each nurse perceives, feels, and thinks differently than any other nurse entering the same nursing situation.

TABLE 15.2 Deliberative Nursing Process Tools

Category	Abbreviation	Example
Anxiety		State Anxiety Inventory (Spielberger, Gorsuch, & Lushene, 1970).
Attitude change		Spouse Questionnaire (Silva, 1979) Spouses' Perception Scale (Silva, 1979)
Emotional state	WI	Welfare Inventory (Eisler et al., 1972)
Nurse-expressed empathy	BTIS SPIRS	Behavioral Test of Interpersonal Skills (Gerrard & Bussell, 1980) Staff–Patient Interaction Response Scale (Gallop, 1989)
Patient-perceived empathy	BLRI	Barrett-Lennard Relationship Inventory (Barrett-Lennard, 1962)
Patient distress	POMS MAACL BPSID	Profile of Mood States (McNair, Lorr, & Droppleman, 1981) Multiple Affect Adjective Check List (Zuckerman & Lubin, 1965) Bockenhauer–Potter Scale of Immediate Distress (Bockenhauer & Potter, 2000) Pain and distress questionnaire (Hall-Lord & Larsson, 2006)
Patient's self-harm incidents	SA	Safety Agreement (Potter et al., 2005)
Nurse-perceived comfort with use of safety agreements		Registered Nurses Evaluation Survey (Potter et al., 2005)
Therapeutic effectiveness	EPPS SII	Edwards Personal Preference Schedule (Edwards, 1959) Social Interaction Inventory (Methven & Schlotfeldt, 1962)
Postoperative physical recovery	RI	Recovery Inventory (Eisler et al., 1972)
Social approval	SD Scale	Social Desirability Scale (Crowne & Marlowe, 1964)

Different tools have been developed and/or used to measure different aspects of Deliberative Nursing Process. These tools facilitate examination of such factors as patient outcomes, nursing process, nurse empathy, and patient-perceived empathy. The instruments have been developed and/or used to test Deliberative Nursing Process qualitatively and quantitatively. Instruments used in different studies explore different aspects of the Deliberative Nursing Process, such as theory description and analysis, use in research, use in clinical practice, and use in administrative practice.

Much of the testing done with Deliberative Nursing Process involves questionnaires and surveys. Examples of tools that have been used for studies involving Orlando's Deliberative Nursing Process are listed in Table 15.2.

SAFETY AGREEMENT INSTRUMENT

One instrument used in the study of Deliberative Nursing Process has been the Safety Agreement. The Safety Agreement instrument, developed by nurses at NHH, was designed to measure patients' risk for self-harm and willingness and the ability to agree to remain safe (see Table 15.2). Most of the agreements are designed in Likert-style format. A question related to a patient's perceived ability to remain safe requires a "yes" or "no" response. In addition, a question seeking to determine how the patient and RN might work together to manage the current risk for self-harm elicits a response from a number of given choices with an "other" option included. The intent of the Safety Agreement is to assist the RN in a deliberative process of determining with the patient the patient's risk for self-harm.

A Safety Agreement was implemented by Potter et al. (2005) at NHH; the agreement was used in a convenience sample, with all patients admitted or considered at risk for self-harm. Patients were asked to self-rate the following areas with the RN: (a) their current harm level, (b) the likelihood of their acting on their thoughts of self-harm, (c) their thoughts about managing the risk with the RN, (d) their willingness to enter an agreement for safety with the RN, and (e) their thoughts about how long they think they can remain safe.

In the context of this study, RNs were given the Registered Nurses Evaluation Survey, which also was in Likert-type format, except one question. RNs were asked to evaluate (a) the number of times they used the Safety Agreement in a 3-month period, (b) if the Safety Agreement assisted them in feeling more comfortable while helping patients at risk for self-harm, (c) if they thought self-harming incidents decreased since implementation of Safety Agreements, and (d) if they had any other comments to share related to use of Safety Agreements. With the use of Safety Agreements, RNs reported improvement in patient responsibility, nurse contact with patients, guidance for safety concerns, discussions with patients related to safety, and time guidelines around issues of safety. Research Application 15.1 describes the design and outcome of this research study implementing Safety Agreements at NHH (Potter et al., 2005).

PAIN AND DISTRESS INSTRUMENT

A study of nursing caregivers (RNs and nursing students) revealed associations between nursing assessments of patient distress according to particular patient and caregiver characteristics (Hall-Lord & Larsson, 2006). The investigators measured patients' pain and distress with a 13-item pain and distress questionnaire to evaluate sensory, emotional, and existential dimensions of distress (see Table 15.2). Caregiver characteristics were assessed using the sense of coherence (SOC) scale, five-factor personality inventory (FFPI), and their degree of experience in nursing. When given the same patient scenarios, Hall-Lord and Larsson (2006) refer to Orlando's assertion that nurses' personality factors contribute to their automatic responses, which is supported in their research. They report that nursing experience and personality factors apparently impacted their assessments and ability to empathize with patients in distress, along with factors of patient age and illness type and severity. Their study supports the need for more reliable pain and distress instruments, and improved self-awareness among nurses, to diminish biases and variability in assessments of patient comfort.

SUMMARY

Ida Jean Orlando developed Deliberative Nursing Process theory at a time of great need and growth within the nursing profession, and as demonstrated in the recent examples, her work continues to be relevant to improving patient outcomes and advancing the nursing profession. Soon after Orlando's original publication, Gowan and Morris (1964) speculated that the nursing shortage of that era and the increased expectations upon nurses led to nurses spending more time designing care than providing care. Results from their study indicated that patients experienced undue delays in receiving care and withheld requests that involved their well-being due to patient perceptions that the nurses were too busy, would disapprove, would not like to be interrupted, or would think the request was not helpful to the patient. Might this same scenario be repeating itself today?

In 1990, the National League for Nursing honored Orlando by reprinting *The Dynamic Nurse–Patient Relationship.* Orlando noted in the Preface to that edition that interest in the United States using her theory had waned (Orlando, 1990, p. viii). Interest and use of the theory may have subsided temporarily, but it never ceased. As noted by Orlando herself, her work has been published in five foreign countries, and there have been numerous publications in recent years related to Deliberative Nursing Process (Potter & Bockenhauer, 2000; Potter & Dawson, 2001; Potter & Tinker, 2000; Schmieding, 1993b, 1999, 2002;

Rosenthal, 1996). Many changes have occurred in nursing. However, the essence of nursing, described so simply yet eloquently by Orlando, has not changed—namely that the nurse–patient relationship involves a dynamic and unique process that evolves between nurse and patient when approached deliberatively and validated with the patient on an ongoing basis.

Deliberative Nursing Process is a nursing theory for all times. The use of Deliberative Nursing Process helps nurses maintain a patient-centered approach when providing nursing care amidst additional and varied expectations of the nurse. Orlando has kept the message of Deliberative Nursing Process clear throughout the years: "It is the nurse's direct responsibility to see to it that the patient's needs for help are met, either directly by her own activity or indirectly by calling in the help of others" (Orlando, 1961, p. 29). Adopting such a clear function promotes effective and efficient nursing practice as has been demonstrated through empirical studies on Deliberative Nursing Process for more than 40 years.

ANALYSIS OF THEORY

Using the criteria presented in Chapter 2, critique the theory of Deliberative Nursing Process. Compare your conclusions about the theory with those found in Appendix A. A nurse scholar who has worked with the theory completed the analysis found in the Appendix.

Internal Criticism	External Criticism
1. Clarity	1. Reality convergence
2. Consistency	2. Utility
3. Adequacy	3. Significance
4. Logical development	4. Discrimination
5. Level of theory development	5. Scope of theory
	6. Complexity

CRITICAL THINKING EXERCISES

1. Scenario: Upon entering a patient's room on the medical unit, the nurse notices the patient's right hand over her heart. The patient has her head down and is sobbing. Give examples of how you, as the nurse, might share each of the following:

   a. Your perceptions

   b. Your thoughts

   c. Your feelings

2. What is the function of "validation" in Deliberative Nursing Process?

3. State three ways using Deliberative Nursing Process is more beneficial in the nurse–patient relationship than using automatic nursing process.

4. Compare and contrast the concept and definition of comfort in Deliberative Nursing Process with the concept of comfort according to other nursing theorists, such as Kolcaba or Leininger.

5. Discuss if/how Deliberative Nursing Process could benefit nursing practice in an intensive care setting, even if patients were unconscious or unable to communicate verbally.

6. Consider Orlando's distinction between the roles of "nursing" and "doctoring" in patient care. Discuss how the same roles do/do not apply to physicians and nurses today.

7. Do you agree with Orlando's assertion that nursing is either "good" or "bad"? If so, why? If not, how would you define excellence in nursing?

WEB RESOURCES

Visit **http://thePoint.lww.com/Peterson3e** for helpful web resources related to this chapter.

ACKNOWLEDGMENTS

Much appreciation is expressed to: Mimi Dye, MSN, ARNP, who completed the critique on Deliberative Nursing Process in the Appendix A and studied Deliberative Nursing Process as a student with the theorist, Ida J. Orlando, MS, RN; Joy L. Potter, who served as research assistant in the 2nd edition, and Dorothy Y. Kameoka, MLS, MSW, RN, who sought out materials for the 1st and 2nd editions. To Rebecca E. Andersen, RN, MSN, who served as research assistant in this 3rd edition, the author extends her gratitude and best wishes for a meaningful journey in nursing.

REFERENCES

Alexander, G. L. (2007). The nurse–patient trajectory framework. In K. Kuhn, et al. (Eds.) *MEDINFO 2007.* Amsterdam: IOS Press.

Allen, D. E., Bockenhauer, B., Egan, C., & Kinnaird, L. S. (2006). Relating outcomes to excellent nursing practice. *Journal of Nursing Administration, 26*(3), 140–147. doi:10.1097/00005110-200603000-00008

Alligood, M. R. (2002). The nature of knowledge needed for nursing practice. In M. R. Alligood & A. Marriner-Tomey (Eds.), *Nursing theory—Utilization & application* (2nd ed., pp. 3–14). St. Louis, MO: Mosby.

Alligood, M. R., & Choi, E. C. (1998). Evolution of nursing theory development. In A. Marriner-Tomey & M. R. Alligood (Eds.), *Nursing theorists and their work* (4th ed., pp. 55–66). St Louis, MO: Mosby.

Andrews, C. M. (1989). Ida Orlando's model of nursing practice. In J. J. Fitzpatrick & A. L. Whall (Eds.), *Conceptual models of nursing: Analysis & application* (2nd ed., pp. 69–87). Norwalk, CT: Appleton & Lange.

Aponte, J. (2009). Meeting the linguistic needs of urban communities. *Home Healthcare Nurse, 27*(5), 324–329. doi:10.1097/01.NHH.0000356786.85750.e9

Barron, M. A. (1966). The effects varied nursing approaches have on patients' complaints of pain. *Nursing Research, 15,* 90–91. doi:10.1097/00006199-196601510-00053

Bezanson, A. (2002). *Theoretical application of Orlando's theory of deliberate Nursing process in an outpatient surgery center.* Unpublished manuscript.

Bochnak, M. A. (1963). The effect of an automatic and deliberative process of nursing activity on the relief of patients' pain: A clinical experiment. *Nursing Research, 12,* 191–192.

Bochnak, M. A., Rhymes, J. P., & Leonard, R. C. (1962). The comparison of two types of nursing activity on the relief of pain. In *Innovations in nurse–patient relationships: Automatic or reasoned nurse action* (Clinical Paper No. 6). New York: American Nurses Association.

Bolden, L. V., & Larrabee, J. H. (2001). Defining patient-perceived quality of nursing care. *Journal of Nursing Care Quality, 16,* 34–60.

Clausen [Cameron], J. C. (1983). Clinical nursing research on the science and art of breastfeeding using a deliberative nursing care approach. *Western Journal of Nursing Research, 5,* 29.

Dracup, K. A., & Breu, C. S. (1978). Using nursing research findings to meet the needs of grieving spouses. *Nursing Research, 27,* 212–216.

Dumas, R. G., & Leonard, R. C. (1963). The effect of nursing on the incidence of postoperative vomiting. *Nursing Research, 12,* 12–15. doi:10.1097/00006199-196301210-00005

Eisler, J., Wolfer, J. A., & Diers, D. (1972). Relationship between need for social approval and postoperative recovery and welfare. *Nursing Research, 21,* 520–525. doi:10.1097/00006199-197211000-00013

Faust, C. (2002). Orlando's deliberative nursing process theory: A practice application in an extended care facility. *Journal of Gerontological Nursing, 28*(7), 14–18.

Gowan, N. I., & Morris, M. (1964). Nurses' responses to expressed patient needs. *Nursing Research, 13,* 68–71. doi:10.1097/00006199-196401310-00023

Haggerty, L. A. (1987). An analysis of senior nursing students' immediate responses to distressed patients. *Journal of Advanced Nursing, 12,* 451–461. doi:10.1111/j.1365-2648.1987.tb01354.x

Hall-Lord, M. L., & Larsson, B. W. (2006). Registered nurses' and student nurses' assessment of pain and distress related to specific patient and nurse characteristics. *Nurse Education Today, 20,* 377–387. doi:10.1016/j.nedt.2005.11.007

Johnson, B. M., & Webber, P. B. (2001). *Theory and reasoning in nursing.* New York: Lippincott Williams & Wilkins.

Jonasson, L. (2009). *Ethical values in caring encounters from elderly patients' and next of kin's perspective.* Linköping University Studies in Health Sciences Thesis No. 107. Linköping, Sweden.

Marriner-Tomey, A. (1998). Introduction to analysis of nursing theories. In A. Marriner-Tomey & M. R. Alligood (Eds.), *Nursing theorists and their work* (4th ed., pp. 3–15). St. Louis, MO: Mosby.

McEwan, M. (2002). Middle-range nursing theories. In M. McEwan & E. M. Wills (Eds.), *Theoretical basis for nursing* (pp. 202–225). Philadelphia, PA: Lippincott Williams & Wilkins.

Meleis, A. I. (1997). *Theoretical nursing: Development & progress* (3rd ed., pp. 343–353). Philadelphia, PA: Lippincott-Raven.

Mertz, H. (1963). A study of the process of the nurse's activity as it affects the blood pressure readings and pulse rate of patients admitted to the emergency room. *Nursing Research, 12,* 197–198.

Orlando, I. J. (1961). *The dynamic nurse–patient relationship.* New York: Putnam.

Orlando, I. J. (1972). *The discipline and teaching of nursing process (an evaluative study).* New York: Putnam.

Orlando, I. J. (1976, August). *The fundamental issue in professional nursing.* Paper presented at the University of Tulsa College of Nursing, Tulsa, OK.

Orlando [Pelletier], I. J. (1983, October). *Comments on ANA's social policy statement of 1980.* Paper presented at Southeastern Massachusetts University, College of Nursing, Honor Society, South Dartmouth, MA.

Orlando, I. J. (1987). Nursing in the 21st century: Alternate paths. *Journal of Advanced Nursing, 12,* 405–412. doi:10.1111/j.1365-2648.1987.tb01349.x

Orlando, I. J. (1990, reissue). *The dynamic nurse–patient relationship.* New York: National League for Nursing.

Orlando, I. J., & Dugan, A. B. (1989). Independent and dependent paths: The fundamental issue for the nursing profession. *Nursing and Health Care, 10,* 77–80.

Pelletier, I. O. (1967). The patient's predicament and nursing function. *Psychiatric Opinion, 4,* 25–30.

Pelletier, I. O. (1976). *The fundamental issue in professional nursing.* Unpublished manuscript, pp. 1–22.

Potter, M. L. (2008, February). *Tribute to a nursing leader: Ida Jean Orlando Pelletier.* New Hampshire Board of Nursing. Retrieved March 11, 2008, from http://www.nh.gov/nursing/general/documents/0208.pdf

Potter, M. L., & Bockenhauer, B. J. (2000). Implementing Orlando's nursing theory: A pilot study. *Journal of Psychosocial Nursing and Mental Health Services, 38,* 14–21.

Potter, M. L., & Dawson, A. M. (2001). From safety contract to safety agreement. *Journal of Psychosocial Nursing and Mental Health Services, 39,* 38–45.

Potter, M. L., & Tinker, S. W. (2000). Put power in nurses' hands: Orlando's nursing theory supports nurses—simply. *Nursing Management, 31,* 40–41.

Potter, M. L., Vitale-Nolen, R., & Dawson, A. M. (2005). Implementation of safety agreements in an acute psychiatric facility. *Journal of the American Psychiatric Association, 11*(3), 144–155. doi:10.1177/1078390305277443

Potter, M. L., Williams, R. B., & Costanzo, R. (2004). Using nursing theory and a structured psychoeducational curriculum with inpatient groups. *Journal of the American Psychiatric Nurses Association, 10*(3), 122–128. doi:10.1177/1078390304265212

Reid-Ponte, P. (1988). *The relationship among empathy and the use of Orlando's deliberative process by the primary nurse and the distress of the adult cancer patient.* Doctoral dissertation, Boston University, Boston.

Rosenthal, B. C. (1996). An interactionist's approach to perioperative nursing. *Association of Operating Room Nurses Journal, 64,* 254–260.

Schmieding, N. J. (1984). Putting Orlando's theory into practice. *American Journal of Nursing, 84,* 759–761. doi:10.2307/3463720

Schmieding, N. J. (1992). Relationship between head nurse responses to staff nurses and staff nurse response to patients. *Western Journal of Nursing Research, 13,* 746–760. doi:10.1177/019394599101300606

Schmieding, N. J. (1993a). *Ida Jean Orlando: A nursing process theory.* London: Sage.

Schmieding, N. J. (1993b). Successful superior-subordinate relationships require mutual management. *Health Care Supervisor, 11,* 52–63.

Schmieding, N. J. (1999). Reflective inquiry framework for nurse administrators. *Journal of Advanced Nursing, 30,* 631–639. doi:10.1046/j.1365-2648.1999.01134.x

Schmieding, N. J. (2002). Orlando's nursing process theory. In M. R. Alligood & A. Marriner-Tomey (Eds.), *Nursing theory utilization & application* (2nd ed., pp. 315–337). St. Louis, MO: Mosby.

Sheldon, L. K., & Ellington, L. (2008). Application of a model of social information processing to nursing theory: How nurses respond to patients. *Journal of Advanced Nursing, 64*(4), 344–398. doi:10.1111/j.1365-2648.2008.04795.x

Stevens-Barnum, B. J. (1990). *Nursing theory: Analysis, application, evaluation.* Glenview, IL: Scott Foresman/Little & Brown.

Tutton, E., & Seers, K. (2003). The concept of comfort. *Journal of Clinical Nursing, 12,* 689–696. doi:10.1046/j.1365-2702.2003.00775.x

Tyra, P. A. (2008). In memoriam: Ida Jean Orlando Pelletier. *Journal of the American Psychiatric Nurses Association, 14,* 231–232. doi:10.1177/1078390308321092

Walker, L. O., & Avant, K. C. (1995). *Strategies for theory construction in nursing* (3rd ed.). Norwalk, CT: Appleton & Lange.

Wills, E. M. (2002). Overview of grand nursing theories. In M. McEwan & E. M. Wills (Eds.), *Theoretical basis for nursing* (pp. 111–124). Philadelphia, PA: Lippincott Wilkins & Williams.

Wooldridge, P. J., Skipper, J. K. Jr., & Leonard, R. C. (1968). *Behavioral science, social practice, and the nursing profession.* Cleveland, OH: Case Western Reserve University.

BIBLIOGRAPHY

Cameron, J. (1963). An exploratory study of the verbal responses of the nurse–patient interactions. *Nursing Research, 12,* 192.

Chapman, J. S. (1969). *Effects of different nursing approaches upon psychological and physiological responses of patients.* Unpublished doctoral dissertation. Case Western Reserve University, Frances Payne Bolton School of Nursing, Cleveland, OH.

Dumas, R. G., & Johnson [Anderson], B. A. (1972). Research in nursing practice: A review of five clinical experiments. *International Journal of Nursing Studies, 9,* 137–149. doi:10.1016/0020-7489(72)90040-5

Dumas, R. G., & Leonard, R. C. (1963). The effect of nursing on the incidence of postoperative vomiting. *Nursing Research, 12,* 12–15. doi:10.1097/00006199-196301210-00005

Dye, M. C. (1963a). Clarifying patients' communication. *The American Journal of Nursing, 63,* 56–59. doi:10.2307/3452729

Dye, M. C. (1963b). A descriptive study of conditions conducive to an effective process of nursing activity. *Nursing Research, 12,* 194.

Elms, R. R., & Leonard, R. C. (1966). Effects of nursing approaches during admission. *Nursing Research, 15,* 39–48.

Farrell, G. A. (1991). How accurately do nurses perceive patients' needs? A comparison of general and psychiatric settings. *Journal of Advanced Nursing, 16,* 1062–1070. doi:10.1111/j.1365-2648.1991.tb03367.x

Faulkner, S. A. (1963). A descriptive study of needs communicated to the nurse by some mothers on a postpartum service. *Nursing Research, 4,* 260. doi:10.1097/00006199-196301240-00037

Forchuck, C. (1991). A comparison of the works of Peplau and Orlando. *Archives of Psychiatric Nursing, 5,* 38–45. doi:10.1016/0883-9417(91)90008-S

Gillis, S. L. (1976). Sleeplessness: Can you help? *The Canadian Nurse, 72,* 32–34.

Hampe, S. O. (1975). Needs of grieving spouses in a hospital setting. *Nursing Research, 24,* 113. doi: 10.1097/00006199-197503000-00009

Kokuyama, T., & Schmieding, N. J. (1995). Responses staff nurses prefer compared with their perception of head nurse responses. *Japanese Journal of Nursing Administration, 5,* 33–38.

Laurent, C. L. (1999). A nursing theory for nursing leadership. *Journal of Nursing Management, 8,* 83–87. doi:10.1046/j.1365-2834.2000.00161.x

Mahaffy, P. P. (1965). The effects of hospitalization on children admitted for tonsillectomy and adenoidectomy. *Nursing Research, 14,* 12–19. doi:10.1097/00006199-196501410-00005

Nelson, B. (1978). A practical application of nursing theory. *Nursing Clinics of North America, 13,* 157–169.

Olson, J. K. (1995). Relationships between nurse expressed empathy, patient perceived empathy, and patient distress. *Image: Journal of Nursing Scholarship, 27,* 323–328. doi:10.1111/j.1547-5069.1995.tb00895.x

Olson, J., & Hanchett, E. (1997). Nurse-expressed empathy, patient outcomes, and development of a middle-range theory. *Image: Journal of Nursing Scholarship, 29,* 71–76. doi:10.1111/j.1547-5069.1997.tb01143.x

Peitchinis, J. A. (1972). Therapeutic effectiveness of counseling by nursing personnel. *Nursing Research, 21,* 138–148.

Pride, L. F. (1968). An adrenal stress index as a criterion measure of nursing. *Nursing Research, 17,* 292–303. doi:10.1097/00006199-196807000-00002

Rittman, M. R. (2001). Ida Jean Orlando (Pelletier): The dynamic nurse–patient relationship. In M. E. Parker (Ed.), *Nursing theories and nursing practice* (pp. 125–130). Philadelphia, PA: Davis.

Schmieding, N. J. (1987a). Problematic situations in nursing: Analysis of Orlando's theory based on Dewey's theory of inquiry. *Journal of Advanced Nursing, 12,* 431–440. doi:10.1111/j.1365-2648.1987.tb01352.x

Schmieding, N. J. (1987b). Analyzing managerial responses in face-to-face contacts. *Journal of Advanced Nursing, 12,* 357–365. doi:10.1111/j.1365-2648.1987.tb01342.x

Schmieding, N. J. (1987c). Face-to-face contacts: Exploring their meaning. *Nursing Management, 12,* 82–86.

Schmieding, N. J. (1988). Action process of nurse administrators to problematic situations based on Orlando's theory. *Journal of Advanced Nursing, 13,* 99–107. doi:10.1111/j.1365-2648.1988.tb01396.x

Schmieding, N. J. (1990a). A model for assessing nurse administrator's actions. *Western Journal of Nursing Research, 12,* 293–306. doi:10.1177/019394599001200303

Schmieding, N. J. (1990b). Do head nurses include staff nurses in problem solving? *Nursing Management, 21,* 58–60. doi:10.1097/00006247-199003000-00016

Schmieding, N. J. (2006). Ida Jean Orlando (Pelletier): Nursing process theory. In A. M. Tomey & M. R. Alligood (Eds.), *Nursing theorists and their work* (6th ed., pp. 431–451). St. Louis, MO: Mosby.

Silva, M. C. (1979). Effects of orientation information on spouses' anxieties and attitudes toward hospitalization and surgery. *Research in Nursing and Health, 2,* 127–136. doi:10.1002/nur.4770020308

Sitzman, K., & Eichelberger, L. W. (2004). *Understanding the work of nurse theorists: A creative beginning.* Sudbury, MA: Jones & Bartlett.

Tarasuk [Bochnak], M. B., Rhymes, J., & Leonard, R. C. (1965). An experimental test of the importance of communication skills for effective nursing. In J. K. Skipper Jr. & R. C. Leonard (Eds.), *Social interaction and patient care* (pp. 110–120). Philadelphia, PA: Lippincott.

Tryon, P. A. (1966). Use of comfort measures as support during labor. *Nursing Research, 15,* 109–118. doi:10.1097/00006199-196601520-00003

Tryon, P. A., & Leonard, R. C. (1964). The effect of patients' participation on the outcome of a nursing procedure. *Nursing Forum, 3,* 79–89. doi:10.1111/j.1744-6198.1964.tb00273.x

Williamson, Y. M. (1978). Methodologic dilemmas in tapping the concept of patient needs. *Nursing Research, 27,* 172–177. doi:10.1097/00006199-197805000-00023

16

Resilience

JOAN E. HAASE

SANDRA J. PETERSON

DEFINITION OF KEY TERMS

Boundaries of resilience	The contextual influences, dimensions, and assumptions that are considered in determining the attributes of resilience
Meaning-based models	Explanatory models focused on the patterns and experiences of illness from a subjective and holistic perspective
Person-focused research	Research to identify the patterns of variables in which resilience naturally occurs, then examining what might contribute to these outcomes; or using cut-off scores on selected variables to categorize adversity subgroups, then examining outcomes in these groups
Positive health research	Efforts to gain understanding of ways individuals sustain or regain optimal health
Protective factors	The individual, family, social, or other contextual factors that enhance resilience processes and outcomes
Quality of life	A sense of well-being
Resilience	General definition: positive adjustment in the face of adversity; context-derived definition: the process of identifying or developing resources and strengths to flexibly manage stressors to gain a positive outcome, a sense of confidence/mastery, self-transcendence, and self-esteem
Risk factors	The individual, family, social, or other contextual factors that impede development of resilience processes and outcomes
Strengths-based research	Research that focuses on individual, family, or community "promise" rather than on risk
Triangulation	Use of quantitative or qualitative research approaches either sequentially or simultaneously to refine, evaluate, and/or extend theory
Variable-focused approaches	Use of multivariate statistics to test for linkages to resilience among measures of adversity, outcomes, and environmental or individual qualities that may protect from or compensate for negative consequences

Contributing Authors: Chin-Mi Chen, National Defense Medical Center, Taipei, Taiwan; and Celeste Phillips-Salimi and Cynthia Bell, Indiana University School of Nursing, Indianapolis, IN.

INTRODUCTION

Researchers and practitioners have long sought answers to questions about psychosocial adjustment to illness, especially chronic conditions. While much research is still guided by pathology and deficit-based models that examine risk, adjustment problems, and developmental delays (Hymovich & Roehnert, 1989), salutogenic, positive health, and strengths-based models are gaining recognition as useful perspectives in nursing and other health care disciplines (Antonovsky, 1979; Hymovich & Roehnert, 1989; Singer & Ryff, 2001; Woodgate, 1999). Theories such as resilience (Rutter, 1979, 1987), hardiness (Kobasa, 1982), self-efficacy, and learned resourcefulness (Bandura, 1977; Rosenbaum, 1983) were developed to explain positive adjustment to illness, based on the belief that such theories may yield information about effective interventions (Forsyth, Delaney, & Gresham, 1984; Garmezy, 1991; Kadner, 1989; Sinnema, 1991). In 2001, the Committee on Future Direction for Behavioral and Social Sciences identified resilience as a research priority for the National Institutes of Health (Singer & Ryff, 2001). The committee highlighted the significance of behavioral and psychosocial processes in disease etiology, well-being, and health promotion. In addition, the committee recommended increased study of the protective factors that are correlates of resilience, such as optimism, meaning and purpose, social and emotional support, and related neurobiological mechanisms that promote recovery and increased survival rates (Singer & Ryff, 2001). These recommendations have been accepted at least to some extent, as indicated by the rapidly increasing number of theory and research reports in the literature. Nurses also recognize the importance of positive health concepts and are increasingly seeing an understanding of resilience as potentially useful to (a) guide development of interventions to enhance positive outcomes; (b) improve outcomes for at-risk populations; (c) prevent poor outcomes; and (d) influence public policy related to individuals, families, and communities.

Resilience is broadly defined as a phenomenon of positive adjustment in the face of adversity. Historically, resilience was most frequently studied in children and adolescents and was characterized by attributes usually identified as positive. Examples of such positive attributes found in early research on resilience include competence (Garmezy, Masten, & Tellegen, 1984; Rutter, 1979); self-esteem (Garmezy, 1981); superior coping (Garmezy, 1991; Murphy & Moriarty, 1976); advanced self-help, communication, and problem-solving skills (Garmezy, 1981; Hauser, Vieyra, Jacobson, & Wertlieb, 1985); tendency to perceive experiences constructively (Werner & Smith, 1982); and ability to use spirituality to maintain a positive vision of a meaningful life (Rutter, 1979; Wells & Schwebel, 1987).

HISTORICAL BACKGROUND

Since the 1970s, shifting perspectives on resilience inquiry have occurred. Two authors' descriptions of these shifting perspectives are especially informative. Richardson (2002) describes resilience research as occurring in three ways:

1. Efforts to describe personal qualities that predict success
2. Resilience as a process
3. Resilience as a motivational life force to be fostered in all individuals

Similarly, Masten (2001) portrays a gradual change in perspectives of resilience, from a view of resilience as an extraordinary occurrence to the current evidence-based perspective that resilience is a commonly occurring phenomenon that is essentially a basic function of adaptational systems.

Positive adaptation research began with studies on the premorbid competence of patients with schizophrenia (Garmezy, 1974; Masten, Best, & Garmezy, 1990). Those studies were precursors to the seminal theoretical and empirical groundwork on resilience done with children of mothers with schizophrenia. The major characteristic of these children was the fact that they thrived despite their high-risk status. After describing children who thrived despite adversity, subsequent studies were directed to understanding individual differences in response to adversity. This effort to understand individual differences was gradually expanded to other contexts, such as childhood exposure to adverse conditions of socioeconomic adversity (Rutter, 1979), abuse (Henry, 2001), urban poverty and community violence (Luthar, Cicchetti, & Becker,

2000), and chronic illness (Wells & Schwebel, 1987). In the early 1990s, researchers began to identify external factors that contributed to development of resilience. Three general classes of protective factors—individual, family, and social—are now generally recognized as influencing resilience development (Rutter, 1987). Currently, in addition to continuing to identify protective factors, researchers are seeking to understand the underlying mechanisms or processes of how the interaction of risk and protective factors influence resilience outcomes (Luthar et al., 2000). There is a strongly emerging priority for research on the biological contributors to or correlates of resilience (Curtis & Cicchetti, 2003). And, there is increasing focus on research examining and fostering resilience with adolescents, while simultaneously on expansion of ages and contexts studied.

DEFINITION OF THEORY CONCEPTS

There is widespread agreement that resilience is a complex, multidimensional construct. Largely because of the complexity of the construct, there is a lack of consensus about terminology, characteristics, or boundaries of resilience. The following sections examine the various perspectives in these three areas from both the general and the nursing literature.

PERSPECTIVES ON RESILIENCE

TERMINOLOGY AND ATTRIBUTES OF RESILIENCE

To adequately define a construct, terminology needs to be consistent. In the case of resilience, even the labels for the phenomenon have been inconsistently used. Labels variously applied to the phenomenon have included resilience, resiliency, and ego-resilience. Researchers currently recommend the term *resilience,* rather than *resiliency,* to describe positive adjustment in face of adversity (Luthar et al., 2000; Masten, 1994). "Resiliency" is not recommended, because it implies a personality trait that is difficult to alter, much like hardiness. The term *ego-resilience* characterizes resilience as a distinct personality trait. Hence, ego-resilience decreases the options for intervention and increases the danger of labeling individuals as innately "inadequate."

There are two generally recognized essential attributes of resilience present in most definitions. These are the presence of (a) "good" or positive outcomes that occur in spite of (b) adverse conditions (Masten, 2001).

Good Outcomes. "Good" or positive outcomes are not consistently theoretically or operationally defined in the literature. Debate centers on what constitutes "good" outcomes and who decides. Additional questions include whether external criteria (e.g., academic achievement), intrapersonal characteristics (e.g., sense of well-being, self-esteem), or a combination of both are defining characteristics of positive outcomes (Masten, 2001).

Paradigmatic approaches also contribute to differences in ways positive outcomes are defined. A pathology-based worldview often defines positive outcomes as the absence of psychopathology or low levels of symptoms or impairments (Masten & Coatsworth, 1998). Developmental and life-span perspectives usually define positive outcomes as those that meet or exceed expectations. More recently, a subtle shift in worldviews has occurred that emphasizes dynamic ecosystems influenced by complex, ever-changing, and interacting forces (Richardson, 2002; Waller, 2001) and the notion that resilience is possibly a common human characteristic—"ordinary magic" (Masten, 2001).

Adverse Conditions. The theoretical and operational definitions of "adverse conditions" are also inconsistent in the literature. Frequently, definitions infer threats or risk factors that occur in contexts such as war, illness, community deficits, or family adversity. Beyond the requirement that such factors negatively affect resilience outcomes, there is no agreement on how such risks should be operationalized. Options include: (a) current or past occurrence; (b) predictors of poor outcomes or status (moderating) variables such as low socioeconomic status; or (c) single-exposure variables or cumulative combinations of factors. Adding to the inconsistency of defining characteristics, risk factors can be continuous bipolar variables classified as either less or more aversive (e.g., mild to severe symptoms) or as negative to positive assets (e.g., low to high economic status and negative to positive coping) (Masten, 2001). In general, much research indicates that risk factors, however operationalized, often co-occur (Masten, 2001).

BOUNDARIES OF RESILIENCE

Boundaries of resilience are the contextual influences (conditions under which resilience exists/varies/ disappears), dimensions (e.g., objective/subjective and physiological/psychological), and underlying assumptions (e.g., growth vs. stability and state vs. trait) that are considered in determining the attributes of resilience. Some boundaries of resilience that need careful explication in theory and research include state/trait/process, psychological/physiological, individual/aggregate, and objective/subjective perspective. Within each of these boundaries, the cross-cultural implications also need thoughtful examination and further research.

Trait/State/Process. Although the definition of resilience as the presence of "good" outcomes that occur in the presence of adverse conditions implies a process, there is no consensus on the issue of resilience as trait, state, or process. Again, the confusion is exacerbated by inconsistent terminology and the inability to draw conclusions of causality (Jacelon, 1997; Pettit, 2000). As indicated above, the term *ego-resiliency*, for example, is frequently used interchangeably with resilience, but the former refers to a set of personal characteristics (traits) that may or may not be specifically linked to adversity (Luthar et al., 2000). In addition, terms such as *resilient children* cause confusion. Although this term implies that resilience is a trait, it is used most often in conjunction with the two coexisting conditions of adversity and positive adaptation, and adaptation is usually conceptualized as a process. Even the terms such as *outcome* and *process* contribute to the confusion, when researchers do not clearly identify a model of resilience that stipulates how the underlying mechanisms in a resilience process may result in specific resilience outcomes. Luthar and Cicchetti (2000) encourage researchers to clearly specify the context to which resilience outcomes apply and to clearly delineate the outcomes by using terms such as *emotional resilience, behavioral resilience,* or *educational resilience.* It would also be helpful, through staged-model specification, to distinguish proximal resilience outcomes, such as self-transcendence and confidence/mastery, from more distal outcomes, such as quality of life, which result from the resilience process and resilience outcomes.

Psychological/Physiological. Psychological concepts associated with resilience have been more widely studied than physiological concepts. Concepts such as self-esteem, self-perception, personality, temperament, intellect, coping, and problem-solving skills are just a few of the psychological concepts that have been studied in relation to resilience. What is not clear is whether these identified psychological variables influence the process and outcomes associated with resilience or whether they are components of resilience (Jacelon, 1997).

Fewer studies have examined physiological dimensions of resilience. Singer and Ryff (2001) identify several positive physiological mechanisms, including those that involve the hypothalamic-pituitary-adrenal (HPA) axis and the autonomic nervous system, which may be linked to positive health and resilience. They further argue for integrative levels of analysis that include the physiological, behavioral, environmental, and psychosocial systems to better understand how each contributes individually and interactively to resilience. Curtis and Cicchetti (2003) provided a thoughtful perspective of the theoretical and methodological considerations for examining the biological contributors to resilience. Specifically, they discuss a transactional organizational theoretical perspective as a framework for including biological considerations. The recent advances in neurosciences and related technology, such as functional magnetic resonance imaging (fMRI), clearly make this avenue of investigation promising.

Individual/Aggregate. Resilience is most often studied in individuals, but to avoid confusion in yet another boundary, it is important for researchers to clarify the level of analysis. At an individual level, family factors have been identified that influence resilience. For example, Hauser et al. (1989) identified both direct and indirect effects of family factors on individual resilience. Family direct effects included household composition and family structure, as well as family atmosphere factors such as patterns of communication, adaptability, and flexibility. Family factors apparently also have an indirect effect on individual and social protective factors, since child personality factors (temperament, attitudes, self-esteem, etc.) and social milieu process are often shaped by family processes.

There are growing bodies of literature focused on additional levels of analysis—resilient families (Hawley & DeHaan, 1996; Patterson, 2002) and resilient communities (Bosworth & Earthman, 2002). At these levels, studies most frequently take a systems approach. The family research on resilience is primarily built on family systems theory, and much of the work was done from a family stress and coping framework. Resilience is equated with family adaptation, that is, the balancing of family demands and capabilities through interaction with family meanings (McCubbin, Balling, Possin, Frierdich, & Bryne, 2002; Patterson, 1995, 2002). Resilience research at the family and community level is increasing and may provide strong significance for public policy decisions.

Objective/Subjective. In a qualitative study of homeless adolescents, Hunter and Chandler (1999) found adolescents who considered themselves resilient. According to the adolescents, being resilient was "surviving." The characteristics self-attributed by the adolescents as being resilient were quite different from the characteristics of resilience found in other literature. Hunter and Chandler's research indicated that resilience in homeless adolescents may be a "process of defense using such tactics as insulation, isolation, disconnecting, denial, and aggression or as a process of survival using such responses as violence" (p. 246). These findings indicate that self-attributed resilience in homeless adolescents seems to lack a positive or good outcome, a key characteristic of resilience in the literature. These findings were further supported in a subsequent study by Hunter (2001) that examined cross-cultural perspectives of resilience in adolescents from New England and Ghana. All the adolescents viewed themselves as resilient, regardless of age, gender, culture, or socioeconomic status. Yet, depending on the presence or absence of consistent, loving, caring, and mentoring adults, there were qualitative differences in how the adolescents overcame adversities. Hunter classified these as two different "forms of resilience": self-protective survival resilience or connected resilience.

Hunter and Chandler's findings imply that if the objective and subjective dimensions of resilience are not carefully delineated, much of what determines the process and outcomes of resilience will be difficult to ascertain. For example, the cognitive appraisal of the adversity, the actions that are taken to deal with the adversity, and subsequent evaluation of how one is dealing with the adversity can all influence how resilience as a process proceeds (Fine, 1991). Further, if the objective and subjective appraisal, actions, and evaluation differ, evaluation of outcomes and development of interventions will be more complex.

One potentially helpful way to delineate the objective/subjective dimensions of resilience is to consider whether resilience may be interpersonally assigned to an individual, much like courage is interpersonally assigned (Haase, 1987). Research indicates that individuals usually do not attribute courage to themselves, unless someone else initially indicates that their behavior could be interpreted as courageous (Haase, 1987). Likewise, it is possible that persons who have resilience require time to reflect on the meaning of their actions. That is, resilience may occur through a process that includes deriving meaning from the experience through interaction with others (Haase, Heiney, Ruccione, & Stutzer, 1999). After interviews were conducted, Hunter and Chandler's findings supported this perspective in that the adolescents' resilience scores increased from baseline measures (Hunter, 2001). A second consideration regarding the subjective perspective is the social desirability of being labeled "resilient." It is possible that a label of being resilient parallels a label such as "honest," in that, when asked, one would not readily deny having such a characteristic.

Cross-cultural Considerations Related to Boundaries. In the midst of adversity, individuals are especially likely to return to cultural tradition to seek solutions (Hwang, 2006, p. 90). Hence, a full understanding of resilience needs to include cultural considerations. Few studies have explicitly examined the cultural boundaries of resilience. As an exemplar of how cultural boundaries may influence resilience, we briefly examine Chinese and Western cultural differences in two concepts that are important to resilience: sense of self and relational self.

The sense of self, a key individual protective factor of resilience, is different in Western and Chinese societies. In Western society, self is individual oriented and reflects the interaction of "I" and "me"

(Mead, 1952). "I" is a subjective perception of individual and "me" is an objective evaluation from others about "me" in certain situations. This individualistic perspective that is more prominent in Western society assumes the importance of opportunity to achieve personal goals, irrespective of group goals (Bedford & Hwang, 2003; Triandis, Bontempo, Villareal, Asai, & Lucca, 1988). In contrast, in Chinese culture, self is noted as interdependent self or relational self that is composed of "great self" (social self) and "small self" (physical self) (Ho, Chen, & Chiu, 1991; Hwang, 1997). "Great self" means an individual has obligations to prevent his or her family or group members from any threats; "small self" refers to an individual's physical self that is independent from others (Bedford & Hwang, 2003). "Small self" is similar to the perspective of self in Western society. The Confucian concept of collectivism advocates that one's life is an inheritance from ancestors of the clan and that this ancestral inheritance perspective fosters expectations from families or group members and overrides individual goals (Bedford & Hwang, 2003; Triandis et al., 1988). In the Chinese culture, then, family or community protective factors may have greater influence as pathways to resilience, and individual protective factors, such as sense of self, may require alignment with family goals to actually serve a protective function. In these cases, positive coping strategies, such as confrontive coping from a Western perspective, may be less positive, and strategies that are less effective in Western culture, such as fatalism in deference to ancestors, may actually have a positive influence on resilience.

Interpersonal relationship is another important concept related to resilience. In Western society, interpersonal interactions hold an assumption of respect for the principles of egalitarianism and independence (Triandis et al., 1988). Thus, interpersonal relationships are based on a decisional choice. In Chinese culture, interpersonal relationships are composed of horizontal and vertical relationships. Horizontal relationships are constructed according to intimacy/distance and vertical relationships are built according to superiority/inferiority (Hwang, 1997). Horizontal relationship indicates interaction within equal family or social positions, such as sibling or peer relationships. Vertical relationship means interaction among hierarchal family or social positions, such as child–parent or student–teacher relationships. The vertical relationship is less emphasized in Western society.

Since both sense of self and interpersonal relationships are culturally different in Western and Chinese societies, how they work to foster resilience is also likely to be different. In Western society, the presentation of self is based on one's interpretation of interactions in specific social situations (Charon, 1998; Mead, 1952). In contrast, in Chinese society, the self is defined not by any situational interpretation, but by person-in-relation status, which is called the "relational self" (Ho et al., 1991). In Chinese society, based on relational self, personal coping strategies, purpose in life, and interpersonal interactions may be more driven by status concerns in social relationships than in Western cultures.

RESILIENCE PERSPECTIVES IN NURSING

Not surprisingly, information in Table 16.1 indicates that there is no greater consensus on definitions, characteristics, or boundaries of resilience in the nursing literature than there is in the literature from other disciplines. The nursing literature on resilience parallels that of the general literature. Although nurses historically have focused more extensively on individual and family strengths than many disciplines, systematic study of resilience by nurses only began in the mid- to late 1980s. A major contribution to understanding resilience from the nursing literature is the focus on resilience in the context of health, an otherwise neglected area in the resilience literature. The articles included in Table 16.1 provide a representative sample of both theoretical and empirical efforts to understand resilience by nurses, including varied populations and approaches to knowledge development.

TERMINOLOGY AND ATTRIBUTES OF RESILIENCE

Most definitions in Table 16.1 include the characteristic of adversity. Some definitions specifically describe the adversity as stress, loss, or illness, while others use more global terms, such as "challenging life condition" (Drummond, Kysela, McDonald, & Query, 2002) or a "disaster" (Polk, 1997). The "good" varies considerably in the definitions, as well. Although several of the definitions use vague terminology, such as "go on with life" (Dyer & McGuinness, 1996) or "spring back" (Jacelon, 1997), other definitions indicate the "good" reflected in processes of adaptation, positive health, and/or well-being (Ahern, 2006;

TABLE 16.1 Nursing Literature on Resilience

Source	Methods of knowledge development	Populations studied	Definition of resilience	Primary boundaries
Ahern (2006)	Rodger's Evolution-ary Model of Concept Analysis	Adolescents	Process of adaptation to risk that incorporates personal characteristics, family and social support, and community resources	Individual, dynamic psychosocial process
Aronowitz (2005)	Grounded theory	Adolescents who previously engaged in risk behaviors and then stopped	(Borrowed) Values, attitudes, and be-havioral dimensions that influence the dynamic, responsive abilities foster-ing health development and adaptation in the face of normal or unexpected challenges (Luthar et al., 2000; Perkins, Luster, & Villarruel, 1998)	Individual, dynamic psychosocial process
Black & Ford-Gilboe (2004)	Cross-sectional, descrip-tive correlational design	Adolescent mothers	(Borrowed) Internal strength that develops in the context of adversity (Kadner, 1989) Resilience operationalized by Resilience Scale (Wag-nild & Young, 1993)	Individual process influenced by familial experiences
Drummond et al. (2002)	Family Adaptation Model Development, using resilience theory (family protective fac-tors) as underpinnings Survey and posttest-only experimental design	Families of children with special needs and families with children in Head Start	(Borrowed) Maintenance of positive adjustment under chal-lenging life conditions (Luthar et al., 2000)	Family processes
Dyer & McGuinness (1996)	Concept analysis	Adults	A process whereby people bounce back from ad-versity and proceed with their lives	Individual psychosocial process with outcome on a continuum

Components: antecedents/exogenous variables	Components: attributes/processes	Components: outcomes	Key relational statements/findings

Risks: internal or external factors	Individual protective factors:
	    Competence
	    Positive coping
	    Sense of humor
	    Connectedness with
	    caring adults
	    Knowledge of health
	    behavior and risks
	Sociocultural protective factors:
	    Connectedness with
	    family
	    Community resources
		Resilience is the outcome of triadic influences of risk, protection, and interventions	A proposed model of resilience includes a continuum of behaviors from risk (internal and external factors) to protection (individual and sociocultural).

Connectedness with caring, competent, and responsible adults
Specific behaviors displayed by adults:
    Modeling
    Monitoring
    Coaching
    Countering
	Feeling competent
	Elevating expectations
		Envisioning a positive future
		Fewer risk behaviors
			Having a connected relationship with a caring, competent, and responsible adult helped the adolescents envision a positive future for themselves and promoted positive health behaviors.

Adversity Income Professional support	Resilience is viewed as an aspect of health potential.	Health-promoting lifestyle practices	Mother's resilience and family health work explained 30.2% of the variance in mother's health-promoting lifestyle practices. Moderate positive correlations were found between mother's resilience and both family health work and mother's health-promoting lifestyle practices.
Presence of vulnerability processes in family life that may create demands in the maintenance of family protective processes	Ongoing development and successful use of protective family processes (appraisal, support, and coping)	Family adaptation	Normative adaptation is managed mostly through use of supports and through positive appraisals in the families.
Adversity and at least one caring, emotionally available person	Prosocial attitude Rebounding and carrying on Sense of self-determination	Outcome a continuum of vulnerability to resilience Toughening effect Sense of having overcome that fosters mastery Enhanced coping	Accessed skills and abilities may occur within the individual or interpersonally through a supportive, caring, and responsive environment.

(continued)

TABLE 16.1　Nursing Literature on Resilience (*Continued*)

Source	Methods of knowledge development	Populations studied	Definition of resilience	Primary boundaries
Felten (2000), Felten & Hall (2001)	Concept analysis	Women older than 85 who experienced illness or loss	The ability to achieve, retain, or regain a level of physical or emotional health after devastating illness or loss	Individual psychosocial state influenced by external factors
Haase (2004), Haase et al. (1999)	Triangulation using qualitative model and instrument generating and quantitative model evaluating studies	Adolescents with chronic illness, primarily cancer	The process of identifying or developing resources and strengths to manage stressors flexibly and gain a positive outcome (i.e., a sense of confidence or mastery, self-transcendence, and self-esteem)	Individual psychosocial process resulting in specific outcomes
Heinzer (1995)	Descriptive, model evaluation	Adults who lost a parent when an adolescent	(Borrowed) The dynamic ability or strength (both physiological and psychological in nature) that enables an individual to recover from or adjust easily to loss or misfortune and to mobilize coping resources (Garmezy et al., 1984)	Individual process Psychological variables studied, but physiological recognized in definition
Hodges, Troyan, & Keeley (2010)	Grounded theory	Acute care nurses	Transformative, intentional desire to persist in an adverse environment of complexity and unpredictability (p. 85)	Individual psychosocial processes
Humphreys (2003)	Descriptive correlation design	Sheltered battered women	(Borrowed) An individual's ability in the face of overwhelming adversity to adapt and restore equilibrium to his or her life and to avoid the potentially deleterious effects of stress (Wagnild & Young, 1993)	Individual psychological process
Hunter (2001), Hunter & Chandler (1999)	Triangulation: Concept clarification through focus groups, phenomenological analysis, and journal writing Cross-cultural comparisons Quantitative analysis using Resilience Scale	Homeless adolescents Adolescents in variety of situational settings across two cultures	State of being that allows a person to overcome adversity without suffering long-term negative consequences	Individual psychological state taking two forms Objective and subjective perspectives on a continuum

Components: antecedents/exogenous variables	Components: attributes/processes	Components: outcomes	Key relational statements/findings
Illness or loss	Environmental factors: frailty, determination, previous experience learning to cope, access to care, cultural-based health beliefs, family support, self-care activities, caring for others, and functioning efficiently External factors: structure of the environmental factors and stress		Resilience is conceptualized as a coiled wire enclosed in a box. External factors of resilience are a configuration of environmental factors within the box and stress.

Social protective:
  Health care resources
  Social integration
Family protective:
  Family atmosphere
  Family support/
  resources
Illness-related risk:
  Illness perspective
  Illness-related distress
	Individual risk:
	  Defensive coping
	  (sustained over time)
	Individual protective:
	  Derived meaning
	  Courageous coping
		Resilience:
		  Self-esteem,
		  self-transcendence, confidence/mastery
		Quality of life:
		  Well-being
			Illness-related risk and social and family protective factors directly affect individual risk and protective factors. All these factors directly or indirectly affect resilience and quality-of-life outcomes.

Time since death of parent Age of adolescent at death Gender Circumstances of death (sudden or expected)	Parental attachment as basis for developing social relationships Adaptive coping	Social competence, global self-worth, perceived health	Adaptive coping consistently predicted outcome variables of resilience. Attachment was not significant.
Unpredictable, challenging, and chaotic work environment	Verifying fit; stage setting, and optimizing the environment		Professional resilience is a synergistic relationship between personal needs and principles and the environment.
Battering experience; physical and psychological distress	Resilience is a pattern of successful outcomes in individuals despite challenging or threatening circumstances.	Less physical and psychological distress	Participants who had higher levels of resilience reported significantly fewer symptoms of physical and psychological distress.
Developmental independence Developed competencies Invincibility Mastery Resourcefulness Perseverance Stress	Connected resilience: self-esteem, self-efficacy, connectedness, trust, competence, ego-resilience, sociability or Survival resilience: psychopathology, maladaption, social and emotional withdrawal, high-risk behaviors, survival tactics of violence		Adolescents without support showed survival and self-protected resilience; those with support showed a connected form of resilience.

(continued)

TABLE 16.1 Nursing Literature on Resilience (*Continued*)

Source	Methods of knowledge development	Populations studied	Definition of resilience	Primary boundaries
Jacelon (1997)	Synthesis of literature on resilience	Children, adolescents, and adults in various circumstances	(Borrowed dictionary definition) Ability of people to "spring back" in the face of adversity	Individual psychological trait and process
Kadner (1989)	Synthesis of literature on resilience in context of mental health services	Vulnerable populations, especially psychiatric	Ability to regain psychosocial equilibrium after a brief fragmentation in response to severe stress	Individual psychological trait, partially physically (genetically) predisposed
Lawn et al. (2011)	Grounded theory	Adolescents and adults who never smoked who came from an environment in which smoking was prevalent	Interaction between internal perspectives and a set of external conditions that allow individual adaptation or resistance to different forms of adversity at various times in life	Individual psychological process influenced by external circumstances
Lothe & Heggen (2003)	Ethnography	Young adult famine survivors in Ethiopia	The ability to return to the original form or position after being bent, compressed, or stretched	Individual psychological trait and process
Mandleco & Peery (2000)	Review of relevant literature on resilience from developmental psychology, child psychiatry, and nursing	Children	Tendency to spring back, rebound, or recoil that involves the capacity to respond and endure or develop and master in spite of life stressors or adversity	Individual psychological state influenced by biological trait
McCubbin & McCubbin (1993, 1996)	Triangulation of qualitative and quantitative approaches for model and instrument development	Families experiencing illness of a family member, usually a child	Positive behavioral patterns and functional competencies individuals and the family unit demonstrate under stressful or adverse circumstances, which determine the family's ability to recover by maintaining its integrity as a unit while insuring, and where necessary restoring the well-being of family members and the family unit as a whole	Dynamic family behavioral and functional process

Components: antecedents/exogenous variables	Components: attributes/processes	Components: outcomes	Key relational statements/findings
Triad of personal, family, and community factors including resources, above-average intelligence, strong sense of self, self-reliance, independence, and positive outlook			Process is labeled "resilition." Trait is labeled resilience.
Stressor as antecedent is implied	Attributes are psychological resources: ego strength, social intimacy, and resourcefulness.	Outcome implied is psychological equilibrium manifested as coping.	The aggregate of psychological resources promotes coping efficacy.
Significant experiences with smoking, involvement in non-smoking environments, and negative experiences with smoking	Internal resilience: self-confidence and self-determination with clears sense of self as different than peers. External factors: wide range of coping strategies and external supports	Healthy life style related to smoking behaviors	There is a dynamic relationship between internal and external influences on resilience. Positive peer interactions are significant external influences.
Internal and external stressors	Faith Hope Having a living relative Having memories of one's past roots	Adaptation	Participants who managed a successful adaptation had the ability to look at their lives with a balanced perspective.
Internal biological factors: general health, genetic predisposition, temperament, and gender Internal psychological factors: cognitive capacity, coping ability, and personality characteristics External within family factors: home environment, parenting practices, and particular family members External outside family factors: supportive individuals and community resources			Interactional or transactional relationship exists with the internal and external factors affecting resilience and between the internal and external factors.
Family experienced stress and hardship	Family developed strengths and competencies in adjustment phase including patterns of family functioning, resources, appraisal, coping strategies, and problem solving.	Restoration and adaptation: well-functioning individual members, family sense of balance and harmony in carrying out tasks and responsibilities and in relationship to the community	Resiliency factors that helped families dealing with cancer recovery included internal family rapid mobilization and reorganization; social support from the health care team, extended family, the community, and the workplace; and changes in appraisal to make the situation more comprehensive, manageable, and meaningful.

(continued)

TABLE 16.1 Nursing Literature on Resilience (*Continued*)

Source	Methods of knowledge development	Populations studied	Definition of resilience	Primary boundaries
Polk (1997)	Concept synthesis for model development using nursing model as philosophical underpinnings	No specific population	The ability to transform disaster into a growth experience and move forward	Individual pattern that is transformative
Rew et al. (2001)	Descriptive/exploratory correlational design	Homeless adolescents	No specific theoretical definition Resilience operationalized by Resilience Scale (Wagnild & Young, 1993)	Individual psychological It is unclear if viewed as state or trait
Rew & Horner (2003)	Author-developed framework	Adolescents	(Borrowed) Resilience represents the interaction between risk factors and protective resources (Rutter, 1987)	Context of health-risk behaviors Dynamic process
Stewart et al. (1997)	Synthesis review of literature on resilience and health	Children	Capability of individuals to cope successfully in the face of significant change, adversity, or risk	Individual physiological and psychological state that changes over time and is influenced by protective factors in the individual and environment
Tusaie & Patterson (2006)	Descriptive, correlational examination of types of optimism to clarify the concept in preparation for developing evidence-based resilience intervention	Rural adolescents	No definition of resilience	Individual Apparently focused on optimism as a mediator
Vinson (2002)	Inner Core Child Resilience Model Development and Testing based on resilience literature synthesis and data-based findings of descriptive correlational study	School-age children with asthma	A combination of personality characteristics, family influences, and available social and cultural supportive environments that permits the epigenetic unfolding of adaptive processes	Individual psychosocial process

Components: antecedents/exogenous variables	Components: attributes/processes	Components: outcomes	Key relational statements/findings
Human and environmental energy field	Dispositional attributes (e.g., physical and ego-related attributes such as competence and sense of self) Patterns of relationships and roles Situational patterns: characteristic approaches to situations or stressors Philosophical pattern of personal beliefs		Transformation manifested as specific dispositional, relational, situational, and philosophical patterns
Homelessness as condition Loneliness, hopelessness, life-threatening behaviors, and connectedness	Resilience may be an adaptive or defense strategy, rather than a protective factor.		Loneliness, hopelessness, life-threatening behaviors, and connectedness were negative predictors of resilience as measured by Resilience Scale.
Sociocultural context of interaction among individual risk and protective factors and family and community contexts	Resiliency is process of interaction of the antecedents that can be influenced by interventions.	Reduction of health-risk behaviors/morbidity and mortality	Model developed that proposes interaction between individual risk and family and individual and community protective factors
Transition, increased stressors	*Protective factors:* *Individual level:* Coping, self-help, self-esteem, intelligence, self-efficacy *Family level:* Positive parent–child attachment, future orientation, rules in the household, social support *Community Level:* Positive school experiences	Maintenance of physiological and psychological health, such as: Global psychosocial adjustment Lack of psychopathology Self-esteem Confidence Intelligence Positive immune response	Relationship of resilience and health is clarified in discussions of risk and protective factors and resilient outcomes, in particular psychological and physical health and health behavior.
Age, sex	Trait, situational, and comparative optimism	Expectation of positive outcomes (implied resilience)	Adolescent optimism is expressed differently when examining the trait, situational, and comparative aspects of the concept.
Exogenous variables: Child characteristics Family environment	Coping patterns, threat appraisal	Quality of life, illness indices	Paths are from family to child characteristics, child characteristics to appraisal, appraisal to quality of life, family to child coping, child coping to illness indices, and child perceived quality of life to illness indices.

(*continued*)

TABLE 16.1 Nursing Literature on Resilience (*Continued*)

Source	Methods of knowledge development	Populations studied	Definition of resilience	Primary boundaries
Wagnild & Young (1990, 1993)	Grounded theory and factor analysis of instrument	Older adults	A personality characteristic that moderates the negative effects of stress and promotes adaptation	Individual trait
Windle (2011)	Synthesis of methodological approaches: concept analysis, literature review using systematic principles, and stakeholder consultation	Not limited	The process of effectively negotiating, adapting to, or managing significant sources of stress or trauma (p. 152)	Individual psychosocial processes influenced by family, community, and political factors
Woodgate (1999), Woodgate & McClement (1997)	Synthesis of resilience literature in context of cancer to develop a model	Adolescents with cancer	Dynamic process involving the development of resources within the individual that allows the individual to gain a positive outcome in the face of significant adversity	Individual, dynamic psychological process

Haase et al., 1999; McCubbin & McCubbin, 1996; Vinson, 2002). Only a few definitions of resilience provide clear descriptions of outcome variables associated with resilience.

Regarding the essential characteristics of adversity and "good" outcomes, there is the same inconsistency in the nursing literature as was found in the general resilience literature. Risk or adversity factors primarily focus on how protective factors of resilience can deter the impact that risk has on resilience outcomes. In some cases, both protective and vulnerability, or risk, factors were listed together. In these cases, one is forced to assume that either the risk factor is the absence of the protective factor identified or that resilience occurs on a continuum of risk to protection. Examples of the risk factors identified in the nursing literature include survival tactics of violence (Hunter & Chandler, 1999); defensive coping and illness-related risks such as uncertainty and symptom distress (Haase et al., 1999); and gender, antisocial behavior, and chronic illness (Stewart, Reid, & Mangham, 1997). Few models specify the mechanisms by which the adversity itself may influence and even contribute to resilience. This is puzzling because individuals often clearly credit the adversity itself as the important factor that influences the outcome. To illustrate, consider Lance Armstrong's quote, "The truth is that cancer was the best thing that ever happened to me. I don't know why I got the illness, but it did wonders for me, and I wouldn't want to walk away from it. Why would I want to change, even for a day, the most important, and shaping event of my life?" (Armstrong, 2000).

The positive factors of resilience reflected in Table 16.1 are numerous. In many cases, where models were specified based on literature synthesis and/or qualitative research to develop a resilience model, the relationship to and among positive factors is clearly described. Taken as a whole, the literature set provides an emerging pattern that may help distinguish positive resilience outcomes from positive outcomes of resilience. Positive resilience outcomes may include:

Components: antecedents/exogenous variables	Components: attributes/processes	Components: outcomes	Key relational statements/findings
Personal competence including self-reliance, independence, determination, invincibility, mastery, resourcefulness, and perseverance Acceptance of self and life including adaptability, balance, flexibility, and balanced perspective of life			The Resilience Scale is of potential use as a measure of internal resources and of the positive contribution an individual brings to a difficult life event.
Biological, psychological, economic, or social stressors. Not if a majority of people would experience no adaptive response leading to negative consequence	Protective factors: (a) individual (e.g., psychological, neurobiological), (b) social (e.g., family cohesion, parental support, (c) community/society (e.g., political capital, institutional and community factors). Competence seen as essential component (p. 157)	Maintenance of normal development or functioning, or better than expected functioning, given exposure to the specific adversity	Resilience experience varies throughout the life span, with different vulnerabilities and strengths emerging from changing life events.
Stressors	*Protective factors:* Self-concept Meaning Coping Social support from family External support from peers	Adaptation (social competence) or maladaptation (depression, low self-esteem)	Resilience is a mediating process initiated by stressors and the results in outcomes on a continuum of adaptation and maladaptation.

- Confidence, self-esteem, and self-transcendence (Haase et al., 1999)
- Self-esteem, self-efficacy, trust, connectedness, competence, and ego-resilience (Hunter & Chandler, 1999)
- Maintenance of physiological and psychological health (Stewart et al., 1997)
- Self-esteem, confidence, intelligence, a toughened effect, hope, mastery, and enhanced coping (Dyer & McGuinness, 1996)
- Social competence, global self-worth, and perceived health (Heinzer, 1995)
- Sense of humor (Ahern, 2006)

Positive outcomes of resilience include:

- Enhanced quality of life conceptualized as well-being (Haase et al., 1999; Hockenberry-Eaton, Kemp, & Dilorio, 1994; Vinson, 2002)
- A sense of having overcome that fosters mastery (Dyer & McGuinness, 1996)
- Psychological equilibrium (Kadner, 1989)
- Global psychosocial adjustment (Stewart et al., 1997)
- Health-promoting lifestyles and less risk-taking behavior (Ahern, 2006; Black & Ford-Gilboe, 2004)

BOUNDARIES OF RESILIENCE

With the exception of the psychological dimension that is identified by all authors, all the other boundaries of resilience, either explicit or implied, are inconsistent. There is no consensus on whether resilience is a trait, state, process, or some combination of these dimensions. Most definitions imply that a change occurs, but there is inconsistency as to whether the resilience change is a return to a steady state or is part of a growth-producing process. Jacelon (1997) explicitly distinguishes and labels resilience as the trait and "resilition" as the process. Only one definition explicitly addresses a time frame (Hunter, 2001; Hunter & Chandler, 1999).

The existence of biological contributions to resilience remains strikingly missing from most of the nursing literature. This gap is reflective of the general state of the science on resilience on biological dimensions. This situation may improve with the advancing technologies that have resulted in a rapidly developing knowledge base in neuroscience (Curtis & Cicchetti, 2003). In nursing, Hockenberry's and Mandleco's works (Hockenberry-Eaton et al., 1994; Mandleco & Peery, 2000) are among the few that consider biological contributions to resilience. In the context of childhood cancer, Hockenberry argued that activation of the endocrine system as a less adaptive response to stress—as indicated by an elevation of both catecholamine and cortisol—could indicate less resilience to the stressors associated with cancer (Hockenberry-Eaton, Dilorio, & Kemp, 1995). Mandleco and Peery (2000) identified four biological factors as possibly affecting resilience: general health, genetic predisposition, temperament, and gender. Research supports that children with resilience are usually quite healthy and have little hereditary or chronic illness. However, hypotheses about gender and temperament need further exploration. Evidence that temperament is a factor of resilience is derived from studies examining infant temperament; however, it is not clear that temperament is biologically based. Regarding gender, although males are more vulnerable to all risk factors, one cannot assume that more vulnerability equates to less resilience.

Resilience was most frequently studied as an individual dimension rather than as a family or community aggregate. In studies focused on individuals, the family or community variables were often included as protective factors that influence outcomes for the individual. In some ways, the state of knowledge on family resilience is further along than individually focused research, in that the limited number of proposed models is more consistently being used and evaluated, and there is more consistency in the ways that family level measures are used.

Nurses studying resilience seem to assume the importance of obtaining subjective indicators. These subjective indicators were obtained as narratives and as self-reported quantitative measures of resilience-related concepts. As indicated in section on "methods," nurse researchers have also developed creative methods for obtaining the personal meanings associated with resilience. Ways of making sense of combined, simultaneous objective, physiological measures as they relate to subjective ratings is not addressed well in either the nursing or the general literature. Since nurses focus on both physiological and psychosocial aspects of health, it would seem logical that nurse researchers would be well positioned to provide leadership in this area.

DESCRIPTION OF RESILIENCE: THE THEORY

There is agreement that models of resilience should include factors generally characterized as "protective." In addition, "risk" factors are also generally identified as influencing resilience processes and outcomes. A major problem in developing theory about resilience is that these protective and risk factors frequently resemble "laundry lists." That is, they lack an explicit description of underlying assumptions or an explicit theoretical framework that describes the mechanisms by which the protective and risk factors are linked to outcomes. Especially lacking are hypothesized paths or the magnitude of their influence on development of resilience. In addition, much confusion relates to whether these protective and risk factors are direct ameliorative effects or, rather, they are interactive effects reserved for individuals who have a particular attribute and who were relatively unaffected by high or low levels of adversity (Luthar & Cicchetti, 2000).

Important components that should be considered in all modeling efforts to understand and enhance resilience are contexts, including culture, psychological and physiological mediating units, and the patterns of mediators in relation to the context (Coyne & Downey, 1991; Freitas & Downey, 1998). Further, there is value in interventions that manipulate mediating variables, such as coping and hope, that have been found to influence resilience outcomes (Singer & Ryff, 2001).

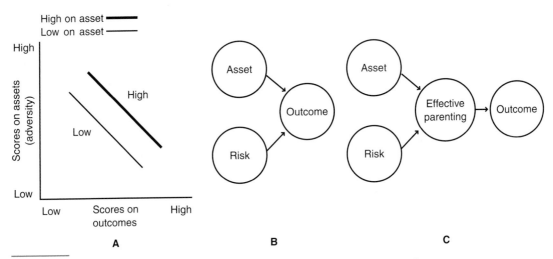

Figure 16.1 Variable-focused research models: (**A**) main, (**B**) direct, and (**C**) indirect effects.

Masten (2001) provides a useful distinction between variable- and person-focused approaches to model development. In variable-focused approaches, multivariate statistics are used to test for linkages among measures of adversity, outcomes, and environmental or individual qualities that may protect or compensate for negative consequences. Models may examine direct, indirect, and interaction effects (Luthar et al., 2000; Masten, 2001). Direct-effects models hypothesize direct effects in multivariate correlational analyses. A direct-effects example is when the relationship of high and low scores on outcomes is directly related to high and low scores on measures of adversity, or when a path diagram directly links specific variables with an outcome. Figure 16.1A and B illustrates the direct effects model. Indirect-effect models are those that hypothesize that the effect of variables, such as adversity or personal characteristics, is mediated by another variable, such as parental styles, as seen in Figure 16.1C. Interaction models hypothesize that the effects of adversity can be modified by individual characteristics or the environment. In general, variable-focused research indicates that adversity does not result in lasting or major effects, unless moderating and mediating systems, such as parent or social protective factors, are compromised (Masten, 2001).

Person-focused research attempts to identify and describe the patterns of variables that naturally occur, often identifying persons with either positive or poor functioning and then examining what might contribute to these outcomes, or using cut-off scores on selected variables to categorize adversity subgroups and then examining outcomes in these groups. These types of person-focused designs often lack comparison low-risk groups, which are important to answer questions of whether resilient children differ from children who are doing well but do not have high-risk characteristics. Masten (2001) also argues for more complex person-oriented models that include both health and maladaptive pathways of development in lives studied over time, giving special attention to turning points. These pathway models have a greater potential for providing intervention frameworks.

APPROACHES TO RESILIENCE KNOWLEDGE DEVELOPMENT IN NURSING LITERATURE

Although there is a relatively small amount of research on resilience in the nursing literature, the work accomplished to date has creatively used a variety of approaches to gain a fuller understanding of resilience. In no other discipline is such a rich combination of approaches to studying resilience found. Several of the articles in Table 16.1 include extensive analyses and syntheses of existing literature on resilience (Ahern, 2006; Dyer & McGuinness, 1996; Jacelon, 1997; Kadner, 1989; Polk, 1997; Stewart et al., 1997; Woodgate, 1999; Woodgate & McClement, 1997), and many of these were used to propose models of resilience in specific health contexts. For example, Woodgate (1999) derived the resilience model as applied to adolescents with cancer based on her synthesis of the literature on resilience within the context of cancer, and Vinson (2002) proposed a model of resilience in children with asthma. Another synthesis article used a nursing metatheory, the Science of Unitary Human Beings, as the underlying framework for developing a resilience model (Polk, 1997). Ahern (2006) used evolutionary concept analysis to specify a model of adolescent resilience that includes potential interventions, and Haase et al. (1999) used a combination of methods to develop the Adolescent Resilience Model (ARM).

In addition to literature synthesis approaches, several articles were data based. Qualitative research approaches used to gain understanding of resilience included grounded theory and phenomenology. Qualitative methods of data collection included open-ended or phenomenological interviews, focus groups, and free-writing exercises. Some authors used triangulation of qualitative and/or quantitative empirical studies to derive models of resilience in the context of health or a specific illness. For example, Haase et al. (1999) used a decision-making process to triangulate qualitative and quantitative approaches for instrument identification or development as well as model testing, and Hunter (2001) conducted concept clarification by triangulating qualitative data collection methods, such as free-writing exercises with quantitative measures of resilience, to conduct a cross-cultural comparison of resilience.

The data-based nursing studies in Table 16.1 fall into three categories of design. First are studies describing characteristics of a sample of participants who were designated, a priori, as having resilience. Examples of such studies are resilience in women older than 85 experiencing illness or loss (Felten, 2000; Felten & Hall, 2001); resilience in homeless adolescents (Hunter & Chandler, 1999); resilience in adult daughters of battered women (Humphreys, 2001); modes of comfort used by a resilient survivor suffering multiple losses and severe, excruciating burn pain (Morse & Carter, 1995); and adolescents who had stopped engagement in risky behaviors (Aronowitz, 2005).

Second are studies of resilience conducted with a specific population, but without a priori designation of participants as being resilient. Examples include resilience studies of adolescents with cancer (Haase et al., 1999); resilience in a sample of adults who lost a parent when they were adolescents (Heinzer, 1995); and resilience in children with asthma (Vinson, 2002). Third, design type includes studies that did not have resilience as a primary focus, but found resilience as an outcome variable. Examples of these studies include a study of women with a cardiac pacemaker (Beery, Sommers, & Hall, 2002) and a study of risk behavior in adolescents with cancer (Hollen, Hobbie, Finley, & Hiebert, 2001). Although these studies fit into Masten's description of variable- and person-focused research, they do not reflect the complexity of design Masten recommended, to include both healthy and maladaptive pathways of development in lives studied over time, giving special attention to turning points (Masten, 2001). By their creative approaches to clarify the patterns/processes/components of resilience, it is clear that studies conducted by nurses are headed in the "right" direction. More complex designs would seem to be a logical next phase. Tusaie and Patterson (2006) did not directly study resilience, but examined to clarify factors that may influence resilience before developing a resilience intervention.

SPECIFIC MODELS OF RESILIENCE

The articles in Table 16.1 that describe literature synthesis and concept analysis of resilience indicate the value that nurse scientists place on carefully developing theory. Models or theories of resilience are being developed that link society to cellular-levels of coping in older adults (Szanton & Gill, 2010; Szanton, Gill, & Thorpe, 2010). Individual-level resilience models include mastery of chronic illness with resilience as an emergent outcome (White, 1995); a "CARE" framework (containment, awareness, resilience, and engagement) for guiding mental health practice (McAllister & Walsh, 2003); the ARM for adolescents with cancer and other chronic conditions (Burns, Robb, & Haase, 2009; Chou & Hunter, 2009; Corey, Haase, Azzouz, & Monahan, 2008; Haase et al., 1999); the Inner Core Child Resilience Model for children with asthma (Vinson, 2002); the resiliency model applied to adolescents with cancer (Woodgate, 1999); a model of resilience in the context of loss of a parent (Heinzer, 1995); a model of resilience in community-dwelling women older than 85, overcoming adversity from illness or loss (Felten, 2000; Felten & Hall, 2001); and a model of adolescent resilience focused on the outcome of reduction of risk behaviors

(Aronowitz, 2005). In addition, a model of resilience in adolescents was proposed by Rew & Horner (2003), adapted by Ahern (2006), and used in working with high-risk teens (Halloran, 2011). Both of these models propose a continuum of risk and protective factors. Many of these models were constructed with the perspectives of those experiencing the adversity taken into consideration. Potential interventions are proposed in three models (Ahern, 2006; Haase, 2004; Rew & Horner, 2003). These models differ in specificity of targeted factors and in potential timing of interventions. Although there is less nursing literature on family or community resilience models, these models are being developed and used in practice with increasing frequency. The Family Resilience Model developed by McCubbin and McCubbin (1996) is supported in the literature on family resilience (Board & Ryan-Wenger, 2000; Smith, 1997; Svavarsdottir, McCubbin, & Kane, 2000; White, Bichter, Koeckeritz, Lee, & Munch, 2002) and has been suggested as a framework for caring for those with chronic pain (West, Usher, & Foster, 2011). Other family models are also being proposed. Drummond et al. (2002) proposed and tested a model of family adaptation that identified family protective factors of appraisal, support, and coping as mediators of adaptation. Appraisal was a key variable predicting adaptation. Community-based models have been considered for drug education of adolescents (Brown, Jean-Marie, & Beck, 2010), bereavement care for the non-bereaved (Kellehear & Fook), and mental health promotion and mental illness prevention (Power, 2010).

Across the models of resilience, the many adversity and positive concepts were inconsistently identified as antecedents, critical components, and outcomes of resilience. Antecedents usually included adversity (e.g., death, loss, illness, stressor[s], and homelessness). Protective factors were modeled as antecedents in only a few studies (Haase et al., 1999; Hunter & Chandler, 1999; Polk, 1997). Across several studies, especially those that viewed resilience as a trait, it was difficult to discern the role or order of resilience-related concepts, such as coping, hope, or mastery. These concepts were alternatively viewed as antecedent and critical component protective factors or as outcomes of resilience. For example, in some articles, coping is viewed as a mediating protective factor, while in others, it is an outcome of resilience. Reflective of the general literature, many protective factors do fall into broad classes of factors classified as individual, social, or family.

It is clear that more work needs to be done to clarify the relationship among concepts that are correlated with resilience and those that influence resilience. To increase explanatory power, this work will most productively be done in longitudinal studies, with models that attempt to capture the full, integrative perspective of resilience.

APPLICATIONS OF THE THEORY

RESEARCH TO DEVELOP A MODEL AND GUIDE THE DEVELOPMENT OF INTERVENTION

The ARM provides one example of how a theoretical model that is grounded in contextual experiences can guide interventions. The context for the ARM was chronic illness in adolescents. Most of the work was done from the perspective of adolescents with cancer; some studies included parent and health care provider perspectives.

To develop the ARM, two series of studies were conducted: (a) model generation studies, using inductive approaches and (b) model evaluation studies, involving instrumentation and exploratory model testing (Haase et al., 1999). The qualitative, model-generating studies provided a basis for the development of the ARM through identification and clarification of salient concepts to be included in the model, and as a qualitative means of evaluating subsequent model testing results. These studies were also guided by the Haase Decision-Making Process for Model and Instrument Development (Haase et al., 1999).

RESEARCH TO EVALUATE INSTRUMENTS

The quantitative model and instrument evaluation studies for the ARM were primarily done using latent variable structural-equation modeling approaches. The studies were done to evaluate the psychometric properties of the instruments used to measure each latent variable, and to develop an appropriate

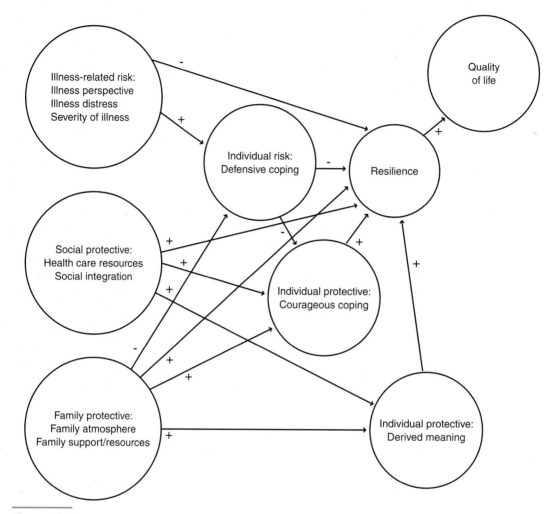

Figure 16.2 The Adolescent Resilience Model.

measurement model. Based on the exploratory studies of the theoretical model, factors were identified that affect the development of resilience. The resulting ARM, as it is being studied longitudinally and guiding interventions, is found in Figure 16.2.

Both protective and risk factors are included in the ARM. These factors with their related variables are highlighted in Table 16.2. Three classes of ARM protective factors are hypothesized to positively affect resilience outcomes. Class I Individual Protective Factors include courageous or positive coping and derived meaning. Class II Family Protective Factors include family atmosphere and support/resources available to the family. Class III Social Protective Factors include health care resources and social integration. Two classes of ARM risk factors are hypothesized to negatively affect resilience. The Class IV Individual Risk Factor is sustained defensive coping. The Class V Illness-Related Factors include illness perspective and illness distress. The outcome factors of resilience include self-esteem, mastery/confidence, and self-transcendence, as well as quality of life, defined as a sense of well-being.

PRACTICE APPLICATIONS OF THE THEORY

Most of the literature is devoted to research, examining the correlations between resilience and health outcomes in a variety of populations. The articles that do address how resilience can be promoted are more frequently found in educational and public health peer-reviewed journals than in nursing journals. Several

TABLE 16.2 Adolescent Resilience Model Latent and Manifest Variables

Latent factor	Manifest variables
I. Individual Protective	
Courageous coping	Confrontive coping
	Optimistic coping
	Supportant coping
Derived meaning	Hope
	Spiritual perspective
II. Family Protective	
Family atmosphere	Adaptability and cohesion
	Parent–adolescent communication
	Perceived social support—family
Family support/resources	Family strengths
	Socioeconomic status variables
III. Social Protective	
Health care resources	Perceived social support—health care provider
	Adolescent support program participation and satisfaction
	Adolescent support program site evaluation
Social integration	Perceived social support—friends
IV. Individual Risk	
Defensive coping	Evasive coping
	Emotive coping
V. Illness-Related Risk	
Illness perspective	Uncertainty in illness
Illness distress	Symptom distress
	Severity of illness
VI. Resilience	
	Confidence/mastery
	Self-transcendence
	Self-esteem
Quality of life	Sense of well-being

articles encourage health care workers to reinforce the resilience strategies of others. Ward et al. (2011) explored the additive and subtractive processes used by nonsmokers to never smoke and by smokers to quit smoking. Herrick et al. (2011) described strength-based approaches to prevent HIV in gay men. Other articles simply provide a description of recommended behaviors to promote resilience, for instance in high-risk teens (Halloran, 2011) and social workers involved in the community (Megele, 2011). In addition to Megele's article identifying strategies to promote resilience in social workers, Aiello et al. (2011) discussed an intervention to build resilience in health care workers who would be required to deal with a viral pandemic and Delport, Strydom, Theron, and Geyer (2011) described a support program for educators working with the HIV/AIDs. This program, referred to as Resilient Educators (REd), included nine modules that consider health promotion, psychosocial impact of the pandemic, stigma, health care, and resilience, providing background information and interactive activities.

There are examples of substantial projects developed to apply a resilience framework for promoting healthy behavior. One such project is an "international and prospective application of resilience in school-based drug education, Project REBOUND [resilience-bound]" (Brown et al., 2010, p. 331). The approach was based on an analysis of literature that found: (a) risk-based education was basically ineffective; (b) protective factors and risk factors are independent phenomena; and (c) resilience is a normative process that can be predicted in relation to caring connected relationships, opportunities for participation and contribution, and high expectations of self (p. 337). The education program developed to influence drug use behavior of young people was based on these three predictors.

The drug education model included a Resilience Education (focused more on protective factors) with Risk Competence informational orientation (focused more specifically on the topic of drug use). Both were used in processional development for educators, counselors, and administrators, which involved six 1.5-day workshops. The workshops were designed to not only introduce them to the curriculum but also assist them to integrate the lessons to be taught into their own lives.

The curriculum was delivered in 90-minute lessons over a 16-week period. One of the first issues introduced was the necessity for authentic presence and openness to learn. Most of the Resilience Education was devoted to protective factors, addressing the importance of connection, participation and contribution, and high expectations for self. Finally, these topics were linked to decisions related to drug behavior. Following the focus on Resilience Education, the remainder sessions were devoted to Risk Competence. In those sessions, individual risk is explored, drug information is provided, critical thinking is facilitated, and self-awareness with special emphasis on strengths is encouraged.

Project REBOUND has been supported by the Mentor Foundation and the European Union. It was developed to be first implemented in Germany and then be adopted throughout Europe and the United States. As it is implemented, evaluation will occur at each step of the program.

INSTRUMENTS USED IN EMPIRICAL TESTING

Measurement is an approach to knowledge development for resilience that is gaining more attention (Ahern, Kiehl, Sole, & Byers, 2006). Windle, Bennett, and Noyes (2011) screened close to 3,000 peer-reviewed articles, published from 1989 to September 2009 to identify published resilience scales. They conducted a methodological systemic review of these scales, applying established quality assessment criteria to evaluate their psychometric properties. Windle et al. identified 15 scales, some with refinements and all self-report instruments; the earliest was published in 1989 and the most recent in 2008. These scales provided measurements for all population age groups, children through older adults. Three scales, all developed for use with adults, were determined to have the best psychometric properties: the Connor-Davidson Resilience Scale, the Resilience Scale for Adults, and the Brief Resilience Scale. At best, the quality of these questionnaires would be considered moderate. All 15 scales are described by target population, mode of completion, number of items, purpose, and quality assessment. In addition, complete references and comments on theoretical background are provided. It was noted that different approaches to measuring resilience has resulted in lack of clarity related to potential risk factors and protective processes, and a number of the scales are in early stages of development and require further validation.

The resilience scale with the widest application is the Resilience Scale (Wagnild & Young, 1993). This scale with a two-factor structure, personal competence and acceptance of self and life, has been used in studies that represent different cultural and age samples (Aroian, Schappler-Morris, Neary, Spitzer, & Tran, 1997; Humphreys, 2003; Hunter & Chandler, 1999; Rew, Taylor-Seehafer, Thomas, & Yockey, 2001).

Most studies using quantitative methods in the (Table 16.1) literature used existing instruments or developed instruments to measure numerous variables in proposed models. However, in many cases, it is not clear whether the instruments were derived from theories that are congruent with the conceptual frameworks or philosophical approaches being used in the studies. Haase et al. (1999) describe one approach to identifying and/or developing instruments that is clearly linked to the emerging ARM theory. Triangulation methods were done in a series of studies to develop and test the ARM and to identify or develop the instruments used to evaluate the model (Haase, 1987; Haase, Britt, Coward, Leidy, & Penn, 1992; Haase et al., 1999; Haase & Rostad, 1994). Decision trees were used to decide on labels and definitions for each model factor and to decide whether to use existing instruments or ones developed to measure the model factors. This iterative process of decision making sought to retain the inductively derived meanings from the qualitative studies while taking advantage of existing theory and instruments. The result was a set of 15 instruments to measure manifest variables—8 existing instruments meeting established criteria for reliability and validity and 7 new instruments. To test the ARM and instruments, latent variable instrument and model-testing studies were done (Haase et al., 1999).

It is clear that additional measurement work is essential to further the science of resilience from a nursing perspective. Cultural considerations in measurement are not well addressed. Measurement in nursing research on resilience needs to consider the issues of boundaries, including trait/process and physiological/psychological. Measurement also needs to focus on differences in resilience based on developmental factors, including age (Research Application 16.1).

Research Application 16.1

Using the Adolescent Resilience Model, interventions can be designed to target specific protective or risk factors to enhance resilience outcomes. Several studies were developed and tested using the ARM. In one study, the ARM was used to guide a music video production (Haase, 2004).

The aims of this study were to (a) test the efficacy of a therapeutic music video (TMV) intervention for AYAs during the acute phase of stem cell transplant (SCT), and (b) qualitatively examine the self-reported benefits of the TMV intervention for AYAs.

For AYAs undergoing SCT, participation in the TMV intervention was hypothesized to directly:

- Decrease illness-related distress
- Improve family environment
- Increase perceived social support
- Decrease defensive coping
- Increase positive coping
- Increase derived meaning

Through improved family environment and perceived social support, the TMV was also hypothesized to indirectly affect:

- Positive coping
- Derived meaning

As a consequence of enhancing these variables, the intervention was expected to:

- Increase resilience
- Increase quality of life

In addition to the efficacy of the intervention for AYAs, it was hypothesized that the TMV intervention was helpful and meaningful to family caregivers. This aim was qualitatively evaluated.

The multisite study design was a two-group, randomized clinical trial. Study participants in the treatment group received the TMV intervention over six sessions, conducted by a board-certified music therapist. In the sessions, participants in the music group selected music and engaged in song writing, music recording, and developing the visual content for a music video. Study participants randomized to the low-dose control group also received six sessions conducted by a board-certified music therapist, focused on discussing content of self-selected audio-recorded books. Sites in five states participated in the study to increase sample ethnic, cultural, and economic diversity.

SUMMARY

The work of nurse scientists to add to the body of knowledge on resilience is considerable, but much work still needs to be accomplished. Areas of strength within the nursing literature include the careful attention to theory, both by clarifying concepts through literature analysis and synthesis and by using qualitative methods that explore experiences of resilience from the perspectives of those who have experienced adversity. The recognition of resilience as a positive health concept and the recognition of resilience as a dynamic process are strengths. To advance the science, much work remains for nurses in collaboration with scientists from other disciplines. Some specific recommendations can be made: (a) continue efforts on measurement issues, so that instruments are context and culturally sensitive, meaning based, and time sensitive; (b) conduct longitudinal, prospective studies of resilience to test integrative models; (c) develop and test interventions planned to manipulate targeted variables that are promising to influence resilience outcomes; and (d) take advantage of the rapid advancements in neurocognitive sciences to include biological markers that may contribute to existing knowledge of resilience.

ANALYSIS OF THEORY

Using the criteria presented in Chapter 2, critique the theory of Resilience. Compare your conclusions about the theory with those found in Appendix A. A nurse scholar who has worked with the theory completed the analysis found in the Appendix.

Internal Criticism	External Criticism
1. Clarity	1. Reality convergence
2. Consistency	2. Utility
3. Adequacy	3. Significance
4. Logical development	4. Discrimination
5. Level of theory development	5. Scope of theory
	6. Complexity

CRITICAL THINKING EXERCISES

1. The ARM has primarily been developed for use in adolescents/young adults with cancer. Identify other populations where this model could be used to guide further research. What issues would you need to consider before applying the model to another population?

2. Develop a potential intervention targeted at one or more of the protective factors in the ARM that may influence resilience and quality of life in adolescents and young adults (AYAs).

3. Describe how the middle range theory proposed in this chapter helps refine your previous conceptualization of resilience.

4. Describe the benefits of meaning-based models or strengths-based research in your area of interest.

WEB RESOURCES

Visit **http://thePoint.lww.com/Peterson3e** for helpful web resources related to this chapter.

REFERENCES

Ahern, N. R. (2006). Adolescent resilience: An evolutionary concept analysis. *Journal of Pediatric Nursing, 21*(3), 175–185.

Ahern, N. R., Kiehl, E. M., Sole, M. L., & Byers, J. (2006). A review of instruments measuring resilience. *Issues in Comprehensive Pediatric Nursing, 29*(2), 103–125.

Aiello, A., Khayeri, M. Y., Raja, S., Peladeau, N., Romano, D., Maunder, R. G., et al. (2011). Resilience training for hospital workers in anticipation of an influenza pandemic. *Journal of Continuing Education in the Health Professions, 31*(1), 15–20. doi:10.1002/chp.20096

Antonovsky, A. (1979). *Health, stress, and coping.* San Francisco, CA: Jossey-Bass.

Armstrong, L. (2000). *It's not about the bike: My journey back to life.* New York: Putnam.

Aroian, K. J., Schappler-Morris, N., Neary, S., Spitzer, A., & Tran, T. V. (1997). Psychometric evaluation of the Russian Language version of the Resilience Scale. *Journal of Nursing Measurement, 5*(2), 151–164.

Aronowitz, T. (2005). The role of "envisioning the future" in the development of resilience among at-risk youth. *Public Health Nursing, 22*(3), 200–208.

Bandura, A. (1977). Self-efficacy: Toward a unifying theory of behavioral change. *Psychological Review, 84,* 191–215.

Bedford, O., & Hwang, K. K. (2003). Guilt and shame in Chinese culture: A cross-cultural framework from the perspective of morality and identity. *Journal for the Theory of Social Behavior, 33*(2), 127–144.

Beery, T. A., Sommers, M. S., & Hall, J. (2002). Focused life stories of women with cardiac pacemakers. *Western Journal of Nursing Research, 24*(1), 7–23; discussion 23–27.

Black, C., & Forol-Gilboe, M. (2004). Adolescent mothers: Resilience, family health work and health-promoting practices. *Journal of Advanced Nursing, 48*(4), 351–360.

Board, R., & Ryan-Wenger, N. (2000). State of the science on parental stress and family functioning in pediatric intensive care units. *American Journal of Critical Care, 9*(2), 106–122; quiz 123–124.

Bosworth, K., & Earthman, E. (2002). From theory to practice: School leaders' perspectives on resiliency. *Journal of Clinical Psychology, 58*(3), 299–306.

Brown, J. H., Jean-Marie, G., & Beck, J. (2010). Resilience and risk competence in schools: Theory/knowledge and international application in Project REBOUND. *Journal of Drug Education, 40*(4), 331-359. doi:10.2190DE.40.4.b

Burns, D. D., Robb, S. L., & Haase, J. E. (2009). Exploring the feasibility of a therapeutic music video intervention in adolescents and young adults during stem-cell transplantation. *Cancer Nursing, 32*(5), E8–E16. doi:10.1097/NCC.Ob)13e318a4802c

Charon, J. M. (1998). The nature of the self. In J. M. Charon (Ed.), *Symbolic interactionism: An introduction, an interpretation, an integration* (6th ed., pp. 72–97). Upper Saddle River, NJ: Prentice-Hall.

Chou, L., & Hunter, A. (2009). Factors affecting quality of life in Taiwanese survivors of childhood cancer. *Journal of Advanced Nursing, 65*(10), 2131–2141. doi:10.1111/j.1365-2648.2009.05078x

Corey, A. L., Haase, J. E., Azzouz, F., & Monahan, P. O. (2008). Social support and symptoms distress in adolescents/young adults with cancer. *Journal of Pediatric Oncology Nursing, 25*(5) 13–18. doi:10.1177/1043454208321117

Coyne, J. C., & Downey, G. (1991). Social factors and psychopathology: Stress, social support, and coping processes. *Annual Review of Psychology, 42,* 401–425.

Curtis, W. J., & Cicchetti, D. (2003). Moving research on resilience into the 21st century: Theoretical and methodological considerations in examining the biological contributors to resilience. *Development and Psychopathology, 15*(3), 773–810.

Delport, R., Strydom, H., Theron, L., & Geyer, S. (2011). Voices of HIV&AIDS-affected educators: how they are psychosocially affected and how REds enabled their resilience *AIDS Care, 23*(1), 121–126. doi:10.1080/09540121.2010.498857

Drummond, J., Kysela, G. M., McDonald, L., & Query, B. (2002). The family adaptation model: Examination of dimensions and relations. *Canadian Journal of Nursing Research, 34*(1), 29–46.

Dyer, J. G., & McGuinness, T. M. (1996). Resilience: Analysis of the concept. *Archives of Psychiatric Nursing, 10*(5), 276–282.

Felten, B. S. (2000). Resilience in a multicultural sample of community-dwelling women older than age 85. *Clinical Nursing Research, 9*(2), 102–123.

Felten, B. S., & Hall, J. M. (2001). Conceptualizing resilience in women older than 85: Overcoming adversity from illness or loss. *Journal of Gerontological Nursing, 27*(11), 46–53.

Fine, S. B. (1991). Resilience and human adaptability: Who rises above adversity? 1990 Eleanor Clarke Slagle Lecture. *American Journal of Occupational Therapy, 45*(6), 493–503.

Forsyth, G. L., Delaney, K. D., & Gresham, M. L. (1984). Vying for a winning position: Management style of the chronically ill. *Research in Nursing & Health, 7*(3), 181–188.

Freitas, A. L., & Downey, G. (1998). Resilience: A dynamic perspective. *International Journal of Behavioral Development, 22*(2), 263–285.

Garmezy, N. (1974). The study of competence in children at risk for severe psychopathology. In C. Koupernik (Ed.), *The child in his family: Children at psychiatric risk* (Vol. 3, pp. 77–97). New York: Wiley.

Garmezy, N. (1981). *Children under stress: Perspectives on antecedents and correlates of vulnerability and resistance to psychopathology.* New York: Wiley.

Garmezy, N. (1991). Resilience in children's adaptation to negative life events and stressed environments. *Pediatric Annals, 20,* 459–466.

Garmezy, N., Masten, A. S., & Tellegen, A. (1984). The study of stress and competence in children: A building block for developmental psychopathology. *Child Development, 55*(1), 97–111.

Haase, J. (1987). The components of courage in chronically ill adolescents. *Advances in Nursing Science, 9*(2), 64–80.

Haase, J. (2004). The Adolescent Resilience Model as a guide to interventions. Special section: Proceedings from the 5th annual state of the science workshop on resilience and quality of life in adolescents. *Journal of Pediatric Oncology Nursing, 21*(5), 289–299.

Haase, J. E., Britt, T., Coward, D. D., Leidy, N. K., & Penn, P. E. (1992). Simultaneous concept analysis of spiritual perspective, hope, acceptance and self-transcendence. *Image: Journal of Nursing Scholarship, 24*(2), 141–147.

Haase, J. E., Heiney, S. P., Ruccione, K. S., & Stutzer, C. (1999). Research triangulation to derive meaning-based quality-of-life theory: Adolescent resilience model and instrument development. *International Journal of Cancer Supplement, 12*, 125–131.

Haase, J. E., & Rostad, M. (1994). Experiences of completing cancer therapy: Children's perspectives. *Oncology Nursing Forum, 21*(9), 1483–1492; discussion 1493–1494.

Halloran, L. (2011). Risky business: Working with high-risk teens to foster resilience. *The Journal for Nurse Practitioners, 7*(5), 426–427. doi:10.10.1016/jnurpra.2011.02.004.

Hauser, S. T., Vieyra, M. A., Jacobson, A. M., & Wertlieb, D. (1985). Vulnerability and resilience in adolescence: Views from the family. *Journal of Early Adolescence, 5*, 81–100.

Hauser, S. T., Vieyra, M. A., Jacobson, A. M., & Wertlieb, D. (1989). Family aspects of vulnerability and resilience in adolescence: A theoretical perspective. In T. Dugan & R. Coles (Eds.), *The child in our times: Studies in the development of resiliency.* New York: Brunner-Routledge.

Hawley, D. R., & DeHaan, L. (1996). Toward a definition of family resilience: Integrating life-span and family perspectives. *Family Process, 35*(3), 283–298.

Heinzer, M. M. (1995). Loss of a parent in childhood: Attachment and coping in a model of adolescent resilience. *Holistic Nursing Practice, 9*(3), 27–37.

Henry, D. L. (2001). Resilient children: What they tell us about coping with maltreatment. *Social Work Health Care, 34*(3–4), 283–298.

Herrick, A. L., Lim, S. H., Wei, C., Smith, H., Guadamuz, T., Friedman, M. D., et al. (2011). Resilience as an untapped resource in behavioral intervention design for gay men. *AIDS and Behavior, 15* (Suppl 1), S25–S29. doi:10.1007/s10461-011-9895-0

Ho, D. Y. F., Chen, S. G., & Chiu, C. Y. (1991). Relational orientation: To find an answer for the methodology of Chinese social psychology. In K. S. Yang & K. K. Hwang (Eds.), *The psychology and behavior of Chinese people* (in Chinese). Taipei: Gui-Guan.

Hockenberry-Eaton, M., Dilorio, C., & Kemp, V. (1995). The relationship of illness longevity and relapse with self-perception, cancer stressors, anxiety, and coping strategies in children with cancer. *Journal of Pediatric Oncology Nursing, 12*(2), 71–79.

Hockenberry-Eaton, M., Kemp, V., & Dilorio, C. (1994). Cancer stressors and protective factors: Predictors of stress experienced during treatment for childhood cancer. *Research in Nursing & Health, 17*(5), 351–361.

Hodges, H. F., Troyan, P. J., & Keeley, A. C. (2010). Career persistence in baccalaureate-prepared acute care nurses. *Journal of Nursing Scholarship, 42*(1), 83–91. doi:10.1111/j.1547-5069.2009.01325.x

Hollen, P. J., Hobbie, W. L., Finley, S. M., & Hiebert, S. M. (2001). The relationship of resiliency to decision making and risk behaviors of cancer-surviving adolescents. *Journal of Pediatric Oncology Nursing, 18*(5), 188–204.

Humphreys, J. (2003). Resilience in sheltered battered women. *Issues in Mental Health Nursing, 24*(2), 137–152.

Humphreys, J. C. (2001). Turnings and adaptations in resilient daughters of battered women. *Image: Journal of Nursing Scholarship, 33*(3), 245–251.

Hunter, A. J. (2001). A cross-cultural comparison of resilience in adolescents. *Journal of Pediatric Nursing, 16*(3), 172–179.

Hunter, A. J., & Chandler, G. E. (1999). Adolescent resilience. *Image: Journal of Nursing Scholarship, 31*(3), 243–247.

Hwang, K. K. (1997). Guanxi and mientze: Conflict resolution in Chinese Society. *International Communication Studies, 7*(1), 17–42.

Hwang, K. K. (2006). Constructive realism and Confucian relationalism: An epistemological strategy for the development of indigenous psychology. In U. Kim, K. S. Yang, & K. K. Hwang (Eds.), *Indigenous and cultural psychology: Understanding people in context.* New York: Springer.

Hymovich, D. P., & Roehnert, J. E. (1989). Psychosocial consequences of childhood cancer. *Seminars in Oncology Nursing, 5*(1), 56–62.

Jacelon, C. S. (1997). The trait and process of resilience. *Journal of Advanced Nursing, 25*(1), 123–129.

Kadner, K. D. (1989). Resilience. Responding to adversity. *Journal of Psychosocial Nursing & Mental Health Services, 27*(7), 20–25.

Kobasa, S. C. (1982). The hardy personality: Toward a social psychology of stress and health. *Social Psychology, 37*, 1–11.

Lawn, S., Hersh, D., Ward, P. R., Tsourtos, G., Muller, R., Winefield, A., et al. (2011). 'I just saw it as something that would pull you down, rather than lift you up': Resilience in never-smokers with mental illness. *Health Education Research, 26*(1) 26–38. doi:10.1093/her/cyq065

Lothe, E. A., & Heggen, K. (2003). A study of resilience in young Ethiopian famine survivors. *Journal of Transcultural Nursing, 14*(4), 313–320.

Luthar, S. S., & Cicchetti, D. (2000). The construct of resilience: Implications for interventions and social policies. *Development & Psychopathology, 12*(4), 857–885.

Luthar, S. S., Cicchetti, D., & Becker, B. (2000). The construct of resilience: A critical evaluation and guidelines for future work. *Child Development, 71*(3), 543–562.

Mandleco, B. L., & Peery, J. C. (2000). An organizational framework for conceptualizing resilience in children. *Journal of Child and Adolescent Psychiatric Nursing, 13*(3), 99–111.

Masten, A. S. (1994). Resilience in individual development: Successful adaptation despite risk and adversity. In E. W. Gordon (Ed.), *Educational resilience in inner-city America: Challenges and prospects* (pp. 3–35). Hillsdale, NJ: Erlbaum.

Masten, A. S. (2001). Ordinary magic. Resilience processes in development. *American Psychologist, 56*(3), 227–238.

Masten, A. S., Best, K. M., & Garmezy, N. (1990). Resilience and development: Contributions from the study of children who overcome adversity. *Development and Psychopathology, 2,* 425–444.

Masten, A. S., & Coatsworth, J. D. (1998). The development of competence in favorable and unfavorable environments. Lessons from research on successful children. *American Psychologist, 53*(2), 205–220.

McAllister, M., & Walsh, K. (2003). CARE: A framework for mental health practice. *Journal of Psychiatric Mental Health Nursing, 10*(1), 39–48.

McCubbin, H., & McCubbin, M. (1996). Resiliency in families: A conceptual model of family adjustment and adaptation in response to stress and crisis. In H. I. McCubbin, A. I. Thompson & M. A. McCubbin (Eds.), *Family assessment: Resiliency, coping and adaptation—inventories for research and practice* (pp. 1–64). Madison, WI: University of Wisconsin System.

McCubbin, M., Balling, K., Possin, P., Frierdich, S., & Bryne, B. (2002). Family resiliency in childhood cancer. *Family Relations, 51*(2), 103–111.

McCubbin, M., & McCubbin, H. (1993). Family coping with health crisis: The Resiliency Model of family stress, adjustment and adaptation. In P. Winstead-Fry (Ed.), *Families, health, and illness* (pp. 3–63). St. Louis, MO: Mosby.

Mead, G. H. (1952). Mind, self and society. In C. W. Morris (Ed.), *Mind, self and society.* Chicago, IL: University of Chicago Press.

Megele, C. (2011). How to . . . develop emotional resilience. *Community Care, 17*(1857), 30.

Morse, J. M., & Carter, B. J. (1995). Strategies of enduring and the suffering of loss: Modes of comfort used by a resilient survivor. *Holistic Nursing Practice, 9*(3), 38–52.

Murphy, L., & Moriarty, A. (1976). *Vulnerability, coping and growth from infancy to adolescence.* New Haven, CT: Yale University Press.

Patterson, J. M. (1995). Promoting resilience in families experiencing stress. *Pediatric Clinics of North America, 42*(1), 47–63.

Patterson, J. M. (2002). Understanding family resilience. *Journal of Clinical Psychology, 58*(3), 233–246.

Perkins, D. E., Luster, T., & Villarruel, F. A. (1998). An ecological, risk-factor examination of adolescents' sexual activity in three ethnic groups. *Journal of Marriage and the Family, 60,* 600–623.

Pettit, G. S. (2000). Mechanisms in the cycle of maladaptation: The life-course perspective. *Prevention and Treatment, 3*(35).

Polk, L. V. (1997). Toward a middle-range theory of resilience. *Advances in Nursing Science, 19*(3), 1–13.

Power, A. K. (2010). Transforming the nation's health: Next steps in mental health promotion. *American Journal of Public Health, 100*(12), 2343–2346.

Rew, L., & Horner, S. D. (2003). Youth Resilience Framework for reducing health-risk behaviors in adolescents. *Journal of Pediatric Nursing, 18*(6), 379–388.

Rew, L., Taylor-Seehafer, M., Thomas, N. Y., & Yockey, R. D. (2001). Correlates of resilience in homeless adolescents. *Image: Journal of Nursing Scholarship, 33*(1), 33–40.

Richardson, G. E. (2002). The metatheory of resilience and resiliency. *Journal of Clinical Psychology, 58*(3), 307–321.

Rosenbaum, M. (1983). Learned resourcefulness as a behavioral repertoire for the self-regulation of internal events. In M. Rosenbaum, C. M. Franks & Y. Jaffe (Eds.), *Perspectives on behavior therapy in the eighties* (pp. 54–73). New York: Springer.

Rutter, M. (1979). Protective factors in children's responses to stress and disadvantage. *Annals of the Academy of Medicine, Singapore, 8*(3), 324–338.

Rutter, M. (1987). Psychosocial resilience and protective mechanisms. *American Journal of Orthopsychiatry, 57*(3), 316–331.

Singer, B. H., & Ryff, C. (2001). *New horizons in health: An integrative approach.* Washington, DC: National Academy Press.

Sinnema, G. (1991). Resilience among children with special health-care needs and among their families. *Pediatric Annals, 20*(9), 483–486.

Smith, S. D. (1997). The retirement transition and the later life family unit. *Public Health Nursing, 14*(4), 207–216.

Stewart, M., Reid, G., & Mangham, C. (1997). Fostering children's resilience. *Journal of Pediatric Nursing, 12*(1), 21–31.

Svavarsdottir, E. K., McCubbin, M. A., & Kane, J. H. (2000). Well-being of parents of young children with asthma. *Research in Nursing & Health, 23*(5), 346–358.

Szanton, S. L., & Gill, J. M. (2010). Facilitating resilience using a society-to-cells framework: A theory of nursing essentials applied to research and practice. *Advances in Nursing Science, 33*(4), 329–343. doi:10.1097/ANS.013e3181fb2ea2

Szanton, S. L., Gill, J. M., & Thorpe, R. J. (2010). The society-to-cells model of resilience in older adults. *Annual Review of Gerontology and Geriatrics, 30*(1), 5–34. doi:10.1891/0198-8794.30.5

Triandis, H. C., Bontempo, R., Villareal, M. J., Asai, M., & Lucca, N. (1988). Individualism and collectivism: Cross-culture perspectives on self-in-group relationships. *Journal of Personality and Social Psychology, 54*(2), 323–338.

Tusaie, K. R., & Patterson, K. (2006). Relationships among trait, situational, and comparative optimism: Clarifying concepts for a theoretically consistent and evidence-based intervention to maximize resilience. *Archives of Psychiatric Nursing, 20*(3), 144–150.

Vinson, J. A. (2002). Children with asthma: Initial development of the child resilience model. *Pediatric Nurse, 28*(2), 149–158.

Wagnild, G. M., & Young, H. M. (1990). Resilience among older women. *Image: Journal of Nursing Scholarship, 22*(4), 252–255.

Wagnild, G. M., & Young, H. M. (1993). Development and psychometric evaluation of the Resilience Scale. *Journal of Nursing Measurement, 1*(2), 165–178.

Waller, M. A. (2001). Resilience in ecosystemic context: Evolution of the concept. *American Journal of Orthopsychiatry, 71*(3), 290–297.

Ward, P. R., Muller, R., Tsourtos, G., Hersh, D., Lawn, S., Winefield, A. H., et al. (2011). Additive and subtractive resilience strategies as enablers of biographical reinvention: A qualitative study of ex-smokers and never-smokers. *Social Science and Medicine, 72*, 1140–1148. doi:10.1016/j.socscimed.2011.01.023

Wells, R., & Schwebel, A. (1987). Chronically ill children and their mothers: Predictors of resilience and vulnerability to hospitalization and surgical stress. *Developmental & Behavioral Pediatrics, 2*(2), 83–89.

Werner, E., & Smith, R. (1982). *Vulnerable but invincible: A longitudinal study of resilient children and youth.* New York: McGraw-Hill.

West, C., Usher, K., & Foster, K. (2011). Family resilience: Towards a new model of chronic pain management. *Collegian, 18*, 3–10. doi:10.1016/jcollegn.2010.004

White, K. R. (1995). The transition from victim to victor: Application of the theory of mastery. *Journal of Psychosocial Nursing and Mental Health Services, 33*(8), 41–44.

White, N., Bichter, J., Koeckeritz, J., Lee, Y. A., & Munch, K. L. (2002). A cross-cultural comparison of family resiliency in hemodialysis patients. *Journal of Transcultural Nursing, 13*(3), 218–227.

Windle, G. (2011). What is resilience? A review and concept analysis. *Reviews in Clinical Gerontology, 21*, 152–169. doi:10.1017/S0959259811000420

Windle, G., Bennett, K. M., & Noyes, J. (2011). A methodological review of measurement scales. *Health and Quality of Life Outcomes, 33*(4), 329–343. doi:10.1186/1477-7525-9-8

Woodgate, R. L. (1999). Conceptual understanding of resilience in the adolescent with cancer: Part I. *Journal of Pediatric Oncology Nursing, 16*(1), 35–43.

Woodgate, R., & McClement, S. (1997). Sense of self in children with cancer and in childhood cancer survivors: A critical review. *Journal of Pediatric Oncology Nursing, 14*(3), 137–155.

17

Shuler Nurse Practitioner Practice Model

BARBARA HOGLUND

LAUREL ASH

DEFINITION OF KEY TERMS

Input phase	The subjective and objective data collection phase of the patient encounter associated with taking in energy and information from the environment.
Throughput phase	The active decision-making phase of the patient encounter that reflects energy and information exchange between the patient and the nurse practitioner (NP); includes problem identification, diagnosing, contracting, planning, and implementation.
Output phase	Evaluation activities related to the patient encounter; the feedback phase alters the next input phase.
Clinical decision making	A dynamic process that begins with the chief complaint and consideration of differential diagnoses followed by identification of a working diagnosis based on the subjective and objective data. Clinical decision making continues throughout the problem identification, diagnosis, contracting, and planning phases of the patient encounter.
Problem judgment	Patient and NP interaction that provides the patient with teaching about the diagnosis and signs/symptoms that require follow-up.
Role modeling	NP characteristics/behaviors that are "role modeled" by the NP and observed by the patient such as fitness state, nutritional status, self-care attitude, and ability to handle stress. If NP characteristics/behaviors do not reflect behaviors that are requested of the patient, patient compliance may be reduced and/or blocked communication may exist.

INTRODUCTION

The role of the nurse is to address the human response to potential and actual health problems. The nurse practitioner (NP) expands the nursing role by adding medical decision-making skills of diagnosis and management of health problems to function in the role of the advanced practice nurse. As a result, the NP utilizes a unique blend of both nursing and medical knowledge and skills when caring for and interacting with patients (American Academy of Nurse Practitioners, 2010). The Shuler Nurse Practitioner Practice Model (SNPPM) integrates essential nursing and medical components to provide a framework for a holistic practice paradigm for NP practice and is appropriate to guide NP curricula and NP research activities (Nicoteri & Andrews, 2003; Shuler & Davis, 1993a).

HISTORICAL BACKGROUND

The SNPPM was first proposed by Pam Shuler in 1991 in response to the need for a model that reflects the dual nursing and medical roles assumed by NPs (Shuler, 1991). While the educational model for NPs incorporates nursing philosophy and theory, NPs often find themselves practicing solely within the framework of the medical model and/or unable to articulate or recognize the existence of theory-based NP practice (Nicoteri & Andrews, 2003). According to Shuler and Huebscher (1998), the SNPPM "equips the NP with a theoretically based guide for patient assessment consistent with the goal of providing primary health care services that are nursing oriented and complementary to medicine" (p. 492). Shuler and Huebscher (1998) suggest that consistent and conscious use of the model will help define the unique contribution of NPs to health care.

In addition to addressing the dual nursing and medical roles of the NP, the model was developed purposefully to encourage a holistic patient assessment that considers multiple dimensions related to the patient's health status; the model is oriented toward wellness and health promotion of concerns that go beyond simply physical needs. As a result, the NP is able to meet the needs of challenging and diverse patients (Shuler, Huebscher, & Hallock, 2001).

CONCEPTS

The SNPPM seeks to provide a framework for "everyday nurse practitioner practice" (Hahn, 1995, p. 43). According to Shuler, Gelberg, and Brown (1994), the model is organized from a systems theory perspective and utilizes Clark's Nursing Wellness Theory and the nursing process framework.

There are three major process components of the model that reflect the systems theory paradigm: inputs, patient/NP throughputs, and patient/NP outputs. The SNPPM is considered an open system, which takes in energy and information during the inputs phase, facilitates patient/NP interaction and negotiation during the throughput phase, and releases energy and information into the environment during the outputs phase. Outputs then alter the inputs (both internally and externally) within the model (Shuler & Davis, 1993a).

The SNPPM integrates the concepts of person, health, nursing, and environment with the NP role. While definitions of each concept are fully described by Shuler and Davis (1993a), the model allows NPs to substitute their own definitions of person, health, nursing, and environment while using the model. Several assumptions associated with the SNPPM are listed in Table 17.1.

TABLE 17.1 Shuler Nurse Practitioner Practice Model Assumptions

1. People are physiological, psychological, social, cultural, environmental, and spiritual beings.
2. People have the right to accept or reject health care.
3. The nurse practitioner (NP) and patient are partners in health care.
4. Health is a dynamic state and wellness is an ongoing process; both are related to physiological, psychological, social, cultural, environmental, and spiritual aspects of the patient.
5. NPs assist patients with wellness, health promotion, prevention, maintenance, and restoration through self-care activities.
6. The NP acts as a role model during patient interaction and can influence the patient's health-related attitudes and behaviors.
7. People can learn to move to a higher level of wellness when facilitated by NPs who are well-grounded in wellness theory and practice.
8. The family can be the greatest single influence on the health behaviors of patients since health beliefs, practices, values, and attitudes are often determined and monitored by this unit.
9. Patient health education can improve health and wellness status.
10. Patient health educator is one of the most important roles performed by the NP.
11. The patient is an active participant in the teaching/learning process.
12. Learning abilities and needs change throughout the lifespan.

Source: From Shuler, P., & Davis, J. (1993a). The Shuler Nurse Practitioner Practice Model: A theoretical framework for nurse practitioner clinicians, educators, and researchers, Part 1. *Journal of the American Academy of Nurse Practitioners, 5*(1), 11–18.

PERSON

The SNPPM builds on other theorists (e.g., Roy, 1970) who believe that humans are holistic in nature, interacting with the changing environment, and trying to maintain stability. The person is capable of healing himself and making personal health decisions.

HEALTH

Health is a dynamic state "related to physiological, psychological, social, cultural, and spiritual aspects of individuals" (Shuler & Davis, 1993a, p. 16). Effective coping and adaptation skills are essential to health, which is considered a personal and a social responsibility. "Wellness, illness, disease prevention, health promotion, self-care, rehabilitation, and education" are encompassed by health (Shuler & Davis, 1993a, p. 16).

NURSING

Nursing is considered to be goal directed, based on science, and interpersonal in nature. Nurses and NPs assess, diagnose, and treat actual or potential health problems, and promote wellness. The NP functions within multidisciplinary teams across a variety of practice settings (Shuler & Davis, 1993a, p. 16).

NP Role: Utilizing a holistic approach, the NP incorporates both nursing and medical knowledge to help move the patient to wellness. Depending on individual patient needs, care provided by the NP will focus on health restoration, health maintenance, and/or wellness activities. In addition, the NP serves as a role model for wellness (Shuler & Davis, 1993a, p. 16).

ENVIRONMENT

The SNPPM recognizes the significance of environment on persons and health. The environment includes geography, access to food, heat, shelter, hazards, and other factors (Shuler & Davis, 1993b).

DESCRIPTION OF THE MODEL: CARE PROCESS

The types of patient visits proposed by the model are: (a) episodic, (b) comprehensive with an existing problem, and (c) comprehensive without an existing problem (Shuler & Davis, 1993a). Although the type of encounter influences the interaction between the patient and the NP, the basic care process includes "inputs": history, objective data, role modeling; "throughputs": identifying problems, diagnosing, contracting, planning, and implementation; and "outputs": evaluation activities. Clinical decision making occurs throughout the input and throughput phases. Shuler and Davis (1993b) describe the care process as follows.

Inputs
- **History (subjective data).** The SNPPM begins with a holistic assessment of the patient including the typical medical history and review of systems data along with nursing components identified by Shuler and Davis as "physiologic and psychologic status needs, social supports/network, cultural/health beliefs, environmental/occupational conditions and spiritual tenets" (p. 76).
- **Objective data.** A comprehensive physical examination and laboratory/diagnostic testing information are gathered in the traditional manner.
- **Role modeling.** A distinctive aspect of the model is NP role modeling. The SNPPM asserts that the patient is continuously observing the NP for his/her commitment to wellness behaviors, including "fitness states, ability to handle stress, nutritional status, self-care attitude, cultural sensitivity, and spiritual awareness" (p. 84). The NP who does not role model healthy behaviors and activities is likely to experience reduced patient compliance toward a healthy lifestyle.

THE SHULER NURSE PRACTITIONER PRACTICE MODEL

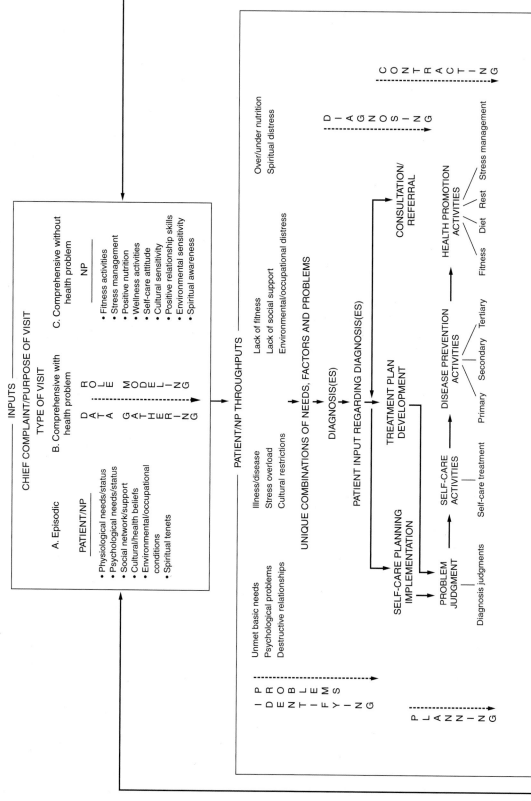

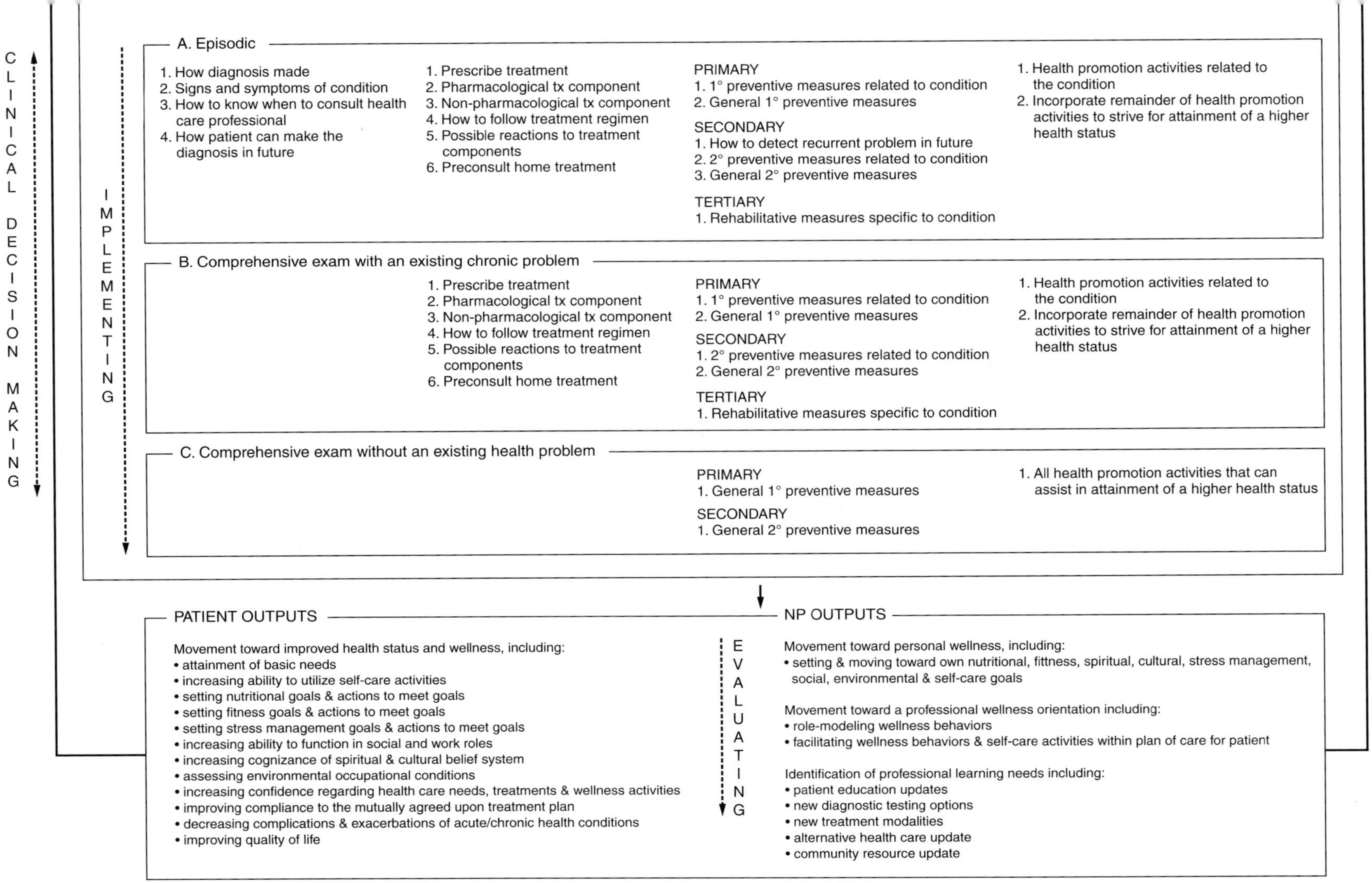

A. Episodic

1. Prescribe treatment
2. Pharmacological tx component
3. Non-pharmacological tx component
4. How to follow treatment regimen
5. Possible reactions to treatment components
6. Preconsult home treatment

1. How diagnosis made
2. Signs and symptoms of condition
3. How to know when to consult health care professional
4. How patient can make the diagnosis in future

PRIMARY
1. 1° preventive measures related to condition
2. General 1° preventive measures

SECONDARY
1. How to detect recurrent problem in future
2. 2° preventive measures related to condition
3. General 2° preventive measures

TERTIARY
1. Rehabilitative measures specific to condition

1. Health promotion activities related to the condition
2. Incorporate remainder of health promotion activities to strive for attainment of a higher health status

B. Comprehensive exam with an existing chronic problem

1. Prescribe treatment
2. Pharmacological tx component
3. Non-pharmacological tx component
4. How to follow treatment regimen
5. Possible reactions to treatment components
6. Preconsult home treatment

PRIMARY
1. 1° preventive measures related to condition
2. General 1° preventive measures

SECONDARY
1. 2° preventive measures related to condition
2. General 2° preventive measures

TERTIARY
1. Rehabilitative measures specific to condition

1. Health promotion activities related to the condition
2. Incorporate remainder of health promotion activities to strive for attainment of a higher health status

C. Comprehensive exam without an existing health problem

PRIMARY
1. General 1° preventive measures

SECONDARY
1. General 2° preventive measures

1. All health promotion activities that can assist in attainment of a higher health status

I M P L E M E N T I N G

E V A L U A T I N G

NP OUTPUTS

Movement toward personal wellness, including:
• setting & moving toward own nutritional, fittness, spiritual, cultural, stress management, social, environmental & self-care goals

Movement toward a professional wellness orientation including:
• role-modeling wellness behaviors
• facilitating wellness behaviors & self-care activities within plan of care for patient

Identification of professional learning needs including:
• patient education updates
• new diagnostic testing options
• new treatment modalities
• alternative health care update
• community resource update

PATIENT OUTPUTS

Movement toward improved health status and wellness, including:
• attainment of basic needs
• increasing ability to utilize self-care activities
• setting nutritional goals & actions to meet goals
• setting fitness goals & actions to meet goals
• setting stress management goals & actions to meet goals
• increasing ability to function in social and work roles
• increasing cognizance of spiritual & cultural belief system
• assessing environmental occupational conditions
• increasing confidence regarding health care needs, treatments & wellness activities
• improving compliance to the mutually agreed upon treatment plan
• decreasing complications & exacerbations of acute/chronic health conditions
• improving quality of life

C L I N I C A L   D E C I S I O N   M A K I N G

Figure 17.1 The Shuler Nurse Practitioner Practice Model. (With permission from P. Shuler.)

Throughputs

- **Identifying problems and diagnosing.** Another unique feature of the SNPPM is that the NP and the patient together determine problems/deficits. These problems/deficits may or may not be related to the determination of the diagnoses made by the NP. The NP considers all the problems/deficits and diagnoses and shares this assessment with the patient to obtain feedback that will assist in determining the plan of care. In this phase, patient input is elicited by clarifying historical and descriptive data to confirm the NP's diagnosis.

- **Contracting and planning.** The process of contracting is ongoing throughout the processes of gathering data, diagnosis (including identifying problems/deficits), and planning of care. Contracting empowers the patient and results in enhanced wellness and self-care behaviors. The plan of care may involve collaboration with other health care providers and may require consultation and/or referral. Treatment of patient problems/diagnoses is planned collaboratively by the patient and NP and includes pharmacologic and non-pharmacologic interventions as indicated; the plan of care seeks to improve current patient status as well as prevent further problems. The nursing components of "physiologic and psychologic status needs, social supports/network, cultural/health beliefs, environmental/occupational conditions and spiritual tenets" are again reviewed and considered as the plan is developed.

  An important component of the contracting and planning phase of the SNPPM is called "Self-care Planning and Implementation," in which four main areas are explored (p. 87). These areas are: (a) problem judgment, which incorporates teaching about the diagnosis and indicators that require follow-up care; (b) self-care Activities, which involves the treatment regimen; (c) disease prevention activities, which are inclusive of primary, secondary, and tertiary prevention; and (d) health promotion activities, which are focused and improving or sustaining wellness.

- **Implementation.** The NP and the patient work together to complete necessary implementation of the goals, which were mutually determined. Pharmacologic and non-pharmacologic actions in addition to disease prevention and health promotion activities are included.

Outputs

- **Evaluation.** The NP evaluates the movement toward improved health status and provides an opportunity for follow-up with the patient. The SNPPM calls this "patient outputs." In addition, the NP conducts self-evaluation activities termed "NP outputs"; the NP identifies professional learning needs important for maintaining the knowledge base essential for providing patient care (i.e., professional wellness), and evaluates his/her own movement toward personal health and wellness.

The SNPPM is depicted in Figure 17.1.

APPLICATIONS OF THE SHULER MODEL IN NURSING PRACTICE, RESEARCH, AND EDUCATION

PRACTICE EXAMPLES

The SNPPM has been described in the literature as a theoretical framework for NP practice in clinical settings such as home care, alternative and complementary care, school-based clinics, clinics for the homeless population, as well as traditional primary care settings (Huebscher & Shuler, 2004; Restrepo, Davitt, & Thompson, 2001; Shuler, 2000; Shuler & Davis, 1993b; Shuler et al., 1995). In diverse clinical settings, use of the model provides a holistic framework that clearly directs NP practice by incorporating medical decision making into a nursing-oriented practice. It is expected throughout a patient encounter that the NP elicits patient input and participation and concludes with patient contracting to facilitate empowerment of the patient and enhance patient behaviors associated with the four areas of treatment plan development: (a) problem judgment, (b) self-care activities, (c) disease prevention activities, and (d) health promotion

TABLE 17.2 Potential Benefits for Nurse Practitioners and Patients Related to Use of the SNPPM

Nurse practitioner outcomes	Patient outcomes
NPs who adopt the SNPPM can: 1. Reflect the combined role of nursing and medicine more consistently 2. Assess their patients more holistically and comprehensively 3. Be more systematic in their approach with patients 4. Be more likely to include patients in the assessment, planning, intervention, and evaluation processes 5. Encourage self-care activities more frequently among their patients 6. Be more likely to included disease prevention and health promotion activities in the treatment plan 7. Become less frustrated when working with patients who have a variety of health and health-related needs 8. Experience an increase in job satisfaction 9. View themselves more readily as members of a holistic multidisciplinary health care team 10. Consult and/or collaborate with diverse members of the multidisciplinary team more readily 11. Be more likely to utilize referral agencies other than health care facilities 12. Be more professionally aware of wellness theory and practices 13. Be more likely to personally participate in wellness activities 14. Be more cost-effective in their practice	Use of the SNPPM with patients can: 1. Ensure inclusion of psychological, social, cultural, environmental, and spiritual aspects of the patient's condition as well as the physical aspects 2. Increase confidence in the patient with respect to his/her health care needs, self-care treatments, and wellness activities 3. Improve the patient's lifestyle by increasing participation in disease prevention and health promotion (wellness) activities 4. Decrease the number of patient follow-up visits 5. Decrease complications and exacerbations of acute and/or chronic health conditions 6. Improve compliance to the mutually agreed upon treatment and/or wellness plan 7. Encourage patients to seek health care early when a problem is beginning to surface 8. Encourage patients to "take charge" of their health care 9. Improve the patient's quality of life by recognizing him/her as a holistic being, encouraging participation in wellness activities and addressing underlying psychological, social, cultural, environmental, and spiritual needs

Source: From Shuler, P. & Davis, J. (1993b). The Shuler Nurse Practitioner Practice Model: Clinical Application, Part 2. *Journal of the American Academy of Nurse Practitioners, 5*(2), 73–88.

activities. Treatment plans are mutually agreed upon between the patient and the NP. Evaluation of the patient response over time is monitored from a holistic perspective. Self-reflection by the NP is also essential for effective practice. Use of the model in practice has the potential to result in multiple benefits for both patients and the NP (see Table 17.2).

RESEARCH EXAMPLES

The Shuler model has provided the framework for investigation of NP clinical practice.

For example, school-based health care services were evaluated using the SNPPM to identify gaps in areas such as data collection processes, development of goals and objectives, intervention strategies, use of consultants and multidisciplinary teams, and the effectiveness of interventions and services delivered (Shuler, 2000).

In a study related to family planning services for homeless women, the Shuler model was used to guide the analysis of chart review data collected from family planning histories on new patients who presented to a clinic designed to meet reproductive needs of homeless women (Shuler et al., 1995). Use of the model assisted in identifying and clarifying risk factors related to unintended pregnancies among homeless women.

EDUCATION EXAMPLES

Education of NP students is perhaps the most valuable application of the SNPPM. Use of the model in NP curricula facilitates productive connections between nursing and medical practices during the formative experiences of NP student development. Use of the Shuler model promotes the use of traditional nursing knowledge and skills while incorporating the medical model approach necessary to conduct a history and physical examination and determine a relevant plan of care. Since NP students are often focused on learning the medical aspects of the NP role (assessment and treatment of conditions), development of the nursing aspects of the NP role (addressing the response to potential and actual problems) requires a more intentional approach. The Shuler model maintains the nursing aspects of the NP role while creating simple, but effective links with medical components required for NP practice. Shuler and Davis (1993b) provide a detailed guide for a history and physical examination associated with a patient encounter that requires a comprehensive examination; the guide identifies components of a history and physical congruent with the medical model approach while clearly presenting additional components related to the nursing domain. Use of the Shuler model ensures the preservation of a nursing orientation in advanced practice nursing (Shuler & Davis, 1993b).

SUMMARY

The SNPPM was developed in 1991 to describe and guide the unique practice of NPs in primary care settings. It emphasizes a holistic patient assessment with an orientation toward wellness and health promotion. Unique to the model is the significance of NP role modeling on the outcome of care. The model fully integrates the medical and nursing aspects of the NP role to guide education, research, and practice.

ANALYSIS OF THEORY

Using the criteria presented in Chapter 2, critique the theory of SNPPM. Compare your conclusions about the theory with those found in Appendix A. A nurse scholar who has worked with the theory completed the analysis found in the Appendix.

Internal Criticism	External Criticism
1. Clarity	1. Reality convergence
2. Consistency	2. Utility
3. Adequacy	3. Significance
4. Logical development	4. Discrimination
5. Level of theory development	5. Scope
	6. Complexity

CRITICAL THINKING EXERCISES

1. Discuss the challenges related to maintaining a nursing philosophy when practicing within the framework of the medical model.

2. Discuss the connection between role modeling of wellness behaviors by the NP and facilitating wellness behaviors among clients.

3. Explore the way systems theory concepts are integrated into the Shuler model. In what ways does a systems theory perspective influence NP practice?

4. The Shuler model provides definitions for the global concepts of person, health, nursing, and environment. At the same time, the model allows the NP to substitute personal definitions for the nursing metaparadigm. If alternative definitions are used, what are the possible effects on the assumptions of the model as outlined in Table 17.1?

5. Explore the benefits of mutually determining problem and deficit areas with the client. What is the significance of collaborating with the client when determining the plan of care?

WEB RESOURCES

Visit **http://thePoint.lww.com/Peterson3e** for helpful web resources related to this chapter.

REFERENCES

American Academy of Nurse Practitioners. (2010). *Scope of practice for nurse practitioners.* Retrieved June 7, 2010 from http://www.aanp.org/AANPCMS2/AboutAANP/About+NPs.htm

Hahn, M. (1995, October). What becomes a nurse practitioner most? The Shuler nurse practitioner practice model. *Advance for Nurse Practitioners,* pp. 43–46.

Huebscher, R., & Shuler, P. (2004). *Natural, alternative, and complementary health care practices.* St. Louis, MO: Mosby.

Nicoteri, J., & Andrews, C. (2003). The discovery of unique nurse practitioner theory in the literature: Seeking evidence using an integrative review approach. *Journal of the American Academy of Nurse Practitioners, 15*(11), 494–500.

Restrepo, A., Davitt, C., & Thompson, S. (2001). House calls: is there an APN in the house? *Journal of the American Academy of Nurse Practitioners, 31*(12), 560–564.

Roy, C. (1970). A conceptual framework for nursing. *Nursing Outlook, 18,* 42–45.

Shuler, P. A. (1991). *Homeless women's wholistic and family planning needs: An exposition and test of the Shuler Nurse Practitioner Practice Model (dissertation).* Los Angeles, CA: University of California.

Shuler, P. A. (2000). Evaluating student services provided by school-based health centers: Applying the Shuler Nurse Practitioner Practice Model. *Journal of School Health, 70*(8), 348–352.

Shuler, P. A., & Davis, J. E. (1993a). The Shuler Nurse Practitioner Practice Model: A theoretical framework for nurse practitioner clinicians, educators, and researchers, Part 1. *Journal of the American Academy of Nurse Practitioners, 5*(1), 11–18.

Shuler, P. A., & Davis, J. E. (1993b). The Shuler Nurse Practitioner Practice Model: Clinical application, Part 2. *Journal of the American Academy of Nurse Practitioners, 5*(2), 73–88.

Shuler, P. A., Gelberg, L., & Brown, M. (1994). The effects of spiritual/religious practices on psychological well-being among inner city homeless women. *Nurse Practitioner Forum, 5*(2), 106–113.

Shuler, P. A., Gelberg, L., & Davis, J. E. (1995). Characteristics associated with the risk of unintended pregnancy among urban homeless women: Use of the Shuler Nurse Practitioner Practice Model in research. *Journal of the American Academy of Nurse Practitioners, 7*(1), 13–22.

Shuler, P. A., & Huebscher, R. (1998). Clarifying nurse practitioners' unique contributions: Application of the Shuler Nurse Practitioner Practice Model. *Journal of the American Academy of Nurse Practitioners, 10*(11), 491–499.

Shuler, P., Huebscher, R., & Hallock, J. (2001). Providing wholistic health care for the elderly: Utilization of the Shuler Nurse Practitioner Practice Model. *Journal of the American Academy of Nurse Practitioners, 13*(7), 297–303.

18

The AACN Synergy Model

SONYA R. HARDIN

DEFINITION OF KEY TERMS

Health care system	The health care system acts as a facilitator or conduit to support patient needs and the power to nurture the professional practice environment of the nurse.
Nurse competencies	The eight competencies of nursing practice as defined by the model are clinical judgment, caring practices, advocacy/moral agency, response to diversity, clinical inquiry, facilitator of learning, collaboration, and systems thinking.
Patient characteristics	Eight patient characteristics have been identified that span a continuum of health to illness: vulnerability, resiliency, stability, complexity, predictability, resource availability, participation in care, and participation in decision making.
Optimal patient outcomes	Patient outcomes include patient satisfaction with care, levels of trust, patient behavior and knowledge, patient functional change, and quality of life.

INTRODUCTION

The American Association of Critical Care Nurses (AACN) has established a vision to create a health care system that is driven by the needs of patients and families where nurses can make optimal contributions in the delivery of care. This vision involved the development of a model that explicates the practice that nurses contribute at the bedside. The model developed was the AACN Synergy Model. The goal of this model was to clearly articulate the competencies brought to patient care by nurses in meeting the needs of patients and families.

HISTORICAL BACKGROUND

During the early 1990s, the AACN Certification Corporation strategically set forth a direction to identify a model that described practice. In 1993, the AACN Certification Corporation, the certifying body of the AACN, established a think tank to draft a document that identified the concepts of nursing practice, most specifically certified practice. The think tank identified 13 patient needs and 9 nurse characteristics. Then in 1995, the AACN Certification Board identified a group of "Subject Matter" experts from across the United States to refine the conceptual model. A revision to the model resulting in eight nurse characteristics and eight patient characteristics occurred.

In February 2002, the Practice Analysis Task Force expanded the assumption to the model to include the following:

■ The nurse creates the environment for the care of the patient. The context/environment of care also affects what the nurse can do.

- There is an interrelatedness between impact areas. The nature of the interrelatedness may change as the function of experience, situation, or setting changes.
- The nurse may work to optimize outcomes for patients, families, health care providers, and the health care system/organization.
- Nurses bring their background to each situation, including various levels of education/knowledge and skills/experience (Practice Analysis Task Force, 2002).

In March 1996, the AACN Certification Corporation appointed an Outcome Think Tank who identified six major quality indicators: (a) patient and family satisfaction, (b) rate of adverse incidents, (c) complication rate, (d) adherence to the discharge plan, (e) mortality rate, and (f) the patient's length of stay (Hardin, 2005). Outcomes derived from the eight patient characteristics include functional changes, behavioral changes, trust, satisfaction, comfort, and quality of life. Outcomes derived from the eight nursing competencies include physiological changes, the presence or absence of complications, and the extent treatment objectives were obtained (Curley, 1998). Outcome data derived from the health care system include readmission rates, length of stay, and cost utilization per case.

DESCRIPTION OF THE THEORY OF SYNERGY MODEL

ASSUMPTION OF THE MODEL

The Synergy Model is based on the following five assumptions:

"1) Patients are biological, social and spiritual entities who present at a particular developmental stage. The whole patient (body, mind, and spirit) must be considered. 2) The patient, family, and community all contribute to providing a context for the nurse-patient relationship. 3) Patients can be described by a number of characteristics. All characteristics are connected and contribute to each other. Characteristics cannot be looked at in isolation. 4) Nurses can be described on a number of dimensions. The interrelated dimensions paint a profile of the nurse. 5) A goal of nursing is to restore a patient to an optimal level of wellness as defined by the patient. Death can be an acceptable outcome in which the goal of nursing care is to move a patient toward a peaceful death" (AACN, 2000, p. 5).

DEFINITION OF THEORETICAL CONCEPTS

There are totally 16 concepts in this model: eight patient concepts and eight nursing concepts (Tables 18.1 and 18.2). The concepts (characteristics) are descriptors that describe the patient and nursing. The eight concepts used to understand patients are resiliency, vulnerability, stability, complexity, resource availability, participation in care, participation in decision making, and predictability. The eight concepts (characteristics) used to describe the practice of nursing are clinical judgment, advocacy, caring practices, collaboration, systems thinking, response to diversity, clinical inquiry, and facilitator of learning. The patient and nurse characteristics are leveled from 1 to 5 and are presented in Tables 18.1 and 18.2.

Patient characteristic levels are based on a five-point Likert scale, ranging from 1 (the worst patient state) to 5 (the best patient state). Nurse characteristic levels are based on a five-point Likert scale with 1 being novice and 5 being expert. Descriptions of levels 1, 3, and 5 have been described by the AACN. Levels 2 and 4 have not been specifically identified in the literature by the AACN. However, the use of the five levels with levels 1, 3, and 5 as benchmarks has been useful to nursing organizations as they develop clinical ladders. Further work has been completed on the nurse characteristics for the advanced-practice role (Becker et al., 2006). Activities of advanced-practice nurses organized by the eight nurse characteristics emerged through a study of practice conducted by the AACN Certification Corporation. While some of these activities overlap with the expert nurse, the study identified four nurse characteristics considered most critical by clinical nurse specialists (clinical judgment, caring practices, facilitator of learning, and clinical inquiry) and two activities most critical by nurse practitioners (clinical judgment and advocacy/moral agency; Becker et al., 2006).

TABLE 18.1 Patient Characteristics and Levels

Characteristic	Definition	Level
Stability	Maintain a steady-state equilibrium	**Level 1—Minimally stable:** labile; unstable; unresponsive to therapies; high risk of death **Level 3—Moderately stable:** able to maintain steady state for limited period of time; some responsiveness to therapies **Level 5—Highly stable:** constant; responsive to therapies; low risk of death
Complexity	Entanglement of two or more systems (e.g., body, family, therapies)	**Level 1—Highly complex:** intricate; complex patient/family dynamics; ambiguous/vague; atypical presentation **Level 3—Moderately complex:** moderately involved patient/family dynamics **Level 5—Minimally complex:** straightforward; routine patient/family dynamics; simple/clear cut; typical presentation
Predictability	Allows one to expect a certain course of events	**Level 1—Not predictable:** uncertain; uncommon patient population/illness; unusual or unexpected course; does not follow critical pathway, or no critical pathway developed **Level 3—Moderately predictable:** wavering; occasionally noted patient population/illness **Level 5—Highly predictable:** certain; common patient population/illness; usual and expected course; follows critical pathway
Resiliency	The capacity to return to a restorative level of functioning	**Level 1—Minimally resilient:** unable to mount a response; failure of compensatory/coping mechanisms; minimal reserves; brittle **Level 3—Moderately resilient:** able to mount a moderate response; able to initiate some degree of compensation; moderate reserves **Level 5—Highly resilient:** able to mount and maintain a response; intact compensatory/coping mechanisms; strong reserves; endurance
Vulnerability	Susceptibility to actual or potential stressors	**Level 1—Highly vulnerable:** susceptible; unprotected, fragile **Level 3—Moderately vulnerable:** somewhat susceptible; somewhat protected **Level 5—Minimally vulnerable:** safe; out of the woods; protected, not fragile
Participation in decision making	Extent to which patient/family engages in decision making	**Level 1—No participation:** no capacity for decision making; requires surrogacy **Level 3—Moderate level of participation:** limited capacity; seeks input/advice from others in decision making **Level 5—Full participation:** full capacity; makes decision for self
Participation in care	Extent to which patient/family engages in aspects of care	**Level 1—No participation:** patient and family unable or unwilling to participate in care **Level 3—Moderate level of participation:** patient and family need assistance in care **Level 5—Full participation:** patient and family fully able to participate in care
Resource availability	Extent of resources the patient/family/community bring to the situation	**Level 1—Few resources:** necessary knowledge and skills not available; financial support and personal/psychological supportive resources minimal **Level 3—Moderate resources:** limited knowledge and skills available; limited financial support and personal/psychological and supportive resources **Level 5—Many resources:** extensive knowledge and skills available and accessible; strong financial, personal, and supportive resources

Source: Adapted from AACN Certification Corporation web site. The AACN Synergy Model for Patient Care (2000). Retrieved September 27, 2007, from http://www.certcorp.org/certcorp/certcorp.nsf/edcfc72ba47aaa708825666b0064bdcf/08482aa8ec2a5b638825666b00654be7?OpenDocument.

TABLE 18.2 Nurse Characteristics and Levels

Characteristic	Definition	Level
Clinical judgment	Clinical reasoning	**Level 1:** collects basic-level data; follows algorithms, decision trees, and protocols with all populations and is uncomfortably deviating from them **Level 3:** collects and interprets complex patient data; makes clinical judgments based on an immediate grasp of the whole picture for common or routine patient populations **Level 5:** synthesizes and interprets multiple, sometimes conflicting, sources of data; makes judgment based on an immediate grasp of the whole picture; helps patient and family see the "big picture"; recognizes and responds to the dynamic situation
Advocacy	Working on another's behalf	**Level 1:** works on behalf of patient; self-assesses personal values; is aware of ethical conflicts/issues that may surface in clinical setting; makes ethical/moral decisions based on rules **Level 3:** considers patient values and incorporates in care, even when differing from personal values; supports colleagues in ethical and clinical issues; moral decision making can deviate from rules **Level 5:** advocates ethical conflict and issues from patient/family perspective; suspends rules; empowers the patient and the family to speak for/represent themselves
Caring practices	Activities that create a compassionate, supportive, and therapeutic environment for patients and staff	**Level 1:** focuses on the customary needs of the patient; has no anticipation of future needs; bases care on standards and protocols **Level 3:** responds to subtle patient and family changes; engages with the patient as a unique patient in a compassionate manner; recognizes and tailors caring practices to the individuality of patient **Level 5:** has astute awareness and anticipates patient and family changes and needs; is fully engaged with and senses how to stand alongside the patient, family, and community; orchestrates the process that ensures the patient's/family's comfort and concerns surrounding issues of death and dying
Collaboration	Working with others in a way that promotes each person's contributions toward achieving optimal outcomes	**Level 1:** willing to be taught, coached, and/or mentored; participates in team meetings and discussions regarding patient care and/or practice issues **Level 3:** seeks opportunities to be taught, coached, and/or mentored; elicits others' advice and perspectives; initiates and participates in team meetings and discussions regarding patient care; recognizes and suggests various team members' participation **Level 5:** seeks opportunities to teach, coach, and mentor and to be taught, coached, and mentored; facilitates active involvement and complementary contributions of others in team meetings and discussions regarding patient care and/or practice issues; involves/recruits diverse resources when appropriate to optimize patient outcomes
Response to diversity	Sensitivity to recognize, appreciate, and incorporate differences into the provision of care	**Level 1:** assesses cultural diversity; provides care based on own belief system; learns the culture of the health care environment **Level 3:** inquires about cultural differences and considers their impact on care; accommodates personal and professional differences in the plan of care; helps patient/family understand the culture of the health care system **Level 5:** responds to, anticipates, and integrates cultural differences into patient/family care; appreciates and incorporates differences, including alternative therapies; tailors health care culture, to the extent possible, to meet the diverse needs and strengths of the patient/family

(continued)

TABLE 18.2 Nurse Characteristics and Levels (*Continued*)

Characteristic	Definition	Level
Clinical inquiry	Ongoing process of questioning and evaluating practice and providing informed practice	**Level 1:** follows standards and guidelines; implements clinical changes and research-based practices developed by others; recognizes the need for further learning to improve patient care; recognizes obvious changing patient situation; needs and seeks help to identify patient problem **Level 3:** questions appropriateness of policies and guidelines; questions current practice; seeks advice, resources, or information to improve patient care; begins to compare and contrast possible alternatives **Level 5:** improves, deviates from, or individualizes standards and guidelines for particular patient situations or populations; questions and/or evaluates current practice based on patients' responses, review of the literature, research, and education/learning
Facilitator of learning	Ability to facilitate learning for patients/ families, nursing staff, other members of the health care team, and community	**Level 1:** follows planned educational programs; sees patient/family education as a separate task from delivery of care; provides data without seeking to assess patient's readiness or understanding; has limited knowledge of the totality of the educational needs **Level 3:** adapts planned educational programs; begins to recognize and integrate different ways of teaching into delivery of care; incorporates patient's understanding into practice **Level 5:** creatively modifies or develops patient/family education programs; integrates patient/family education throughout delivery of care; evaluates patient's understanding by observing behavior changes; sets patient-driven goals for education
Systems thinking	Knowledge and tools that enhance the nurse's ability to manage whatever environmental and system resources exist for the patient/family and staff	**Level 1:** uses a limited array of strategies; does not recognize negotiation as an alternative; sees patient and family within the isolated environment of the unit; sees self as key resource **Level 3:** develops strategies based on needs and strengths of patient/family; is able to make connections within components; sees opportunity to negotiate but may not have strategies; recognizes how to obtain resources beyond self **Level 5:** develops, integrates, and applies a variety of strategies; has a global or holistic outlook; knows when and how to negotiate and navigate through the system; anticipates needs of patients and families as they move through the health care system; uses untapped and alternative resources as necessary

Source: Adapted from AACN Certification Corporation web site. The AACN Synergy Model for Patient Care (2000). Retrieved September 27, 2007, from http://www.certcorp.org/certcorp/certcorp.nsf/edcfc72ba47aaa708825666b0064bdcf/08482aa8ec2a5b638825666b00654be7?OpenDocument.

PATIENT CHARACTERISTICS

Each patient brings a unique set of characteristics to the health care situation. Among many characteristics that are present, eight are consistently seen in acute and critically ill patients. These eight characteristics are consistently assessed by nurses in variable levels given each patient situation. They should be assessed in the patient as well as other patterns that are unique to the given circumstances of the patient. *Resiliency* is the patient's capacity to return to a restorative level of functioning using compensatory coping mechanisms. The level of resiliency is often dependent upon the patient's ability to rebound after an insult. This ability can be influenced by many factors including age, comorbidities, nutritional status, and compensatory mechanisms that are intact. *Vulnerability* is the level of susceptibility to actual or potential stressors that may adversely affect patient outcomes. Vulnerability can be impacted by the patient's physiological/genetic make-up or health behaviors exhibited by the patient, such as risk factors. *Stability* refers to the patient's ability to maintain a steady state of equilibrium. Response to therapies and nursing interventions can impact the stability of the patient. *Complexity* is the intricate entanglement of two or more systems. Systems refer to either physiological or psychological states of the body or family dynamics or environmental interactions with the patient. The more systems involved, the more complex are the patterns displayed by the patient. *Resource availability* is influenced by the extent that resources are brought to the context by the patient, family, and community. The resources can present as pharmaceutical, technical, fiscal, personal, psychological, social, or supportive in nature. A greater potential for a positive outcome exists when a patient has more resources. *Participation in care* is the participation by the patient and the family who are engaged in the delivery of care. Patient and family participation can be influenced by health status, educational background, health literacy, resource availability, and cultural background. *Participation in decision making* is the level of engagement of the patient and the family in comprehending the information provided by health care providers and acting upon this information to execute informed decisions. Patient and family engagement in clinical decisions can be impacted by the knowledge level of the patient, his or her capacity to make decisions given the insult, cultural background (i.e., beliefs and values), and the level of inner strength during a crisis (AACN Certification Corporation, 2002).

Nurse Characteristics

The nurse characteristics can be considered competencies that are essential for providing care to the acute and critically ill. All eight competencies reflect an integration of knowledge, skills, and experience of the nurse. The competencies include clinical judgment, advocacy, caring practices, systems thinking, facilitation of learning, collaboration, response to diversity, and clinical inquiry. *Clinical judgment* is the clinical reasoning that is used by a health care provider in the delivery of care. It consists of critical thinking and nursing skills that are acquired through a process of integrating formal and experiential knowledge. The integration of knowledge and experience brings about the clinical decisions made during the course of care for patients, groups, and communities. *Advocacy* is working on another's behalf when the other is not capable of advocating for him/ herself. The nurse serves as a moral agent in identifying and helping to resolve ethical dilemmas within the clinical setting. *Caring practices* are the constellation of nursing interventions that are unique to the needs of the patient and the family. Caring behaviors include compassion, vigilance, engagement, and responsiveness to the patient and the family. *Collaboration* is the nurse working with others to promote optimal outcomes. The patient, family, and members of various health care disciplines collaborate by working toward promoting the needs and requests of patients. *Systems thinking* is the tool and knowledge that the nurse uses to recognize the interconnected nature within and across the health care system. The ability to understand how one's decision can impact the whole is integral to systems thinking. The nurse uses a global perspective in analyzing problems, making decisions, and negotiating for the patient and the family internally and externally to the health care system. *Response to diversity* is the sensitivity to recognize, appreciate, and incorporate differences into the provision of care. Nurses need to recognize the individuality of each patient while observing for patterns that respond to nursing interventions. Nurses should be open to the patient's spiritual beliefs, ethnicity, family configuration, lifestyle values, and the use of alternative and complementary therapies. *Clinical inquiry* is the ongoing process of questioning and evaluating practice, providing informed practice, and innovating through research and experiential learning. Clinical inquiry evolves as the nurse moves from novice to expert. At the expert level, the nurse enhances, deviates, and/or individualizes standards and guidelines to meet the needs of patients, families, groups, and communities. *Facilitator of learning* is understood as the nurse facilitating learning among patients, families, communities, and staff through tailored educational programs. The educational level of the audience should be considered in the design of the plan to educate. Creative methods should be developed to ensure patient and family comprehension and to make informed decisions. Each nurse and patient characteristic is understood on a continuum from 1 to 5. The level of each patient characteristic is critical in identifying the competency required of the nurse (AACN Certification Corporation, 2002).

RESEARCH

The Synergy Model is useful in identifying optimal patient outcomes given evidence-based nursing interventions (Kaplow & Hardin, 2007). Optimal outcomes can be measured through the use of numerous instruments. For example, as the nurse begins managing the transition of the patient from one setting

TABLE 18.3 Instruments for Measuring the Characteristics of Resilience

Instrument	Description	Reference
Modified Resilience Scale for Adolescents (READ)	23-item five-point Likert scale that measures personal competence, social competence, structured style, family cohesion, and social resources	Soest, T., Mossige, S., Stefansen, K., & Hjemdal, O. (2010). A validation study of the resilience scale for adolescents (READ). *Journal of Psychopathology Behavior Assessment, 32,* 215–225.
The Resilience Scale (RS)	25-item scale on personal competence and acceptance of self and life	Wagnild, G.M. & Young, H.M. (1993). Development and psychometric evaluation of the resilience scale. *Journal of Nursing Measurement, 1,* 165–178.
Ego-Resilience Scale (ER89)	14-item scale on flexibility, curiosity, generosity, and social skills	Block, J. & Kremen, A.M. (1996). IQ and ego-resiliency: Conceptual and empirical connections and separateness. *Journal of Personality and Social Psychology, 70,* 349–361.
Trauma Resilience Scale	9-item questionnaire with a seven-point Likert scale	Madsen, M.D. & Abell, N. (2010). Trauma Resilience Scale: Validation of protective factors associated with adaptation following violence. *Research on Social Work Practice, 20*(2), 223–233.

to another, the outcome of transition without complications is established. The nurse can use numerous research-developed risk-screening instruments to improve postdischarge problems. Or, if the nurse is managing an organ donor, pathways have been developed by the United Network for Organ Sharing to guide the decisions and actions in managing donors. Such pathways have been researched and/or reached through clinical consensus (Kaplow & Hardin, 2007).

Evidence-based practice is based upon clinical inquiry of scientists in the field or developed protocols through clinical evidence. The integration or the translation of research findings into practice is a skill set within the characteristic of clinical inquiry (Titler, 2004). The tools evolved from evidence-based practice and hence clinical inquiry have supported the decision making of nurses. Through evidence-based practice, interventions and outcomes can be identified.

Further research with the model needs to be conducted to validate the model within other practice settings and patient populations. One approach is to identify questions surrounding the concepts of the model and then to identify instruments that can be utilized to measure the concepts. Table 18.3 displays four instruments that measure the patient characteristic of resilience. Although these instruments have not been utilized extensively within critical care settings, the potential exists to design interventional studies to evaluate strategies to improve resilience.

Studies are needed on the nursing characteristics described in the model. How these characteristics impact optimal patient outcomes will require the use of existing instruments and the design of new measurements. Table 18.4 displays instruments that can be utilized to measure the nurse characteristic of collaboration. A number of scales have been developed to measure nurse collaboration and interdisciplinary collaboration. However, these scales have not been utilized in research studies in the setting of critical care.

Using the Synergy Model as the framework for nursing research, which is designed to examine the characteristics of the patient and the nurse is limited in the literature. Quantitative measurement of the characteristic in descriptive studies and studies designed to test an intervention that affects the characteristics is needed to facilitate optimal patient outcomes.

TABLE 18.4 Instruments for Measuring the Nurse Characteristic of Collaboration

Instrument	Description	Reference
Nurse–Physician Collaboration Scale	51-item five-point Likert scale	USHIRO R. (2009). Nurse–Physician Collaboration Scale: Development and psychometric testing. *Journal of Advanced Nursing, 65*(7), 1497–1508.
ICU Nurse–Physician Questionnaire (ICUN-P-Q)		Shortell, S. M., Rousseau, D. M., Gillies, R. R., Devers, K. J., & Simons, T. L. (1991). Organizational assessment in intensive care units (ICUs): Construct development, reliability, and validity of the ICU nurse–physician questionnaire. *Medical Care, 29*(8), 709–726.
Relational Coordination		Gittell, J. H., Fairfield, K. M., Bierbaum, B., Head, W., Jackson, R., Kelly, M., Laskin, R., Lipson, S., Siliski, J., Thornhill, T., & Zuckerman, J. (2000). Impact of relational coordination on quality of care, postoperative pain and functioning, and length of stay: A nine-hospital study of surgical patients. *Medical Care, 38*(8), 807–819.
Interprofessional Collaboration Scale	14-item questionnaire with a four-point Likert scale	Kenaszchuk, C., Reeves, S., Nicholas, D., & Merrick Zwarenstein, M. (2010). Validity and reliability of a multiple-group measurement scale for interprofessional collaboration. *BMC Health Services Research, 10*, 83. Published online March 30, 2010. doi:10.1186/1472-6963-10-83

NURSING EDUCATION

Using the Synergy Model to facilitate the learning of patients, families, communities, and staff has been discussed in the literature (Hardin, 2004; Kaplow, 2002; Zungolo, 2004). Teaching can be enhanced by using the patient and nurse competencies to design care. The patient should be analyzed through identifying data points associated with each of the patient characteristics. Nursing interventions from each of the eight nursing competencies should be chosen to address the patient characteristics. Developing courses or curriculums can be accomplished with the Synergy Model as a framework. An example of the model being used has been described as the framework for the Duquesne University School of Nursing (Zungolo, 2004). In this school, each nurse characteristic has been used as a thread in the undergraduate curriculum across four years of study. The nurse characteristic of caring practices is to be demonstrated in freshman year as care of self and caring processes; sophomore year as initiating caring practices; junior year as integrating caring into one's practice; and senior year as displaying a caring attitude in all aspects of one's practice. The graduate curriculum is guided by the three spheres of influence along with the Synergy Model. Table 18.5 displays the three spheres of influence (Moloney-Harmon, 1999) for the clinical nurse specialist and the content in a graduate curriculum.

TABLE 18.5 Synergy Model in Graduate Education

Nurse–patient sphere	Nurse–nurse sphere	Nurse–system sphere
Establish and maintain outstanding relationships with patients	Establish ways to maximize the use of personnel and enhance patient safety	Analyze the political, economic, and financial realities of the health care industry

Source: Adapted from Zungolo, E. H. (2004). The Synergy Model in educational practice: A guide to curriculum development. *Excellence in Nursing Knowledge.* Retrieved October 3, 2006, from http://www.nursingknowledge.org/Portal/main.aspx? pageid = 3507&ContentID = 56394.

The Synergy Model has been used to revise and update critical care graduate programs such as the one provided by Marymount University in Arlington, VA, to prepare clinical nurse specialists (Cox & Galante, 2003). The eight nurse competencies became the framework for the courses with the instructor preparing a lecture on each competency and then a seminar focused on specific content areas that could be discussed in relationship to the content. For example, during week six, the instructor provided a lecture on collaboration and then had content in the seminar on hypovolemic shock, acute inflammatory diseases, and dysrhythmias. The clinical component of the course ensured integration and application of the Synergy Model as students were expected to learn the role of the critical care clinical specialist and to apply the eight nursing characteristics. The students used the nurse characteristics in a journal for reflecting on the experiential knowing of working in the role of a clinical nurse specialist (Cox & Galante, 2003).

NURSING PRACTICE

The Synergy Model is a model of practice. Practice is driven by the characteristics and needs of the patient. Nurses respond to the needs of the patient through nurse characteristics. When the patient and nurse characteristics are matched to facilitate optimal outcomes, synergy occurs (Pacini, 2005). The eight nursing competencies represent nursing practice. However, the core of nursing is *clinical judgment,* which is grounded in the nursing process of assessment, planning, intervention, and evaluation. Making decisions to act or not act is intervention. These decisions come about through the integration of knowledge and critical thinking skills such as distinguishing relevant data from the irrelevant, recognizing patterns and relationships, determining desired outcomes, and continuously evaluating.

Advocacy is doing for the patient that which he cannot do so for himself in that he lacks the knowledge or ability due to alteration in physiological systems. Nurses advocate through their pursuit of supporting the patient's right to self-determination and autonomy, and being a "protective shield" when the client is unable to advocate for himself (Hanks, 2005, p. 76).

The characteristic of *caring practices* includes interventions of spiritual support for end of life (Levey, Danis, Nelson, & Solomon, 2003), promotion of a "healing environment" (Rex Smith, 2006, pp. 44, 45), and the use of listening and therapeutic communication skills. Nurses intervene by providing an unconditional positive regard and nonjudgmental stance toward the patient, and creatively using self to engage in healing practices (Hardin & Kaplow, 2005).

Given the increasing complexity required in the care of patients, *collaboration* is a critical nurse characteristic. Individuals collaborating together are successful when (a) there is a compelling, shared drive or goals; (b) individuals with unique competencies will contribute to successful outcomes; (c) members operate within a formal structure, with defined roles that facilitate collective/collaborative work; and (d) there is mutual respect, tolerance, and trust. Individuals must be willing to take on different roles within a group and be honest and open with their ideas and concerns. There are times when an individual should be a follower and when he/she should be a leader.

Systems thinking is used to address the most challenging patient and organizational problems in health care. This nurse characteristic allows one to understand reality through the relationships among the system's parts, rather than the parts themselves. Long-term ramifications from a decision and a more accurate picture of reality, so that you can work with a system's natural forces, allow achievement of results desired.

Response to diversity is a characteristic that requires the nurse to approach each situation with an open mind and the ability to use respect when faced with requests or practices that are not understood. Providing culture-specific care is a stance that promotes healing. Nurses must first examine their own biases and values while providing sensitive care to others. To understand another, the nurse must seek knowledge about his or her culture. Assessing the needs of the patient and the family requires the skill of obtaining relevant cultural data to promote optimal patient outcomes (Campinha-Bacote, 2002).

Questioning to uncover best practices or innovative strategies to meet the needs of patients and families is a form of *clinical inquiry.* "Clinical inquiry is the ongoing process of questioning and evaluating practice, providing informed practice based on available data, and innovating through research and experiential learning" (Curley, 1998, p. 66). Nurses must remain knowledgeable of the new scientific information for applying the best research evidence while respecting the patient's and family's values (Titler, 2004).

Facilitator of learning is a characteristic that uses "teaching moments" throughout the time care is provided. Strategies to improve outcomes or to ensure informed decision making require the nurse to educate patients and families. Besides patients and families, nurses must continually work with new nurses who arrive on the unit as orientees. Psychomotor, critical-thinking, and clinical decision-making skills are role modeled, taught, and facilitated (Kaplow, 2002). Whether the nurse is working with a new orientee or patients and families, taking the lead in providing the knowledge and skills for the delivery of care is an aspect of this competency.

The use of the model in practice has been articulated with victims of intimate partner violence (IPV; Cox, 2003). These individuals are typically highly vulnerable and display a maladaptive resiliency, variable stability depending on the degree of physical and psychological injury, and low levels of resource availability. In providing care to victims of IPV, the nurse must possess a moderate to high level of all nurse characteristics. Advocacy and caring characteristics are needed at a high level to enhance prevention and to screen for IPV in a safe environment. At minimum, moderate levels of clinical inquiry, response to diversity, systems thinking, collaboration, facilitator of learning, and clinical judgment are needed to facilitate the best possible level of wellness (Cox, 2003).

USE OF THE THEORY IN A SYSTEM

Clarian Health Partner is the first hospital system in the United States to integrate the AACN Synergy Model for Patient Care in an organization. Nurses hired into the system are as an Associate Partner, Partner, or Senior Partner. These three levels correlate with the three levels of the nurse characteristics and differentiated practice principles (Kerfoot, 2004). In this organization, the model is used to simplify the needs of the patient. From the orientation of the nurse, to the clinical ladder, to job descriptions and documents, the model provides the framework for this organization. The integration of this model into an organization is an exemplary example of advancing accountability and professionalism in the workplace (Kaplow & Hardin, 2007).

The Synergy Model is being utilized nationally in hospitals on the journey to magnetism (Kaplow & Reed, 2008). A professional model of practice is a requirement for Magnet designation. The model must be integrated throughout the system and guide improvement in outcomes. A major step in the process is to embrace the model by designing job descriptions and clinical ladders that promote clinical advancement. This will require staff nurses and leadership of an organization to reach consensus on the level of integration of the model into expectation of job performance.

SUMMARY

The Synergy Model resonates with clinicians because it describes a practice where nurses achieve optimal patient outcomes with patients and families. The mutuality and reciprocal nature of the relationship between nurses and patients are very unique. This uniqueness emerges due to the intimacy from being the primary caregiver and overseer of care across the continuum of care. The nurse is the one constant in the trajectory of disease that has the ability to detect subtle changes due to the intense length of care over time. The use of the Synergy Model enhances the nurse's understanding of the contribution that is brought to the patient and the family through the discipline of nursing.

ANALYSIS OF THEORY

Using the criteria presented in Chapter 2, critique the Synergy Model. Compare your conclusions about the theory with those found in Appendix A. An experienced nurse has completed the analysis found in the Appendix.

Internal Criticism	**External Criticism**
1. Clarity	1. Reality convergence
2. Consistency	2. Utility
3. Adequacy	3. Significance
4. Logical development	4. Discrimination
5. Level of theory development	5. Scope of theory
	6. Complexity

CRITICAL THINKING EXERCISES

1. In today's health care environment, how is it possible to attempt to match patient characteristics to specific nurse competencies in order to optimize patient outcomes?

   • How is this accomplished in the acute care setting?

2. Apply the Synergy Model to a patient scenario that you have been the care provider.

3. Redesign a staff nurse job description to reflect the Synergy Model.

4. As a nursing leader on a patient care unit, how would you introduce the staff to the Synergy Model?

WEB RESOURCES

Visit **http://thePoint.lww.com/Peterson3e** for helpful web resources related to this chapter.

REFERENCES

AACN. (2000). *Assumptions Guiding the AACN Synergy Model for patient care.* Retrieved September 27, 2007, from http://www.certcorp.org/certcorp/certcorp.nsf/vwdoc/SynModel?opendocument#Assumptions%20Gu

AACN Certification Corporation. (2002). *The AACN Synergy Model for patient care.* Retrieved July 2010, from http://www.certcorp.org/certcorp/certcorp.nsf/vwdoc/SynModel?opendocument#Assumptions%20Gu

AACN Practice Analysis Task Force. (2003). *History of AACN Certification Corporation.* Retrieved July 2010, from http://www.certcorp.org/certcorp/certcorp.nsf/vwdoc/AboutUs

Block, J., & Kremen, A. M. (1996). IQ and ego-resiliency: Conceptual and empirical connections and separateness. *Journal of Personality and Social Psychology, 70,* 349–361.

Cox, C. W., & Galante, C. M. (2003). An MSN curriculum in preparation of CCNSs: A model for consideration. *Critical Care Nurse, 23*(6), 74–80.

Gittell J. H., Fairfield K. M., Bierbaum B., Head W., Jackson R., Kelly M., et al. (2000) Impact of relational coordination on quality of care, postoperative pain and functioning, and length of stay: A nine-hospital study of surgical patients. *Medical Care, 38*(8), 807–819.

Hanks, R. G. (2005). Sphere of nursing advocacy model. *Nursing Forum, 40*(3), 75–78.

Hardin, S. R. (2004). Using the Synergy Model with undergraduate students. *Excellence in Nursing Knowledge.* Retrieved July 2010, from http://www.nursingknowledge.org/Portal/main.aspx?pageid=3507&ContentID=56388

Hardin, S. R., & Hussey, L. (2003). AACN Synergy Model for patient care case study of a CHF patient. *Critical Care Nurse, 23*(1), 73–76.

Hardin, S. R., & Kaplow, R. (2005). *Synergy for clinical excellence: The AACN Synergy Model for patient care.* Sudbury, MA: Jones & Bartlett.

Kaplow, R. (2002). Applying the Synergy Model to nursing education—The Synergy Model in practice. *Critical Care Nurse, 22*(3), 77–81.

Kaplow, R., & Hardin, S. R. (2007). *Critical care nursing: Synergy for optimal outcomes.* Sudbury, MA: Jones & Bartlett.

Kaplow, R., & Reed, K. D. (2008). The AACN Synergy Model for patient care: A nursing model as a force of magnetism. *Nursing Economics, 26*(1), 17–25.

Kerfoot, K. (2004). Synergy from the vantage point of a chief nursing officer. *Excellence in Nursing Knowledge.*

Retrieved from July 2010, http://www.nursingknowledge.org/Portal/main.aspx?pageid=3507&ContentID=56442

Kenaszchuk, C., Reeves, S., Nicholas, D., & Merrick Zwarenstein, M. (2010). Validity and reliability of a multiple-group measurement scale for interprofessional collaboration. *BMC Health Services Research, 10,* 83. Published online March 30, 2010. doi:10.1186/1472-6963-10-83

Levy, M., Danis, M., Nelson, J., & Solomon, M. Z. (2003). Quality indicators for end-of-life in the intensive care unit. *Critical Care Medicine, 31,* 2255–2262.

Madsen, M. D., & Abell, N. (2010). Trauma resilience scale: Validation of protective factors associated with adaptation following violence. *Research on Social Work Practice, 20*(2), 223–233.

Moloney-Harmon, P. (1999). Contemporary practice of the clinical nurse specialist. *Critical Care Nurse, 19*(2), 101–104.

Pacini, C. M. (2005). Synergy: a framework for leadership development and transformation. *Critical Care Nursing Clinics of North America, 17*(2): 113–119, ix.

Rex Smith, A. (2006). Using the Synergy Model to provide spiritual care in critical care settings. *Critical Care Nurse, 26*(4), 41–47.

Shortell S. M., Rousseau D. M., Gillies R. R., Devers K. J., & Simons T. L. (1991). Organizational assessment in intensive care units (ICUs): Construct development, reliability, and validity of the ICU nurse-physician questionnaire. *Medical Care, 29*(8), 709–726.

Soest, T., Mossige, S., Stefansen, K., & Hjemdal, O. (2010). A validation study of the resilience scale for adolescents (READ). *Journal of Psychopathology Behavior Assessment, 32,* 215–225.

Titler, M. G. (2004). Understanding synergy: The model from the perspective of a nurse scientist. *Excellence in Nursing Knowledge.* Retrieved July 2010, from http://www.nursingknowledge.org/Portal/main.aspx?pageid=3507&ContentID=56400

Ushiro, R. (2009). Nurse–physician collaboration scale: Development and psychometric testing. *Journal of Advanced Nursing, 65*(7), 1497–1508.

Wagnild, G. M., & Young, H. M. (1993). Development and psychometric evaluation of the resilience scale. *Journal of Nursing Measurement, 1,* 165–178.

Zungolo, E. H. (2004). The Synergy Model in educational practice: A guide to curriculum development. *Excellence in Nursing Knowledge.* Retrieved July 2010, from http://www.nursingknowledge.org/Portal/main.aspx?pageid=3507&ContentID=56394

3 Pain: A Balance Between Analgesia and Side Effects

SHIRLEY M. MOORE

INTERNAL CRITICISM

1. *Clarity.* The terms used and the ideas conveyed in this theory are easy to understand. All terms are defined using words that are common to practicing nurses. The most unique idea expressed in the theory is the major concept of "a balance between analgesia and side effects" as a way to think about pain management. A clear definition is given of this new conceptualization of pain management. In addition, all the propositions are expressed clearly and provide a coherent and comprehensive conceptualization.

2. *Consistency.* The description of this prescriptive theory is consistent in the use of concepts and definitions. The use of the terms and propositions are consistent with those used in other prescriptive theories. For example, the proposition specifying that nurses use appropriate multimodal interventions for pain management is prescriptive because it suggests that specific decisions and actions on the part of the nurse are likely to produce a particular outcome. In addition, consistent with prescriptive level theory, the propositions can be easily tested, using randomized controlled trials.

3. *Adequacy.* This theory presents a comprehensive approach to acute pain management. The theory addresses the affective and sensory dimensions to be considered in the management of acute pain and, as such, represents a more comprehensive approach than other current theories of acute pain management. The theory can be considered in its entirety or regarded as discrete steps in the pain management process. Despite the comprehensive and prescriptive nature of the theory, the number of propositions is manageable for the reader.

4. *Logical development.* The description of the theory clearly chronicles the historical evolution of knowledge about pain management and explains this theory's unique contributions to the field. The theory deductively incorporates previous knowledge and theoretical perspectives of pain management and is consistent with them. For example, the gate control theory of pain can be used to explain the mechanics of effect. This theory is also an exemplar of the utility of developing middle range theory inductively from clinical practice guidelines. The arguments of the theory are well supported and the conclusions are logical.

5. *Level of theory development.* In this prescriptive theory, specific choices and actions of the nurse to promote a balance between analgesia and side effects are posed. The theory is supported by some research; it has been tested in randomized controlled trials. Dr. Good has conducted research on the effects of nonpharmacological adjuvants as part of pain management. Knowledge about the behavioral and social cognitive mechanisms in some of the propositions of the theory is less developed. For example, little is known about the best ways to engage in goal setting for pain management, or timing the amount of information to provide for a patient when soliciting patient participation in acute pain management. In addition, more research is needed about how the propositions may be influenced by cultural orientation.

EXTERNAL CRITICISM

1. *Reality convergence.* This theory is clearly reality based. It addresses the two dimensions of pain management, affective and sensory, that nurses observe in their clients. The assumptions of the theory represent the real world, a clinical reality to which every nurse can relate.

2. *Utility.* Acute pain management is a common problem in nursing. This is a pragmatic theory that nurses in practice and clinical researchers can easily use. Nurses can use this theory to generate testable hypotheses, both at the bedside and in full-scale research studies. Some hypotheses have been generated from this study, and the author describes empirical findings generated from them. The author suggests examples of additional hypotheses that can be tested. The theory can be used by practicing nurses to guide assessment and interventions with individual patients, as well as to guide quality assurance for groups of patients.

3. *Significance.* This theory has high significance. Symptom management is a central function of nurses, and managing pain is particularly important. Findings from studies testing the relationships posed in the propositions of this theory will have an immediate impact on nursing care and patients.

4. *Discrimination.* This theory is unique in that it is the only theory of pain management that focuses on the balance between analgesia and side effects. The theory has precise and clear boundaries, and the author has defined boundaries, clearly describing the phenomena that are addressed and not addressed by the theory. For example, the theory does not address acute pain management in children or management of chronic pain.

5. *Scope of theory.* The scope of this theory clearly meets the criteria for a middle range theory. It is broad enough to be applicable across a number of situations requiring acute pain management, yet narrow enough to be prescriptive for use with individual patients. It is middle range in that the propositions are abstract enough to be testable using research, but concrete enough to be directly applied in practice.

6. *Complexity.* Pain management is a complex idea. Thus, any theory that comprehensively addresses the phenomenon of pain management has the potential to be very complex and not easily understood. Dr. Good, however, has done an outstanding job of developing a parsimonious, easily understood theory. The clear descriptions of the terms, the commonly used language employed in labeling and describing the concepts, and the logical presentation of the propositions make this an easily understood theory despite the complexity of the underlying phenomenon. The use of diagrams of the propositions further reduces the complexity of the theory description.

ABOUT THE AUTHOR

Shirley M. Moore, RN, PhD, FAAN, is Edward J. & Louise Mellon Professor of Nursing and associate dean for Research at Frances Payne Bolton School of Nursing, Case Western University, Cleveland, Ohio. She has taught nursing theory and knowledge-development courses at all levels of the nursing curriculum. Dr. Moore is a nurse researcher who, as principal investigator, has had multiple projects funded by the National Institute of Nursing Research. She has authored several articles on middle range theory development, including Good, M., & Moore, S. (1996). Clinical practice guidelines as a source of middle range theory: Focus on acute pain. *Nursing Outlook,* *44*(2), 74–79.

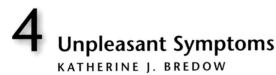

4 Unpleasant Symptoms

KATHERINE J. BREDOW

INTERNAL CRITICISM

1. *Clarity.* The descriptions of the five main components of the Theory of Unpleasant Symptoms (TOUS) are clearly stated. They are described in the text and defined in the Definition of Key Terms. Focusing on unpleasant symptoms (UPSs) as part of the lived experience, the theorists set out to design a model to explain the experience of UPSs as they occur in a dynamic clinical situation. Management techniques

also emerged as a common factor in the author's early discussions on the development of the TOUS. Consideration should be given to including management techniques as a component of the model.

2. *Consistency.* The components are consistently used throughout the explanation of the theory. Development of the components are detailed in the references to the theorists' own symptom models (dispense and fatigue) and others symptom models (SIM and the Model of Symptom Management), and have been refined, as hypothesis testing in clinical practice and research has yielded new information. In the description of the theory, there are three influencing components: physiological, psychological, and environmental factors. In the Definition of Key Terms, situational factors are the third influencing factor, of which environmental factors are a subset. Throughout the rest of this chapter, the terms are used in a congruent manner.

3. *Adequacy.* The theory explanation is succinct. The historical development of the theory was insightful and led to an understanding of the author's intent to make the symptom experience dynamic and more reflective of the real world. The theorists' goal was to construct a model to help the nurse understand all symptoms and their management. The focus of this theory is to understand the experience of UPSs. This is done by identifying antecedent factors, UPSs, and their influence on performance. It is suggested that an understanding of these components and their interrelationships will help the nurse to identify possible UPS-management interventions. Although inferred, it is not clearly stated where the management factor fits into the model. The diagram of the model is helpful in understanding the interrelationship of the factors.

4. *Logical development.* The theorists systematically set out to construct a theory to help the nurse to understand all symptoms and how to manage them. TOUS origins are founded in clinical observations, review of symptom literature, and collaboration with experts in theory development. It logically follows a line of thought of previous symptom work, expanding on it to build a theory that accounts for the antecedent factors, the dynamic experience of one or multiple symptoms, the performance, and their interrelationships. The use of established reliable and valid tools to measure some UPSs supports the logical foundation of TOUS. The examples of TOUS theory-based research helps to establish the usefulness and applicability to the nursing practice and research.

5. *Level of theory development.* TOUS fits the criteria of a middle range theory because it limits its scope and does not attempt to address all of the factors of the nursing metaparadigm. It provides a framework from which nurse researchers can generate hypothesis and research questions to better understand the dynamic experience of unpleasant symptoms.

EXTERNAL CRITICISM

1. *Reality Convergence.* TOUS presents a comprehensive, holistic, and dynamic view of the unpleasant symptom experience. The underlying assumptions of TOUS ring true. Managing the care of people experiencing UPSs is a part of the real world of nursing. Increasing insight into the reality of the unpleasant symptom experience provides direction for management of the unpleasant symptoms that the patients experience.

2. *Utility.* The theory supports the development of research questions and the study of the five components of TOUS. It has been applied to various populations experiencing UPSs and to caregivers distressed by their experience of UPSs in those they care for. Examples are given for both acute and chronic experiences of UPSs. Consideration of the research results led to a refinement of the TOUS. The interaction among components and their interrelationships with the other components were incorporated into the TOUS to make its utility even stronger.

3. *Significance.* Research conducted from hypotheses generated from the TOUS had a significant impact on the care that the nurses provided to patients. Since most clinical nurses deal in their practice with populations that experience UPSs, this theory offers a means of investigating the whole experience of health-threatening changes to patients perceived as normal functioning. It can be useful in gaining an understanding of the UPSs and management strategies.

4. *Discrimination.* The author tells the story of the development of the theory. The theorists constructed a unique theory that combined the essential components identified in earlier single-symptom models, to build a more inclusive, interactive dynamic theory for understanding the whole of UPSs. No other middle range theory addresses the multiple concepts of UPSs at the same time in one encompassing model. Because of the inclusion of situational factors, which are broad and have no clear boundaries, the TOUS is not as discriminating as it could be if it had not included this influencing factor. Moreover, the inclusion of culture and language, which have few definitive parameters, into the quality of symptoms makes the TOUS a less discriminating theory.

5. *Scope of theory.* The theory is useful for investigating one or many UPSs. The scope of the TOUS can range from simple to complex, depending on the number of UPSs and variables the investigator chooses to study. Antecedents or influencing factors have the capability of being broad and all-encompassing, and a thorough assessment of all of these factors may be difficult.

6. *Complexity.* Initially, the TOUS seems succinct, logical, and practical. However, if it is applied to a complex, chronically ill patient with multiple problems, the task of considering all of the possible influencing factors, their interrelationships, and their congruent relationship to the various UPSs quickly becomes very complex. This is not to downplay the importance of a thorough assessment, but the more unpleasant symptoms that are entered into the model, the more complex it becomes.

ABOUT THE AUTHOR

Kate Bredow, MA, RN, is a practicing school nurse, where she sees a variety of unpleasant symptoms in her patients every day. Her research experience dealt with the unpleasant symptom of sleep deprivation in the postpartum period.

---

5 Self-Efficacy
MARJORIE SIMPSON

INTERNAL CRITICISM

1. *Clarity.* Self-efficacy is a clearly defined theoretical framework, with main concepts that include efficacy and outcome expectations as the sources of self-efficacy. Theoretical clarity is supported by the well-defined constructs within the framework and their relationship to each other, with self-efficacy preceding and impacting human behavior. The constructs and concepts incorporated into the self-efficacy theoretical framework are unique to the theory, and, therefore, their meanings are less likely to be misinterpreted.

2. *Consistency.* The relationships between the constructs included in self-efficacy remain consistently defined throughout the theoretical framework. In addition, the theme of causative capabilities as a belief that generates courses of action consistently serves as the foundation for the theory. Based on this premise, the theory of self-efficacy builds on the understanding that each individual's beliefs and past experiences influence his or her behavior.

3. *Adequacy.* The self-efficacy framework adequately explains and predicts behavior. Individuals with higher levels of self-efficacy for a specific behavior are more likely to attempt that behavior. The concept of outcome expectations offers an explanation for failure of an individual to attempt or adopt a behavior. According to the theory, the belief that a behavior will produce a worthwhile outcome is necessary for an individual to execute the behavior, regardless of the level of self-efficacy. The completeness of the theory to predict behavior and explain situations when behaviors are not adopted supports the adequacy of the framework.

4. *Logical development.* The theory of self-efficacy was derived deductively from social cognitive theory, a model proposing that personal and environmental factors influence behavior. A basic assumption of this model is that individuals are human agents and have the ability to exercise control over their lives. This is congruent with other behavior change theories, and supports the logical development of the self-efficacy framework. In addition, the self-efficacy framework proceeds in a logical fashion. Efficacy and outcome expectations are always antecedents to behavior and are reinforced when a behavior is successfully executed. In addition, the theory supports that enactive attainment is a strong influence over behavior and explains why self-efficacy for one behavior can be carried over to a different but similar behavior. These conclusions are logical and have been supported by previous nursing research.

5. *Level of theory development.* The self-efficacy theoretical model has been adapted and used in nursing research for many nursing interventions. Since the theory of self-efficacy accounts for new behaviors as well as lack of behavior change, it is predictive and can be used to explain an individual's responses to an intervention in both research and clinical settings. Therefore, self-efficacy as a middle range theory has been developed to a level that allows for purposeful nursing actions.

EXTERNAL CRITICISM

1. *Reality Convergence.* An underlying assumption of the theory of self-efficacy is that most human behavior is determined by both intrinsic and extrinsic factors. Intrinsic factors include an individual's beliefs, and extrinsic factors include environmental influences that can be affected by an individual's actions. The influence of intrinsic and extrinsic factors on how people behave is reflected throughout nursing practice, and nurses frequently implement formal and informal interventions to alter these factors. For example, a rehabilitation nurse may demonstrate and instruct a patient in the use of adaptive equipment, and offer counseling or verbal persuasion to impact the patient's behavior. The actions of the nurse are altering the patient's self-efficacy for the use of adaptive equipment. In addition, addressing other physiological responses to illness, such as the unpleasant symptoms of pain and fatigue, is central to nursing and alters self-efficacy. Therefore, the theory of self-efficacy is grounded in reality and reflects the real world of nursing practice.

2. *Utility.* Core concepts that are central to the nursing profession include the interaction between the nurse, the patient, health, and the environment. This interaction often involves the nurse intervening to alter the intrinsic factors of the patient and the extrinsic environmental factors to facilitate behavior change and improve the patient's health. The self-efficacy theoretical framework is one that can generate researchable hypotheses on the interaction between these core nursing concepts and can predict the outcomes of interventions, particularly those addressing the management of chronic illnesses and health promotion. Thus, it is useful in both research and practice.

3. *Significance.* Behavior change is an element that is essential to nurses in all specialties. The theory of self-efficacy is significant to the nursing profession because it offers a framework to generate hypotheses and conduct research to test behavioral change interventions. The research results derived from the self-efficacy framework can directly impact the way nurses practice. Self-efficacy measures can be used in clinical settings to identify individuals with low self-efficacy, and nurses can then develop approaches to increase self-efficacy to promote certain behaviors.

4. *Discrimination.* The self-efficacy theory can be used to generate and test hypotheses that are unique to the diverse nursing profession. Since the framework is flexible, it can be adapted by all nursing specialties to the specific behaviors and conditions that are central in research and practice. Self-efficacy is operationalized using scales that measure strength and magnitude of self-efficacy for a specific behavior, as defined by the nurse researcher. The self-efficacy theory, therefore, is not only able to differentiate nursing from other disciplines, but is also able to distinguish and define the parameters of nursing specialties.

5. *Scope of theory.* The scope of the theory of self-efficacy is narrowly focused on the elements that influence behavior. Although the concept of behavior is comprehensive, the four sources of efficacy and outcome expectations account for all of the factors that influence behavior. Therefore, self-efficacy is a middle range theory with a framework that is practical and applicable to all behavior-focused nursing research and practice.

6. *Complexity.* The theory of self-efficacy is complex enough to account for all intrinsic and extrinsic factors that influence human behavior. However, it is parsimonious enough that the relationships between the constructs within the theory are easily understood. The theoretical framework clearly defines and explains the concepts self-efficacy and behavior, as well as the constructs that include outcome expectations and the four sources of efficacy expectations. These variables that are incorporated into the theory are precise enough that they are easily understood and extensive enough to account for all human behavior.

ABOUT THE AUTHOR

Marjorie Simpson, MS, CRNP, is a doctoral student and clinical instructor in the School of Nursing at the University of Maryland, Baltimore, Maryland. Her research for her dissertation is on self-efficacy expectations in performance of restorative-care activities for nursing assistants. She has recently coauthored an article on measurement related to her research topic: Resnick, B., & Simpson, M. (2003). Reliability and validity testing self-efficacy outcome expectations scales for performing restorative care activities. *Geriatric Nursing, 24*(2), 2–7.

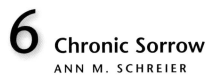 Chronic Sorrow

ANN M. SCHREIER

INTERNAL CRITICISM

1. *Clarity.* The descriptions of the key concepts of the theory are clearly described and easily understood by the reviewer. The definition of chronic sorrow identifies it as a pervasive, permanent, periodic, and potentially progressive experience. The key concepts of loss, disparity, trigger events, and management methods are clearly defined, as well as the proposed relationship between these concepts. The theory is useful in understanding and anticipating various individuals' reactions to trigger events, such as the anniversary of a cancer diagnosis.

2. *Consistency.* The author consistently maintains the definitions of the key terms of loss experience, disparity, trigger events, and management methods. These key terms are congruent with the described research studies.

3. *Adequacy.* This theory explains what chronic sorrow is, as well as some of the common loss experiences that lead to chronic sorrow. However, it does not address why some individuals who have a loss experience do not experience chronic sorrow. In the example of bereaved individuals, 97% of the bereaved had symptoms of chronic sorrow (Eakes, Burke, & Hainsworth, 1999). Given that few of the subjects did not experience the symptoms labeled as chronic sorrow, the theory does address the experience of loss adequately. Future studies could examine whether there are predictors of those who will not experience chronic sorrow. Do individuals who do not experience chronic sorrow have different personality characteristics, or receive different health care interventions at the time of the loss? Another area that is open to future research is the identification of other conditions that commonly lead to chronic sorrow.

4. *Logical development.* The theoretical model of chronic sorrow is logically developed from the 10 qualitative studies conducted by the Consortium for Research on Chronic Sorrow. Because of the excellent base of qualitative studies, the theory aids in the understanding of the loss experience. With this research, the authors are able to draw conclusions and make arguments that are well supported by clinical and research data.

5. *Level of theory development.* The theory is appropriate to a middle range theory because it has a scope that is limited to the explanation of a single phenomena, that of response to loss.

EXTERNAL CRITICISM

1. *Reality convergence.* In clinical work with oncology patients, the theory makes sense of the reactions that nurses see, for example, in patients with a recurrence of the diagnosis of cancer, or to the stress patients experience when awaiting results from routine diagnostic tests during the remission period.

2. *Utility and discrimination.* Researchers could generate hypotheses based on the theoretical model. For instance, an appropriate hypothesis might be that parents of diabetic children, who participate in a six-week support group, will demonstrate less discomfort from chronic sorrow than parents who do not participate in a support group. In addition, the author's work on an assessment instrument and its inclusion in this book clearly enhance the utility of the theory for both research and clinical practice. The theory of chronic sorrow is unique and specifically addresses grieving needs and the experience of loss.

3. *Significance.* This theoretical model lends itself to research on effectiveness of interventions for both caregivers and patients. In addition, the model can be used to determine what conditions are more likely to trigger an exacerbation of chronic sorrow and begin a chronic sorrow experience. With this knowledge, nurses will be able to anticipate needs and respond to these needs in an effective manner.

4. *Scope of theory.* The concepts and hypothesized relationships can easily be applied in clinical settings, and the score is narrow enough to fit the expectations of a middle range theory.

5. *Complexity.* The major concepts include loss experience, disparity, trigger events, chronic sorrow, and management methods. The conceptualization of the model is easily displayed in Figure 6.1 (theoretical model of chronic sorrow). Since the model is logical and cyclical, this figure enhances the reader's understanding of the relationship between the variables. The model clearly delineates the subconcepts of internal versus external management, ineffective versus effective management, and discomfort versus increased comfort, as well as where appropriate intervention by nurses and other health care providers can occur. There are a limited number of variables, and the number appears to be sufficient to explain the phenomena. The description accompanying the theory is succinct and readily understood.

REFERENCE

Eakes, G. G., Burke, M. L., & Hainsworth, M. A. (1999). Chronic sorrow: The lived experience of bereaved individuals. *Illness, Crisis, and Loss, 7*(1), 172–182.

ABOUT THE AUTHOR

Ann M. Schreier, RN, PhD, is an assistant professor of nursing in the Department of Adult Health, East Carolina University, Greenville, North Carolina. She has served as a consultant and clinical director at the Hospice Society in Bethesda, Maryland. She has received external funding to conduct nursing research in the areas of self-care and chronicity. She also has several research-related publications in the areas of self-care, pain control, and patient education.

7 Social Support
JOANN P. WESSMAN

Dr. Schaffer presents several social support theories in her chapter. The present critique is focused on the body of middle range social support theories that she presents. Therefore, some criteria for the critique have been modified.

INTERNAL CRITICISM

The present critique will focus on clarity, consistency, adequacy, and level of theory development. The issue of logical development will not be considered inasmuch as this criterion is specific to one particular theory.

1. *Clarity.* The lack of a clear definition of social support is cited and evident throughout the chapter. Specifically, definitions lack the clarity to differentiate if social support encompasses interactions where (a) negative consequences occur for the provider or recipient, or (b) support providers are in "formal" categories such as professionals. It is unclear from the chapter discussion if social support can be considered to have occurred when it is not the intention of the provider to be helpful, but, indeed, support inadvertently is given. The author gives clear examples that differentiate meaning among emotional, information, instrumental, and appraisal kinds of support. But the uses of the subconcepts structure and function are not so clear.

2. *Consistency.* The lack of consistent use of the construct social support is identified in this chapter. When definitions vary widely, as they do, interpretations, principles, and methods will likewise lack consistency. The section on "Clinical Applications," particularly the use of social support as nursing intervention, highlights the diversity in conceptualizations of social support.

3. *Adequacy.* How adequate is the body of theories reviewed? Certainly, the lack of definitional clarity and inconsistent use of definitional qualities diminishes adequacy. Yet, given these limitations, the robust nature of the concept, social support, is evident throughout the discussion. Of course, some definitional areas are ambiguous and inconsistent. However, the collection of theories reviewed does permit the nursing community to enter into meaningful dialog about the nature of social support. In this sense, the body of current theories possesses at least a degree of adequacy—meaningful conversations are evoked.

4. *Level of theory development.* It is interesting to note that among the theories of social support are the elements of factor-isolating, explanatory, predictive, and prescriptive levels. Each theory cited attempts definition of the concept. Identification of variables related to social support, such as perceptions, timing, motivation, duration, direction, life stage, and source, offers a sense of factor-relating level of theory (explanation). The variability among instances of social support can be explained, at least to some degree, by these variables. We get a sense of explanation as to why not all instances of social support look identical, and relationships within the construct social support begin to emerge. Some social support theorists such as Norbeck clearly are mapping out relationships that can predict the outcomes of nursing interventions aimed at enhancing social support. Clinical situations where social support interventions should be prescribed in a defined manner (predictive and prescriptive theory) are being identified.

EXTERNAL CRITICISM

Each of the six specific criteria of external criticism will be approached from the view of the body of several social support theories available to the nurse in practice and research applications. At times, specific social support theories will be isolated.

1. *Reality convergence.* Several of the social support theories converge well with "real world" nursing experiences. Chronically ill clients thrive when surrounded by supportive families and communities. Nursing's systems succeed when embedded in nurturing broader societal structures.

    The idea inherent in the buffer theory that social support modulates life stressors is one threaded throughout nursing literature. Design of care structures and referrals to the type of caregiving facilities is shaped, in part, by the social supports available to the client to modulate stressors.

    Norbeck's model for using social support as intervention to improve health outcomes "rings true" with common nursing practices. Nurses routinely include family in client education programs because they expect family members to reinforce learning. Nurses often suggest support groups for clients experiencing complex, intense, and/or prolonged health challenges, believing that the group will be a source of healing and growth.

    Many other examples could be given. Social support theories have a high degree of reality convergence with lived nursing experiences.

2. *Utility.* How useful are present social support theories when applied in practice and research? Dr. Schaffer offers several specific examples to support the utility of social support theories for nursing. Table 7.2 offers specific clinical applications of social support theories that, in shaping meaningful interventions, reduce client stress and promote effective client coping. Examples are offered on individual, dyadic, group, community, and systems levels. Clearly, social support theories are useful in a variety of clinical situations.

The examples of social support instruments described in Table 7.3 demonstrate the ability to operationalize social support theories in a way useful for research. The availability of specific instruments to measure social support in a valid and reliable manner is both useful and crucial to the researcher conducting quantitative studies. Schaffer and Lia-Hoagberg's study of the effects of social support on prenatal care and health behaviors of low-income women demonstrates the usefulness of present social support theories in guiding research. Present social support theories clearly are "birthing" useful instruments and studies.

3. *Significance.* Dr. Schaffer supports well her strong assertion that middle range social support theories are of significance to nursing. Social support influences health status, health behavior, use of health services, and health outcomes. Current social support theories help to explain this influence in a manner that permits meaningful intervention. The theories offer a way to apply the nursing process in the arena of interpersonal relationships of the client with supportive "others." Theories place the client within a relevant social context. Social support theories reflect the tradition within nursing to view the individual or family as an integral part of a rich fabric of relationships that define and reflect health.

4. *Discrimination.* The lack of definitional clarity and inconsistent use of the term *social support* among various theories adversely reflects on these theories' ability to discriminate social support from other related concepts. Perhaps this is the greatest limitation of the body of theories taken as a whole. (Individually, each social support theory may discriminate at a commendable level.)

Norbeck's work reflects a strong attempt to develop social support theory in a manner that is unique to nursing. But many of the theorists are not nurses, and do not aim to develop the construct in a manner that discriminates nursing applications from those of other disciplines. This lack of discrimination is also a limitation of many social support theories.

5. *Scope of theory.* The social support theories discussed by Dr. Schaffer clearly are of appropriately circumscribed scope to be considered middle range theories. Their application to practice situations is direct because of this limited scope. Yet the theories are broad enough to encompass a specific type of interpersonal relationships at several levels from the individual to a given society.

6. *Complexity.* The complexity varies among the present social support theories. Some develop a limited number of variables and some, an extensive array. Dr. Schaffer notes that Brown's theory of social support develops one broad factor; in contrast, the model of Barerra is multidimensional. The lack of definitional consensus among social support theories creates an artificial complexity that functions in a negative manner.

SUMMARY

The present body of social support theories lacks a clear definition of the phenomenon. Like clarity, the criterion of consistency is not met. Even with these limitations, there is a sense in which the theories are adequately serving nursing to influence practice and research. Among the theories are elements of factor-isolating, explanatory, predictive, and prescriptive levels of theory development.

Looking at the criteria for external criticism, a positive picture is seen. There is strong reality convergence with the "real world" of nursing. The theories are proving to be useful both to practice and to research. Significance seems evident when looking at social support theories from the perspective of health status, health behaviors, use of health services, and health outcomes. Scope of theories seems clearly to be midrange. Only discrimination is a criterion unmet, and complexity, a criterion difficult to assess.

RELEVANT WORKS

Norbeck, J. S. (1981). Social support: A model for clinical research and application. *Advances in Nursing Science,* *3*(4), 43–59.

Schaffer, M. A., & Lia-Hoagberg, B. (1997). Effects of social support on prenatal care and health behaviours of low-income women. *Journal of Obstetric, Gynecologic, and Neonatal Nursing, 26*(4), 433–440.

ABOUT THE AUTHOR

Joann P. Wessman, RN, PhD, is a professor at Bethel University, St. Paul, Minnesota. She teaches nursing theory development and analysis at the graduate level. She has served as dissertation or thesis advisor to doctoral and master's students using middle range theory. Her recent research is in faith/health integration in church-affiliated frail elderly.

8 Caring

CECELIA I. ROSCIGNO

INTERNAL CRITICISM

1. *Clarity.* In Swanson's Theory of Caring, the structural components of the theory and the descriptions of their relations are made straightforward and easy to comprehend. In her theory, Swanson clarifies that the environment resembles an ecological model with nested levels both within and outside the individual and explains how these environments interact with each other in both directions. This conceptualization clarifies that the client and the environment may be one in the same in some nursing practice settings.

2. *Consistency.* The structural components described, the definitions of those components, and the descriptions of their relations are clearly and consistently used throughout Swanson's publications on her theoretical work.

3. *Adequacy.* This theory presents a comprehensive and yet prescriptive approach to the nursing process that is consistent with nursing's values and mission. The theory addresses the parts of the process in relation to seeing the whole person in the context of his or her environments. The theory provides the discrete steps that lead to the whole process. Despite the comprehensive nature of the theory, the clear description of the necessary structural components makes it understandable and applicable.

4. *Logical development.* The Theory of Caring clearly describes the historical evolution of caring as a human attribute and describes how a caring interactional process between the nurse and his or her client(s) are particularly relevant to the nursing discipline or any discipline within health care. This is because all health care fields have at their core the altruistic values of service to society and promotion of health, which makes it necessary to take client's existential and sociocultural contexts into consideration. The theoretical model incorporated previous knowledge and yet, was also contrasted to extant descriptions of nursing's helping and caring role. The final conceptualization was later empirically tested by the theorist in her own research and further explicated in her publications. For example, in a more recent publication, Swanson explains how her process of caring can be used to create healing environments that consider the whole person. The theorist's theoretical model is well supported by literature and the conclusions remain logical, consistent, and supported by some empirical evidence.

5. *Level of theory development.* The theory as currently conceptualized would be a middle range nursing theory that could be considered prescriptive. The theory has been used by the theorist and others to develop and test intervention programs. Further investigation is required to determine if the interventions provide more than increased client satisfaction but actually influence overall health and well-being.

EXTERNAL CRITICISM

1. *Reality convergence.* The Theory of Caring is clearly reality based beyond the discipline of nursing. It addresses the dimensions of human interaction that demonstrate a caring attitude. In fact, when developing and refining the theory, Swanson went beyond nursing—or any professional-based literature—using a literary meta-analysis to refine and explain the structural components of the theory and how they related. This gave the theory both clinical and social authenticity and makes it applicable to broader human interactions of any kind meant to be caring. In dissertation research, both children and parents describe the interactions they encountered following the child's traumatic brain injury, and across subjects, their descriptions of caring converge with the structures and meanings that Swanson described in her theory.

2. *Utility.* Since the structural components and their relationships are clearly explained, this theory can be used by nurses to generate testable questions or hypotheses, both at the bedside and for research generation. The theorist, herself, created a randomized controlled intervention program for couples following miscarriage. Other junior investigators have recently used it to guide their early programs of research inquiry and to develop preliminary intervention programs. The theory is also being instituted clinically in several health care settings, to guide health care interactions and intervention programs. More research is needed to validate whether guidance by this theory improves health care practitioner interactions or whether intervention programs guided by this theory improve clients' health-related outcomes or a more holistic sense of their own well-being. This latter outcome can be more difficult to capture in research. In practice, the theorist, herself, noted some limitations of capturing this caring process, especially with practitioners of various levels of expertise. She noted that novice nurses might be so focused on new tasks that they might miss the wholeness of the caring process described in Swanson's theory. She also noted that more experienced nurses may embed their caring processes in such an elaborate set of advanced skills that acknowledgment of the process could potentially be overlooked in an investigation.

3. *Significance.* Swanson's theory is both relevant and has tremendous significance to both the science and practice of nursing. This theory ties the key disciplinary values into the principles for framing what are ideal nursing research phenomena and what may guide improved professional interactions with clients. From a research perspective, this theory recognizes and incorporates that nursing is a human science that sees humans as wholes and advocates for understanding each person's health in terms of this whole. This theory also recognizes that both nursing practice and nursing research strive to understand the unique life existence of each person in order to appreciate the unique meanings the person may attach to his or her nurse–client interactions, social–environmental interactions, and ultimately definitions of health and well-being. From a practice perspective, this theory points out that nurses need to clearly recognize how their interactions can influence the ecological environments, health, and overall well-being of the clients they serve in their practice and vice versa.

4. *Discrimination.* This theory is not the only theory of caring in nursing. Since caring is a universal concept to humans, the theory does not have precise and clear boundaries. In addition, caring is a concept that is not unique to the profession of nursing alone. Other health care professions also have an altruistic and caring charge to their values. Thus, this theory has begun to be adopted in a variety of health care settings and across health care disciplines. Its appeal to the caring nature of all human interactions makes this theory have even broader societal implications, but does not limit its significance to the nursing profession.

5. *Scope.* The scope of this theory clearly meets the criteria for a middle range theory. It is broad enough to be applicable across a number of situations requiring caring interactions both professionally and nonprofessionally. However, the detail with which Swanson describes the processes of informed caring makes it prescriptive enough for application to individual situations, even to laypersons. The structural components of this theory are abstract enough to be testable, but are also concrete enough to be applicable to the clinical practice setting.

6. *Complexity.* Caring in the context of human interactions can be a complex and abstract idea, which could easily be difficult to understand. However, Dr. Swanson has presented comprehensible descriptions of the structural components and a logical presentation of how these components interrelate to each other. She makes it clear that with each client, the nurse must learn his or her uniqueness and use that to apply the nursing process. Swanson also uses a diagram to aid in illuminating this model.

> **ABOUT THE AUTHOR**
>
> **Cecelia I. Roscigno, MN, PhC, RN, CNRN**, is a predoctoral research fellow and doctoral student at the University of Washington, Seattle, Washington. She is currently conducting a research study to learn children's perspectives of their life following a traumatic brain injury.

9 Interpersonal Relations

SONJA J. MEIERS

KATHLEEN SHERAN

INTERNAL CRITICISM

1. *Clarity.* This theory is rather complex when all aspects are considered. The major concepts are clearly defined and readily understandable, but numerous. The major concepts are nurse–patient relationship, phases of the nurse–patient relationship, roles of the nurse, psychobiological experiences, and psychological tasks. All concepts are generally at a high level of abstraction. The role and importance of the nurse's self-understanding in the therapeutic relationship is clearly outlined.

2. *Consistency.* The theory is consistent and congruent in defining concepts throughout the original work. The focus on the nurse–patient relationship as central to practice and the concept of how the nurse intervenes are consistent with a theory based on interpersonal relations. Phases of the nurse–patient relationship, as originally defined, have been subsequently altered. This alteration has been from the defined phases of orientation, identification, exploitation, and termination, to the orientation, working, and resolution phases, with identification and exploitation now considered subphases of the working phase. Concepts of anxiety, tension, unmet needs, frustration, and conflict are consistently presented as targets for the counseling role of the nurse. The worldview is phenomenological in nature and reinforced throughout the theory.

3. *Adequacy.* The theory is adequate in its ability to transfer to settings that allow the nurse time and opportunity to interact with the patient. Since the major foundations of the theory are deducted from disciplines other than nursing, the uniqueness is not found in the body of knowledge but, rather, in the therapeutic role of the nurse in interaction with the patient. Current weaknesses are its emphasis on the individual patient to the exclusion of family and community, the absence of pathophysiology, and a narrow set of cultural assumptions surrounding interpersonal interaction.

4. *Logical development.* Both inductive and deductive methods are used in development of the theory. The works of Freud, Havighurst, Sullivan, Maslow, and Rogers formed the deductive integration base for the hypothesis statements. In addition, and most beneficial to nursing, Peplau's inductive approach is a well-formulated theory development process, where observation of nursing practice with patients has resulted in identification of concepts of interest. Theoretical relationships between concepts are clearly presented in the statements of assumptions throughout the historical development of the theory. Within the theory, the role of the nurse is to facilitate the individual in his or her movement through the steps of the nursing process.

5. *Level of theory development.* This middle range theory is at the descriptive level. Classification of the phases of interpersonal relations between the nurse and patient is its focus. Specifically, interactional phenomena and intrapersonal and interpersonal phenomena of nursing situations and psychosocial phenomena are described.

EXTERNAL CRITICISM

1. *Reality convergence.* The basic underlying assumptions ring true and represent the real world of nursing, particularly in the specialty of psychiatric nursing. Definitions of major tradition domains of nurse, patient, health, and environment are similar to those used in practice. Elements of developmental psychology, humanistic psychology, and learning theory used in the theory are widely accepted premises within the discipline of nursing. The influence of Freud regarding the unconscious motivation of the patient as important to the nurse's role of assisting patients with management of anxiety is evident. These deductions from Freud, Sullivan, and others as they pertain to the nurse–patient interpersonal process are generally accepted, but may not be commonly understood or applied by the nurse generalist. The behaviorist perspective does provide an alternative and popular view of therapist–patient relationships.

2. *Pragmatic.* The theory can be operationalized in nursing practice settings that value the primacy of the interpersonal process intended to be therapeutic. It is most helpful for viewing and understanding the patient's psychobiological needs and provides a method for assessing and intervening with these issues. The theory is applicable as a framework to teach the essential elements of therapeutic communication in nursing education.

3. *Utility.* This theory has not yet generated large numbers of research studies, though it meets the criteria of empirical adequacy for a middle range theory. Research that has been completed focuses on factors that influence the development of the nurse–patient relationship. Since many of the practice aspects of the theory have been inductively derived, instrument development has been limited. Therefore, measurement of variables within the theory has not been broadly achieved. Further demonstration of the link between the nurse–patient relationship, symptom relief, and the ultimate well-being of patients is needed.

4. *Significance.* The theory meets the criterion of significance for the discipline. The theory has been published, unchanged, since 1952 and continues to be useful, specifically in contemporary mental health nursing. Other nurse scientists have expanded the use in areas such as therapeutic milieu, crisis, and family theory. The frequency of reference to the importance of and phases of the nurse–patient relationship in nursing textbooks and empirical studies attests to its continued utility.

5. *Discrimination.* Although the theorist is clear in distinctions between professional nursing practice and medicine in original works, there is not clear distinction between the important content of the nurse–patient relationship and the physician–patient relationship. The basic theory is easily applicable to a variety of helping professions and, though contributing its focus on the interaction to disciplinary development in nursing, is not limited uniquely to nursing.

6. *Scope of theory.* The theory is broad and can be applied in many practice domains, especially those nursing roles that assist the patient with interpersonal or intrapersonal difficulty. It does not provide concepts about pathophysiological or biological phenomena.

7. *Complexity.* The theory has breadth, life, and fluidity. The core of the theory is parsimonious (the relationship between the nurse and the patient). However, the theory describes several important related concepts that explain how to understand the nurse–patient interaction, creating complexity. If these concepts are considered part of the Theory of Interpersonal Relations, it meets the criterion for complexity. Application of the theory requires that the nurse be able to be both inductive and deductive when reasoning.

ABOUT THE AUTHORS

Sonja J. Meiers, PhD, MS, RN, is an associate professor and director of the Graduate Program at Minnesota State University, Mankato. Theory development is one of her areas of research interest.
Kathleen Sheran, MS, RN, CNS, is an assistant professor at Minnesota State University, Mankato. Her education, practice, and teaching background is in psychiatric–mental health nursing, all of which have made use of Peplau's Theory of Interpersonal Relations.

10 Attachment
SANDRA J. PETERSON

INTERNAL CRITICISM

1. *Clarity.* The main constructs of attachment theory are presented as attachment, internal working models, and patterns of attachment. These are clearly defined and further described with subtypes. What remains somewhat unclear is the nature of the relationship between caregiver and child as it relates to the development of specific patterns of attachment. The specific behaviors of the primary caregiver that elicit a healthy attachment experience care appear vague.

2. *Consistency.* Consistency exists in the description and use of the theory as long as the focus is on caregiver–child relationships. When applied to other relationships, clarity is compromised.

3. *Adequacy.* Though the origins of the theory can be traced to the mother–child relationship and most of the work with the theory explored this relationship, more recently, as evidenced by examples from the professional literature described in the chapter, the theory has been applied to individuals across the lifespan. In addition, the theory has been used to consider relationships other than the mother–child, for instance, counselor–client and husband–wife. There is certainly potential for further theory development with an expanded focus of attachment throughout the lifespan and in caring relationships other than mother–child.

4. *Logical development.* The theory was derived from the work of Freud, especially as it relates to his consideration of object relations and secondary drive. The integration of medicine, ethology, learning theories, developmental biology, and psychology, though credited as contributing to the development of the theory, is less obvious. Animal behavior was used as a means of confirming theory precepts. Further refinement of the theory occurred as a result of the work of Ainsworth, who through her research contributed the description of five patterns of attachment. The later work on the theory proceeded logically from the original work.

5. *Level of theory development.* The theory as described does not provide propositional statements, so it is difficult to identify the theory as more than factor isolating (descriptive). There are implied elements of the theory that suggest that it could be labeled as factor relating (descriptive—explanatory). The nature of the mother–child relationship is seen as determining the degree to which the child experiences healthy attachment.

EXTERNAL CRITICISM

1. *Reality convergence.* Attachment is an obvious human need. As noted in the chapter, though not clearly related to Maslow's hierarchy of needs, attachment may be implied a basic need. Attachment could be considered an aspect and integration of the human needs for safety and security and love and belonging.

2. *Utility.* Though the propositional statements of attachment theory are not delineated, the body of research seems to indicate that the theory can generate testable hypotheses. The Care Index is one means of measuring the parent–child interaction that has been developed for and used to explore the caring or comfort behaviors of mothers and the responses of their children.

3. *Significance.* The theory of attachment would be of most use to nurses involved with young families, particularly as it relates to parent education and early detection and intervention with children in stressful environments. In addition, there appears to be growing interest in application of the theory with individuals of all ages and in the context of the counseling relationship. The theory is being used to better understand the centrality of human relationships as an element essential for health throughout the lifespan.

This critique of the theory of attachment is based on the description provided by Dr. Klett in Chapter 10.

4. *Discrimination.* As a borrowed theory, it will not generate hypotheses unique to nursing. As noted by Bowlby who originally proposed the theory, attachment is derived from multiple disciplines. See comments included in "Internal Criticism," under "Logical development." Other theories that consider interpersonal relationships, for instance, Peplau's theory, might generate similar hypotheses, particularly if applied to attachment in the counseling relationship. The difference is the degree of focus on this element of human relationships.

5. *Scope of theory.* Attachment theory can be legitimately considered a theory in the middle range. The number of concepts is limited but not overly specific, providing parameters for understanding a phenomenon of interest to nursing but not of the discipline in its totality. Because attachment is considered a basic human need, it can be applied to the person domain of nursing's metaparadigm.

6. *Complexity.* Though the number of concepts included in the theory is not excessive, the nature of the mother–child relationship and the effect of that relationship on the developing child are inherently complex. The factors that influence attachment are multidimensional; there are both individual care and socially contributing factors, adding to the complexity of the theory.

ABOUT THE AUTHOR

Sandra J. Peterson, RN, PhD, is past chair of nursing and professor emerita, Bethel University. Her clinical background is in psychiatric-mental health nursing. As a nurse educator, for over 30 years, she has taught nursing theory courses to both undergraduate and graduate students.

---

11 Modeling and Role-Modeling
MARTHA SOFIO

INTERNAL CRITICISM

1. *Clarity.* The theory is easy to understand. The language is simple and the concepts are clearly defined and used with consistency throughout the theory. The coined concept of affiliated individuation is one that does not immediately generate semantic clarity for the reader; however, it is clearly defined in this framework. It calls for further validation and concept analysis. The concept of self-care has a meaning in this framework that varies greatly from its general use, or use in other nursing theories. The concept of self-care knowledge as a subconscious component of person requires validation.

2. *Consistency.* Concepts remain consistently defined throughout the theoretical content. The concept of adaptation as an equilibrium level on a continuum of health and illness is consistent with the interpretation of person as a system adjusting in response to environmental stimuli. Stress is consistently presented as response to a stressor, and adaptation as a holistic response to experienced stressors. Other conceptual definitions of nurturance, object attachment, unconditional acceptance, self-care, holism, and health remain constant throughout the theory. The worldview is that of holistic human experience as related to mind–body interaction; however, it is not proposed to the extent of person/environment unity. The conceptualization of holism is addressed with consistency in reference to both client and nurse.

3. *Adequacy.* This theory is adequate in that its concepts and principles transfer readily into a variety of practice settings. The authors do not specify clinical situations for the use of this theory, and it is readily applicable to the care of individuals in almost all clinical settings. It is challenging, however, to extrapolate it to situations of family assessment and intervention. Because of the major use of theories from other disciplines, its exclusive differentiation for nursing is questionable.

4. *Logical development.* The theory evidences logical development. Deductively using different external theoretical bases in the description of person, the author systematically presents theoretical

relationships. Initially, theories are presented supporting how people are alike, followed by theoretical support for how people are different. These theoretical bases are then described in relationships called "linkages," which offer rich ground for hypothetical deductive research and development of nursing interventions. The theoretical bases and linkages are synthesized to aid in developing a conceptualization of the client's world, the process of which is called modeling. The nursing process is explicated through the use of role-modeling the developed model of the client's world. Specific interventions are subsumed under five generalized aims, all oriented to fulfilling the purpose of the model. All logical steps of the nursing process are intact.

5. *Level of theory development.* This theory is at the explanatory level. It provides clarity as to how to develop a model of the client's world and proposes that use of that unique model in the role-modeling process will facilitate the client's adaptation. It is in this sense that role-modeling or nurturance provides the basis for predictive and prescriptive nursing theory development.

EXTERNAL CRITICISM

1. *Reality convergence.* The basic premises of the theory easily converge with reality. The principles of growth and development, basic human needs, and adaptation to change and loss are commonly understood and generally accepted. The theory purports to be holistic, and the understanding of mind–body–spirit interaction is widely accepted within the discipline. The conceptualization of mutual goal planning is congruent with the values system of today's practitioners. The conceptualization of self-care knowledge, however, where the client knows what made him ill and what will make him better, might offer some difficulty in this regard.

2. *Utility.* The theory fulfills the criterion of utility. It readily gives the practicing nurse a framework with which to view the client, and from which to facilitate the client's plans for care. Detailed processes for collecting, aggregating, analyzing, and synthesizing data are provided. The theory easily lends itself to curricular development and student education. Adaptive potential, self-care, affiliated individuation, role-modeling, and multiple other conceptualizations offer important subject matter for the execution of nursing research.

3. *Significance.* The theory addresses essential issues in nursing, namely those of client assessment and intervention. Its most significant foci are those of mind–body interaction and mutual goal planning, which compel the nurse to respectively envision the client holistically and to empower him or her. The theory proposes multiple content areas supportive of research in the development of the discipline's body of knowledge.

4. *Discrimination.* A major limitation of the theory is its lack of capacity to discriminate nursing from other health professions and its interventions from other care-tending acts. It would be possible for a physician, psychologist, or social worker to implement this theory. The boundaries are open, and the extant acts and practices can flow inside or outside the discipline.

5. *Scope.* The theory is broad in scope and can be used in diverse practice domains.

6. *Complexity.* The theory is not parsimonious. It is complex and composed of multiple descriptive and explanatory components. The subject matter is rich and presented in great depth. The concept of person is dominant and the interrelationship of theoretical variables is numerous.

ABOUT THE AUTHOR

Martha Sofio, MS, RN, assistant professor at Metropolitan State University, St. Paul, Minnesota, is a certified nurse practitioner and certified hypnotherapist who studied with Helen Erickson. She teaches in both the graduate and the undergraduate nursing programs at Metropolitan State University. Modeling and Role-Modeling is the theoretical foundation of its undergraduate curriculum.

12 Comfort

LINDA WILSON

INTERNAL CRITICISM

1. *Clarity.* The criterion of clarity is evaluated by how clearly the theory is presented and how easily it is understood by the reader (Barnum, 1990). Comfort Theory is clearly presented in the literature and can be easily read and understood by any reader. Through her program of research and numerous publications, Dr. Kolcaba clearly presents the development and evolution of the Comfort Theory.

2. *Consistency.* The criterion of consistency is evaluated by examining the definitions and repeated use of the terms of a theory (Barnum, 1990). Comfort Theory has several key concepts that are defined throughout the literature. In every publication, these key concepts are clearly and uniformly defined.

3. *Adequacy.* The criterion of adequacy is evaluated by how the theory accounts for the specialty to which it applies (Barnum, 1990). Comfort Theory can be applied to all populations. The three senses of comfort (ease, relief, and transcendence) and the contexts in which they occur (physical, social, psychospiritual, and environmental) account for comfort care with any patient.

4. *Logical development.* The criterion of logical development prescribes that the reasoning and conclusions of a theory be clearly presented (Barnum, 1990). Throughout the literature, the ongoing development of Comfort Theory is clearly presented in a reasonable and valid manner. In each of her publications, Dr. Kolcaba presents the theory and the logical reasoning that supports its evolution.

5. *Level of theory development.* To assess the level of theory development, the researcher needs to evaluate the research that has been completed using the theory (Barnum, 1990). At the time of this author's dissertation research (1998–2000), comfort and Comfort Theory had been clearly defined in the literature; therefore, studies testing explanatory theory using a correlational design were in order. Since that time, Dr. Kolcaba has published the development of the middle range Theory of Comfort. Comfort Theory meets the description of a middle range theory because it consists of several well-defined concepts and can be viewed as both general and complex (Fawcett & Downs, 1992).

EXTERNAL CRITICISM

1. *Reality convergence.* The criterion of reality convergence can be evaluated by examining the principles, interpretations, and method of a theory (Barnum, 1990). Both the concept of comfort and the Comfort Theory have practical application to many populations. The essential principles and assumptions of Comfort Theory are clearly defined in the literature by Dr. Kolcaba and can easily be applied to any patient population. The logical development and presentation of the theory allows for easy interpretation and application of the theory in nursing research. Dr. Kolcaba's perception of the nursing world presents the patient and family who are cared for holistically.

2. *Utility.* The criterion of utility refers to the usefulness of the theory by nursing in any practice setting (Barnum, 1990). Comfort Theory can be applied to patients of all ages and in any practice setting. During dissertation research, this author was able to easily apply Comfort Theory to the population of hospitalized medical patients.

3. *Significance.* The criterion of significance is met if the theory contributes to the further development of nursing knowledge, and if it addresses essential nursing issues (Barnum, 1990). Comforting patients is a fundamental part of nursing care because comfort is a desired and expected patient outcome. Comfort

Theory provides the basis for comfort care by presenting the three senses (ease, relief, and transcendence) and contexts (physical, social, psychospiritual, and environmental) in which the outcome of comfort occurs.

4. *Discrimination.* The criterion of discrimination is evaluated by the ability of the theory to differentiate nursing from other health professions and other caring acts (Barnum, 1990). Nurses care for patients holistically and in four contexts of human experience (physical, social, psychospiritual, and environmental) from which the outcome of comfort occurs.

5. *Scope of theory.* The criterion of scope of theory evaluates if the theory is broad or limited in scope (Barnum, 1990). The Theory of Comfort is broad in scope because it can be applied to patients of all ages and in various practice settings.

6. *Complexity.* The criterion of complexity allows the researcher the opportunity for explanation and interrelationship of multiple variables (Barnum, 1990). Comfort Theory allows the researcher the opportunity to examine comfort through the three senses of comfort (ease, relief, and transcendence) and the four contexts (physical, social, psychospiritual, and environmental) in which the outcome of comfort occurs. Any or all of these variables can be measured at one time. In addition, Comfort Theory posits relationships between nursing interventions, patient comfort, health-seeking behaviors, and institutional integrity. Any or all of these relationships can be tested through nursing research.

REFERENCES

Barnum, B. J. (1990). *Nursing theory: Analysis, application, evaluation.* Glenview, IL: Scott Foresman/Little, Brown.

Fawcett, J., & Downs, F. S. (1992). *The relationship of theory and research* (2nd ed.). Philadelphia, PA: Davis.

ABOUT THE AUTHOR

Linda Wilson, RN, PhD, CPAN, CAPA, BC, is an education specialist for Nursing Continuing Education and Perianesthesia at Thomas Jefferson University Hospital in Philadelphia. Dr. Wilson used the Comfort Theory during her dissertation research, while studying adult hospitalized medical patients.

---

13 Health-Related Quality of Life

LYNNE PLOETZ

INTERNAL CRITICISM

1. *Clarity.* The detailed description of Wilson and Cleary's model of health-related quality of life (HRQOL) allows the reader to develop a clear understanding of the components and concepts involved in the theory. With a focus on patient outcomes, the authors (both physicians) indicate that health measures exist on a continuum of increasing complexity. They spell out five domains: biophysiological factors, symptoms, functioning, general health perceptions, and overall quality of life. They explain the health concepts involved in each level and relate these to general health perceptions and overall quality of life. In addition, they discuss the role of patient preferences and the emotional or psychological factors involved in HRQOL (Wilson & Cleary, 1995).

2. *Consistency.* The terminology used by Wilson and Cleary (1995) in explaining and discussing HRQOL is consistent throughout their paper. Since they are medical doctors, their terminology is congruent with nursing terminology and can readily be understood by nurses.

3. *Adequacy.* The questions asked by HRQOL are highly relevant to nursing research and practice, and exist on both individual and global scales. Using Wilson and Cleary's model, HRQOL thoroughly addresses the issues relevant to one's health perceptions and quality of life.

4. *Logical development.* Wilson and Cleary (1995) provide a well-researched argument that proceeds logically from their initial discussion on the role of HRQOL in research outcomes and how this can be used to improve patient outcomes. They identify the lack of a conceptual model of how different types or levels of patient outcomes relate to each other and to overall HRQOL, and propose a model that considers five main factors and their relationship to each other in determining overall HRQOL. The systems-type model flows logically from the description of these factors to define causal relationships between the factors.

5. *Level of theory development.* HRQOL is sufficiently defined and narrow to be considered an explanatory middle range theory. The practical nature of the theory allows the researcher to develop testable hypotheses regarding HRQOL in different patient populations.

EXTERNAL CRITICISM

1. *Reality convergence.* The HRQOL theory immediately "makes sense" to the nurse. This theory provides a framework for better understanding the relationship of illness and nursing interventions to patients' quality of life.

2. *Utility.* The HRQOL model is useful for nurses in both research and practice. Nurses in any discipline can identify hypotheses that can be tested by using the HRQOL model.

3. *Significance.* HRQOL is highly significant to nursing research and practice. As patients live longer with chronic illness because of improved diagnostics and therapeutics, research into nursing interventions that improve HRQOL becomes even more significant.

4. *Discrimination.* Since HRQOL is a multidisciplinary concept, boundaries could extend beyond nursing practice. When HRQOL is used as a framework for nursing research, care must be taken to provide clear boundaries regarding nursing interventions.

5. *Scope.* This model is sufficiently narrow in scope that research can focus on individuals as well as groups. However, studies could be designed that allow a broader scope, if desired.

6. *Complexity.* The HRQOL model by Wilson and Cleary is quite complex, with five determinants, each having multiple variables. However, the model allows the researcher to identify specific variables for study. Control of extraneous variables is necessary in any research study, and the thorough explanation of variables in the model would facilitate identification and control of those considered extraneous.

REFERENCE

Wilson, I. B., & Cleary, P. D. (1995). Linking clinical variables with health-related quality of life: A conceptual model of patient outcomes. *Journal of the American Medical Association, 273*(1), 59–65.

ABOUT THE AUTHOR

Lynne Ploetz, RN, BS, is the president and CEO of Matrix AdvoCare Network, Minneapolis. She is a nurse entrepreneur who works to improve her patients' health-related quality of life through innovative nursing practice. Ms. Ploetz is certified in gerontological nursing by the American Nurses Credentialing Center and is a certified case manager through the Commission for Case Management Certification. Several years ago, she started a geriatric case management company, Matrix AdvoCare Network. Today, she employs 20 registered nurses, care consultants throughout Minnesota, who provide health advocacy, and care consulting services to frail elderly and people with mental and physical disabilities.

14 Health Promotion
MADELEINE J. KERR

INTERNAL CRITICISM

1. *Adequacy.* The model broadly describes several factors that have relationships to health-promoting behavior. In comparison to some other models, the Pender Health Promotion Model is broader, in that the model includes a number of intrapersonal factors (such as perceived barriers to the behavior), interpersonal factors (such as social norms), and situational influences (such as availability of healthful options). A possible gap is the model's focus on individual health promotion. The model has implications for the health promotion of families and communities; however, use of multiple models would be ideal to address these populations. Tests of the initial Health Promotion Model in 38 studies have accounted for considerable variance in health-promoting lifestyle and several specific behaviors, such as exercise. The revised Health Promotion Model needs to be tested empirically.

2. *Clarity.* The phenomenon that the model seeks to explain is health-promoting behavior. This phenomenon has multiple definitions, but Pender's definition carefully circumscribes the limits of this phenomenon. Some readers may struggle with the concept, particularly in light of the traditional medical model with which so many nurses are familiar. While Pender offers that one major distinguishing feature between health promotion and health protection is motivation for the behavior, these may not be easily distinguished in practice. For instance, a client may engage in exercise for the dual benefits of increasing energy and avoiding cardiovascular disease and obesity. It is not clear how these dual motivations may affect the model.

    Pender's model is presented in a language and style that is easily understood by nurses and other health professionals. A schematic illustrates relationships between concepts. She provides clear definitions of terms. Relationship statements are established in Pender, Murdaugh, and Parson's (2002) *Health Promotion in Nursing Practice* (4th ed.).

3. *Consistency.* Model terminology in definitions corresponds with use in relationship statements and throughout the description of the theory.

4. *Logical development.* The revised model includes clearly established assumptions, concepts, and relationships. Each of these is clearly labeled and presented to the reader.

    The theoretical foundations of the model are attributed to several well-established theories of behavior. These theories include Feather's Expectancy Value Theory and Bandura's Social Cognitive Theory. Concepts that did not receive empirical support in the initial Health Promotion Model were dropped in the revised model. The rationale for each of the model revisions is explained, and detailed results of previous model-testing empirical studies are clearly presented in *Health Promotion in Nursing Practice* (4th ed.).

5. *Level of theory development.* The model represents a middle range theory in which it addresses a specific phenomenon. It is intended for use in providing health promotion services to clients.

EXTERNAL CRITICISM

1. *Reality convergence.* Pender's model describes phenomena of interest to nurses and includes a variety of factors that are well known to experienced health professionals, such as client perceptions of barriers and benefits. The theory has been supported in a number of model-testing studies.

2. *Utility.* The theory can be operationalized to provide interventions in real-life settings. For example, Lusk, Kerr, Ronis, and Eakin (1999) used the Pender Health Promotion Model to identify factors influencing

workers' use of hearing protection. This information was subsequently used to develop an educational intervention that increased this health behavior 20% from baseline. The model also is potentially useful for individually tailoring behavior change interventions to individuals with interactive computer communications.

Research shows the model to be useful for explaining and predicting client behavior in several important areas, including exercise and nutrition. The model has only recently begun to be used in the design of interventions, but may prove useful in guiding nurses to design cost-effective strategies to improve client health. The model provides a "framework for understanding the dimensions on which health promotion interventions can be based" (Pender et al., 2002, p. 75). However, the model does not guide the nurse using the framework in methods to develop interventions.

3. *Significance*. Health promotion as a phenomenon has enormous potential for the discipline of nursing. A change in focus from disease prevention to health promotion expands the role of nursing in society and has the potential for greatly enhancing the well-being of the society. Investment in diagnosis and treatment of disease has been the dominant model of health care until recently. However, the limitations of this model are now recognized more than ever, while the role of health behavior as a determinant of health is growing in recognition. The economic and nontangible advantages of investing in health promotion are gaining popularity in business and government. Since health behavior is a large and growing concern, having far-reaching consequences for the health and prosperity of society, the Health Promotion Model has great potential significance.

4. *Discrimination*. The Pender Health Promotion Model is unique within nursing, although it does bear some resemblance to theories of health behavior in the social and psychological sciences. However, its unique approach-oriented nature distinguishes it from other theories of health behavior that have an avoidance orientation. The model provides a framework for discriminating which concepts are relevant to specific health behaviors. Much work remains to be done to determine how the model can be applied to different behaviors, and in various cultural, developmental, and gender-based populations. The model focuses more on health promotion for individuals than on families, communities, and society.

5. *Scope*. The espoused scope of the theory is health-promoting behavior. Health-promoting behavior is directed toward increasing the level of well-being and self-actualization of a given individual or group (Pender et al., 2002, p. 34). Examples of health-promoting behavior provided by the authors include physical activity, nutrition, stress management, and social support. This range of behaviors is appropriate to middle range theory. However, the authors also describe the application of the model to health behavior beyond the scope of health promotion (e.g., use of hearing protection and environmental tobacco-smoke exposure). The success of the model in describing and explaining these client behaviors suggests that the model may have a scope of application beyond its original intent.

6. *Complexity*. The Pender Health Promotion Model uses relatively few (11, to be exact) concepts to address the complex phenomenon of health-promoting behavior. Relationships between even this small number of concepts are potentially large, however, because a single factor may have multiple relationships to other factors within the model. The authors seem to have achieved a balance between thoroughness and parsimony.

REFERENCES

Lusk, S., Kerr, M., Ronis, D., & Eakin, B. (1999). Applying the health promotion model to development of a worksite intervention. *American Journal of Health Promotion, 13*(4), 219–226.

Pender, N., Murdaugh, C., & Parsons, M. (2002). *Health promotion in nursing practice* (4th ed.). Upper Saddle River, NJ: Prentice Hall.

ABOUT THE AUTHOR

Madeleine J. Kerr, PhD, RN, is an associate professor in Public Health Nursing at the University of Minnesota School of Nursing, Minneapolis. She applied Pender's Health Promotion Model to the study of construction workers' hearing health behavior, and to the design of computer-based tailored educational interventions to promote the use of hearing protection devices. She has also conducted one of the first cross-cultural tests of the Health Promotion Model with Mexican-American workers.

15 Deliberative Nursing Process
MIMI DYE

INTERNAL CRITICISM

1. *Clarity.* The theory demonstrates clarity in its specific definition of easily understood terms and in its specific use of those terms as they are involved in the flow of communication and activities inherent in the Deliberative Nursing Process.

2. *Consistency.* The theory demonstrates consistency because the definition, use of terms, and formulation remain the same throughout.

3. *Adequacy.* The theory demonstrates adequacy because its scope includes any professional communication relevant to meeting patient needs at any level within and throughout the health care system. Implicit in the theory is that the nurse will validate the needs of a patient who is mute, cognitively impaired, or cognitively compromised, by means other than direct verbal communication, such as observations by the nurse or information provided by significant others.

4. *Logical development.* The theory demonstrates logical development from its premises to its product or outcome because the flow of ingredients explicitly used in the Deliberative Nursing Process reasonably leads one to the product or outcome, that is, improvement in the patient's immediate behavior.

5. *Level of theory development.* Since this theory is a situation-producing or prescriptive theory, it is Level IV theory. For instance, the nurse's greater understanding of the patient's need for help results in alleviating the patient's distress more effectively.

EXTERNAL CRITICISM

1. *Reality convergence.* The theory begins with the premise that the patients may have the needs that they may not be able to express or meet without professional nursing assistance. Therefore, it is the responsibility of nurses to explore with patients whether or not they have such needs, and whether or not their nursing activities meet those needs. This theory includes using the Deliberative Nursing Process in any communication relevant to patient needs anywhere in the health care system. Essentially, it involves the patient as a crucial member of this communication system. Meeting patient needs is widely accepted in nursing.

2. *Utility.* Since the theory offers the Deliberative Nursing Process as an explicit way of keeping communication clear and has as its purpose ascertaining and meeting patient needs, it is useful to the administrators as well as to the practitioners. It is useful to the educators because it can be taught and practiced within the educational system. It is also useful to the researchers because its variables lend themselves to research. The theory, therefore, has a high degree of utility for the nursing profession.

3. *Significance.* Since the theory focuses on nurse–patient communications and communications within the health care system relevant to meeting patients' health care needs, specifically, responding to and relieving patients' immediate distress, the theory addresses the essential core issue in nursing— responding to and meeting patients' needs that cannot be met without professional nursing assistance. The theory contributes to nursing knowledge by offering the Deliberative Nursing Process, designed to ascertain and meet patients' needs and relieve patients' immediate distress. The theory can be taught. Its variables lend themselves to research. Therefore, the theory has immense significance for the nursing profession.

4. *Discrimination.* The theory constructs a system of nursing practice for nurses to fulfill a distinct professional function wherever they practice. The theory is inclusive for nurses in administration, education,

and clinical practice in all specialties. The unique professional nursing function is to ascertain and meet patients' immediate needs for help when patients are unable to do so without professional nursing assistance. The product or outcome of this function is to relieve patients' distress. Therefore, this theory differentiates nursing from health professions.

5. *Scope of theory.* The scope of the theory is broadly applicable because it includes nursing communications relevant to meeting patients' health care needs in all specialties, wherever and however nurses are practicing, whether in administration, education, practice, or research.

6. *Complexity.* The theory offers a balance between parsimony and complexity. It is parsimonious in that its elements are few and include only those needed to describe and explain the theory. It is complex because communication between and among people can be complex and the dynamics of relationships including nurse–patient relationships can be complex.

ABOUT THE AUTHOR

Mimi Dye, MSN, ARNP, is a former student and longtime friend of Ms. Orlando. She has recently served as a consultant to the New Hampshire Hospital Orlando Project.

---

16 Resilience

MARSHA L. ELLETT

INTERNAL CRITICISM

1. *Clarity.* According to the Adolescent Resilience Model (ARM), resilience may occur as a result of a process that includes deriving meaning from an adverse experience through interaction with others. The ARM is parsimonious, given the widespread agreement among researchers that resilience is a complex, multidimensional construct. The concepts of the model are named but are not explicitly defined. They are operationalized clearly by instruments derived from decision trees for the qualitative work. Three classes of protective factors—individual, family, and social—are hypothesized to positively affect resilience outcomes. The individual protective factors include courageous or positive coping and derived meaning. The familial protective factors include family atmosphere and support/resources available to the family. The social protective resources include health care resources and social integration. Two classes of factors are hypothesized to negatively affect resilience: individual risk factor and illness-related stress factors. The individual risk factor is sustained defensive coping, and the illness-related stress factors include illness perspective and illness distress. The outcome factors of resilience include self-esteem, mastery/confidence, and self-transcendence, as well as quality of life, defined as a sense of well-being.

2. *Consistency.* There is consistency between the text and the model (Fig. 16.2) in the social and family protective factors. However, the illness-related stress factors, including illness perspective and illness distress, in the text are referred to as symptom-related risk in the model and include illness perception, symptom distress, and severity of illness. This inconsistency in wording between the text and the model is somewhat confusing. In addition, the only outcome variable depicted in the model is quality of life, so the relationships of self-esteem, mastery/confidence, and self-transcendence to quality of life are unclear.

3. *Adequacy.* The strength of the ARM is that it is an emerging model grounded in contextual experiences. It appears that defensive coping is an individual risk factor only if it is sustained. Progression to courageous coping can occur, which is positively related to resilience. Further refinement of the concepts will occur with continued use of the model.

4. *Logical development.* The ARM was developed first through qualitative studies that allowed the identification and clarification of concepts to be included in the model. Next, quantitative structural equation modeling was used to identify relationships among concepts. Then, qualitative methods were again used to evaluate these identified relationships.

5. *Level of theory development.* The ARM is only beginning to be used to guide nursing interventions; therefore, it is an emerging middle range theory.

EXTERNAL CRITICISM

1. *Reality convergence.* The assumptions underlying the ARM were not specifically stated as such; however, one assumption may be that persons with resilience require time to reflect on the meaning of their actions. Thus, Haase and colleagues state that resilience may occur through a process that includes deriving meaning from the experience through interaction with others. The ARM appears to reflect the real world of nursing and makes inherent sense to this reader. This model's ability to guide interventions is just beginning to be tested. The one described study testing the ARM aims to test the efficacy of a therapeutic music video intervention for adolescents and young adults during the acute phase of stem cell transplant. This indicates that the model has the potential to be useful in real-life settings.

2. *Utility.* The researchers state that several studies are currently being developed using the ARM, but only the study mentioned was described. In this study, the ARM was being used to generate hypotheses.

3. *Significance.* Any model that can guide nursing interventions to enhance resilience outcomes in adolescents and young adults faced with cancer would be highly significant.

4. *Discrimination.* Whether the ARM will guide hypothesis generation that could not be generated by other models of resilience is not known presently. At this time, the boundaries of resilience are inconsistent.

5. *Scope of theory.* The scope of the ARM currently is narrow in that it is being studied in chronically ill adolescents, mostly those with cancer, and is being tested in practice. If the initial intervention research is successful, the reader can see expanding the scope of this model slightly to include adolescents with other serious chronic illnesses and then, later, to chronically ill participants in different age groups facing different developmental tasks. The ARM has the potential to become more global in time with continued refinement.

6. *Complexity.* Given that resilience is a complex, multidimensional construct, the ARM is parsimonious, with few concepts that can be fairly easily understood without lengthy descriptions or explanations.

RELEVANT WORKS

Haase, J. E., Heiney, S. P., Ruccione, K. S., & Stutzer, C. (1999). Research triangulation to derive meaning/based quality of life theory: Adolescent resilience model and instrument development. *International Journal of Cancer Supplement, 12*, 125–131.

ABOUT THE AUTHOR

Marsha Ellett, DNS, RN, is an associate professor at Indiana University School of Nursing, Indianapolis, and a pediatric clinical nurse specialist. She teaches pediatrics in both the baccalaureate and the master's programs (Pediatric Clinical Nurse Specialist Program). Her research has focused on enteral tube placement in children and colic in infants. It is through her association with her colleague, Joan Haase, that she became familiar with the Adolescence Resilience Model. She identifies the model's utility to the practice of her specialty, in work with young people with chronic illnesses, such as Crohn's disease, ulcerative colitis, and chronic aggressive hepatitis.

17 Shuler Nurse Practitioner Practice Model
MARJORIE WEBB

RUTH STAUS

INTERNAL CRITICISM

1. *Clarity.* The Shuler Nurse Practitioner Practice Model (SNPPM) depicts a step-by-step process for the nurse practitioner (NP)–patient interaction. Application of the three-step process of NP–patient interaction is somewhat complex; however each phase of the process is clearly defined. In addition, each component of each phase is defined clearly as well.

2. *Consistency.* Throughout the description of the model, definitions of terms remain consistent. The general definitions of nursing and the NP role, person, health, and the environment remained consistent from the authors' publications in 1993 and 2001.

3. *Adequacy.* The authors' goal for this model was to give NPs a way to retain their nursing identity while working within a health care system based in the biomedical model. The SNPPM is adequate in that it provides the NP the ability to simultaneously develop both nursing and medical diagnoses during the same patient visit. In addition to illness and/or disease, topics such as physiological needs, social support, environmental issues, and spiritual distress are addressed during the NP–patient interaction.

4. *Logical development.* The SNPPM has developed logically from abstract concepts within the grand theories to concrete definitions that NPs can use in practice.

5. *Level of theory development.* Shuler and Davis (1993a; 1993b) have noted a number of problems with applying grand nursing theory to NP practice including: (a) a viewpoint that is too broad and abstract, (b) abstract language that is not congruent with the language used in clinical practice, and (c) it describes nursing as it should be instead of the "messy reality" of daily clinical practice. The SNPPM utilizes concrete language to describe the NP role and define concepts within the model. This concretization of definitions makes the model more congruent with the definition of a middle range theory. Currently, the model is both descriptive and prescriptive.

EXTERNAL CRITICISM

1. *Reality convergence.* The basic assumptions of the SNPPM are fundamentally sound and represent the real world of nursing practice in the advanced practice NP role. Shuler and Davis utilized the grand nursing theories to operationally define the concepts of person, health, nursing, and the environment. In addition, the model is based on the General Systems Model of input, throughput, and output.

2. *Utility.* The model is useful for practice, teaching, and research. The model can be used for most types of NP–patient interaction. It has definite practical applications for the instruction of NP students. In addition, the model framework is useful for hypotheses and the generation of new knowledge.

3. *Significance.* The results of research performed using this model will have a very real impact on NPs' day-to-day practice. A holistic, prevention-focused approach to patient care is fostered by the use of SNPPM (Shuler et al., 2001). The model addresses essential elements of the NP–patient interaction in such a way as to describe the actual interaction and prescribe various outcomes of the interaction. A unique feature of the model is the focus on NP self-care as a fundamental component of patient care.

4. *Discrimination.* The SNPPM is unique to advanced practice nursing in that it is the only current model that addresses the dual nursing and medical role of the NP. The model has clear boundaries within its framework. The areas of nursing and medicine that are blended by the NP are clearly defined. It would

be difficult to use other middle range theories in the advanced practice setting in the way that the SNPPM can be used.

5. *Scope.* The model remains within the scope of middle range theory. The definitions are concrete and were formulated to operationalize easily. The SNPPM can be used in a variety of NP practice settings but maintains its identity in middle range theory.

6. *Complexity.* The model is complex but each concept and phase is well defined. The complexity of the model does not detract from the usefulness of the model; NP practice is complex and not simply defined.

REFERENCES

Shuler, P. A., & Davis, J. E. (1993a). The Shuler nurse practitioner practice model: A theoretical framework for nurse practitioner clinicians, educators, and researchers, part 1. *Journal of the American Academy of Nurse Practitioners*, 5, 11–18.

Shuler, P. A., & Davis, J. E. (1993b). The Shuler nurse practitioner practice model: Clinical application, part 2. *Journal of the American Academy of Nurse Practitioners*, 5, 73–88.

Shuler, P. A., Huebsch, R., & Hallock, J. (2001). Providing wholistic health care for the elderly: Utilization of the Shuler nurse practitioner practice model. *Journal of the American Academy of Nurse Practitioners*, 13, 297–303.

ABOUT THE AUTHORS

Marjorie Webb, DNP, RN, ACNP-BC, is an assistant professor in the College of Nursing and Health Sciences at Metropolitan State University in St. Paul, Minnesota. As chair of the BSN-DNP committee, she worked together with Dr. Staus to implement the SNPPM as the instructional core of the BSN-DNP program. Dr. Webb also practices at the United Heart and Vascular Clinic in St. Paul, Minnesota and her research interests include heart failure associated with pacemaker-induced dyssynchrony.

Ruth Staus, DNP, RN, ANP-BC, is an assistant professor in the College of Nursing and Health Sciences at Metropolitan State University in St. Paul, Minnesota. She utilizes the SNPPM in her Adult Nurse Practitioner practice at Edgerton Wellness Center and Love Grows Here Wellness Center. Dr. Staus has 27 years of experience in clinical geriatrics and has conducted regional and national award-winning applied clinical research in the area of healthy aging and holistic approaches to caring for aging adults.

18 The AACN Synergy Model

AMY REX SMITH

INTERNAL CRITICISM

1. *Clarity.* The contents of The AACN Synergy Model are understood with ease because the terminology is commonly used by nurses. The language accurately reflects acute care and critical care specialty practice. For example, patients are called patients, a word that both recognizes nurses' caring role and holds an appreciation of patients' vulnerability when critically ill. Further review of the descriptions of the eight patient characteristics demonstrates respect for patient individuality and empowerment of patients (to the extent that they are able) and of their families.

2. *Consistency.* Each component of the model is used in a consistent manner throughout the model, with no evidence of any inconsistencies. The relationships within the model are direct, such as the nurse–patient relationship, and as such are uncluttered, which supports consistency.

3. *Adequacy.* This model was developed to describe nursing practice in the hospital setting: 24-hour-a-day nursing care provided in a high-technology, complex, and often chaotic environment. It adequately captures the salient factors present in the setting.

4. *Logical development.* The process of the development of this model is described in this chapter in great detail. The model is unusual because it was developed by and for a specialty discipline, critical care nursing, rather than for all nursing situations. Despite the long history of prestigious certification in critical care nursing—the CCRN—leaders in the specialty recognized the need to move beyond using a task checklist and the medical perspective of physiological systems for the certification examinations. The process of model development was serial groups of carefully selected nurse leaders using a reflective and iterative process. This provided many checks and balances.

5. *Level of theory development.* The AACN Synergy Model was designed as a broad conceptual model of nursing. As such, it provides a starting point for middle range theory development (Fawcett, 2005). In general, its strength is in how it describes the real practice world of critical care nursing. In addition to the excellent description, the model provides a framework for patient assessment and a structure to guide development of nurse expertise. It also attempts to prescribe good matches between nurses and patients, and because it posits that "synergy" occurs when these good matches happen, it could be seen as prescriptive. However, synergy, defined in the model as it is commonly understood as "something more than the sum of the parts," is not a measurable outcome and there is no way to tell if it has occurred or not. In this way, the model does not try to prescribe or predict any specific outcomes, only general measures not linked to any specific set of interventions. It only tells the "what is" and describes the ideal "what is."

   As middle range theories are derived from the model, specific interventions and outcomes will be identified.

EXTERNAL CRITICISM

1. *Reality convergence.* The AACN Synergy Model is well matched to the real world of clinical nursing practice. It is meant to be used in the real world of the hospital environment and focuses attention exclusively on nurses and their patients.

2. *Utility.* The model is inherently useful. The model can be used every time a charge nurse makes a patient care assignment. It can also be used to design a curriculum to help nurses move from novice to expert and it can help to focus preceptors as they mentor new nurses on inpatient units. The model can be used to organize initial and ongoing patient assessments. Its use as a conceptual framework for research and theory development is only in the beginning stages, but the potential for its use in research is impressive. One of the reasons it has not been well used in research is that it is still new, and it is difficult to study nurse–patient pairing. Thus far, most synergy-based studies focus on patients or nurses, not both. The challenges of developing research designs that are congruent with basic ideas of the model are a crucial next step for AACN members.

3. *Significance.* It is significant that the model is used for the certification examination of both patient care nurses (CCRNs) and advanced-practice nurses (CCNSs). As such, the model reflects certified practice. The model can be used to address a clinical issue, such as providing a structure for providing spiritual care in the intensive care unit (ICU; Rex Smith, 2006).

4. *Discrimination.* The boundaries of this model appear to be well delineated, because they are clearly contained within the hospital setting. Consistent with all conceptual frameworks, however, the broad utility of the model is evident. The model has begun to be extended to the outpatient setting. Specifically, Hardin and Hussey (2003) presented a synergy model–based case study of advanced-practice nurse intervention with a congestive heart failure (CHF) patient in an outpatient clinic. So, the boundaries as originally described in the model may be more fluid than the originators perceived.

5. *Scope of theory.* All four concepts of the nursing metaparadigm are addressed by this conceptual model: It includes the patient, the nurse, the environment, and the health outcomes. This gives it a broad

scope, broader than the middle range theories included in this book. Its scope is limited only by being designed for hospital-based nursing practice in acute care and critical care settings. Because of the focus on the nurse–patient relationship, the scope of the model is actually broader than it was originally conceived. In addition to the outpatient case study described previously, many of the nurse practitioner master's degree students at the University of Massachusetts, Boston have selected this model for their final comprehensive paper.

6. *Complexity.* The model is less complex than many of the other nursing conceptual models. It is elegant in its simplicity, with a clear focus on the nurse–patient relationship. The synergy model guides users to identify when optimal nurse–patient matches occur and what needs to be done to create matches when they have not yet occurred.

REFERENCES

Fawcett, J. (2005). *Contemporary nursing knowledge: Analysis and evaluation of nursing models and theories* (2nd ed.). Philadelphia, PA: Davis.

Hardin, S., & Hussey, L. (2003). AACN synergy model for patient care case study of a CHF patient. *Critical Care Nurse, 23*(1), 73–76.

Rex Smith, A. (2006). Using the synergy model to provide spiritual care in critical care settings. *Critical Care Nurse, 26*(4), 41–47.

ABOUT THE AUTHOR

Amy Rex Smith, DNSc, APRN, BC, is an associate professor at the University of Massachusetts, Boston, where she coordinates the acute care/critical care clinical nurse specialist track. She is a board-certified advanced-practice nurse (clinical nurse specialist in adult health nursing). She maintains a clinical practice on a medical intermediate care unit at Brigham and Women's Hospital in Boston. She has a special interest in spiritual care of hospitalized patients. She has published using the AACN Synergy Model and is doing research using it as a conceptual framework.

Burke/Eakes Chronic Sorrow Assessment Tool©

The questions below are asked about the effects that certain life events or situations may have on people over a period of time so that helping professionals can better meet their needs. In answering these questions, please focus on the impact that these life events or situations continue to have on your life. There are no right or wrong answers. You do not have to answer any or all of the questions and can stop without penalty of any kind. Thank you for taking the time to answer these questions.

DEMOGRAPHICS/BACKGROUND

1. Which of the following best describes your situation? (Please check only one)
   (a) _____ Parent of disabled child (please specify the disability). _____
   (b) _____ Person with a chronic condition (please specify the condition). _____
   (c) _____ Caregiver of someone with a chronic or life-threatening illness (please specify the condition). _____
   (d) _____ Bereaved person (please specify the relationship of deceased to you). _____

2. I have been dealing with this situation/loss for _____ years (please write in number of years).

3. Please provide the following information about yourself:
   (a) Sex: _____ male _____ female
   (b) Age: _____ years
   (c) Marital status: _____ single _____ married _____ widowed _____ divorced _____ separated
   (d) Religion: _____ Protestant _____ Catholic _____ Jewish _____ Other (please write in): _____
   (e) Ethnic origin: _____ Caucasian _____ Hispanic _____ African American _____ American Indian _____ Asian
       Other (please write in): _____
   (f) Please indicate your highest completed level of education:
       a. Less than high school
       b. High school graduate
       c. Associate/technical degree
       d. Bachelor's degree
       e. Master's degree
       f. PhD/MD or equivalent
   (g) Total family income per year from all sources before taxes:
       a. Below $5,000
       b. $5,001–10,000
       c. $10,001–15,000
       d. $15,001–20,000
       e. $20,001–25,000
       f. $25,001–30,000
       g. $30,001–40,000
       h. Over $40,000

DISPARITY

4. Even though some time may have passed since you began dealing with your situation/loss, you may still be coping with some ongoing issues and reactions. Please read the following statements and indicate if this is true for you. Remember, there are no right or wrong answers.

    (a) I recognize the hole this situation/loss has created in my life.   ❏ True   ❏ False

    (b) I think about the difference this situation/loss has made in my life.   ❏ True   ❏ False

    (c) I experience changes in my life as a result of the situation/loss.   ❏ True   ❏ False

    (d) I feel its effects in bits and pieces.   ❏ True   ❏ False

GRIEF-RELATED FEELINGS

The following are feelings you may have experienced as a result of your situation/loss.

5. At those times when you experience these feelings associated with your situation/loss, please indicate how upsetting they are for you. Remember, there are no right or wrong answers.

	Have not Experienced	Have Experienced but not Upsetting	Have Experienced, Somewhat Upsetting	Have Experienced, Very Upsetting
(a) Sad				
(b) Anxious				
(c) Angry				
(d) Overwhelmed				
(e) Heartbroken				
(f) Other (please specify):				

CHARACTERISTICS OF CHRONIC SORROW (PERVASIVE, PERMANENT, PERIODIC, POTENTIALLY PROGRESSIVE)

The questions below ask more about the feelings you may experience related to your situation/loss. Please mark the extent to which each statement below is true for you.

6. In describing my feelings about my situation/loss, I:

    (a) Have ups and downs   ❏ True   ❏ False

    (b) Feel their effects on other parts of my life   ❏ True   ❏ False

    (c) Feel them more strongly now than at first   ❏ True   ❏ False

    (d) Believe they will impact me the rest of my life   ❏ True   ❏ False

TRIGGERS

There may be certain times when you tend to experience the feelings associated with your situation/loss. Please read the following statements and indicate which are true for you.

7. These feelings about my situation/loss come up when I:

(a) Have to seek medical care	❑ True	❑ False
(b) Realize all the responsibilities I have	❑ True	❑ False
(c) Compare where I am now with where others are in their lives	❑ True	❑ False
(d) Think of all I now have to do	❑ True	❑ False
(e) Meet someone else in the same situation	❑ True	❑ False
(f) Experience the anniversary of when this began	❑ True	❑ False
(g) Have a "special day" such as a birthday or holiday	❑ True	❑ False

(h) Other (please specify): _____

INTERNAL COPING MECHANISMS

The statements below are things you may have found helpful to you in managing the feelings associated with your situation/loss. Please indicate which is true for you.

8. It helps me deal with my feelings when I:

	Never Tried	Have Tried, but not Helpful	Have Tried, Somewhat Helpful	Have Tried, Very Helpful
(a) Keep busy				
(b) Take one day at a time				
(c) Talk to someone close to me				
(d) Pray				
(e) Exercise				
(f) Count my blessings				
(g) Work on my hobbies				
(h) Express my feelings				
(i) Go to church, synagogue, or other place of worship				
(j) Talk with others in similar situations				
(k) Take a "can do" attitude				
(l) Talk with a minister, rabbi, or priest				
(m) Talk with a health professional				
(n) Focus on the positive				

(o) Other (please specify): _____

EXTERNAL COPING MECHANISMS

The following questions are to find out how helping professionals can assist people who are dealing with situations/losses such as yours. Please indicate which is true for you. Remember, there are no right or wrong answers.

9. It helps me deal with my feelings when helping professionals:

	Never Tried	Have Tried, but not Helpful	Have Tried, Somewhat Helpful	Have Tried, Very Helpful
(a) Listen to me				
(b) Recognize my feelings				
(c) Answer me honestly				
(d) Allow me to ask questions				
(e) Take their time with me				
(f) Provide good care				

(g) Other (please specify): _____

Friends and family may also be helpful to you as you deal with the feelings associated with your situation/loss. Please read the following and indicate which is true for you.

10. It helps me deal with my feelings when family and friends:

	Never Tried	Have Tried, but not Helpful	Have Tried, Somewhat Helpful	Have Tried, Very Helpful
(a) Listen to me				
(b) Have a positive outlook				
(c) Accept my feelings				
(d) Provide emotional support				
(e) Offer a helping hand				
(f) Acknowledge my situation/loss				

(g) Other (please specify): _____

Thank you for answering these questions. Please return the questionnaire at this time.

General Comfort Questionnaire

Thank you VERY MUCH for helping me in my study of the concept COMFORT. Below are statements that may describe your comfort right now. Four numbers are provided for each question; please circle the number you think most closely matches what you are feeling. Relate these questions to your comfort *at the moment you are answering the questions.*

	Strongly Agree			Strongly Disagree
1. My body is relaxed right now.	4	3	2	1
2. I feel useful because I am working hard.	4	3	2	1
3. I have enough privacy.	4	3	2	1
4. There are those I can depend on when I need help.	4	3	2	1
5. I do not want to exercise.	4	3	2	1
6. My condition gets me down.	4	3	2	1
7. I feel confident.	4	3	2	1
8. I feel dependent on others.	4	3	2	1
9. I feel my life is worthwhile right now.	4	3	2	1
10. I am inspired by knowing that I am loved.	4	3	2	1
11. These surroundings are pleasant.	4	3	2	1
12. The sounds keep me from resting.	4	3	2	1
13. No one understands me.	4	3	2	1
14. My pain is difficult to endure.	4	3	2	1
15. I am inspired to do my best.	4	3	2	1
16. I am unhappy when I am alone.	4	3	2	1
17. My faith helps me to not be afraid.	4	3	2	1
18. I do not like it here.	4	3	2	1
19. I am constipated right now.	4	3	2	1
20. I do not feel healthy right now.	4	3	2	1
21. This room makes me feel scared.	4	3	2	1
22. I am afraid of what is next.	4	3	2	1
23. I have a favorite person(s) who makes me feel cared for.	4	3	2	1
24. I have experienced changes that make me feel uneasy.	4	3	2	1
25. I am hungry.	4	3	2	1

	Strongly Agree			Strongly Disagree
26. I would like to see my doctor more often.	4	3	2	1
27. The temperature in this room is fine.	4	3	2	1
28. I am very tired.	4	3	2	1
29. I can rise above my pain.	4	3	2	1
30. The mood around here uplifts me.	4	3	2	1
31. I am content.	4	3	2	1
32. This chair (bed) makes me hurt.	4	3	2	1
33. This view inspires me.	4	3	2	1
34. My personal belongings are not here.	4	3	2	1
35. I feel out of place here.	4	3	2	1
36. I feel good enough to walk.	4	3	2	1
37. My friends remember me with their cards and phone calls.	4	3	2	1
38. My beliefs give me peace of mind.	4	3	2	1
39. I need to be better informed about my health.	4	3	2	1
40. I feel out of control.	4	3	2	1
41. I feel crummy because I am not dressed.	4	3	2	1
42. This room smells terrible.	4	3	2	1
43. I am alone but not lonely.	4	3	2	1
44. I feel peaceful.	4	3	2	1
45. I am depressed.	4	3	2	1
46. I have found meaning in my life.	4	3	2	1
47. It is easy to get around here.	4	3	2	1
48. I need to feel good again.	4	3	2	1

Available at www.uakron.edu/comfort. No permission needed.

Code # _____   Date _____   Time _____

Comfort Behaviors Checklist

How is patient acting right now?
Please circle best response. *NA* = not applicable

	NA	No	Somewhat	Moderate	Strong
Vocalizations					
1. Complaining	0	1	2	3	4
2. Awake	0	1	2	3	4
3. Moaning	0	1	2	3	4
4. Content sounds/talk	0	1	2	3	4
5. Crying/shouting	0	1	2	3	4
Motor Signs					
6. Peaceful	0	1	2	3	4
7. Agitated	0	1	2	3	4
8. Rapid pacing	0	1	2	3	4
9. Fidgety	0	1	2	3	4
10. Muscles relaxed	0	1	2	3	4
11. Rubbing an area	0	1	2	3	4
12. Guarding	0	1	2	3	4
Behaviors					
13. Anxious	0	1	2	3	4
14. Accepts kindness	0	1	2	3	4
15. Likes touch/hand holding	0	1	2	3	4
16. Appears depressed	0	1	2	3	4
17. Able to rest	0	1	2	3	4
18. Able to eat	0	1	2	3	4
19. Calm, at ease	0	1	2	3	4
20. Purposeless movements	0	1	2	3	4

	NA	No	Somewhat	Moderate	Strong
Facial					
21. Grimaces/winces	0	1	2	3	4
22. Relaxed expression	0	1	2	3	4
23. Wrinkled brow	0	1	2	3	4
24. Appears frightened or worried	0	1	2	3	4
25. Smiles	0	1	2	3	4
Miscellaneous					
26. Unusual breathing	0	1	2	3	4
27. Focuses mentally	0	1	2	3	4
28. Converses	0	1	2	3	4
29. Awakens smoothly	0	1	2	3	4

If this is the *only* comfort/pain instrument being used, ask the patient:

30. Do you have any pain? No_____ Yes _____ [Please rate your pain from 1 to 10, with 10 being the highest possible pain.] _____ (rating)

31. Taking everything into consideration, how comfortable are you right now? [Please rate your total comfort from 1 to 10, with 10 being the highest possible comfort.] _____ (rating)

Other open-ended comments

(Change in medication use, recent injury, recent decline in functional status, staff reports of comfort/discomfort, changes in appetite, ambulation, etc.)

Adapted by K. Kolcaba from: Volicer, L. (1988). Management of advanced Alzheimer's dementia/the comfort checklist. In L. Volicer (Ed.), *Clinical management of Alzheimer's disease*. Rockville, MD: Aspen Publications.

Scoring of the Behaviors Checklist

1. *Subtract* number of "not applicable" (NA) from 29, to obtain **total answered**.

2. *Multiply* total answered (step 1) by 4, to obtain **total possible score**.

3. *Reverse code* numbers 1, 3, 5, 7, 8, 9, 11, 12, 13, 16, 20, 22, 23, and 25 to obtain **raw comfort responses**.

4. *Add* **raw comfort responses** (step 3) for all questions not marked NA, to obtain **actual comfort score**.

5. *Divide actual comfort score* (step 4) by *total possible score* (step 2) and round to two decimal places. (If the third decimal place is 5 or greater, round the second decimal place up to the next number.)

6. Report score as a **2-digit number** (rounded percent without the % sign or decimal). *Higher scores* indicate *higher comfort.*

PEDIATRIC ASTHMA QUALITY OF LIFE QUESTIONNAIRE WITH STANDARDIZED ACTIVITIES (PAQLQ(S))

SELF-ADMINISTERED

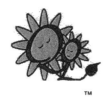

™

For further Information:

Elizabeth Juniper, MCSP, MSc
Professor
20 Marcuse Fields,
Bosham,
West Sussex,
PO18 8NA, UK
Tel: + 44 (0) 1243 572124
Fax: + 44 (0) 1243 573680
E-mail: juniper@qoltech.co.uk
Web: www.qoltech.co.uk

JANUARY 2001

PEDIATRIC ASTHMA   PATIENT ID _____

QUALITY OF LIFE QUESTIONNAIRE(S)

SELF-ADMINISTERED   DATE _____

Please complete **all** questions by circling the number that best describes how you have been during the **past week as a result of your asthma**.

How **bothered** have you been during the last week doing:

	Extremely Bothered	Very Bothered	Quite Bothered	Somewhat Bothered	Bothered a Bit	Hardly Bothered at All	Not Bothered
1. Physical activities (such as running, swimming, sports, walking uphill/upstairs, and bicycling)?	1	2	3	4	5	6	7
2. Being with animals (such as playing with pets and looking after animals)?	1	2	3	4	5	6	7
3. Activities with friends and family (such as playing at recess and doing things with your friends and family)?	1	2	3	4	5	6	7
4. Coughing?	1	2	3	4	5	6	7

In general, **how often** during the last week did you:

	All of the Time	Most of the Time	Quite Often	Some of the Time	Once in a While	Hardly Any of the Time	None of the Time
5. Feel frustrated because of your asthma?	1	2	3	4	5	6	7

PEDIATRIC ASTHMA   **PATIENT ID** _____

QUALITY OF LIFE QUESTIONNAIRE(S)

SELF-ADMINISTERED   **DATE** _____

	All of the Time	Most of the Time	Quite Often	Some of the Time	Once in a While	Hardly Any of the Time	None of the Time
6. Feel tired because of your asthma?	1	2	3	4	5	6	7
7. Feel worried, concerned, or troubled because of your asthma?	1	2	3	4	5	6	7

How **bothered** have you been during the last week by:

	Extremely Bothered	Very Bothered	Quite Bothered	Somewhat Bothered	Bothered a Bit	Hardly Bothered at All	Not Bothered
8. Asthma attacks?	1	2	3	4	5	6	7

In general, **how often** during the last week did you:

	All of the Time	Most of the Time	Quite Often	Some of the Time	Once in a While	Hardly Any of the Time	None of the Time
9. Feel angry because of your asthma?	1	2	3	4	5	6	7

How **bothered** have you been during the last week by:

	Extremely Bothered	Very Bothered	Quite Bothered	Somewhat Bothered	Bothered a Bit	Hardly Bothered at All	Not Bothered
10. Wheezing?	1	2	3	4	5	6	7

In general, how **often** during the last week did you:

	All of the Time	Most of the Time	Quite Often	Some of the Time	Once in a While	Hardly Any of the Time	None of the Time
11. Feel irritable (cranky/ grouchy) because of your asthma?	1	2	3	4	5	6	7

PEDIATRIC ASTHMA   PATIENT ID _____

QUALITY OF LIFE QUESTIONNAIRE(S)

SELF-ADMINISTERED   DATE _____

Page 3 of 5

How **bothered** have you been during the last week by:							
	Extremely Bothered	Very Bothered	Quite Bothered	Somewhat Bothered	Bothered a Bit	Hardly Bothered at All	Not Bothered
12. Tightness in your chest?	1	2	3	4	5	6	7

In general, **how often** during the last week did you:							
	All of the Time	Most of the Time	Quite Often	Some of the Time	Once in a While	Hardly Any of the Time	None of the Time
13. Feel different or left out because of your asthma?	1	2	3	4	5	6	7

How **bothered** have you been during the last week by:							
	Extremely Bothered	Very Bothered	Quite Bothered	Somewhat Bothered	Bothered a Bit	Hardly Bothered at All	Not Bothered
14. Shortness of breath?	1	2	3	4	5	6	7

In general, **how often** during the last week did you:							
	All of the Time	Most of the Time	Quite Often	Some of the Time	Once in a While	Hardly Any of the Time	None of the Time
15. Feel frustrated because you could not keep up with others?	1	2	3	4	5	6	7
16. Wake up during the night because of your asthma?	1	2	3	4	5	6	7
17. Feel uncomfortable because of your asthma?	1	2	3	4	5	6	7

PEDIATRIC ASTHMA   PATIENT ID _____

QUALITY OF LIFE QUESTIONNAIRE(S)

SELF-ADMINISTERED   DATE _____

Page 4 of 5

	All of the Time	Most of the Time	Quite Often	Some of the Time	Once in a While	Hardly Any of the Time	None of the Time
18. Feel out of breath because of your asthma?	1	2	3	4	5	6	7
19. Feel you could not keep up with others because of your asthma?	1	2	3	4	5	6	7

In general, **how often** during the last week did you:

	All of the Time	Most of the Time	Quite Often	Some of the Time	Once in a While	Hardly Any of the Time	None of the Time
20. Have trouble sleeping at night because of your asthma?	1	2	3	4	5	6	7
21. Feel frightened by an asthma attack?	1	2	3	4	5	6	7

Think about all the activities that you did in the past week:

	Extremely Bothered	Very Bothered	Quite Bothered	Somewhat Bothered	Bothered a Bit	Hardly Bothered at All	Not Bothered
22. How much were you bothered by your asthma during these activities?	1	2	3	4	5	6	7

PEDIATRIC ASTHMA   PATIENT ID _____

QUALITY OF LIFE QUESTIONNAIRE(S)

SELF-ADMINISTERED   DATE _____

Page 5 of 5

In general, **how often** during the last week did you:							
	All of the Time	Most of the Time	Quite Often	Some of the Time	Once in a While	Hardly Any of the Time	None of the Time
23. Have difficulty taking a deep breath?	1	2	3	4	5	6	7

DOMAIN CODE:
Symptoms: 4, 6, 8, 10, 12, 14, 16, 18, 20, 23
Activity Limitation: 1, 2, 3, 19, 22
Emotional Function: 5, 7, 9, 11, 13, 15, 17, 21

Index